Vaccination: a History

From Lady Montagu to Genetic Engineering

Éditions John Libbey Eurotext
127, avenue de la République
92120 Montrouge, France.
Tél. : 01 46 73 06 60
e-mail : contact@jle.com
http://www.jle.com

John Libbey Eurotext Limited
42-46 High Street
Esher
KT109KY
United Kingdom

ISBN : 978-2-7420-0775-2

Illustration on cover

Painting by Gaston Mélingue (1879) : "The first vaccination – Dr. Edward Jenner". Donated by the Fasquelle family to the *Académie nationale de Médecine*. Three main characters can be seen: James Phipps, sitting in an armchair, Edward Jenner inoculating the vaccine and, on the right, Sarah Nelmes, who just provided the "matter" and is placing a dressing on her own hand. Most probably, it is James' father, an agricultural day labourer, who is holding the child during the operation. The other figures are harder to identify. Katherine Jenner could be standing behind the armchair, and James' mother could be at Sarah Nelmes' right. The decor resembles Chantry Cottage, Jenner's house with its trellis.

(Reproduced with the kind permission of the *Académie nationale de Médecine*.)

Unless otherwise specified, the illustrations in this book come from a personal collection.

Vaccination: a History

From Lady Montagu to Genetic Engineering

Hervé Bazin

John Libbey EUROTEXT

Acknowledgements

I would like to thank, first of all Dominique Latinne, Thomas P. Monath, Andy Morgan, Pierre-Paul Pastoret, Stanley Plotkin, Jose Esparza and Michael Watson who read, and often read and reread, and commented all or parts of this work despite the magnitude of the task. Their opinions and corrections have been very valuable, and I am deeply endebted to them. I am very grateful to Agnès Jacob and Chantal Vezin, who translated and edited this book with skill, patience and great care.

I would also like to thank the numerous individuals who provided information and documents, thereby enriching my knowledge of the subject, my brothers, sisters-in-law or brothers-in-law: Charles and Annick, Gabriel and Andrée, Eric and Bernadette, Jean-François and Irène, Guy and Christiane, Daniel and Mireille, as well as friends and acquaintances Jean Bellot, Fernand Blaze, Bruno Bonnemain, Daniel Boutin, André Dubail, Maurice Durand, Jacques and Niquette Keller, Jacques Noury, Jean Rigoulet, Francis Thiaucourt, François Vallat...

Thanks are also owed to the staff of the *Bibliothèque Nationale de France* and the libraries of the *Muséum d'Histoire naturelle*, of the *Ecole nationale vétérinaire d'Alfort*, of the *Faculté de Médecine de Paris*, of the *Académie des Sciences*, of the *Université Catholique de Louvain* and, most particularly, of the *Académie nationale de Médecine* (BANM), where I could always count on the generous and valuable help on the entire staff, and particularly that of Laurence Camous, Irmine Casy, Damien Blanchard, Gildas Bouric and Jérôme van Wijland.

To my wife Jacqueline,
my children and children-in-law:
François and Caroline, Berthe and Christophe, Cécile and Yvon,
and my grandchildren: Alice, Noé, Antoine, Léon and Victor.

Contents

Foreword

The great French positivist philosopher, Auguste Comte, wrote that "one does not know science completely as long as one does not know its history". Thus, to understand the science of vaccination one must know its roots, which now reach back in time at least three centuries.

Prof. Hervé Bazin has now provided us with a detailed and comprehensive history of vaccination, first published in French and now in this English translation. That vaccination which has influenced the health of billions on this planet, saving more lives than any intervention except the provision of clean water, is inadequately known, a deficiency which this book will help to correct. Although the medical science, now called vaccinology (a term invented by Jonas Salk and the French industrialist Charles Mérieux), uses the same tools of microbiology, molecular biology, and epidemiology that are used by other branches of medicine, it is singular in that its goal is to prevent disease, rather than to treat it.

It is fitting that the first target of vaccination was smallpox, one of the four Horsemen of the Apocalypse, known for its contagiousness and high mortality. Bubonic plague may have had a higher mortality in its pulmonary form, but smallpox was more perennial. Although it is unclear whether the practice of variolation arose in the Middle East or in China, certainly it was an old practice, probably born from the observation that people seldom suffered smallpox twice and perhaps also from the protection afforded to important people against large doses of poison by prior administration of small amounts.

Voltaire in his *Lettres philosophiques* famously and amusingly wrote about the use of variolation in the Caucasus in order to preserve the beauty of Circassian women, and George Washington resorted to variolation to protect the American army during the War of Independence against Great Britain, despite the risk that soldiers would die or be disabled.

In the light of the importance given to prevention of smallpox one can understand the efforts to find another less dangerous method of prevention. It appears that Jenner had predecessors with respect to the identification of cowpox as a vaccine against smallpox, but Jenner was a scientist, and as such was able to prove the value of cowpox and thus to convince other scientists and politicians to use it. As is well known, Napoleon Bonaparte was one of those quick to realize its value.

We do not know, and may never know, the origin of the virus strain used by Jenner, as modern studies show that it is a poxvirus not identical to any other, but capable of inducing immune responses that act against *variola*. As Hervé Bazin shows, the years between Jenner and Pasteur saw much controversy about vaccination, primarily due to non-standardization of vaccine production and administration. Out of this controversy arose the first anti-vaccination groups, still active today and still opposed to "interfering with nature".

Hervé Bazin also shows that during those years, practices akin to variolation or vaccination were tried against many diseases, although little was known about the microbes that caused the diseases.

Pasteur arrived on the scene just as microbiology was beginning to emerge. The ability to obtain pathogens in pure culture was the key that opened the way to modification of those pathogens. Prof. Bazin recounts in detail how the idea of vaccination came slowly to Pasteur as he worked on chicken cholera caused by the bacterium we now call *Pasteurella multocida*. Was it a stroke of genius to challenge chickens that had been exposed to aged cultures of the organism with fresh cultures, or was it an accident? Difficult to say, but it is just that trait of making the right choices that makes certain people geniuses. The idea that the chickens inoculated with attenuated bacilli would be protected was not obvious, and Hervé Bazin is right to quote Emile Roux, who said "Science appears calm and triumphant when it is finished, but science in the course of being done is only contradiction and torment, hope and disappointment".

A short time later, Pasteur started work on rabies. Prof. Bazin is particularly good at describing how the attenuation of rabies virus gradually was obtained through numerous detailed experiments in animals. The decision to try to vaccinate humans exposed to rabies was not taken lightly, and the story of Josef Meister, told and retold by many prior writers, emerges here as a clinical trial undertaken in the light of much animal data and anguished reflection. I did not know that a Commission on Rabies had been set up before the first human trials at the request of Pasteur, and that the deliberations of the Commission prepared the way for those trials.

In the last part of the book, Hervé Bazin covers the developments that have taken place since the late 19th Century. Perhaps the most important was the incorporation of immunology into vaccinology, allowing us to know what vaccines do to protect us. Not surprisingly, it becomes clear that the scientific discoveries that are giving us multiple new vaccines against bacteria, viruses, and probably soon parasites, have their origins in events that took place long ago. The dramas that surrounded the development of the two polio vaccines remind us that the character of scientists has effects on their discoveries, and that scientific controversies are no less heated than those in other fields, but with outcomes that are possibly more important. Raymond Queneau has remarked that "the truly important history is that of inventions".

It is only in recent years, with the advent of molecular biology, that vaccine development has substantially changed from the methods used by Pasteur and his collaborators. The fact is that we can now make almost any antigen of interest, either by isolation from the microbe or by *de novo* synthesis. The problem that remains is to learn more about the pathogenesis of disease and the relationship between the microbe and the host.

The merit of this book is its historical accuracy, its investigation and description of the fits and starts, the successes and failures and the complexities of historical events, even when they take place in science or perhaps particularly when they take place in science. It is only by knowing the context in which these events took place that we can understand the immense endeavor that is now modern vaccinology, and it is this context that Hervé Bazin has given us.

Stanley Plotkin, MD

Emeritus Professor of Pediatrics, University of Pennsylvania

Emeritus Professor of the Wistar Institute

Introduction

In October 1347, twelve galleys set anchor in Messina, a seaport on the Sicilian coast, facing continental Italy.

A crowd quickly gathered, attracted by the unusual sight. Unfortunately, there was not much to see: only a few rather dirty and emaciated people saying they came from Caffa, in the Crimea. For several months Caffa had been besieged by Tartar invaders. But the Tartars had been forced to end their siege, having fallen prey to a plague that was decimating their ranks.

However, before leaving they took the time to hurl some corpses over the walls of the city, using catapults. An early form of bacteriological warfare! The Ancients were aware of the contagious nature of certain diseases, and there is reason to presume that the Tatars knew perfectly well what they were doing. The consequences of their actions were quickly apparent. The plague spread through the city, and then throughout Europe, carried by people already infected who were running as fast and as far as possible to avoid it. The epidemic returned to Caffa in 1356, eight years after it had left the city; this time, the disease seemed less virulent, and eventually subsided. Pope Clement VI spoke of 26 million victims, meaning that one out of three or four Europeans was killed. It was certainly "*the most impressive epidemic recorded in history*"[1]. The Spanish influenza might have caused comparable casualties, but on a world-wide scale.

Many diseases caused by pathogenic agents have brought devastation to our cities: smallpox, cholera, leprosy, diphtheria, tuberculosis, poliomyelitis, AIDS; and to our rural areas: rinderpest, foot-and-mouth disease, bovine pleuropneumonia, sheeppox and many others! The incalculable suffering and despair caused by infectious diseases has remained unchanged. From a personal point of view, it matters little whether a loved one dies during an epidemic of great or small proportions! In the words of Lamartine, in *Méditations poétiques*, where he laments the loss of his beloved Elvire, killed by... phthisis, or pulmonary tuberculosis:

> "*What are these vales, towers, cottages to me?*
> *Vain things whose charm for me has long abated?*
> *Streams, rocks, woods - places loved and solitary.*
> *Sometimes, when one person is missing, the whole world seems depopulated!*"

How has humankind fought infectious perils? The identification of certain infectious diseases was no doubt an important turning point. Smallpox was probably one of the first diseases to be identified, due to its easily recognizable pustules, although it was sometimes confused with chicken pox. The contagiousness of the two diseases is thought to have been recognized at about the same time. Local containment measures were taken, such as isolation or quarantine, even sanitary barriers enforced by troops... with orders to shoot to kill[2], or more or less massive destruction of animals in the case of an epizootic[3].

---

1. Nysten, 1858, p. 1064.
2. Howard, 1801; Vicq-d'Azyr, 1776.
3. Bouley, 1856, t. 1, p. 1; Vallat, 2006.

The observation that contagious diseases do not recur in the same subject was another major breakthrough. But it was not known how to make use of this fact in the active prevention of infectious diseases.

Awareness of this fact was very likely first used to create natural contagion by voluntarily bringing together infected individuals with healthy individuals, especially children. Inoculation (variolation) was the next step; it introduced an active method of disease prevention. What incited these measures? What diseases were the first to "benefit" from them?

Three diseases seem to compete for this privilege: smallpox in humans and contagious pleuropneumonia or rinderpest in bovines. The earliest texts known are Chinese, dating back to the end of the sixteenth century or, more probably, to the seventeenth century. They concern smallpox inoculation[4], but there could well have been oral transmission of similar practices concerning smallpox, rinderpest or contagious bovine pleuropneumonia in Africa.

4. Leung, 1996, p. 57.

I
Prehistory

1
Smallpox or Variola

"For centuries, prior to Jenner's discovery of vaccination in 1798, small-pox had been regarded as the king of fatal diseases."
Eugene Foster, 1888[1].

Why should smallpox be the subject of a special discussion, in a book on the history of vaccination? Today, over thirty years since smallpox has disappeared from the planet, it is interesting to take a closer look at this disease. In the Western world, it is safe to say that not one doctor in a thousand is likely to have seen a case of smallpox. The disease was eradicated world-wide in the 1970s, and in developed countries well before that. Smallpox was at the origin of the idea of active protection against infectious diseases through variolation, and later through Jennerian vaccination, which led to its eradication... Thus, the disease played a crucial role in the fight against infectious diseases, giving it special status among them. Moreover, it is the only human infectious disease that has disappeared, eradicated by man through considerable and admirable collective effort.

Variola was given the name "small" pox to differentiate it from the "great pox", "Pox" or "French pox", as syphilis was called, and from "chicken" pox, or varicella.

Variola was a particularly terrifying disease. Around the year 900, Rhazes (al-Razi) entitled the first chapter of his treatise on smallpox: "*On the causes of smallpox & why all men, except one or two, are attacked by this disease.*"[2] In fact, this incidence varied depending on the time and place concerned... One thing is certain: the disease was extremely widespread. It was a terrible affliction, sometimes killing a quarter to one third of those infected, and when it did not kill, it left its victims disfigured or maimed! The mortality rate depended on the particular epidemic: "*Timoni claims that in Constantinople, sometimes one out of two sufferers died. Hofman speaks of an epidemic that killed eighteen out of twenty of its victims.*"[3] By contrast, Jenner describes a particularly benign epidemic: "*About seven years ago a species of small-pox spread through many of the towns and villages of Gloucestershire: it was of so mild a nature, that a fatal instance scarcely ever heard... I never saw nor heard of an instance of its being confluent.*"[4] There was a

1. Foster, 1888, vol. VI, p. 478.
2. Rhazes, about 900 (1778), p. 1.
3. de la Condamine, 1759a, p. 23.
4. Jenner, 1798 (1800b), p. 44.

time when smallpox killed or maimed a predictable and almost constant percentage of humans. It is believed that "*Europe, in the century preceding the discovery of vaccination, lost in deaths from small-pox 50,000,000 of her population*"[5].

The Arrival of Smallpox in the Western World

Smallpox appeared on the European continent after having wrought its ravages in other lands, probably since very ancient times. The Egyptian mummy of Ramses V (who died in 1157 B.C.) bears traces that could be attributed to this disease.

But according to most authors, it first emerged in the year of the birth of Mahomet, in 570 or 572[6]. Rhazes was the first to describe the disease and its treatment[7]. It was probably the crusades that brought smallpox to Europe from Asia; European colonizers were responsible for its spread at least through the Americas.

Many hypotheses were put forth as to the nature of this disease. For a long time, the most common theory concerned an innate smallpox germ that most people carried from birth. The evacuation of the smallpox germ after a first infection was thought to explain the fact that a second infection almost never occurred. Popular wisdom also held that contracting smallpox at some point in life was necessary for good health. In this regard, Cothenius raises the question: "*... is it necessary for the development of this germ to take place in the human body for health to acquire all the solidity & consistence of which it is capable? Or is this a new disease, born under a foreign sky, & which could spare human beings, whose constitution and health would not suffer the least prejudice as a result?*"[8] This idea of the loss of susceptibility to catching smallpox still existed in 1888: "*One attack of variola usually destroys the susceptibility of the individual to the disease during the remainder of his life.*"[9] The concept of an active defence of the body against infectious diseases only appeared with Metchnikoff[10] and Behring[11]. Its acceptance required some time.

The hypothesis of an infectious agent emerged during the first half of the 18th century; hesitant at first, it became more solid over time. The contagiousness of smallpox was a strong argument in favour of the "virus" theory. In 1768, Paulet spoke of a seed "*... consisting of pus & scabs, that can attach itself, seep into upholstery, bedding, clothing, metals, &c... We are therefore dealing with a foreign entity that enters the body of an animal, where it finds fluids and a substance allowing its reproduction... Only beings that can replicate themselves could produce such a phenomenon; they must then be vegetable or animal seeds*"[12]. However, the germ theory took a long time to be accepted, and this was still not the case in 1799, when Webster wrote: "*From the date of the earliest historical records, the opinions of men have been divided on the subject of the causes and origin of pestilential diseases... In the history of opinions on this mysterious subject, there is a remarkable distinction between the ancients and moderns. The*

5. Foster, 1888, vol. VI, p. 478.
6. Paulet, 1768, t. 1, p. 77.
7. Rhazes, about 900 (1778).
8. Cothenius, 1774, p. 156.
9. Foster, 1888, vol. VI, p. 478.
10. Metchnikoff, 1887, p. 321.
11. Behring, 1890a, p. 1113.
12. Paulet, 1768, t. 1, pp. 143 & 276.

ancients derived most of their knowledge and science from personal observation, as they had very few books and little aid from the improvements of their predecessors. The philosophers of antiquity, attentive to changes in the seasons and to the revolution of the heavenly bodies, attempted to trace pestilential diseases to extraordinary vicissitudes in the weather, and to the aspects of the planets. Modern philosophers and physicians, on the other hand, unable to account for pestilence on the principle of extraordinary seasons, and disdaining to admit the influence of the planets to be the cause, have resorted to invisible animalculae, and to infection concealed in bales of goods or old clothes, transported from Egypt or Contantinople, and let loose, at certain periods, to scourge mankind and defoliate the earth."[13]

One characteristic of smallpox was its extremely contagious nature; it infected rich and poor alike. The disease took a heavy toll on many royal families. Great Britain's royal family was no exception; the disease killed Queen Mary and left her husband, King William III of England (1650-1702), disfigured. Louis XV, King of France, died of smallpox in 1774! His agony was so terrible that it made many French people reconsider and accept variolation, the only method of protection known at the time.

The existence of tiny, invisible beings had been suspected for a long time, but nothing was known about their nature. "*The only known factor in the origin of smallpox is contagion...*"[14].

For a long time, fermentation phenomena (bread, wine, vinegar...) were supposed to be the origin of smallpox. In Anglo-Saxon countries, this theory was judged to offer (from 1844 to about 1900-1910) an explanation as to the cause of all infectious diseases. Proposed by Farr of the British Registrar-General's Department, it classified all these diseases under the heading "zymotic diseases" (*see Glossary*)[15].

Modern viral classification has placed the smallpox virus with pathogens that can be separated with ultrafiltration membranes. Viruses were discovered thanks to Chamberland-Pasteur or Berkfeld filters that made it possible to separate bacteria blocked by a filter from the viruses that pass through it. A Russian, Dimitri Ivanowski, isolated the tobacco mosaic virus; later, two Germans, Loeffler and Frosch, isolated the foot-and-mouth disease virus, the first filterable agent of an animal disease. A few years later, the yellow fever virus was isolated by Reed and his associates. The real, although still approximate, nature of the smallpox virus only became known in the 1930s[16].

Smallpox is caused by a virus of the Poxvirus family. Its genetic make-up consists of a single, double-stranded deoxyribonucleic acid (DNA) molecule. Later, two varieties of variola virus were identified, one causing the benign form or "alastrim" (*Variola minor*), the other causing the severe form (*Variola major*). Smallpox viruses are distinctive, and are related to numerous other viruses which confer variolic diseases to various animal species, such as cattle (cowpox), ovines (sheeppox), monkeys (monkeypox), etc. These diseases have been classified into a single category for some time.

13. Webster, 1799, vol. 1, p. 9.
14. Black's Medical Dictionary, 1914, p. 694.
15. Black's Medical Dictionary, 1914, p. 857.
16. Fenner, 1988, p. 69.

Ordinary Smallpox

Smallpox has been extremely well described. "*Before going any further, let us note that four stages are to be distinguished in smallpox: 1) the invasion period with rising fever, called boiling; 2) the eruptions; 3) the period of suppuration; 4) drying-up or scab formation.*"[17]

The various types of variolic viruses have approximately the same incubation period of about nine to ten days. This is followed by an invasion period: "*When the physician comes to examine a patient, he can immediately judge reasonably well what type of illness he is witnessing, by the frequent sighs and the moaning of the patient seized by a fear without name, the pains in his stomach region, with an urge to vomit, pain and frequent stabbing in his back and kidneys, a painful, general fatigue with violent chills that no external source of heat can disperse, constant somnolence and loss of appetite.*"[18] The patient often experiences intense anxiety and intermittent delirium. In ordinary or discrete smallpox, this state lasts two or three days, and is followed by a period of appeasement.

The eruption stage follows. "*As this period approaches, the patient, particulary if the eruption is to be copious, experiences a sensation of distention about the head, face, eyes, and mouth, frequently imagines that the whole cutaneous surface is greatly swollen. Towards the end of the third day, or more commonly on the morning of the fourth, and after a series of symptoms such as have been described, the eruption begins to appear.*"[19]

A rash ("the eruptions") then appears on the face, first on the chin, then on the forehead and cheeks, spreading to the neck, the trunk and the lower limbs. The rash first takes the form of small, red spots of varying sizes, spaced out over the skin. These are the macules. "*They are usually of a pinkish colour at first, but can often be rather colourless, being very hard to see, except in the light of day, or by looking at the skin horizontally with a candle that anyone can hold and point as he pleases, without having a degree from an Academy...*"[20]. These small spots will become papules, then superficial vesicles on about the sixth day, with a slightly raised centre. At first, the papules fill with clear fluid which gradually becomes more or less opaque, and is yellowish-white in colour. Smallpox is said to be ordinary when the pustules are separated by a distance at least equal to their diameter. These pustules appear as small, spherical, whitish spots. They continue to develop for three or four days, becoming round and firm to the touch. They are surrounded by a rather wide, reddish circle. The pustules on the oral, pharyngeal and laryngeal mucosa, as well as those on the eyelids and the eyes, and even on the preputial or vulva mucosa, determine to a great extent the severity of symptoms and, in most cases, the degree of pain experienced by the patient. This stage is associated with local inflammatory swelling, and with the recurrence of very painful general symptoms, such as fever (often called the second fever), muscle aches and even delirium.

The dessication stage follows: the blisters burst and the pus they contain dries up forming yellowish, then brownish-black scabs. The scabs fall off, taking pieces of epidermis with them, and causing more or less intense itching. The skin recovers an almost normal appearance in a few weeks, but irregular, white scars dotted with black remain at the places where the scabs fell off.

17. Société de médecins (Society of Physicians), 1772, t. 6, p. 435; Copland, 1856, p. 883.
18. Thornton, 1808, p. 2.
19. Fisher, 1834, p. 9.
20. Fouquet, 1772, p. 102.

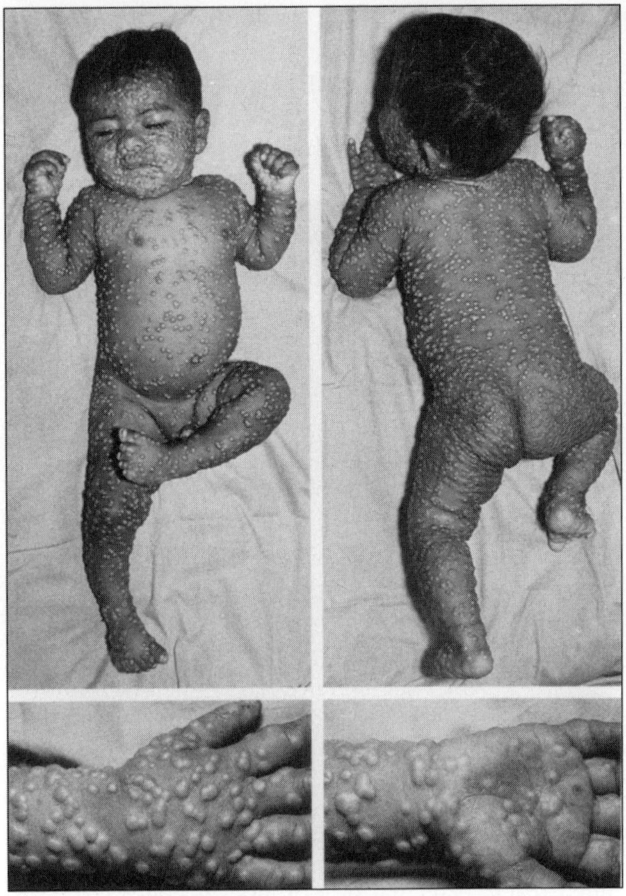

Figure 1. Child with ordinary or benign smallpox. (Reprinted courtesy of the WHO.)

Various Forms of Smallpox

Ordinary smallpox, also called benign, discrete or common, lasts between eleven and twenty-one days. The disease causes much suffering, even in its lightest forms. Unfortunately, the disease also occurs in much more severe forms. The confluent form starts with symptoms rather similar to those of ordinary smallpox, but very quickly the symptoms take on acute or very acute intensity. In the eruptive stage, the face becomes red, swollen and shiny; macules appear and they are soon transformed into whitish, almost continuous blisters. The mucosa are even more seriously affected, and the patients suffer a loss of speech. The stage of "*suppuration is always accompanied by severe swelling of the face, that completely erases the features; the eyes, nose, cheeks, lips, neck and ears are hideously deformed. No other disease distorts the face to this extent. The swollen eyelids remain closed for 5 or 6 days; the nostrils are obstructed by the swelling and by scabs; the gaping mouth is dry, black, fetid; the lips, dried out, fungous, bleeding and twisted by the swelling, let saliva dribble out abundantly. It must be added that the patient has great difficulty breathing, that he is in a continuous state of sub-delirium and agitation, prostrated in his bed but making repeated attempts to leave it.*

In short, he offers one of the most lamentable, the most horrible spectacles a doctor can ever see."[21]

In most cases, death occurs between the eleventh and the fifteenth day. When the patient survives, he can often have complications and sequelae like blindness, motor paraplegias, boils and facial scars that can make him frightening to see[22].

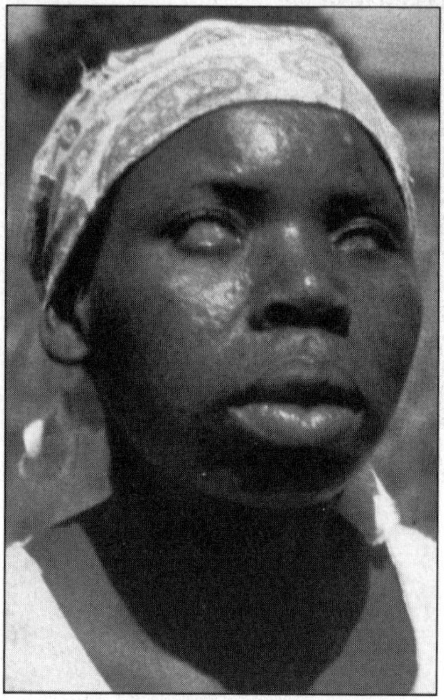

Figure 2. Young woman from Zaïre, cured of smallpox but bearing its sequelae: she is completely blind and her face is covered with scars. (Reprinted courtesy of the WHO.)

Haemorrhagic smallpox, also called black, petechial or scorbutic, is characterized by eruptions accompanied by blood, mixed with serosity or not, in the pustules. Its rapid development ends in death in the great majority of cases. The fulminant form, always fatal, progresses so rapidly that the pustules hardly have time to appear.

Treatments

Two competing treatments existed. Fouquet depicts the earliest in picturesque terms: "*I remember*, he says, *that when I was a child in Montpellier* (France) *I saw people with smallpox being wrapped in red sheets, or being kept in beds surrounded by curtains of the same material, in a way similar to what is still being done in Japan. Superstition dictated that live toads be hidden under the bed, because they were thought to have the power to attract and absorb all the venom of the disease, just as in Rivière's time a sheep or a lamb was placed in bed beside a sick child, based on the same belief, to say nothing of the great care taken to keep the patient's room almost always*

21. Balzer, 1885, p. 341.
22. Councilman, 1907, p. 250.

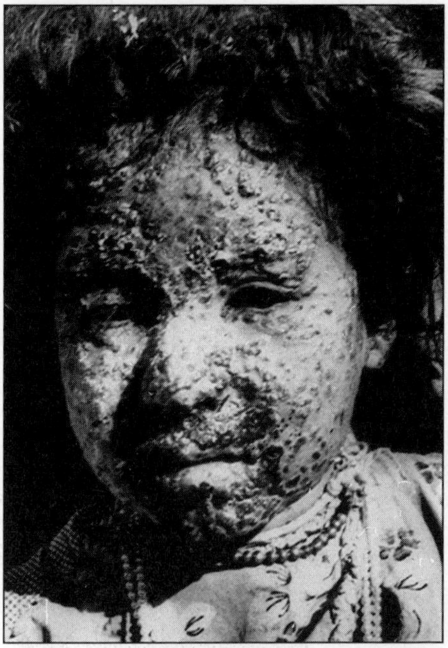

Figure 3. A case of smallpox in Afghanistan, during the final years (around 1950-1970) that this disease could be found on the planet. (Reproduced with permission of WHO.)

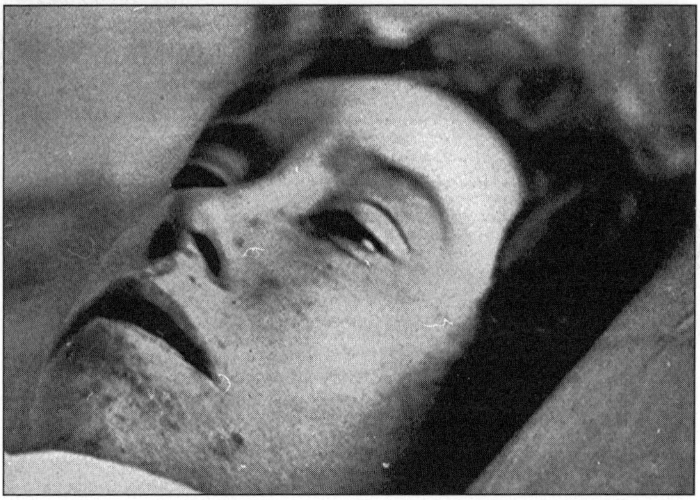

Figure 4. Toxic or haemorrhagic smallpox, the most dangerous type of smallpox, characterised by a profound weakness and also by the absence of pustules. From Riketts and Byles (Heagerty, 1924).

hermetically closed, and to heat the air with stoves in which scents burned continually..."[23]. This "heat" method was gradually abandoned and replaced with a so-called "cold" method that will be described later.

23. Fouquet, 1772, p. 16.

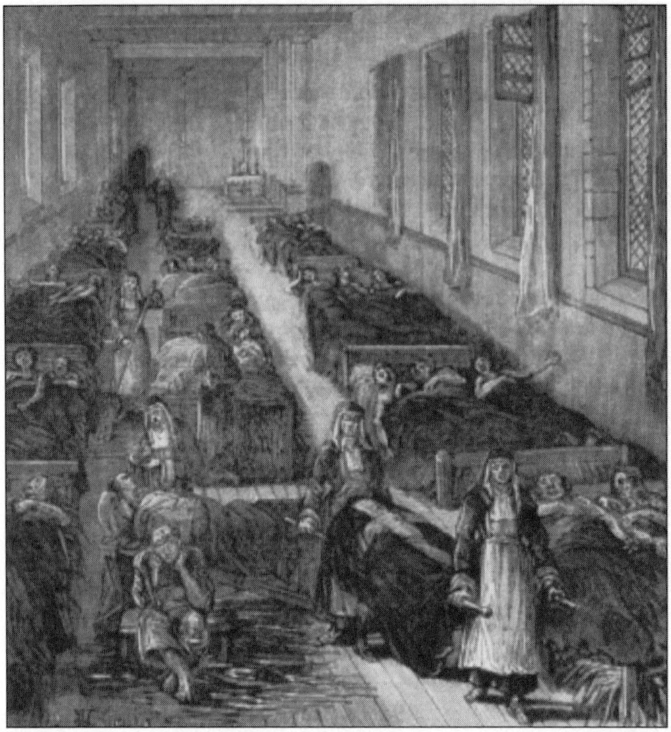

Figure 5. Smallpox patient's room at the Hôtel-Dieu Hospital in Paris, 1718, as depicted by an engraving of the period. The article accompanying this illustration gives an accurate description of the hygiene of the times: "*To have several children with smallpox sleep together in the same bed has the most serious consequences... There is nothing more unhealthy than the habit, among simple people, of having the children keep the same clothes on for the entire duration of this disgusting disease, for fear that they will catch cold when their clothes are changed...*". The author, writing around 1900, believed that this practice had disappeared in private homes, but persisted in hospitals (Clerc)[24].

Extent of Mortality Due to Smallpox

At the start of the eighteenth century, mortality due to smallpox was still very high, especially in big cities. According to Petit, one smallpox victim out of seven was killed by the disease[25], but at times "a bad" epidemic could kill one sufferer out of three. "*In England deaths from smallpox formed one-tenth of the entire mortality; in France 30,000 died of it yearly* (out of a population of about 20 millions); *and in Prussia alone in one year (1796) there were 26,646 deaths.*"[26] The figures for fatalities and infirmities were high: "*The fact is that over thirty thousand people in France fall victim to ordinary smallpox each year, & that the disease mutilates, mains or disfigures an even greater number.*"[27] In

24. Clerc, around 1900, p. 169.
25. Petit, 1766a, p. 79.
26. Councilman, 1907, p. 250.
27. de la Condamine, 1764, p. 51.

terms of the overall population, the death rate was between one out of seven and one out of fourteen, depending on the author cited.

"*The annual loss of lives by Small Pox in Great Britain and Ireland in the latter period* (end of the eighteenth century) *was separately calculated by two able physicians (Sir Gilbert Blane, Bart. and Dr. Letsom), and the result laid before a* Committee *of the* House *of* Commons. *The one estimated the numbers at 34,260. Adding that he believed those deaths to be under the truth. The other phycician made them amount to 36,000. But this immense and increasing consumption of human lives was not the sole evil produced by this distemper: for a considerable portion of the survivors were pitted and disfigured; some lost one of their eyes, a few became totally blind, and others had their constitution impaired, and predisposed to a variety of complaints, which were productive of future distress, and sometimes to death. These additional calamities cannot be reduced by calculation; but as the mortality for Small Pox was continually on the increase, these concomitant evils must have been so likewise.*"[28]

"*No complete statistics of American cities for the period before the introduction of vaccination can be obtained. The data contained in the accompanying table are compiled from the most reliable historical sources, with references to the prevalence of small-pox in Boston. After the settlement of the colony at Plymouth, in 1620, small-pox appeared frequently in Massachusetts, among the Indian tribes and the English settlers. Such epidemics occurred in 1631, 1633, 1639, 1677, 1678 (from 700 to 800 died in this year), 1702 (213 died, which was about 4.4 per cent of the population)... In 1730, with a population of 15,000 people, 4,000 were sick, and about 500 died.*"[29]

Table I. Number of smallpox cases, patients disfigured, maimed or dead, in France, between 1815 and 1885, based on yearly vaccination reports.
Only data for years ending in 0 and 5 is presented.
No report was published for 1870; the 1871 report seems to contain the figures for 1870-1871.

Year	Departments providing reports/number and (%)		Smallpox cases	Maimed, disfigured	Deaths
1815	56/76	(73.7%)	37,630	3,625	4,626
1820	79/84	(94.0%)	38,254	3,221	4,823
1825	52/86	(60.5%)	26,571	2,245	3,369
1830	32/86	(37.2%)	9,764	831	1,340
1835	54/86	(62.8%)	13,336	1,486	1,893
1840	71/86	(82.5%)	14,285	1,412	2,316
1845	61/86	(70.9%)	7,777	866	1,181
1850	63/86	(73.2%)	13,755	1,669	1,677
1855	67/86	(77.9%)	23,112	1,988	3,143
1860	58/89	(65.1%)	13,755	1,494	1,662
1865	72/89	(80.8%)	25,993	4,089	4,166
1871	70/87	(80.4%)	221,417	24,004	58,236
1875	48/87	(55.1%)	4,103	374	698
1880	59/87	(67.8%)	17,579	1,433	2,997
1885	48/87	(55.1%)	8,948	1,005	1,727

28. Moore, 1815, p. 300.
29. Abbott, 1889, vol. VII, p. 509.

We can conclude that variolation as it was practiced at the time did not stop the devastation caused by smallpox in Western societies.

The introduction of Jennerian vaccination changed outcomes, while at the same time living conditions in Western countries improved.

Throughout most of the nineteenth century, the variola virus remained present everywhere in France, as is evidenced by the considerable number of cases recorded. The Annual Reports of the Central Committee for Vaccination or of the Academy (Royal, Imperial and finally National) of Medicine reproduce the statistics submitted by departmental prefects. Although they remain incomplete, they give an indication of the extent of this plague. Up to 1813, French data is sparse. Between 1813 and 1885, France saw an average of 10,000 to 20,000 smallpox cases per year, with the numbers showing a gradual decline...

Table II below gives mortality rates due to smallpox in England and Wales over a period of 10 years, and includes a major epidemic (1871).

Table II. Mortality rates due to smallpox in England and Wales.

Year	1860	1861	1862	1863	1864	1865	1866	1867	1868	1869	1870	1871
Deaths	2,749	1,320	1,628	5,964	7,684	6,411	3,029	2,513	2,052	1,565	2,580	22,907

It is clear that considerable fluctuations existed in the extent of epidemics; the one of 1871 ended in mid 1872. The combined population of England and Wales at the time was about 20 millions inhabitants[30]. These figures were more or less the same in all European countries. They may not be very precise, but they provide a good indication of the situation. After the introduction of Jennerian vaccination, between 1811 and 1887, mortality due to smallpox, in Boston, fluctuated from 0.06 for 1,000 inhabitants in 1811 to 2.95 in 1872, 1.21 in 1873, followed by a drastic decrease of 0.003 to 0.012 reached in 1887[31], a decrease due perhaps to a successful vaccination campaign following the 1871-1872 smallpox epidemic... Interest in vaccinations faded quickly as the threat became more remote...

These statistics, albeit approximate, clearly show that even in the case of an effective preventive method such as Jennerian vaccination, obtaining all the benefits it could provide depended on correct application. Complete world-wide eradication of smallpox only became possible thanks to the collective will and effort of the member countries of the WHO.

30. Haydn's Dictionary of Popular Medicine, 1874, pp. 416 & 570.
31. Abbott, 1889, vol. VII, p. 509.

2
Lady Montagu Brings Variolation from Turkey: 1721...

Announcement of Variolation in the Western World: circa 1700

At this point in history, medicine was emerging from a long period when it had accepted the theories of the Ancients without question, be they good or bad. Now, learned minds were introducing new ideas... Between 1751 and 1772, the Encyclopaedists publish their work, which exerted great influence all over Europe.

One fact, already known, was that a person who had contracted smallpox once could not have it again, except in very rare cases. Those who were pockmarked, on whose faces the disease had left its distinctive, indelible mark, were not going to have it again. Therefore, they could tend to smallpox sufferers without being in danger of catching the disease. This observation had probably led to the practice of "variolation", which consisted of transmitting the disease to a healthy person by using "matter" from an infected person chosen, theoretically, because his smallpox was mild. The intention was to transmit a benign form of smallpox at a convenient time, to someone prepared for this operation, to induce in this individual a state refractory to an "attack of smallpox". This procedure seemed surprising: "*It appears at first extraordinary to think of giving a disease to a healthy person, & there need be, most certainly, very good reasons to come to this decision: these reasons are found in the character of small-pox, the circumstances influencing the outcome of the disease, & the success of the inoculation.*"[1] The procedure was called inoculation or insertion. Today it is called variolation. Prior to Jennerian vaccination, the word "inoculation" referred essentially to smallpox and, more rarely, to animal diseases like sheeppox or cattle plague.

Accounts of variolation in China apparently reached England in 1700, through a letter from the merchant Joseph Lister to London physician Martin Lister. Records indicate that a certain Dr. Clopton Havers reported on it at a meeting of the Royal Society on February 14, 1700. One or two other reports apparently circulated in Europe[2]. The most descriptive account of variolation in China is probably that of the Jesuit priest d'Entrecolles (1726), who described how the Chinese had been practicing it for a long time: "*It* (smallpox inoculation) *is called Tchung-teou, planting the small Pox. This method seems to have appeared a little over a century ago; they do not make one or two incisions like in Europe, to introduce the variola virus in the blood immediately. Instead, scabs from a benign case of small Pox are taken, crushed, & mixed with musc to make pellets that are used when needed. When parents want to inoculate a child, they place a few pellets in his nostrils, & the small Pox soon breaks out. For while here (in Europe) only one inoculated person in two or three hundred dies, & even less when much care is taken & the subjects are clean, it seems that in China it is considered fortunate to lose only one in ten.*"[3] Later,

1. Société de médecins (Society of Physicians), 1772, t. 6, p. 451.
2. Miller, 1957, p. 48.
3. d'Entrecolles, 1726 (1756), p. 288.

missionaries asserted that this practice went back to the 17th or even to the end of the 16th century, if not to the Song dynasty, that is, about 590 AD, but no proof of this exists. It seems that the procedure was never applied on a large scale[4].

In Hindustan, inoculation is said to have been practiced since early Antiquity by Brahmins, in the religious context of a vegetarian diet, observance of principles of hygiene, and prayer. The custom is said to have spread along African coasts to Tripoli, Tunis, Algiers, where the incision on the subject was performed "*on the back of the hand between the thumb and the first finger, ...*"[5], and even as far as Senegal. In Egypt and Syria, variolation was known in the eighteenth century[6].

In Europe, numerous testimonials confirm that bringing together children who had never had smallpox with several others who had it was customary in Holland, Germany, Italy, Sweden, Denmark, South Wales, and in France in the Perigord region. But no details are given, except that this popular practice of inoculation was generally called "buying the smallpox". In Northern Scotland, the old women of the Highlands often infected children by putting them to bed with wool strands soaked in smallpox matter tied to their wrists[7]. It was a kind of natural inoculation.

Authors give examples that concern various continents[8]. It is possible that these testimonials are all true, and we can ask ourselves why the official medical establishment of the era was apparently remained unaware of this protection technique... On the other hand, rumour has it that inoculation started in Circassia, to protect the beauty of young girls destined for the harems of the rich in Constantinople, who bought them from their parents[9]. "*In any case, it was in this country* (Circassia) *that a commercial impetus or, if we prefer maternal concern, gave rise to the idea of inoculating small-pox before the age when it usually appears, in the hope of reducing its virulence through prevention.*"[10] This source could be right, but it remains uncertain. As to the young girls of Circassia, their fate can also be seen in a different light. Speaking of the origins of inoculation (variolation), Joseph Duffour wrote: "*Since time immemorial, these beautiful women of Georgia and Circassia, whose most seductive traits and enchanting forms allowed them to offer the sovereigns of Turkey and Persia all the charms of voluptuous pleasure, owe this preference they obtain over the women of other nations to the inoculation customary in their country.*"[11] It is not certain that all the women granted this privilege were delighted with their fate! The undisguised truth is that their parents sold them, when they were still children, uneducated but variolated, to intermediaries, like puppies certified "vaccinated". They were trained, and then sold to rich harem owners. Many authors considered this commerce to be abject: La Condamine, Dezoteux, Husson and Monteils, but other historical commentators, most notably Voltaire, do not mention this custom[12]!

Around 1700, while Greece was under Turkish domination, there was an important Greek colony in Constantinople (modern-day Istanbul). During a smallpox epidemic,

4. Leung, 1996, p. 65; Moore, 1815, p. 218.
5. Caffem Aga, 1756, p. 138.
6. Volney, 1787, p. 222.
7. Moore, 1815, p. 218; Roux, 1765, p. 9; Creighton, 1894, p. 471.
8. Anonymous, 1914, p. 9.
9. Montagu, 1991.
10. Bousquet, 1833, p. 151.
11. Duffour, 1808, p. iij.
12. Voltaire, 1727 (1817), p. 18.

a Greek woman inoculated 4,000 people, a number that seems very high, since the Turks were not very interested, or not at all, in this operation. Around 1703, the success of these inoculations practiced in Constantinople attracted the attention of Dr. Emmanuel Timone, a Greek physician, graduate of the University of Padua, with a degree from Oxford and practicing in Turkey. In 1713 he sent his observations of the situation to Dr. Woodward, who later published them in *Philosophical Transactions*. Apparently, inoculation was practiced by "*old women who, with no medical training whatever, encroach on our rights by practicing it*"[13]. An early example of corporate protectionism!

The literature provides accounts of two of these Greek inoculators: one from Philippopolis, representing the classical technique, and the other from Thessalonica, using another technique that combined religion with medicine.

The first, from Philippopolis, refused Timone's invitation to meet him in his house, so that he went to see her where she lived. "*I submitted to her several questions that I thought her competent to answer... In regard to origin, she did not know... As to her manner of proceeding to inoculate, a manner she shared with most of the others who practiced the same trade, here it is: 1°. She prescribed to the person she was to inoculate, a Purgation appropriate to his temperament & his strength. 2°. She recommended that the person abstain from meat, eggs, wine & other liqueurs producing a heating effect, for five or six days before the procedure. 3°. She advised staying in a well-closed Room, & in moderate heat. 4°. She chose a child of healthy temperament, who had natural small-pox of the distinctive type & not confluent, and went to see him on the tenth day of eruption. Using a triangular needle, she pierced some of the pustules on his legs & shins, & by squeezing them with her fingers she caused pus to come out, that she received in a glass vessel or a vessel of some other material, which she took care to keep warm by placing against her breast. Once this was done, she hastened to proceed with the operation; she made the injections in the same places of the body from which she extracted the variolous matter, mixing it with the blood from the injection, using a blunt silver needle; after this, she covered the wounds with acorn shells or some similar thing, & made a bandage over them, for fear that the rubbing of clothing might disturb the mixing of the blood with the virus. This dressing only stayed in place 5 to 6 hours, after which she removed it. Finally, she prescribed not just the diet above, but recommended a diet of vegetables & barley or flour stock only for 30 days & more. After the 3rd, 4th or 5th day the eruption appeared... it was usually limited to 15 or 20 pustules, more or less, rarely 30: what is more, this eruption was so untroublesome, that at times the Patient barely noticed his indisposition, & that neither his sight nor his features suffered any accident...*"[14].

A variation of this method was practiced by the Thessalonica inoculator, who "*says that this method is not a human invention, but that it was revealed by the Virgin, so that in order to sanctify it, she accompanies each step of her procedure by a Sign of the Cross, and by some Prayers she murmurs, & through which she gives the operation an air of respectable Mystery; and, aside from her salary, she requests a few candles to be placed before the Altar & the Statues of the Virgin*"[15].

At about the same time, the government of Venice named signor Pylarini, a physician, Consul of Smyrna (modern-day Izmir). After having studied inoculation in Turkey as early as 1701, in 1715 he published a little book describing this method; the book was

13. Timone, 1714 (1756), p. 12.
14. Timone, 1714 (1756), p. 13.
15. Timone, 1714 (1756), p. 16.

also reviewed in *Philosophical Transactions* in London. In 1717, in Montpellier (France), Boyer[16] defended a doctoral thesis on the insertion of smallpox. A Greek student named Antoine Le Duc wrote another thesis on the subject at the University of Leiden in 1722. He himself had been inoculated, at a young age, in his native city, Constantinople. In that city, as well as in Smyrna, it was the Greeks and the Armenians who were the first to take advantage of prevention by inoculation; next, it was used by Europeans living in these cities[17].

Around 1727, in his traveller's accounts, de la Motraye wrote: "*Because I saw no one (among Circassians) marked by the small-pox, it came to my mind to enquire if they had some secret to preserve themselves from the ravages that this enemy of beauty was causing in so many Nations: they told me that they did, & said that their secret was to inoculate it, or communicate it to those they wanted to preserve, by taking pus from someone who had it & mixing it with their blood through incisions made on them.*"[18] Circassia is the region now called Chechnya. "*Circassians are Muslim or schismatic Greek orthodox. The men are brave & ugly; the women beautiful and seductive with foreigners. They offer hospitality & sell their daughters.*"[19] "*Kleeman, a traveller of the XVIII century, tells us that he saw Circassians at the Kaffa market selling girls for prices as high as 6 or 7,000 Turkish piasters*"[20], very approximately the equivalent of 20,000 to 25,000 euros.

Accounts of smallpox inoculation no doubt reached France quite early, but they were ignored. "*The Latin treatise of Timoni, Physician of the Great Lord, on Greek inoculation, reprinted in the travels of Motraye, was brought to France by Lord Sutton, Ambassador of England to the Ottoman Empire, upon his return from Constantinople, before the first experiments made in London on criminals. Cardinal Dubois, then Secretary of State, entrusted Mr. Humin, now Minister to the King of Poland, Duke of Lorraine, with translating it into French: it was read at the Regency Council (1715-1723), & the subject was to be discussed, but more pressing matters caused the subject to be forgotten.*"[21] No official action was taken.

Lady Mary Wortley Montagu

It is often difficult to decide exactly what priority should be granted a particular person in the discovery of a method. Who introduced variolation in the Western world? The physicians Timone and Pylarini certainly contributed to this initiative. But who was the first to variolate in Europe? Roux points to an interesting sequence of events: "*I find in the observations of Mr. Eller, page 150, that in 1720, this knowledgeable Physician, while in Paris, learned from a Greek named Carraza the method being used in Constantinople to inoculate the small-pox. He made the experiment on a beggar boy seven years old...* (Back) *in his country, Mr. Eller, at the request of Prince d'Anhalt Bernbourg, inoculated two children of his first officers and two or three children of bourgeois families of the city of Bernbourg, with equal success.*"[22] Afterwards, Eller apparently stopped variolating because his status, defined by contract, of physician to the King in Berlin forbade all contact with persons

16. Domenjon, 1801, p. 26.
17. Ranby, 1751 (1756), p. 225.
18. de la Motraye, 1727? (1756), p. 6.
19. Roman, 1773, p. 237.
20. Pietkiewicz, 1834, p. 355.
21. de la Condamine, 1758 (1759b), p. 3.
22. Roux, 1765, p. 16.

infected with smallpox[23]. This could have been the first variolation performed by a physician in Western Europe, before the first British attempts.

In Europe, the most decisive contribution was made by a woman of character, Lady Mary Wortley Montagu, whose husband was the British ambassador to the Ottoman Empire, in Constantinople, between 1716 and 1718. Having accompanied her husband to Constantinople, curiosity and a marked spirit of independence made Lady Montagu walk through the city and learn the local customs. Wearing a veil was very useful for preserving her anonymity.

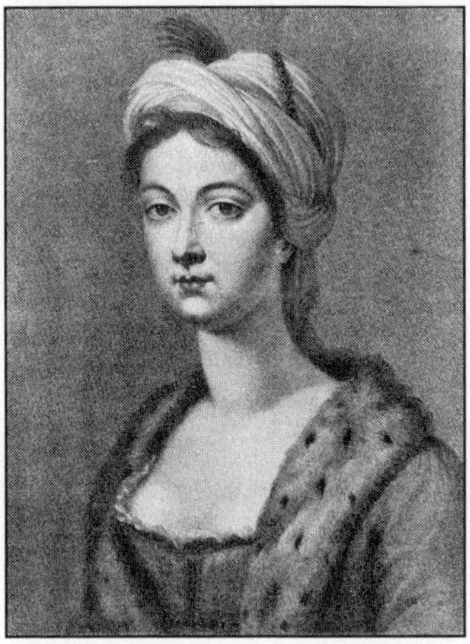

Figure 1. Portrait of Lady Montagu from "*La Défense contre la variole*" by Dr. Rondelet, *La Médecine Internationale Illustrée*, May, June and July, 1907. (Author's document.)

This is how she came to learn about the practice of inoculation. In a letter dated April 1, 1717, she gave a very interesting description of inoculation as she had seen it performed: "*A propos of distempers, I am going to tell you a thing that will make you wish yourself here. The small-pox, so fatal and so general amongst us, is here entirely harmless by the invention of engrafting, which is the term they give it. There is a set of old women, who make it their business to perform the operation, every autumn, in the month of September, when the heat is abated. People send to one another to know if any of their family has a mind to have the small-pox* (inoculated); *they make parties for this purpose, and when they are met (commonly fifteen or sixteen together) the old woman comes with a nut-shell full of the matter of the best sort of small-pox, and asks what vein you please to have opened. She immediately rips open the vein that you offer to her, with a large needle (which gives you no more pain than a common scratch) and puts into the vein as much matter as can lie upon the head of her needle, and after that, binds up the little wound with a hollow bit of shell, and in this manner opens four or five veins* (obviously, not veins but little wounds). *The Grecians have commonly the superstition of opening one in the middle of the forehead, one in each arm, and one on the breast, to mark the sign of the cross; but this has a very ill effect, all these wounds leaving little scars, and is not done by those that are not superstitious, who choose to have them in the legs, or that part of the arm that is concealed. The children or the young patients play together all the rest of the day, and are in perfect health to the eighth. Then the fever begins to seize them, and they keep their beds two days, very seldom three. They have very rarely above twenty or thirty* (pustules) *in their faces, which never*

23. Miller, 1957, p. 67.

mark, and in eight days time they are as well as before their illness. When they are wounded, there remains running sores during the distemper, which I don't doubt is a great relief to it. Every year thousands undergo this operation, and the French Ambassador says pleasantly that they take the small-pox here by way of diversion, as they take the waters in other countries. There is no example of any one that has died in it, and you may believe I am well satisfied of the safety of this experiment, since I intend to try it on my dear little son. I am patriot enough to take pains to bring this useful invention into fashion in England, and I should not fail to write to some of our doctors very particularly about it, if I knew any one of them that I thought had virtue enough to destroy such a considerable branch of their revenue, for the good of mankind. But the distemper is too beneficial to them, not to expose all their resentment, the hardy weight that should undertake to put an end to it. Perhaps, if I live to return, I may, however, have courage to war with them. Upon this occasion, admire the heroism in the heart of, Your friend, &c. &c."[24]

She asked the surgeon attached to the Embassy, "doctor" Maitland, to inoculate her 6-year old son, probably with the help of a Greek woman inoculator, and this was done in March 1718. Since her husband was away, she did not solicit his opinion. In a letter dated April 18, 1718, she wrote him: "*Your son is very well, I cannot help telling you, although you do not often enquire after him.*"[25]

Few detailed figures exist concerning the number of the inoculations made in Constantinople: two sons of Lord Sutton's secretary were inoculated before returning to Europe, in 1716[26], the three children of the secretary of the French Ambassador, the Marquis de Chateauneuf[27] and Antoine Le Duc, future physician with a degree from Leiden, and probably many others that remain unknown.

When she returned to London, at the start of the reign of George I, in 1721, a smallpox epidemic was sweeping the country. Lady Mary summoned Maitland and asked him to inoculate her daughter Mary, who was 3, in April 1721, in the presence of several physicians of the Royal Court. Maitland was not enthusiastic. He had retired to Hertford, just North of London. He requested beautiful weather similar to the weather in Constantinople at variolation season, and above all, the presence of two physicians during the operation. A *priori*, he did not wish to be solely responsible for this variolation. And yet, most authors considered that responsibility in case of an incident associated with variolation lay with the parents: physicians recommended prevention and explained the risks of the operation, parents made the decision. Lady Mary did not like physicians, as her letter (April 17, 1717) clearly shows. She refused to provide the witnesses, but an apothecary - an old family friend - and two or three doctors followed the development of the artificially induced smallpox, as this fell into their field of competency, and not that of the surgeon Maitland. The operation was performed on May 11, 1721 (first official inoculation in England), with complete success.

One of the physicians who visited the little girl, Dr. James Keith, was so impressed with the attempt that he asked Maitland to inoculate his son, the only one of his children who had not yet succumbed to smallpox. Word of these two inoculations soon spread throughout the city[28].

24. Wortley, 1763, t. II, p. 59.
25. Montagu, 1991, p. 198.
26. Miller, 1957, p. 51.
27. Gandoger de Foigny, 1768, p. 22.
28. Moore, 1815, p. 228.

The King of England, George I, showed great interest in the procedure; his daughter-in-law, Caroline Princess of Wales, was even more interested, after the serious case of smallpox which had afflicted her oldest daughter Anne. She wanted to protect her other children. Exercising caution, the College of Physicians proposed to conduct an experiment on six criminals, three men and three women destined to be hanged. But an unlooked-for obstacle occurred; the surgeon (Mr. Maitland) refused to perform the operation. For notwithstanding his former success (the daughter of Lady Mary), he dreaded a failure; and of being stigmatised for doing the work of the executioner[29]. He was finally persuaded to conduct the experiment for love of the royal family. The inoculation took place on August 9, 1721, at Newgate prison, under the direction of Sir Hans Sloane and Dr. John George Steigherthal, before about twenty-five doctors, surgeons and pharmacists, including members of the College of Physicians and the Royal Society. The results were as expected[30], but one of the prisoners, Evans, had lied. He had already had an attack of smallpox, but did not say so and the variolation did not take. Of course, this was proof of the validity of the method. Shortly after the inoculation of the Newgate prisoners, Dr. Richard Mead, renowned London physician, obtained permission to inoculate smallpox, using the Chinese method, to Elisabeth Harrison, a young prisoner. She became very ill, much more so than the subjects of the first experiment. Despite this, all the tests were positive and all the prisoners were liberated on September 6, 1721, as a reward for their cooperation. The variolated prisoners were certainly those who had gained the most, because for them the alternative would have been hanging. This trial gave rise to no unfavourable commentary: "*Neither the legality nor the morality of this unprecedented act was questioned...*"[31]. At least one of the prisoners found employment tending smallpox patients: "Mr. *Maitland, quoted by Kirkpatrick, has told us that one of the criminals inoculated at Newgate, upon his liberation, tended many, that is, about twenty smallpox sufferers, without having a new attack.*"[32]

It was thought prudent to conduct another experiment, this time on five (eleven, according to Moore) children of the St James parish. These were poor children (orphaned or abandoned), who mattered little compared to the children of royalty. The experiment was conclusive once more. In the meantime, Maitland successfully inoculated several people in London. All these inoculations were performed before witnesses intended to convince others. In 1722, the Princess of Wales, Caroline, had her two children, Amelia, 11, and Carolina, 9, inoculated[33]. Moore specifies that it was Amyand, the royal surgeon, who performed the operation on the two princesses, under the authority of Sir Hans Sloane[34]. In fact, the Sergeant-surgeon Amyand handled the lancet and Maitland indicated the site of the incision and placed the infectious matter on the small wounds. Amyand made the dressings. "*Finally, all of Europe knows that in 1721 the Princess of Wales, now Queen of England, had inoculation practiced, under the direction of Dr. Hans-Sloane, on her children, the Duke of Cumberland, alive today, the departed Queen of Denmark, & the Princess of Hesse-Cassel; the Prince of Wales the eldest had had the small-pox; the wife of this Prince has since had inoculation practiced on her three*

29. Moore, 1815, p. 230.
30. Petit, 1766a, p. 18.
31. Moore, 1815, p. 229.
32. Kirkpatrick, 1754 (1756), p. 255.
33. Diderot, 1756, p. 755; Roman, 1773, p. 62.
34. Moore, 1815, p. 235.

youngest sons, brothers of the reigning King of England... Can one desire more brilliant testimony in favour of this method? Persons of this rank are exposed to the eyes of the Universe."[35] The method was called the Byzantine operation[36]. News of the smallpox inoculation spread quickly, but candidates were few. Claude Amyand inoculated his two children, Lord Bathurst's six children, Count Berkeley's two children, and then those of Lord Townshend; finally, two others were inoculated by Maitland, but very soon passionate opposition to the method arose.

What was Lady Mary Wortley-Montagu's role in the spread of this medical novelty? There are those who believe she played a major role, such as Tissot, Dezoteux, Valentin and the author of the article on variolation in the *Encyclopaedia Britannica*. Others, like Miller, disagree. In fact, although the variolation of her daughter Mary was undoubtedly a triggering factor, it was not decisive. The acceptance of the method in Great Britain, then in the Western World, was accomplished by physicians, mainly Sloane, and many others, with the subsequent help of scientists like La Condamine or Daniel Bernouilli, philosophers like Voltaire and clergymen of various faiths. History is never simple...

The Entry of Smallpox Inoculation in the Western World

In 1721, variolation was also introduced in New England (the East Coast of North America, south of Quebec) by the preacher Cotton Mather who had studied medicine before theology, and by Zabdiel Boylston, practicing physician. A smallpox epidemic was rampant among the 11,000 inhabitants of Boston, as recorded by Webster[37]. It started in May with one fatality, eight in June, eleven in July, twenty-six in August, one hundred in September, four hundred and eleven in October, two hundred forty-nine in November, and then returned to a "normal" smallpox death rate in December: a total of 850 (or 842) deaths for 5,989 (or 5,759) smallpox sufferers[38]. Mather, who had read texts on inoculation in the Middle-East, persuaded Boylston to inoculate his own 6-year old son and two Negro slaves, Jack and Jackey, the first 36 years old and the second 2 and a half. The operation was performed on June 26, 1721[39], at the start of the epidemic, and only forty-six days after the inoculation of Lady Mary's daughter. It is generally accepted that variolation was established in England and spread from there to New England[40]. This is plausible from a historical perspective, but it is inaccurate. In fact, inoculation was transmitted directly from Asia to America, based on written testimony. On July 19, Boylston had already inoculated ten people, with the consent of religious authorities, although civil authorities were opposed to the practice[41]. However, according to Blake, even though Boylston was aware of the danger of contagion associated with these inoculated persons, he made no effort to isolate them, which could explain subsequent events[42].

35. Roux, 1765, p. 17.
36. Moore, 1815, p. 234.
37. Webster, 1799, vol. 1, p. 227.
38. Abbott, 1889, vol. VII, p. 509; Blake, 1959, p. 60.
39. Fitz, 1911, p. 11.
40. de la Condamine, 1763 (1764), p. 5.
41. Dixon, 1962, p. 226.
42. Blake, 1959, p. 67.

Antagonism between those in favour and those against very quickly became virulent, so much so that Mather had to stay hidden in his house: "*... he remained hidden for fourteen days, unbeknownst to his family with the exception of his wife... One evening, while his wife and children were sitting in the parlor, a lighted hand grenade was thrown into the room, but the fuse striking against some of the furniture fell off before an explosion could take place, and thus providentially their lives were saved.*"[43] Boylston inoculated 242 people during the epidemic. La Condamine points out that problems arose: "*The Magistrate intervened, party loyalties were ignited, the operation was only permitted with restrictions resembling a prohibition.*"[44] In fact, for each inoculation a request had to be submitted to municipal authorities, and specific permission had to be obtained, all of which is quite understandable. At the time, quarantine was favoured as a form of smallpox protection whenever possible. Inoculated persons had the same status as smallpox patients: that is, they had to be submitted to isolation in quarantine.

The First Wave of Inoculations in England: 1722-1730, and on the Continent

After the first inoculations practiced at Court, they continued throughout the country, but at a very slow pace. The first physician to practice inoculation, independently of the Maitland-Sloane tandem, was Dr. Thomas Nettleton, who had already inoculated forty people in Yorkshire by the end of 1721 or the beginning of 1722[45].

In the Spring of 1722, shortly after the first successful experiments, the deaths after inoculation of little Spencer, son of the Count of Sunderland, and of one of Lord Bathurst's domestics planted doubt as to the safety of the operation, and most probably discouraged potential inoculators. Surgeon Legard Sparham headed the anti-inoculists by publishing, in 1722, "*Reasons against the practice of inoculating the small-pox*", in which he denies that there is a difference between natural and inoculated smallpox, also called artificial[46]. Dr. William Wagstaffe, member of the College of Physicians and of the Royal Society, published a "*Letter to Dr. Freind; Showing the danger and uncertainty of inoculating the small-pox*", written in 1721 or 1722[47]. In it, he makes assertions, pell-mell, about inoculation as a fashion in English high society, the rather harmless nature of smallpox, which does not kill more than one person in a hundred, the questionable nature of the inoculated infection, the absence of certainty that the same person could not have natural smallpox twice... Time and experience eventually clarified all these points of contention. Of course, at the time, discussion of these issues had no solid basis, and anti-inoculists could expound their ideas freely.

The first attack against inoculation formulated on a religious basis might have been that of Mr. Wortley's chaplain[48], but this is not certain, since Lady Mary makes no mention of it. However, on July 8, 1722, Reverend Edmund Massey preached a thunderous sermon against inoculation in the name of faith and Providence: "*Remembering*

43. Thacher, 1828 (1967), p. 185.
44. de la Condamine, 1754 (1755), p. 9.
45. Jurin, 1722-1723 (1756a), p. 43; Moore, 1815, p. 233.
46. Miller, 1957, p. 102.
47. Miller, 1957, p. 308; Catalogue, 1756, p. 277.
48. Tissot, 1754, p. 79.

then our text, I shall not scruple to call that a Diabolical Operation, which usurps an Authority founded neither in the Laws of Nature or Religion, which tends in the case to anticipate and banish Providence out of the World, and promotes the encrease of Vice and Immorality."[49] This sermon was widely approved and reproduced in numerous texts. Later, purely medical arguments were to be used to counter those of morality. In this context, some altogether far-fetched ideas started to circulate... Some of them are unexpectedly original: "*We have seen, and we still see today, bigots & old women who decry this practice* (smallpox inoculation), *because it comes from the Land of the Infidel, as if with the small-pox Mahometism was inoculated as well.*"[50] Opposition gave rise to counter-opposition. On the one hand, Drs. John Arbuthnot, John Crawford and Samuel Brady took the trouble to answer Wagstaff. On the other hand, from a religious point of view, Reverend Massey's position was not shared by others: "*If, he says* (Mr. Amyand) *theologian Massay preached that this practice* (inoculation) *was diabolical, & attempted to prove that the Demon had given the small-pox to Job through inoculation, risum teneatis amici, the Bishop of Salibury who had his son inoculated, & several other defenders of the cause who followed his example have proven that it was defying God not to use the means Providence made known for the preservation of life...*"[51].

By the end of 1722, at least 182 inoculations had been performed: 61 by Nettleton, 57 by Maitland... a very distinguished clientele but, after all, very limited compared to the population of the United Kingdom at the time, which was about 7.5 million people[52]. However, the number of unfortunate events, true or reported, was growing. Clouds were gathering on the horizon: "*Two young English gentlemen, inoculated in 1723, succumbed to excesses in the interval between insertion and eruption, & paid this inadvertence with their lives.*"[53] They were then rumoured to be at the origin of the smallpox epidemic that ravaged London that year, which is unlikely, since the disease was endemic in large cities. The subject became so controversial that, around 1723, Jurin, Secretary of the Royal Society, was lamenting: "*The disputes that have arisen on the subject of inoculation have been carried so far that it is difficult to write about the subject without being dragged, despite oneself, into a quarrel, although one is only proposing facts, or drawing inevitable conclusions, with the greatest impartiality and the greatest concern for the truth.*"[54] In 1729, the English Parliament forbade inoculation (partially or completely? It is not clear).

In 1723, de la Coste (often written Delacoste), a French physician, back in France after a voyage to England, contributed to bringing the news to the French. Several famous physicians had responded favourably to the enquiries of the Regent, the Duke of Orleans, regarding inoculation. It seemed likely that it could be tried in Paris. But in December 1723, the death of the Regent, a person open to new ideas, changed the climate at the Court. Inoculation was forgotten, despite the dread inspired by smallpox.

Events in Faculty of Medicine in Paris added to the problem: on December 30, 1723, a thesis against inoculation was defended[55], under the direction of Mr. Claude de la

49. Massey, 1722, p. 15.
50. de la Coste, 1723 (1756), p. 197.
51. de la Coste, 1723 (1756), p. 155.
52. Quid, 2007.
53. Roman, 1773, p. 176.
54. Jurin, 1724 (1756b), p. 80.
55. Duvrac, 1723 (1755).

Vigne de Frecheville, doctor-regent at the Paris Faculty of Medicine. The ideas presented are striking but very doubtful: "*Wastaf mentions thirteen French soldiers inoculated at Cremone, all in the prime of their youth, all of good temperament, all having enjoyed perfect health henceto; six had great difficulty recovering, & it was not without inflammatory tumors that occupied a long time the throat and the tonsels; three were subjected to surgery to no avail, & four others died.*"[56] This episode was apparently witnessed by Dr. Dolhonde, "*passionate antagonist of inoculation in Boston*"[57]. Dr. Lawrence Dalhonde (or Dolhonde), from France, is referred to as practicing medicine in Boston in the first third of the eighteenth century[58].

Another victim of the harm caused by inoculation, still according to Dr. Dolhonde, is described as follows: "*A Moscovite soldier of the Almanza army, who was inoculated without effect & died six weeks later, frenetic, & with ulcerated lungs.*"[59] Dolhonde's eyewitness testimony to an event having occurred twenty-five years earlier (in 1696 or 1697, which seems very surprising), was presented before the Boston magistrates, repeated by Wagstaff in England, then by Duvrac in France. How was it that news of the inoculation of French soldiers at Cremone was not reported directly to Paris? What is the reason for this indirect transmission through Boston and London? In 1828, in his "*History of Medicine in America*", Thacher gives in a footnote the English translation of Dr. Laurence Dolhonde's French testimony. It is clear that Dolhonde did not know the history of the arrival of inoculation in Europe. The misfortunes of the Moscovite soldiers would have had to occur at Almaza in 1707! Thacher describes Dolhonde's testimony as obvious lies[60].

Even stranger moral considerations are presented in Duvrac's thesis: "*The inoculation, if it were received among us, could be the cause of many crimes. Does a Father want to be rid of his child? The inoculation provides him with an easy means of doing so. Does a dishonoured maiden fear that her shame be known? The inoculation provides her with a sure means of destroying its fruit.*"[61] La Condamine resumes his argument: "*This thesis bears the mark of a work of the passions. It is a violent & unfounded oration, whose aim is to excite morality & religion against the new method.*"[62] However, at the time, this thesis provoked a great deal of commentary, generally very unfavourable to inoculation: "*At the Paris Faculty of Medicine, it was viewed as a criminal practice, as deadly magic; inoculators were called executioners and impostors; those inoculated were called credulous fools.*"[63] Rumours of bad results seen in England or elsewhere, true or false, delivered the last blow to discredit inoculation. A dissertation by Hecquet (1724), entitled "*Raisons de doute contre l'inoculation*" ("Reasons for caution regarding the inoculation")[64], in which he calls it an operation of magic, made its proscription inevitable. Hecquet is also the person "*who describes as foolhardy* (sic) *the invention of tree grafting*"[65], which in his opinion was also unnatural.

56. Duvrac, 1723 (1755), p. 29.
57. Catalogue, 1756, p. 282.
58. The Colonial Society of Massachusetts, 1980, p. 73.
59. Catalogue, 1756, p. 271.
60. Thacher, 1828 (1967), p. 42.
61. Duvrac, 1723 (1755), p. 30.
62. de la Condamine, 1754 (1755), p. 12.
63. Husson, 1800, p. 4.
64. Catalogue, 1756, p. 286.
65. de la Condamine, 1759a, p. 5.

In France, like in Great Britain, morality was invoked on the side of the "for", just as on that of "against". Theologians, "*respectable for their brilliance, & the refinement of their conscience*" expressed doubts about authorising "*in good conscience among Christians, the giving of an evil for bringing forth the good*"[66]. But it would be a mistake to think that all members of the clergy were opposed to this novelty. In 1723, de la Coste wrote: "*Since in a conference I had at the Sorbonne about five weeks ago with* Mr. *the Dean & nine of their most famous Physicians (who treat me with all the politeness & mildness that learned persons must always maintain in their disputes;) I had the satisfaction to see them finally conclude, that it would be judicious, in view of being useful to the public, to conduct experiments on this practice. It is true that the greater number insisted that these experiments be conducted on criminals: but some were also of the opinion that seeing the example of the good success of this practice in Turkey and in England, it was justified to conduct experiments indifferently on all sorts of persons; provided that it is done with all the prudence required by such a serious endeavour.*" And clergymen even insisted on the usefulness of practicing these experiments while keeping in mind that children are to be given preference as inoculation subjects[67]. Finally it was agreed that experiments would be carried out on condemned prisoners, but this decision was never put into practice in France, at least at the time.

The influence of the English Court over the Court of Hanover led Prince Frederick Lewis, Duke of Gloucester, grandson of George I, to be inoculated himself. The journey made by Charles Maitland to Hanover on May 10, 1724, to inoculate this prince shows that the operation was rather rare. The patient's artificial smallpox was severe, causing over 500 pustules. Fortunately, neither his eyes nor even his face suffered harmful consequences. Maitland inoculated the eight children of Baron von Schulenburg a few days later. It was a long trip to make for a small number of inoculations. Between 1721 and 1728, 897 inoculations were practiced in Great Britain, New England and Hanover (ruled by George I), with a mortality rate of about one in fifty.

The defenders of inoculation had to face their adversaries armed only with vague statistics based on far-away results obtained in Constantinople or in Boston. Verifiable data was collected by Dr. James Jurin, Secretary of the Royal Society, from inoculators, who were required to supply the names of the inoculated subjects, their ages, addresses, manner of proceeding, number of days of illness, description of eruptions, type of smallpox produced and the final outcome, all of which had to be certified by credible witnesses[68]. A wide cooperative movement emerged, and Jurin received a great volume of mail. His annual report for 1824 indicates a mortality rate of 1 in 48, to 1 in 60, and includes an analysis of the problems encountered. Jurin showed the benefits of inoculation using relatively reliable statistics. Despite this, much effort was needed to persuade opponents of inoculation to admit Jurin's evidence. In 1727, Jurin left his position as Secretary of the Royal Society, and also stopped his work on inoculation. This work was continued by Dr. John Gaspar Scheuchzer, who published the activities covering 1727 and 1728. Upon his death, the project ended definitively.

66. de la Coste, 1723 (1756), p. 140.
67. de la Coste, 1723 (1756), p. 152.
68. Jurin, 1725, p. 32.

Between 1729 and 1738, there were practically no inoculations in England. They started again in 1743[69]. "*We know that inoculation was suspended & almost forgotten in England since 1729 until 1743, and that it recovered probably never to know such a setback again.*"[70] Contemporary literature on the subject indicates that inoculation was similarly forgotten in the whole of the Western World.

In 1732, La Condamine described the Circassian method in the account of his voyage to the East, an account he presented to the Academy of Sciences of Paris. This news aroused only some slight interest in limited circles, and remained without consequence. Some years later, in 1745, returning from a ten-year voyage in the Amazon river region, La Condamine presented to the same Academy an account of his travels in which he insisted on the use of inoculation in this region: "*One can see that in Para this disease* (smallpox) *is even more deadly for the Indians of the missions, recently brought out of the forest, & who go naked, than to the Indians wearing clothes, who were born or have been living for a long time among the Portugese. The first, a sort of amphibian Animals* (sic), *as often in the water as on land, hardened from childhood to the injury of air, likely have skin that is more compact than that of other men, & it seems that this alone can make the eruption of the small-pox more difficult in them... In any case, a Savage Indian just out of the forest, naturally attacked by this disease, is usually a dead man; but why is this not so for the artificial small-pox? Fifteen or twenty years ago* (1725-1730), *a missionary from the Carme Order, from the environs of Para, seeing all the Indians die one after the other, & having learned by reading a gazette the secret of the Inoculation which was much talked about at that time in England, thought it prudent that by using this remedy, he would render at least doubtful a death that was only too certain with ordinary remedies... This cleric was the first in America who had the courage to execute this. He had already lost half of his Indians, and many others fell ill daily. He dared to insert the small-pox to all those who had not yet been attacked by it, & he no longer lost a single one; another Missionary of the Black River followed his example with the same success.*"[71] Unfortunately, La Condamine adds that in 1743, when he travelled for several months through the region, another smallpox epidemic was raging and no one thought of using inoculation again.

Revival of Inoculation in Anglo Saxon Countries, circa 1738

Faced with the threat of a serious smallpox epidemic coming from Africa, in 1738, in Carolina (United States), the Boston inoculations practiced in 1722 were remembered, and about a thousand people underwent the operation. Eight or nine deaths resulted, while the epidemic was killing one out of five smallpox sufferers. Dr. Kirkpatrick himself inoculated eight hundred people, with a mortality of one percent. He published a booklet on inoculation first in Charleston, his hometown at the time, then in London in 1743, where he had come to seek his fortune[72]. He already understood the shortcomings of the operation, long before the Suttons or Gatti: too much inopportune

69. de la Condamine, 1764, p. 3.
70. Editeur, 1756, p. 135.
71. de la Condamine, 1745, p. 477.
72. Kirkpatrick, 1754 (1756), p. 245.

preparation, too much inoculation of "matter". Another reason for the return to inoculation was a very deadly smallpox epidemic in Middlesex, in 1738. Nearly 2,000 people were inoculated; only two pregnant women died, and they had been advised against being inoculated[73]. Mead published a translation of the works of Rhazes on smallpox, accompanied by his own text on the subject, in which he contested the idea that inoculated subjects can have an attack of smallpox. He also added that inoculation preserved the beauty of Circassian girls, a point designed to attract the attention of English mothers and incite them to have their daughters inoculated[74].

Inoculation was once again a subject of interest in England. The first decree making it compulsory for children entering hospitals to be inoculated was issued in 1743, at the Foundling Hospital of London, founded in 1739 to house abandoned children. News favourable to inoculation was again received with interest. "Mr. *Maty reports a fact that appears at first very favourable to inoculation: he says that in Boston, in 1752, 1,974 persons were inoculated, & that only 24 died; others, 1,509 in number, refused to submit to the operation, were infected with the natural small-pox, and 452 of them died.*"[75] In 1742, Boston had 16,382 permanent inhabitants[76]. But Cothenius remarked that in Maty's two groups the inhabitants were not comparable because those who were variolated represented strong-minded individuals, while the others were weak, timid people.

Rumours favourable to inoculation, but *a priori* impossible to prove, were circulating: "*But a planter of St. Christopher's inoculated three hundred persons without the loss of one. For it is singular that in those days all inoculations performed by private gentlemen, monks, and old women, were uniformly successful: and empirics afterwards were equally fortunate: none lost patients from inoculation, except the regular members of the Faculty.*"[77]

Although Moore's comment shows disillusionment, it is indicative of the excessive zeal displayed for a long time by the accredited physicians and surgeons of the era.

Nevertheless, inoculation was more and more appreciated in England. Thanks to donations and endowments, a hospital for smallpox patients was established near London, in 1746 (as attested by an anonymous text dated 1747). The June 1747 issue of *Gentleman's Magazine* reports the opening of the Hospital for Small-Pox, also called the Small-pox and Inoculation Hospital; this institution had a separate building dedicated to inoculations[78]. On the occasion of the hospital's opening, Monsignor Isaac, Bishop of Worcester, gave a sermon to solicit donations, at the same pulpit of the St. Andrew Holborn church, where thirty years earlier Massey had condemned inoculation. "*To the King's Most Excellent Majesty. Sir! It would be a Defect both in Gratitude and Duty, if the first Discourse from the Pulpit in Favour of INOCULATION, was not most humbly inscribed to your Majesty. The Nation, among numerous other Instances of paternal Regards, stands obliged to Your Majesty's Goodness and Resolution, for the Introduction and Progress of the salutary Practice.*"[79]

73. Monteils, 1874, p. 126.
74. Moore, 1815, p. 247.
75. Cothenius, 1774, p. 168.
76. The Colonial Society of Massachusetts, 1980, p. 8.
77. Moore, 1815, p. 247.
78. Anonymous, 1747, p. 270.
79. Isaac, 1752, p. A2.

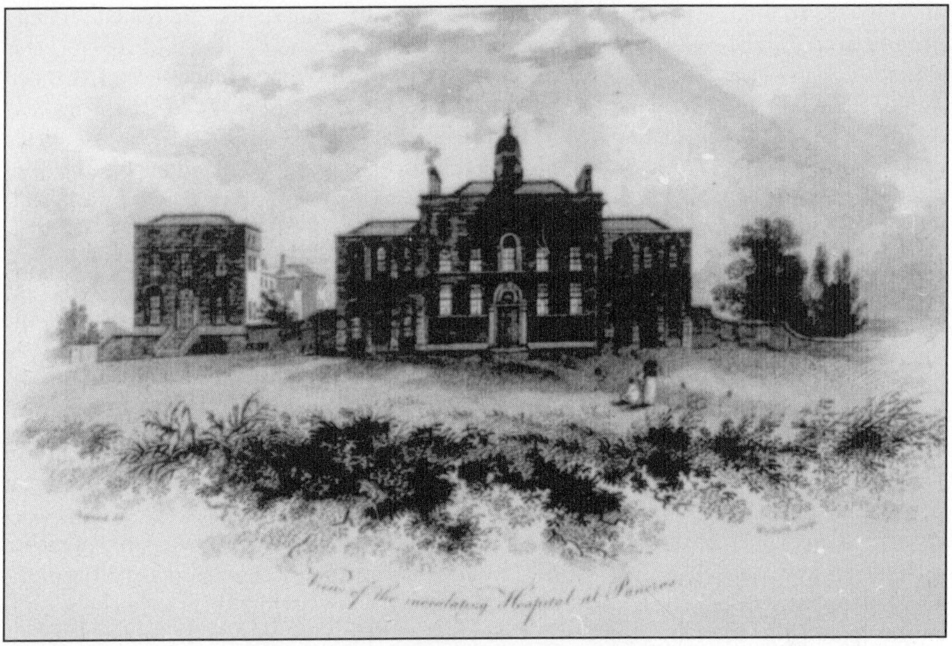

Figure 2. *"View of the Inoculating Hospital at Pancras"* (1806) by William Bond, published by Robert John Thorton. William Woodville was the director of this hospital and a great expert on inoculation (variolation) of smallpox. After some time, Woodville became an enthusiastic supporter of the new vaccine. In 1800, he himself brought the vaccine to the French, first to Boulogne-sur-Mer, and then to Paris. (Reproduced with permission of the Wellcome Institute Library, London.)

Inoculation did involve some economic problems. The rich had to pay the inoculator, and the process took time: two to four weeks of easy or not-so-easy "preparation", ten to fourteen days of real sickness and about a month of convalescence. Only the wealthiest people could afford two or three months of inactivity. The poor could obtain free inoculation in the suburbs of some big cities, but to earn a living and feed their families, they had to return to work as fast as possible, thus taking the risk of contaminating their families. People were not rushing to be admitted to inoculation hospitals! According to several stories, some inoculated patients left the hospitals at night to avoid the stones thrown by passers-by. One legally authorised establishment near Boston (US) was burned down[80]. In England, variolation had now gained a place, but it only concerned a very small fraction of the population and this would remain so until Sutton's work exerted its influence.

The Situation in Continental Europe, Particularly in France

Information from Great Britain and New England was influencing public opinion on the Continent. Attitudes gradually changed, with the help of certain great men such

80. Miller, 1957, p. 168.

as Voltaire. In his eleventh Philosophical Letter, he comments: "*It is inadvertently affirmed in the Christian countries of Europe, that the English are Fools and Madmen. Fools because they give their Children the Small-Pox to prevent them from catching it; and Madmen because they wantonly communicate a certain and dreadful Distemper to their Children, merely to prevent an uncertain Evil. The English, on the other side, call the rest of the Europeans cowardly and unnatural. Cowardly because they are afraid of putting their children to a little pain; unnatural because they expose them to die one time or other of the Small-Pox.*"[81] There were some people who were inoculated in France, in Hungary, in Italy, but certainly very few. In 1748, Tronchin, a physician from Geneva, who was then inspector of the College of Physicians of Amsterdam, inoculated his own son. Soon afterwards, he inoculated nine people in Amsterdam. Several doctors followed his example, but inoculation was only minimally accepted in the Netherlands. Some people preferred the preparation followed by natural contamination... that is, by contact with a smallpox sufferer.

The great Dr. Boerhaave rather favoured inoculation, but he did not practice it. "*In 1752,* Mr. *Butini wrote a little treatise on inoculation, that I* (La Condamine) *had great difficulty in finding when I wrote my first dissertation in 1754. It had not been noticed at all in Paris...*"[82]. Butini reported the first inoculations in Geneva, an operation introduced by Counsellor Calendrini, physicist and geometrician. Support from non-medical scientists was often decisive... or, at least, very useful. In France, La Condamine spared no effort in promoting this practice. He was one of the major artisans of this renaissance. On April 24, 1754, he read a first "*Mémoire sur l'inoculation de la petite vérole*" (Dissertation on the Inoculation of the small-pox), on the occasion of the reconvening of the French Academy of Sciences. This work was much talked about in France and in other countries, since at that time French was a common language between European nations. As a result, Tronchin inoculated a nephew of his in Geneva. Guiot, a Genevese inoculator, records thirty-three inoculations between the first variolation, performed in September 1750, and the month of November 1752.

Among the first three persons inoculated, two were daughters of State Counsellors. No serious accident occurred[83]. In Switzerland, inoculation spread from Geneva to other cities. Jean Bernouilli, from Basel, had his three sons inoculated, and de Haller from Bern, his daughter. Tissot, physician with medical degrees from Geneva and Montpellier, practicing in Lausanne, brought immense credit to inoculation by publishing *L'Inoculation justifiée* (Justification for the Inoculation), a work intended for the general public[84].

Attitudes in France toward inoculation started to change. In 1755, in the *Journal de Médecine, Chirurgie et Pharmacie*, an anonymous author proposed that a large survey be conducted, in the whole country, on smallpox and variolation: "... *Physicians and Surgeons would be invited to send the exact & certified list of patients who died or were saved from the Small-Pox in each circonscription. A Form in which they would be asked to enter details...*"[85]. It was an ambitious project, similar to Jurin's, but it was never

81. Voltaire, 1727 (1817), p. 18.
82. Valentin, 1802, p. 11.
83. Guiot, 1819, p. 387.
84. Tissot, 1754.
85. Anonyme, 1755, p. 314.

implemented... In the same year, as a result of rumours in Paris that the inoculation had caused the deaths of several distinguished persons in London, the Royal College of Physicians of London decided to counter these rumours by declaring itself in favour of inoculation[86]. In March 1755, "Mr. *Hosty, physician on the Paris Faculty of Medicine, went to London with recommendations from the Ministry, in view of learning particularly all things concerning the practice of Inoculation. During his stay in England, he witnessed 252 operations...*"[87]. Hosty published the account of his observation mission in England. He defended inoculation in these terms: "*I could not find, in all of London, a single physician, Surgeon or Apothecary opposed to the inoculation...*"[88].

Even before Hosty returned to France, on April 1, 1755, on the insistence of Turgot and his brother, an inoculation took place: it was that of a 4-year old child, with the consent of his mother, "*a woman of the people*". Turgot himself had wished to be inoculated at the same time as the child, but he could not because he was called away to Bordeaux[89]. A courageous adult opted for inoculation and chose Tenon, surgeon at La Salpêtrière, to perform the operation: "*The doctrine of Inoculation had only been discussed speculatively in France up to that time, & no one had yet availed himself of the new preservative. Mr. the Knight of Chateleux, twenty years of age, convinced of the advantages of the English method, animated by love of the public good, gave the example, & and was inoculated on May 14 (1755). The operation had a happy outcome, & the patient was perfectly healed at the end of the month...*"[90]. At his induction speech into the Académie Française in 1775, the famous naturalist Buffon told him: "*Alone, without advice, in the prime of youth, but convinced by maturity of reason, you made the experiment that was still feared... I was also able to witness your success... You say: I am saved and my example will save many others.*"[91] The Knight (later Marquis) François-Jean de Chastellux wrote two texts on inoculation in 1764. Other sources maintain that the first inoculation in France was practiced in Lyon in 1754[92].

On April 8, 1759, La Condamine wrote to Tronchin: "*Inoculations are sure to make their way here. Mr. Hosty is preparing five to six subjects and a few surgeons who rouse my suspicions inoculate on the quiet.*"[93] Obviously, the number of inoculated subjects remained small. La Condamine worked ceaselessly for years to promote the method. Armed with the caution worthy of a diplomat, he managed to avoid mishaps. He was accused of going to Rome to ask the Pope for a papal edict in favour of inoculation. After having given a copy of one of his dissertations on inoculation to Cardinal Valenti, prime minister to Pope Benoît XIV, Valenti had it translated into Italian and published. On the occasion of a second audience, he gave La Condamine six copies of this translation, saying: "*... if the approval of the Holy seat is awaited to introduce it in France, this will suffer no difficulty. My only answer was to bow deeply. I had no mission to accept this offer, & I feared that accepting it might multiply the obstacles rather than remove them.*"[94] La Condamine did not, in fact, want to mix religion with inoculation.

86. Anonymous, 1914, p. 47; Dezoteux, 1799, p. 55.
87. Gandoger de Foigny, 1768, p. 48.
88. Hosty, 1755, p. 337.
89. de la Condamine, 1758 (1759b), p. 15.
90. Gandoger de Foigny, 1768, p. 48.
91. Tronchin, 1906, p. 111.
92. Valentin, 1802, p. 11.
93. Tronchin, 1906, p. 374.
94. de la Condamine, 1764, p. 176.

A book entitled "*The Inoculation practiced in the ecclesiastic State*" was publicized and commented upon in a Roman newspaper: "A *famous Catholic theologean, of strict morality, Father Berti, a Dominican of Florence, consulted by Cardinal Corsini on the question of the inoculation, concluded for the affirmative. This consultation I have in my possession took place on December 30, 1756.*"[95]

An unexpected attack that left its mark came from Dr. Cantwell, Irish physician who had studied in Montpellier and practiced in Paris. In his "*Faits concluans contre l'inoculation*" (Conclusive Proof against Inoculation) he points out the dangers of communicable diseases: "*It is possible to transmit scrofula with artificial small-pox... It is possible to communicate syphilis by inoculating the small-pox... One can die of natural small-pox long after having submitted to the artificial...*"[96]. The College of Physicians of London "*in extraordinary assembly upon publication of this work, publically certified the advantages of the artificial small-pox... His* (Cantwell's) *blindness was cruelly punished by the loss of his only daughter, a charming maiden in the flower of her youth.*"[97] After this, transmission of other infectious diseases with the smallpox inoculation became a subject of concern.

On March 12, 1756, unaware of these disputes and especially of an anonymous pamphlet (written by d'Astuc, respected Paris physician very much in view at the time) entitled "*Doutes sur l'inoculation*" (Doubts about the Inoculation), the Duke of Orleans had his children inoculated: Monsignor Duke of Chartres (the future Philippe Egalité) and Mademoiselle de Montpensier. This inoculation was carried out by Tronchin himself, who had made the journey from Geneva to Paris for this purpose. When the father of the children had talked of his intention to Louis XV, who was to die of the disease a few years later, the King replied: "*You are the master of your children*"[98], not a very encouraging answer. As for Tronchin, he received expressions of esteem, as well as fifty thousand pounds, and a few gold boxes and various jewels[99], which made it worth his while to have endured the hardships of the voyage across the snow-covered Jura Mountains in February.

On September 15, 1758, before the public assembly of the Academy of Sciences, La Condamine presented a second dissertation on the inoculation of the smallpox, describing its history since 1754[100]. His presentation aroused great interest. Physicians, learned men, clergy and even ordinary people expressed favourable or unfavourable opinions, praise or reservations. In the sphere of science, where certainly it is often the rule, the scholars Bernouilli and d'Alembert did not reach the same conclusions! Bernouilli, physician and geometrician, saw the problem from the viewpoint of pure mathematics; d'Alembert, on the other hand, took into consideration the notion of time, concluding that the probability of dying of so-called "natural" smallpox was perceived as occurring in a more or less distant future, while that of "artificial" (variolation) smallpox was, much closer, inside a period between two weeks and a month. "*This is, without a doubt,* Mr. *d'Alembert adds, what makes so many persons among us, & particularly so many mothers, disinclined to favour inoculation.*"[101] Mathematics and common sense diverged, but during an epidemic the time factor became identical and

95. de la Condamine, 1758 (1759b), p. 41.
96. Cantwell, 1758, p. 208.
97. de la Condamine, 1763 (1764), p. 9.
98. Tronchin, 1906, p. 112.
99. Tronchin, 1906, p. 117.
100. de la Condamine, 1758 (1759b).
101. d'Alembert, 1761, p. 73.

the only difference was the risk taken, which was much smaller for the inoculated smallpox than for the natural disease. D'Alembert did not consider this point, which in any case was difficult to evaluate.

Strangely, during these controversies, no one mentioned the important difference in the suffering caused by natural smallpox and that caused by artificial smallpox. D'Alembert discusses some social considerations that are obvious to us today: "*This supposition leads him* (d'Alembert) *to observe that we have too often confused the interest that the State, in general, can have in inoculation, with that which individuals can have in it. For instance, it is certain that the State would gain from inoculation, if we consider this principle: the State considers all citizens indifferently; & by sacrificing one victim out of five, it matters little to it who this victim will be, as long as the other four are saved; but for each individual, the foremost interest is his own particular preservation.*"[102] Despite everything, Tronchin's article in Diderot and d'Alembert's *Encyclopédie* is clearly in favour of the inoculation of artificial smallpox[103]. In most countries, the desirability of possible population growth, linked with the use of variolation (and later Jennerian vaccination), created a positive impact on the attitude of national leaders. For nations, an increase in the number of citizens meant more soldiers and more taxes; for the Church, more worshippers.

Opinions were very divergent. Many texts against inoculation were anonymous and intemperate: "*L'inoculation de la petite vérole déférée à l'Eglise et aux magistrats*" (The inoculation of small-pox deferred to the Church and the magistrates) consisted of a series of categorical statements: "*Review of the main grievances... The inoculation can serve as a pretext for several crimes... It puts a sword in the hands of fools & madmen. It came into being, & it is nourished by greed. The Church can repress it...*"[104]. Time does not seem to change certain attitudes.

In France, Excesses, Prohibition and Clamour

Dr. Gatti, a young professor at the University of Pisa, stopped in Paris on his way to England. He had seen inoculation practiced in Constantinople, and he had inoculated in Italy. Very quickly, he "conquered" Paris and became the fashionable inoculator in that city[105]. According to Creighton, Gatti was the first to practice the "new inoculation", before the Suttons and Dimsdale[106], and this could in fact be true. Because he advocated the simplification of preparation and of the inoculation itself, he became the target of denigration and was accused of not transmitting artificial smallpox, but only a skin rash with no relation to the disease. To prove the safety of his inoculations, Gatti deposited twelve thousand francs in a bank: "*Gatti had entrusted 12,000 francs to Bataille, Receiver General of finances, at Place Vendôme, in Paris, for six years, for anyone who could prove true reinfection. No one claimed the money.*"[107] By 1763, Gatti had inoculated 97 persons, a sufficient number to establish his renown.

---

102. d'Alembert, 1761, p. 79.
103. Tronchin, 1765, p. 755.
104. Anonyme, 1756, pp. 1 & 208.
105. Dezoteux, 1799, p. 77.
106. Creighton, 1889, p. 136.
107. Dezoteux, 1799, p. 271.

But some recently inoculated individuals escaped his vigilance and went out into the city while still contagious. "... *One distinguished inoculated person, who showed himself at the opera and the Tuileries, caused an outrage...*"[108]. It was said that this is what started the smallpox epidemic that reigned in Paris at the end of 1762 and the beginning of 1763. The King's advisors and their counsel, Mr. Omer Joly de Fleury, asked for Parliament intervention: "*The Inoculation of the small-pox, known in some foreign countries, seems to have been accepted for some time amongst us... A general outcry is heard, either against inoculations, or against those who, while awaiting the effect of the inoculation they received, do not take precautions in society. This imprudent conduct can have the most serious consequences... We believe, Messieurs, that no one is better qualified to consider these opinions than the Faculties of Theology & of Medicine of this University... The only observation we have left to make at the Court regarding this matter, is the consideration that since the opinion of the Faculty of Theology can depend greatly upon the judgement given by the Faculty of Medicine, on the usefulness or danger of the Inoculation, it would be advisable that the Faculty of Medicine express an opinion first on all matters under its competence, & that the Faculty of Theology only contribute an opinion after having learned those of persons in a position to observe, & apt to judge the merits or inconveniences of Inoculation experiments...*"[109]. On June 8 or 19, 1763, Parliament ordered that all inoculations within its jurisdiction be stopped, until the Faculties of Theology and of Medicine of Paris had delivered their judgement. Inoculations could be performed only outside cities, and the persons inoculated had to remain in isolation for six weeks after the operation. In itself, the stopping of the procedure seems reasonable. It was temporary and served as a precaution. However, the decision led to a veritable unleashing of passions. Battles were fought in the press through exchanges of commentary. "*These little battles were only the prelude to more serious & much more important action. Defenders and opponents of the inoculation were light troops involved in skirmishes while awaiting a decisive battle. Finally, the long-awaited day arrived. The medical profession entered the combat. Divided into two camps, the attack started with the anti-inoculists...*"[110].

In effect, the Faculty of Medicine named a commission composed of twelve members. Soon, they divided into equal camps and published separate reports. In the course of four sessions, between August 29 and October 24, 1764, Mr. Guillaume-Joseph de l'Epine read "*Un rapport de six des douze Commissaires nommés par la Faculté de Médecine de Paris*" (A Report of six of the twelve commissioners named by the Faculty of Medicine of Paris), against inoculation[111]. The report expounds on four main points: "*That the inoculated small-pox is not always benign... Inoculated small-pox can have the most serious consequences, just as the natural small-pox... Inoculated small-pox in particular has specific associated mishaps... Finally, that it is possible to die from the inoculated small-pox...*"[112]. The arguments to support these claims were long and meticulous. The discussion soon became inflamed around the examples or testimony chosen: old facts often false or unverifiable that led to interminable quarrels.

On November 21, 1763, Cochu presented his report entitled "*Observations sommaires au sujet de l'inoculation de la petite vérole*" (Summary observations on the subject of the

108. Gandoger de Foigny, 1768, p. 62.
109. Dufranc, 1763.
110. Gandoger de Foigny, 1768, p. 69.
111. de l'Epine, 1765.
112. de l'Epine, 1765, p. 84.

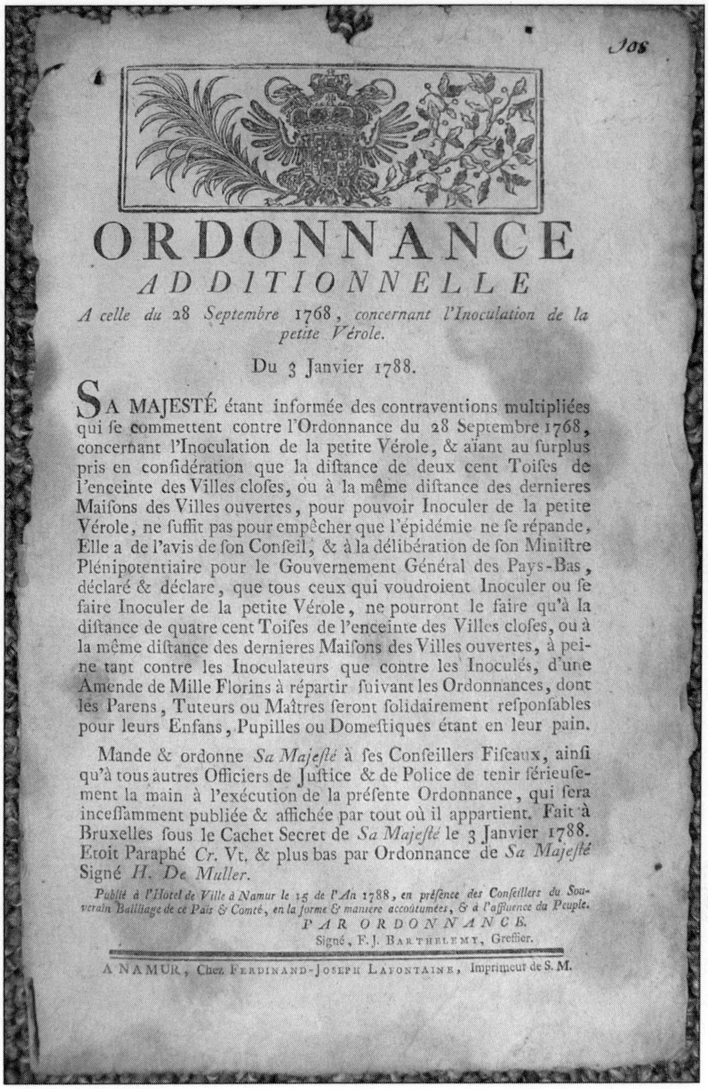

ORDONNANCE
ADDITIONNELLE

A celle du 28 Septembre 1768, concernant l'Inoculation de la petite Vérole.

Du 3 Janvier 1788.

SA MAJESTÉ étant informée des contraventions multipliées qui ſe commettent contre l'Ordonnance du 28 Septembre 1768, concernant l'Inoculation de la petite Vérole, & aïant au ſurplus pris en conſidération que la diſtance de deux cent Toiſes de l'enceinte des Villes cloſes, ou à la même diſtance des dernieres Maiſons des Villes ouvertes, pour pouvoir Inoculer de la petite Vérole, ne ſuffit pas pour empêcher que l'épidémie ne ſe répande, Elle a de l'avis de ſon Conſeil, & à la délibération de ſon Miniſtre Plénipotentiaire pour le Gouvernement Général des Pays-Bas, déclaré & déclare, que tous ceux qui voudroient Inoculer ou ſe faire Inoculer de la petite Vérole, ne pourront le faire qu'à la diſtance de quatre cent Toiſes de l'enceinte des Villes cloſes, ou à la même diſtance des dernieres Maiſons des Villes ouvertes, à peine tant contre les Inoculateurs que contre les Inoculés, d'une Amende de Mille Florins à répartir ſuivant les Ordonnances, dont les Parens, Tuteurs ou Maîtres ſeront ſolidairement reſponſables pour leurs Enfans, Pupilles ou Domeſtiques étant en leur pain.

Mande & ordonne *Sa Majeſté* à ſes Conſeillers Fiſcaux, ainſi qu'à tous autres Officiers de Juſtice & de Police de tenir ſérieuſement la main à l'exécution de la préſente Ordonnance, qui ſera inceſſamment publiée & affichée par tout où il appartient. Fait à Bruxelles ſous le Cachet Secret de *Sa Majeſté* le 3 Janvier 1788. Etoit Paraphé *Cr. Vt.* & plus bas par Ordonnance de *Sa Majeſté* Signé *H. De Muller.*

Publié à l'Hotel de Ville à Namur le 15 de l'An 1788, en préſence des Conſeillers du Souverain Balliage de ce Pais & Comté, en la forme & maniere accoûtumées, & à l'affluence du Peuple.

PAR ORDONNANCE.

Signé, F.J. Barthelemy, Greffier.

A NAMUR, Chez Ferdinand-Joseph Lafontaine, Imprimeur de S. M.

Figure 3. Variolated individuals were contagious and there was a risk that they could contaminate persons who were not immune. In many cities, authorities took measures to prevent this danger. In 1788, in Namur (Belgium), the minimal distance of variolation from walled-in cities or from the last houses of open cities was changed from 200 to 400 "toises" (about 800 meters), subject to heavy penalty. (Author's document.)

small-pox inoculation)[113]. Cochu tended to be against inoculation, but advocated tolerance. On September 5, 1764, Mr. Antoine Petit presented "*Un premier rapport en faveur de l'inoculation*" (A first report in favour of the inoculation), on behalf of the opposing camp[114]. On one side, six opposed; on the other five in favour and one tolerant. Where did each camp find arguments for its position? "*This is not a question*

113. Cochu, 1763 (1765).
114. Petit, 1764 (1766a).

of theory; &, to clarify the facts, eye witnesses have to be found. Where can they be found other than in the countries where the insertion is practiced? Among foreign universities, I see only Oxford, Cambridge, Edinburgh & Dublin; those of Leiden, Hanover, Gottingen, Basel, Coppenhagen, Uppsala, Pisa, Lucca & perhaps Padua that could supply facts or reasoning based on experiences to which they were witness."[115] Therefore, requests for information were sent all over Europe, to the places where inoculation was practiced; traces of these requests remain in texts found outside France: "*The learned Commissioners, named by the Paris Faculty of Medicine to examine the advantages and disadvantages of the small-pox inoculation, sent in 1764 some questions on this important subject to Dr. Alexandro Monro the father, in Edinburgh. The testimony of this famous man...*"[116]. A substantial amount of mail arrived in response to these requests, allowing the commissioners and the members of the Faculty to form an objective opinion on the inoculation. Other documents were read, including the one written by A. Petit in 1766, entitled "*Un second rapport en faveur de l'inoculation*" (A second report in favour of the inoculation), which essentially refutes the arguments of the first report of the anti-inoculists[117]; and in 1767, de l'Epine's report "*Un supplément au rapport des six commissaires de la Faculté de Médecine de Paris qui ont conclu contre l'inoculation*" (A supplement to the report of the six commissioners of the Paris Faculty of Medicine who concluded against the inoculation), a 164-page document[118]. The more time passed the more heated the arguments in these reports became, each side accusing the other of wanting to mislead the reader... All of these texts were published long after they were written.

Discussions reached an impasse; in order to break it, advice was solicited from the Assembly of Physicians of the Faculty of Medicine. "*Each member of the Faculty is asked to submit his opinion in writing. The members cannot do this without becoming aware of the debate. It is now their duty, and an honour, to study the question.*"[119] The outcome of a first vote showed the Faculty of Medicine to favour tolerance of the practice of inoculation. After this favourable vote, a second vote, on September 11, produced identical results, but took place in a stormy atmosphere[120]. Partisans and opponents of inoculation attacked each other fiercely. There were reports and counter-reports, and an unfortunate incident came about to complicate the situation. "*A child of three was inoculated in Besançon; the disease followed its ordinary course until the fourth day of the eruption; at that stage, developments that could not be controlled caused the death of the child on the thirty-first day after the operation.*"[121]

In fact, an inquiry carried out locally showed very quickly that the tragedy was due to the technique employed. "*The inoculator pinches the skin, and snips the fragment with scissors. He applies over the wound a scab of small-pox, a piece of gauze & a bit of cotton, both soaked in variolous matter; this is his technique, which will seem new to you and specific to him alone.*"[122] Dezoteux, a young physician and Surgeon-Major of the King's regiment, with the Besançon garrison, who revealed the cause of the tragedy in order to

115. de la Condamine, 1764, p. 45.
116. Haygarth, 1786, p. 144.
117. Petit, 1766b.
118. de l'Epine, 1767.
119. de la Condamine, 1764, p. 36.
120. de la Condamine, 1764, p. 160; Gandoger de Foigny, 1768, p. 72.
121. Gandoger de Foigny, 1768, p. 73.
122. Dezoteux, 1763 (1765a), p. 11.

defend inoculation, was attacked by the local inoculator and his supporters. His efforts to defend himself produced dozens of letters, explanatory documents, brochures, certificates, dissertations, excerpts from a personal diary, open letters and letters sent to persons at the Academy of Dijon, particularly Dr. Maret[123].

In the meantime, in Paris, the battle was reaching a climax. There too, dissertations, examinations, observations, clarifications, research and reflections followed one another. Moreover, official reports were printed at the expense of the Faculty of Medicine, to be distributed to members. Finally (as confirmed by Dezoteux), on January 15, 1768, four and a half years after the parliamentary decree, a third assembly of the Paris Faculty of Medicine declared the practice of insertion (inoculation; variolation) "*admissible*"[124]. According to Guersant and Blanche, the Faculty of Medicine rendered its decision by a vote of 52 against 26[125]. Other authors indicate that the decision kept being postponed and was never really made. A minority of the Faculty of Medicine of the University of Paris is no doubt responsible for this tarrying. The majority of members made the right choice, but only after endless hesitation...

The opinion of the Faculty of Theology seems to have been forgotten in the dispute, although La Condamine speaks of a: "*... question resolved affirmatively as early as 1723 by nine Sorbonne doctors consulted, & since then by a large number of other Catholic and Protestant doctors, French and foreign...*"[126]. But the position taken by the nine Sorbonne physicians, when reported by La Condamine, dates back forty-one years... In fact, the opinion of this Faculty is still not known and probably never will be.

Improvement of the Variolation Technique by the Suttons: 1760 - 1763

Inoculation as it was practiced in Europe between 1721 and the arrival of Sutton's method was very dangerous. It was, undeniably, at the limit of the tolerable. "*However, the manner of inoculating still had considerable drawbacks... inoculation was practiced in about the same manner still; until* Mr. *Sutton, without being a medical Doctor, nor a graduate of any University, but endowed with good sense & wisdom, discovered a new manner of treating inoculation, much superior to the old, & whose advantages have been confirmed by the greatest success.*"[127] Robert Sutton, the father of the dynasty, was a farmer said to have been apprenticed with a surgeon in his youth. He was apparently not practicing this profession when he himself was inoculated, in a most unpleasant fashion. His knowledge led him to reflect seriously on the manner of operating. He revolutionised the field of inoculation. "*Being in possession of such a superior manner of inoculating... Mr. Sutton fortunately had several very intelligent & very educated sons, to whom he taught his method & everything that could ensure its success. One of his sons, Mr. Daniel Sutton, was the first to leave his father's home; & he was also the one who perfected his father's method even more, contributing to the great fame it has enjoyed since. In 1763 he came to live near Chelmsford, in Essex county, ten leagues* (about 50 km) *from London.*"[128]

123. Dezoteux, 1765b.
124. Gandoger de Foigny, 1768, note in the Warning to the Reader.
125. Guersant, 1846, tome 30, p. 393.
126. de la Condamine, 1764, p. 78.
127. Power, 1769, p. 10.
128. Power, 1769, p. 12.

Daniel Sutton left his father's house in Debenham, in Suffolk, and opened a practice in a poor region with bad climate. Mistrust regarding inoculation was great. Fortunately, he also had a talent for treating natural smallpox. He was even able to bring about unexpected cures: "Mr. *Daniel Sutton started by inoculating the poorest population; the advantages of the new method (that I shall also call that of the Suttons or Suttonian) persisted; & these inoculations, despite being performed in such an unhealthy region, had the desired success, so that the people inoculated, full of satisfaction at having been inoculated so happily, did not cease to give him the highest praise...*" Daniel Sutton's affairs prospered: "*He had taken a large house so that he might provide shelter to those who would wish to stay with him during the Inoculation; one year later, in 1764, so many came that he was forced to take another house, next to his own, to have more room. His house, which had twenty-four beds, had become too small for all those who wanted to be inoculated; & these two houses, which contained more than fifty* (beds), *were constantly full of people of all ages & sexes. The eagerness with which people came from everywhere, often obliged* Mr. *Sutton to inoculate fifty, sixty, & sometimes up to a hundred persons at once; but what is hardest to believe is the prodigious number he inoculated one day at Malden, a small seaport in Essex county. It was the month of August, many people had gathered in this place for the harvest, and* Mr. *Sutton inoculated up to 470 in the same day.*"[129]

The fact that the Suttons were achieving such excellent results led to a following of new inoculators to whom the Suttons taught their methods for a fee (100 pounds), on condition that they kept the technique secret and that they performed inoculations in regions far removed from their own, so as not to compete with them. The price of an inoculation, which included the preparation, the insertion and post-operative care, was 10 pounds per patient (as a reference, Jenner paid 600 pounds for the house he bought in 1785), and 25 pounds for wealthy patients.

The Suttons had immense success, and achieved great renown. In 1766, after thirteen years of activity, Daniel Sutton had apparently inoculated twenty thousand persons, "*without losing a single one by the Inoculation...*"[130]. Still according to Power, one of their disciples, the Suttons and their followers had already inoculated seventy thousand people by 1769, an immense number... representing enormous financial gain at 10 pounds minimum per inoculation.

Robert and Daniel simply returned to the ancient practices of the inoculators who performed variolation in the Midde East; they imposed great (?) cleanliness and the precepts of the famous English physician Sydenham. Thus, the Suttons practiced a much healthier preparation based on exercise, fresh air and light meals. A "Suttonian" variolation could take place in any season. The inoculation started with a preparation: "*... I would say therefore that in the Suttonian method, we prepared the persons we were to inoculate, by nutrition, a vegetarian diet & purgations...*"[131]. After the preparation, the actual inoculation: "*The Inoculator dipped in ordinary water the tip of a lancet loaded with dried variolous pus. Once the pus was diluted, he made one or two punctures on one of the child's arms... so that they were very superficial; I never saw blood appear.*"[132] They also administered pills and powders with secret contents, before and after the inoculation.

129. Power, 1769, p. 15.
130. Power, 1769, p. 47.
131. Power, 1769, p. 53.
132. Gardane, 1774, p. 11.

Afterwards, they administered a local treatment on the pustules, and anti-phlogistics (general anti-inflammatories), as recommended by Rhases, Sydenham and Boerrhave. In a short time, all Western inoculators started to variolate using the Suttons's method: "*But Hauquins* (anyone at all), *not knowing the secret of the Suttons, simply imitated their inoculations, prescribed a healthy died to the Patients, let them breathe fresh air, & succeeded just as well.*"[133]

The Suttons had developed a so-called cold treatment of the smallpox, more efficient than the hot treatment used by their contemporaries: "*Thus at the same period we do not keep the patients in their room, and certainly not in their bed, unless special circumstances require it; which almost never happens. We bring them into the fresh air & allow them to go about their business...*"[134]. This last point could account for certain very regrettable cases of contagion. In fact, the danger was the same for patients with natural smallpox and those with smallpox inoculated by variolation. However, this treatment could have suited those who could not spare much time and, above all, it had become less dangerous in a population almost entirely variolated or rendered immune by the "natural" disease itself.

The financial aspect of the Suttonian method must not be forgotten as precised by Power: "*I hope that I will be dispensed from giving any details on this subject, as well as on the subject of the other remedies we employed in the course of our treatment... but amongst all my regrets on this subject, being constrained by my commitments to him* (Daniel Sutton), *I cannot act otherwise.*"[135] Gardane quotes several inoculators, a Devonshire shepherd, Mr. Gatti and Mr. Jauberthou in Paris, who obtained comparable results, using light punctures and fresh air, without the pills and powders used by the Suttons[136].

In practice, at the site of Suttonian punctures, on about the third day, a red spot that became circular and prurient appeared. On the fifth day, this spot changed into a vesicle that kept growing and then filled with pus. At the same time, general symptoms appeared: chills, fever, muscle aches, vomiting, insomnia; in short, symptoms resembling those of true smallpox. The eruption stage was characterized by the appearance of "pustules" similar to those of smallpox, but most often limited in number. Suppuration started about the fourteenth day, with severe lymphangitis taking the form of inflammation of the variolated arm, accompanied by adenopathy (inflammation of lymph nodes). Dessication of the buttons started a short time later. With time, as the inoculators acquired experience, complications became rarer. Inoculation was not yet a routine procedure, but real progress had been made and smallpox was no longer inevitably the fearsome disease it had once been.

Variolation Gains Ground Gradually: the Period after the Suttons

Despite the Paris Parliament's suspicious attitude, and especially the hesitation shown by the Faculty of Medicine of Paris, the inoculation became accepted in France as elsewhere. It was practiced, in limited numbers, in Lyon by Grassot, in Montpellier by

133. Gardane, 1774, p. 17.
134. Power, 1769, p. 60.
135. Power, 1769, p. 61.
136. Gardane, 1774, p. 19.

Vigarous, in Nimes (78 between 1757 and 1764) by Razoux[137], in Marseilles and Toulon, Bordeaux, Nantes, Rennes, Strasbourg, Besançon, Aix... In 1754, La Condamine presented his first dissertation to the King of Poland, the Duke of Lorraine, who, on the advice of the Royal College of Medicine of Nancy, authorised inoculation in his Kingdom[138].

Dr. Goëtz, a fervent advocate of the inoculation, provides his own statistics: in 1766, two children were inoculated; in 1767, one child; in 1768, three; in 1769, two; in 1770, two. Obviously, these numbers are small, but Goëtz specifies that these are children "*of the utmost distinction*", which changes everything in terms of prestige and perhaps of fees[139]. Sometimes, an exceptional event took place: "*In the autumn of 1768, the insertion was practiced with great success at the Royal Military School, & its success caused the King to have the inoculation given to the students of de la Flèche College. It was upon the King's orders that* Mr. *Gatti inserted the small-pox at that College in March 1769, to 122 Subjects. Out of this number, 112 had the small-pox without the least accident, & ten did not have it at all, despite being inoculated with it up to ten times, & being left almost six weeks in the midst of the contagion.*"[140]

Toward 1768, the "Suttons", represented by family members and disciples, arrived in France. A nephew of Daniel Sutton, practicing on the outskirts of Paris, was called to the bedside of Louis XV when the latter was near death. Neither reckless nor a fool, he refused to ruin his reputation for a lost cause since the King had a clear case of confluent smallpox. Mr. Worlock, who claimed to be Daniel Sutton's father-in-law, also set up residence outside of Paris: "*He* (Mr. Worlock) *rented an isolated house, outside of Paris, with fresh air near Mont-Louis, called P. Lachaise. It had comfortable apartments & pleasant garden.*"[141] Worlock has been traced to Rennes, Nantes, Abbaye de Fontevrault, and Rochefort... where, according to his own published accounts, he accomplished remarkable feats[142]. His successes were so highly appreciated that the French government entrusted Dr. Gardane with learning the method and broadcasting it[143].

On June 18, 1774, the future King Louis XVI, his brothers and the Countess of Artois were inoculated by Richard, Inspector General of military hospitals, with the help of Mr. Jauberthou, under the supervision of Mr. Lieutaud and Mr. de Lassone, in the best conditions, to prevent the infection of persons in their entourage. "... *It is to be hoped that in the practice of inoculation, the care & caution Louis XVI demonstrated at Marli are always taken; this benevolent monarch... chose, for his inoculation, one of the most isolated castles, & ... he ordered at the same time all those who had not yet had the small-pox, to remove themselves from the Court during the inoculation.*"[144] The children of the French royal family benefited from the inoculation fifty years after those of England! Mlle Rose Bertin, renowned fashion designer, used the occasion to launch her "*Pouf à l'inoculation*" (inoculation ottoman) hairstyle! Unfortunately, because of the recent death of Louis XV in May 1774, and the deep mourning which followed, the Court could

137. de la Condamine, 1764, p. 152; Domenjon, 1801, p. 35.
138. de la Condamine, 1758 (1759b), p. 12.
139. Goëtz, 1770, p. 247.
140. Roman, 1773, p. 194.
141. Worlock, 1770, p. 3.
142. Worlock, 1770, p. 14.
143. Gardane, 1774.
144. Duhaume, 1776, p. 299.

not adopt this fashion[145]. The dead King spoiled the party! However, far from the Court, a comedy entitled "*The Inoculation Party*" was playing at the Italian Theatre. "*The inoculation has become the most interesting subject of conversation in high society.*"[146]

Variolation enjoyed local success in particular regions of France, specifically in Auxois and Franche-Comté[147]. Traces of inoculation in the Auxois region seem hard to find. But there is ample testimony concerning inoculation in Franche-Comté. In 1765, Dezoteux wrote: "*At about the same period I had finally convinced Girod, a Besançon physician, to learn the practice of inoculation. A favourable occasion arose; he seized upon it, and that was the start of the immense services he has rendered since to his province, Franche-Comté at the time.*"[148] Intendant de Lacorée was going to provide Girod with efficient and valuable assistance. In 1776, the local government established an annual Fund to remunerate surgeons who inoculated children when a smallpox epidemic was declared in their region. Between 1765 and 1776, 17,000 people were inoculated; between 1776 and 1781, 5,250 and in 1882, 1,705, for a total of 23,955 people. Losses were one out of 300 to 350 inoculated subjects, but after analysis of the causes of mortality, the losses are only one out of 600.

In Tuscany and in the Papal State, inoculation arrived between 1750 and 1757. Soon it spread throughout Italy, but few people benefited from it[149].

In Venice, in 1769, the Senate issued a decree stating that all orphan children in the different hospitals of the Republic would be inoculated in the spring of 1770.

The Duke of Parma had lost the Infanta Louise-Elisabeth of France, his wife, and four years later, the Archduchesse Marie-Elisabeth, his daughter, both killed by smallpox. The Duke decided to have his only son, Prince Ferdinand, inoculated; he made his request to Tronchin, the most highly reputed inoculator of the era. On October 23, 1764, the Prince was inoculated and the operation went very well, at least for him. "*The Abbot Condillac, tutor of the young Prince had the courage and zeal to stay quarantined with him, although he was not certain that he had had the small-pox; he soon became infected, & his love for his venerable student almost cost him his life.*"[150] A *Te Deum* was sung, and Tronchin received the title of first physician to the young Prince. He was also made a citizen of Parma. It was decided that a medal would be engraved with his image, but in fact only a gilded plaster medal was coined. One can be grateful and thrifty at the same time!

In Austria, the great Van Swieten did not take a position on the matter, following the publication of a book against the use of inoculation, by "*Mr. de Haën, Aulic Counselor to their Imperial Majesties, Professor at the University of Vienna in Austria*"[151]. Haen's long argument against the inoculation starts with: "*These are then the principal questions, to which I request positive answers: I If the law of God permits the Inoculation? II If more people can be saved by this method than by the rules that Medicine teaches us independently of the Inoculation? III If it has been proven that almost all men must have the small-pox? IV*

145. Larousse, 1865, t. IX, p. 706.
146. Roman, 1773, p. 65.
147. Tronchin, 1906, p. 138.
148. Dezoteux, 1799, p. 85.
149. Dezoteux, 1799, p. 97.
150. Roman, 1773, p. 136.
151. de la Condamine, 1758 (1759b), p. 42.

If it is certain that the inoculation, followed or not by the small-pox, confers lifelong protection from it?"[152] Haen's answer to all these questions was obviously "no".

Smallpox had broken out numerous times at the Court of Austria, a fact which worried Marie-Thérèse: "*The Queen-Empress had the inoculation given to the two young Archdukes, her sons, & to the Archduchess Thérèse, her granddaughter, on September 13, 1768... at the Castle of Schonbrun. On September 20, the Te Deum was sung, in the presence of the inoculated Archduchess and Archdukes. In the evening, fireworks were launched under their windows...* Mr. *Ingenhauss, who was fortunate enough to be chosen to give the artificial small-pox to the two princes and to the young princess, received from the Queen-Empress a thousand gold sovereigns, a golden snuffbox bearing the portraits of their Imperial Majesties, a magnificent ring, the title of Court Physician, 5,000 florins in salary, 2,000 of which were transferable to his future wife. The little girl who provided the pustule to be inserted received 24 ducats, & her father an annuity which she inherits.*"[153] Ingenhauss later became known in England as Jenner's first competitor. In fact, in the summer of 1768, the Empress ordered the inoculation of sixty-five (sixty, according to Boutry) little boys and little girls at the Meydling Hospital, before having the operation practiced on her children by the Dutch physician Jugenhouse (Boutry's spelling). The honourability of the young "matter" donor's family was ascertained. Everything went well[154].

"*The Empress Catherine II submitted, on October 10, 1768, to the insertion of the small-pox, in Czarskozelo. Dr. Dimsdale, a British physician, was her inoculator, & he could not obtain that the First Physician be informed of the Empress's project, nor that he should be present during the operation. The Court was only informed after the eruption. Back in Petersbourg, this courageous Princess had the inoculation given, in her presence & with matter taken from her, to the Great Duke, her son... Dr. Dimsdale received from her Imperial Majesty 10,000 pounds sterling, 1,000 for his voyage back to England, & 500 pounds sterling as an annuity.*"[155] He also received a hereditary title of nobility, and that of First Physician to the Empress. It is said that as a precaution, Dimsdale requested that a horse-drawn carriage be always ready for him in case something went wrong during the development of the Empress's artificial smallpox.

In Prussia, inoculation started around 1765. Dr. Hosti was called to Brussels in 1768 to inoculate several persons. "*A few important persons of the Spanish nation came to France to be inoculated. Among this small number, we count the children of the Duke of Infantado, who were inoculated by citizen Dezoteux, near Paris, in 1785... In Madrid, the contagion was deadly enough to finally persuade the King to have three of his children inoculated* (1798). *Following the successful operation, he issued an Order making it compulsory to introduce inoculation in hospitals, houses of charity and other establishments directly under the King's jurisdiction.*"[156]

In Scandinavian countries such as Sweden and Norway, La Condamine's writings spread the idea of the inoculation. In Norway, it was introduced in 1759 by a physician called Honoré Bonnevie. The King of Sweden sent Dr. Schulz to England to learn about inoculation; the physician returned completely instructed in the use of the

152. de Haen, 1757, p. 249.
153. Roman, 1773, p. 201.
154. Boutry, 1903, p. 305; Dezoteux, 1799, p. 101.
155. Roman, 1773, p. 202.
156. Dezoteux, 1799, p. 105.

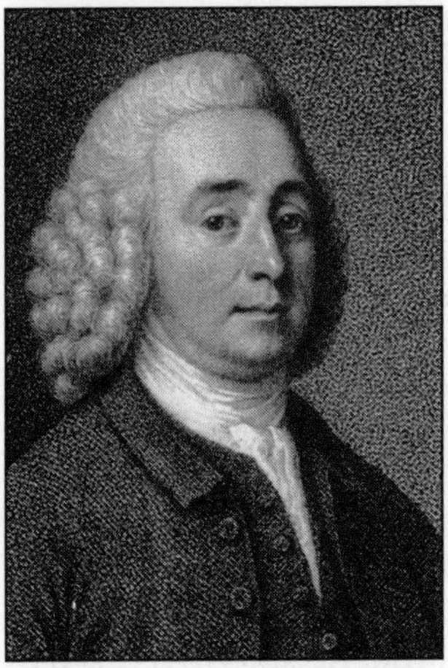

Figure 4. Thomas Dimsdale (1712-1800) was a famous English physician who inoculated the Empress Catherine of Russia and the Grand Duke Paul in 1768. In 1780 he was elected a member of the House of Commons. He was successfully operated on to remove a cataract in 1784, and ended his life amongst friends in Hereford where he had been born 88 years before. From the *European Magazine*, engraved by Redley, published by J. Sewell Cornhill, 1st September 1802. (Author's document.)

method. In 1760, the College of Health hired the Swedish to build an inoculation hospital, and the Order of Freemasons had two hospitals built; their inspection was entrusted to Dr. Schulz. The hospitals were located in Stockolm and Christiana (Oslo). In 1769, the Swedish royal family was successfully inoculated by Dr. Boecz[157]. Inoculations were performed in Copenhagen, in private offices and in hospitals. Prince Frederic of Denmark was inoculated in 1769.

Dr. Louis Valentin, who had just "*spent seven or eight years in the French Cape* (today's Haitian Cape, north of Haiti) *and in the United States of America, where he himself inoculated and had inoculation practiced on a great number of subjects, while employed by our Republic as chief physician...*"[158], recounts how the inhabitants of North America protected themselves from smallpox epidemics by the application of strict rules of hygiene and quarantine. Inoculations were authorised in case of serious threat of a smallpox epidemic, provided they were also performed in the neighbouring states.

Was it Wise to Be Variolated in the Eighteenth Century?

It was not easy to evaluate the risk/benefit ratio of the inoculation compared to natural contagion; several hard-to-assess parameters were involved: in big cities, smallpox was endemic and the risk of contamination was great in public places such as churches... In the countryside, smallpox epidemics were followed by the total disappearance of the virus. During periods of calm, it was difficult to predict the return of an epidemic. In certain rare cases, a veritable pandemic threatened the inhabitants of cities and countryside alike. In short, the situation was fluctuating and not easily foreseeable.

Preparing candidates for the inoculation was considered important. The idea was to bring the person to his optimal state of health, so as to ensure the best "physiological" response to inoculation. In case of problems after the inoculation, the fact of having provided good preparation or not could protect the inoculator against blame and legal

157. Dezoteux, 1799, p. 97.
158. Dezoteux, 1799, p. 15.

repercussions. This left the door open to all kinds of excesses. Jenner himself describes the preparation to inoculation he received in his youth: "*There was bleeding till the blood was thin; purging till the body was wasted to a skeleton; and starving on vegetable diet to keep it so.*"[159] Not a very appealing picture, although it might be seen as a caricature. Fifty years would have to pass before the West would return to primitive preparation, which was less dangerous.

The inoculation technique also underwent numerous changes, sometimes beneficial to the patient, but most often unfavourable. According to Paulet, it was Emmanuel Timone who effected the change in the inoculation technique, about 1700, for his European clients living in the Orient. Instead of the punctures made by the Greek women of Constantinople, he favoured incisions. Maitland was also accused by Paulet of having replaced punctures with incision in both arms "*to give it a more pronounced aspect, & make it look more like a surgical procedure*"[160]. It must be said that, to her credit, Lady Mary Wortley-Montagu tried in vain, and as early as 1722, to stop this European surgical deviation from the initial Middle-Eastern technique. Lady Mary published a text in *The Flying-Post* or *Post-Master* entitled "A *plain Account of the Inoculation of Small-Pox by a Turkey Merchant*"[161], in which she berates the physicians who distorted the original Constantinople inoculation: "*Out of compassion to the numbers abused and debuted by the knavery and ignorance of physicians, I am determined to give a true account of the manner of inoculating the small pox as it is practised at Constantinople with constant success, and without any ill consequence whatever. I shall sell no drugs, nor take no fees, could I persuade people of the safety and reasonableness of this easy operation. Tis no way my interest (according to the common acceptation of that word) to convince the world of their errors; that is, I shall get nothing by it but the private satisfaction of having done good to mankind, and I know no body that reckons that satisfaction any part of their interest.*" Lady Mary's judgement concerning inoculation as it was performed in England at the time is absolutely relevant, but her high social position prevented her from entering into a public controversy. Her intervention ended there!

Another point of disagreement was the responsibility of inoculating in case of contamination within a person's family.

Finally, the fear of unhappy consequences of the inoculation was always present in people's minds. Mortality related to inoculation continued to diminish thanks to better knowledge of the method. In the 1720s, it was 1 out of 50, with peaks, according to Jurin and Scheuchzer's statistics: "... *out of fifty-eight children two years of age who were inoculated, six died*"[162], which is 10%! Just before 1800, when the Jennerian method of vaccination appeared, the figures cited are 1 fatality for 400 inoculated subjects, 3 for 1,000; 5 for 1,000. In 1799, Woodville himself refers to a mortality rate of one out of 600, among the last 5,000 inoculated patients in his own hospital[163].

In truth, inoculation encountered serious problems even in its period of maturity, at the end of the eighteenth century. Valentin describes some of them, occurring about 1795, during general inoculations, in North America. In Norfolk, there were 64

159. Baron, 1838, t. 1, p. 123.
160. Paulet, 1768, t. 1, p. 198.
161. Halsband, 1953, p. 390.
162. Thornton, 1808, p. 51.
163. Woodville, 1799 (1889), p. 109.

fatalities out of 700 inoculations. The text is not very explicit, but death was probably due to gangrene at the point of inoculation, either in the arm or the leg. The same author recounts that in 1760 "*a small-pox epidemic having spread in Charleston (South Carolina), it was decided to conduct general inoculation: fifteen hundred persons were inoculated in one day; but five hundred died*"[164]. It is possible that these variolations were practiced during the incubation period of the smallpox, or that additional infections were present.

Very early, the potential risk of transmitting infectious diseases with the inoculated smallpox was a topic of concern. "*How can we convince people, even those with limited discernment, that if a venereal, schrophulous or scorbutic affection is present in the blood with the small-pox virus, the latter can be separated out without being at all tainted by the others, & that it can be inserted with the same confidence as the virus of simple Varicella?*"[165]

Inoculation eventually acquired an official place in France. In 1799, the "*Faculty of Medicine founded an inoculation clinic. Two of its members, citizen Pinel, professor of internal pathology, physician at the hospice of La Salpétrière, and citizen J.J. Leroux, associate professor of internal medicine, performed inoculations for the instruction of students who were admitted to the small-pox ward.*"[166] A report submitted to the Faculty of Medicine of Paris, describing the inoculation clinic, was written by Pinel and Leroux on Fructidor 29th, year 7* (September 15, 1799). It was the first establishment of its kind created in Paris, intended to allow the working classes to benefit from the inoculation, and to train physicians to become inoculators. Seventeen girls, ten of them from the "Orphan Hospice", and three boys were inoculated in a local of the "*Maison nationale des femmes*" hereafter the Salpêtrière Hospital. The results were favourable. However, Pinel and Leroux had certain grievances. First, the room was cold and humid; several smallpox patients were being treated there at the start of the inoculation session. The complaint ended with a plea: "*We have not forgotten that the official intention of the Faculty, which we dare predict, will become that of the government, is that the small-pox inoculation, associated to the principles of medicine, should be generally practiced by all those worthy of exercising the art of healing, and that the entire French population, informed of what is in its true interest, might benefit from the advantages it provides.*"[167]

To be inoculated against the smallpox during periods when it was not highly endemic was an act of courage at the beginning of the eighteenth century, and an act of prevention at the end of that century. However, during epidemics and depending on the virulence of the causal agent involved, in time it became simply a matter of common sense.

Smallpox Inoculation: a Medical Revolution

The introduction of the smallpox inoculation had implications for the entire medical profession. Some physicians became fashionable as inoculators, and gained fame and fortune: the English physician Dimsdale, the Swiss Dr. Tronchin, the Dutch physician

* French Revolutionary Calendar.

164. Valentin, 1802, p. 26.

165. de Ponsard, 1776, p. 65.

166. Dezoteux, 1799, p. 393.

167. Dezoteux, 1799, p. 430.

Ingenhousz, the Italian Dr. Gatti and many others... and even individuals who were not physicians, like the Suttons. Many others worked quietly, like Girod, whose well-earned glory came late. Finally, scholars like La Condamine, the Bernouillis, etc. found satisfaction in defending it.

Variolation was a major subject of interest in the eighteenth century among the intellectual elite. No other prevention technique had given rise to so many discussions, pamphlets and letters of contestation that were sometimes quite acrimonious. The *Journal de Médecine, Chirurgie et Pharmacie* (one of the best known at the time) dedicated about one tenth of its content to it for most of the eighteenth century. Opposing voices were also being heard. Paulet, a knowledgeable physician, advocated the eradication of smallpox through hygiene: quarantine and disinfection. "*If men want to rid themselves entirely of this disease* (smallpox), *they must concentrate all their attention on the allure of the inoculator, the nurse, the washerwoman, the skin, the bedding & the clothing of the patient*."[168] Paulet's recommendations for avoiding contagion are clear and detailed. He adds some observations concerning sheeppox, which are just as judicious. But his injunctions were not taken into consideration; their application would have been too constraining.

Controversy about the inoculation forced physicians to start comparing groups of individuals. Thus, the assessment of morbidity in inoculated populations compared to populations that were not inoculated was an important step forward. From that point on, the problem of "natural" death among inoculated subjects was submitted to questioning: "*There have in truth been a few examples of children who died during the inoculation; but would it not be an excessive injustice to blame it for the event? Who would dare to affirm that a hundred normally constituted children, & in the best of health on the first of January 1777, will all be alive on December 31 of the same year?*"[169]

According to Arthur Boylston, the inoculation provided the occasion for the first modern clinical study, conducted by an English physician, William Watson, working at the Hospital for the Maintenance and Education of Exposed and Deserted Children, better known as the Foundling Hospital. The study was very innovative. Boerhaave and many other physicians prescribed the use of antimony and of mercury salts to smallpox sufferers and to inoculated subjects. Watson took thirty-one children living in identical conditions, and divided them into three groups. He inoculated each of them in the same manner. The first group (five boys and five girls) received a mercury potion and Jalap (a laxative) before and after the operation. Watson administered to a second group, similar to the first, three senna infusions and rose syrup, a mild laxative. Finally, eleven boys were inoculated with no other treatment. Watson's brilliant idea, according to Boylston, was to count the pustules of each patient and to compare their number per group. Counting the number of pustules of each inoculated subject was very common at the time, and even served to assess the malignity of natural smallpox, and above all of inoculated smallpox, since the first texts written by Timone and Pylarini. The new idea was the comparison of different groups based on one or more parameters. Because laxative administered with antimony and mercury could prevent proper absorption of these substances, Watson conducted another experiment to avoid this bias, using inoculum from ripe pustules. In a third experiment, he used natural smallpox pus from pustules having reached the end of the maturation stage, while the

168. Paulet, 1768, t. 1, p. 351.
169. de Ponsard, 1776, p. 11.

other trials had used early lesions. Based on these experiments, Watson concluded that, on the one hand, mercury did not contribute to the effects of a mild laxative and that, on the other hand, inoculum from an early or ripe pustule is preferable to inoculum from a pustule having entered the stage of dessication. Boylston submitted Watson's data to a modern statistical test and demonstrated that none of the pretreatments used showed a significant difference compared to absence of premedication and, in addition, that the three inoculums produced smallpox of the same malignity[170]. Watson was clearly ahead of his time as far as experimental methods were concerned. In his 1774 report on the secret of the Suttons, Gardane wrote: "*At the same time, Mr. Watson, Physician at the Inoculation Hospital in the English Capital, oversaw the inoculation of a certain number of children prepared with Sutton's remedies, & an equal number given simple injections without any preparatory remedy; he obtained the same results on one side & the other.*"[171]

Much commentary and discussion concerned the morality of inoculation, and sometimes produced surprising conclusions. Aside from the view that inoculation might be contrary to the will of God, a view still held by certain populations of Holland and the United States and perhaps elsewhere, the question of a physical or moral parental obligation to inoculate one's children arose. Some curious opinions were expressed on the subject: "*I can forgive families with many children, & without means, for letting nature take its course and perhaps delivering some of these unfortunate children from the misery awaiting them, & for neglecting precautions whose omission has not yet been declared a criminal act. But I find no excuse for those who are preparing the most brilliant future for their children, for not using a safe means of stopping the blow that can put an end to this future.*"[172] Tissot, who wrote these words, was a well-known Lausanne physician, son of the priest of the church of Pampigni. The same author makes a strange comparison: "*The first* (argument in favour of inoculation), *is the advantage of being delivered from the fear of the small-pox. In the words of* Mr. *Maty, the emancipation of the slaves pales in comparison with the emancipation afforded to the great number of people who, before suffering of this dreadful disease, lived in constant terror, & were often made inapt to render useful services to their closest friends, or to go about their own affairs.*"[173] The point of view changes perhaps with one's position: master or slave.

Finally, at the end of the eighteenth century, the situation was clear: in continental Europe, the number of inoculated people was small. "*Since the beginning of the last century, when the inoculation brought from Asia was introduced in Europe, the most distinguished physicians have attempted, thanks to their talents and great knowledge, to spread this salutary method: all their efforts only served to have it adopted by the wealthy classes of society. We have not yet succeeded, despite all the means of persuasion we used, despite the clearest successes, to make access to it easy for the working classes of the countryside and for artisans in the cities... In the end, the method has almost not utility for the people.*"[174] This was true, because the working classes in question were more inclined to think about the present than about the future.

---

170. Boylston, 2002, p. 1326.
171. Gardane, 1774, p. 18.
172. Tissot, 1754, p. 155.
173. Tissot, 1754, p. 152.
174. Vigarous, 1801, p. 2.

The effects of variolation on populations were very difficult to evaluate. This is why careful consideration was given to the recommendation issued in 1857 by the Board of Health, a public health agency in England, the country where variolation was most widely practiced. The recommendation was based partly on Dr. Heberden's conclusions, written in 1801: "*The inoculation of the small-pox having been first used in England since the beginning of the eighteenth century, and having been now for many years generally adopted by all the middle and higher orders of society, it becomes an interesting inquiry to observe, from a review of the last hundred years, what have been the effects of so great an innovation upon the mortality occasioned by that disease. But however beneficial inoculation prove to individuals, or indeed to the nation at large, the Bills of Mortality incontestably shew that in London more persons have died of the small-pox since the introduction of that practice. The poor, who have little care of preserving their lives beyond the getting their daily bread, make a large part of mankind. Their prejudices are strong, and not easily overcome by reason. Hence while the inoculation of the wealthy keeps up a perpetual source of infection, many others, who either cannot or do not choose to adopt the same method, are continually exposed to the distemper. And the danger is still increasing by the inconsiderate manner in which it has lately been the custom to send into the open air persons in every stage of the disease, without any regard to the safety of their neighbours. It is by these means that, while inoculation may justly be esteemed one of the greatest improvements ever introduced into the medical art, it occasions many to fall a sacrifice to what has obtained the distinction of the natural disease. This must always be an objection against making any great city the place for inoculation, until the practice is become universal amongst all ranks of people. Out of every thousand deaths in the Bills of Mortality* (of London), *the number attributed to the small-pox during the first thirty years of the nineteenth century, before inoculation could yet have had any effect upon them, amounted to seventy-four. During an equal number of years at the end of the century, they amounted to ninety-five. So that, as far as we are enabled to judge from hence, they would appear to have increased in a proportion of above five to four.*"[175] The same arguments and conclusions can be found in the writings of John Cross, who quotes Sir Gilbert Blane's work, based on mortality rates due to smallpox over 15-year periods, between 1706 and 1818, in London[176].

Heberden's conclusions are close to those observed by other authors: disinterest of the poor in variolation, given their daily cares ; obvious danger of contamination by variolated individuals who felt well and ignored isolation and quarantine rules to be followed by variolators and their variolated patients. The final comparison between the beginning and the end of the nineteenth century is highly debatable, because conditions of analysis had changed in the meantime. However, these figures clearly indicate the lack of decrease of mortality due to smallpox in the city of London after years of variolation.

The General Board of Health added: "*Thus, even assuming an unanimous willingness to adopt inoculation to operate, there must inevitably remain against it this twofold objection (1) that it would directly destroy a certain, though small, proportion of those submitted to its performance; and (2) that to the very considerable number of persons, temporally or permanently ineligible for the operation, it would occasion a greatly increased danger of contracting the natural disease.*"[177]

175. Heberden, 1801, *in* General Board of Health, 1857, p. ix.
176. Cross, 1820, p. 213.
177. General Board of Health, 1857, p. ix.

After all these years, these points are still valid. But both risks have been considerably reduced, as the history of vaccination has shown. Mankind's ideas about infectious diseases have also evolved. Who would dare to propose, today, a vaccine that would kill a fiftieth to a tenth of those who received it? And yet, there were candidates!

The example of variolation inspired various other ideas. The use of different types of "lymph", each one corresponding to an identified infectious disease, was a tempting notion. Attempts were made to protect men and animals by inoculating them with each-other's viruses. This was risky but acceptable if the disease in question was dreadful enough. In humans, the procedure was most often used with caution... In veterinary medicine, this rudimentary method was widely used, with variable results (*see Chapter 4*).

3
Smallpox Vaccination and its Uses from Jenner to Pasteur: 1796... to 1880-1900

Eighteenth century variolation prepared the medical profession and an influential echelon of society to accept the idea of active and individual prevention of infectious diseases. This practice was a first step on Jenner's road to vaccination.

The Birth of Vaccination

Edward Jenner was a surgeon whose only diploma was a Scottish medical doctorate (from the University of Saint Andrews), not recognized in England. He practiced medicine and surgery legally, thanks to some years of apprenticeship and nothing else. The two years he spent as John Hunter's boarding pupil had no legal value. Back in Berkeley, Jenner began to practice surgery; at the time, a surgeon was considered a second-rate physician, having no doctorate, and relying solely on his reputation to acquire patients. Smallpox inoculation (variolation) was part of his medical practice. He used the Suttonian method, established in the 1760s, whose application was extending to new population groups, including those with a modest income, the rural population that constituted most of his clientele in Berkeley. Jenner himself had been variolated at the age of 8[1]. Thus, he was familiar with smallpox and inoculation. He also knew about cowpox and its transmission to humans. During his apprenticeship, he had heard, and reportedly never forgotten, the remark of a young milkmaid: "*I cannot take that disease* (smallpox), *for I have had the Cow Pox.*"[2]

As part of his Berkeley practice, Jenner variolated the local peasant populations. He soon noticed that some people remained resistant to the inoculation he gave them: "My *attention to this singular disease* (cowpox) *was first excited by observing that among those whom in the country I was frequently called to inoculate, many resisted every effort to give them the small Pox. These patients I found had undergone a disease they called the Cow Pox, contracted by milking Cows affected with a peculiar eruption at their teats.*"[3]

In effect, many of these individuals attributed this resistance to the fact that they had previously suffered from cowpox. Common lore considered smallpox and cowpox to be related and mutually exclusive: "*People had noticed that these spots* (of cowpox) *were transmitted to the farm girls who milked the cows infected with this disease; and it became apparent that people who had contracted it were not vulnerable to small-pox infection.*"[4]

Husson, Jenner's French contemporary, records this interesting observation of human nature: Jenner learned that "*when farmers rent servants, they give preference to those who*

1. Baron, 1838, t. 1, p. 121.
2. Baron, 1838, t. 1, p. 122.
3. Jenner, 1801 (1998), p. 5.
4. Husson, 1803b, p. 2.

have had small-pox. There were no doubt two reasons for this: the first was the desire to avoid the presence of such a disgusting and contagious disease as small-pox in one's home; the second was that because individuals who had already had smallpox and bore its characteristic marks on their faces, were unlikely to contract cow-pox, there was no risk that they would pass it on to the animals, who would then infect each-other, reducing milk production"[5]. Paradoxically, immunity to smallpox was used as protection against cowpox, and not the reverse, at least in Gloucestershire.

However, Jenner encountered opposing evidence that troubled him: one bout of cowpox, or what had been taken for that disease, did not always protect against natural or artificially induced smallpox. But he was intelligent enough not to be deterred by this initial obstacle. He made a close study of cowpox, a disease category that included several affections of the cow udder. What was needed was to distinguish protective cowpox or "true cowpox" from other forms of the disease, *i.e.* "spurious cowpox" that did not provide protection. Here, Jenner was faced with another problem: the true cowpox transmitted to humans did not always provide immunity against smallpox. He discovered that cowpox lymph taken from the cow in the early stage of the disease gave humans a classic form of cowpox, while lymph taken at a more advanced stage only transmitted ulcers probably caused by ordinary pathogenic agents, and produced more serious side effects. Therefore, true cowpox was the cowpox induced by vesicle lymph taken at an early stage of the disease[6].

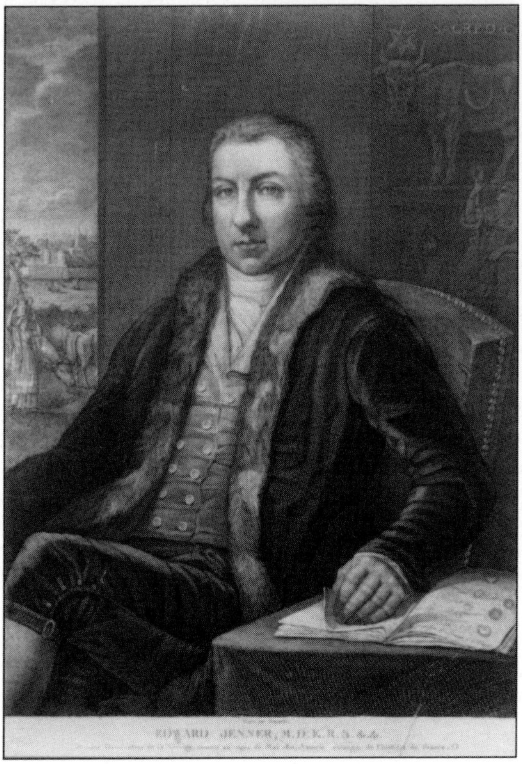

Figure 1. In 1811, two etchings measuring 32 by 36 cm were offered for sale in France, one of Dr. Edward Jenner, the other of Mr. de la Rochefoucault-Liancourt, for 25 francs in Paris and 30 francs in the provinces. Here, Jenner is portrayed against a rural background with bovines, his hand over an etching showing cowpox inoculations on different days. (Author's document.)

5. Husson, 1800, p. 12.
6. Moore, 1817, p. 4.

Although cowpox is a relatively benign disease in cows, it had economic consequences. Jenner describes it as follows: "*This disease has obtained the name of the Cow Pox. It appears on the nipples of the Cows in the form of irregular pustules. At their first appearance they are commonly a palish blue, or rather of a colour somewhat approaching to livid, and are surrounded by an erysipelatous inflammation. These pustules, unless a timely remedy by applied, frequently degenerate into phagedenic ulcers, which prove extremely troublesome. The animals become indisposed, and the secretion of milk is much lessened*"[7]. Husson describes the disease as having four stages, like smallpox: the infection stage is characterized by loss of appetite: "*The cows move their lips in a way similar to the mouth movement made by men when they are blowing out the smoke of tobacco; this is why people say the cows are smoking... Milk secretion is much reduced... the eyes are dark, melancholy; fever appears... the eruption period begins. Pustules appear on the udders, especially around the teats... Eruption stops on the fourth or fifth day after it first appeared... The maturation period begins... In the fourth stage, called dessication...*"[8].

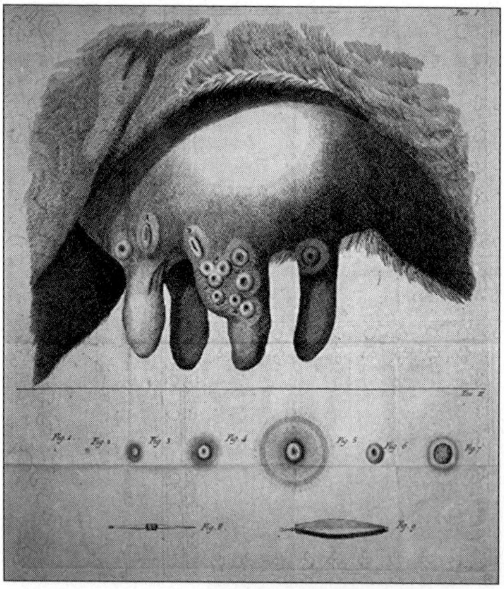

Figure 2. Cowpox/vaccine. Explanation of Tables. Table I: drawing of a cow tift, with smallpox pustules. AA: pustules produced at the graft* site. aaaa: natural pustules. Table II: Fig. 1: graft mark. Fig. 2: first indication of infection, obtained after the fourth or fifth day (the time indicated can vary depending on extent of infection). Fig. 3: development of pustule on day 6. Fig. 4: pustule on day 8. Fig. 5: pustule with erysipelas areola, on day 11, starting to retreat from the centre toward the periphery. Fig. 6: dried out pustule on fifteenth day. Fig. 7: suppuration crust. Fig. 8: needle used to inoculate. Fig. 9: tweezers to carry the thread to the graft site. (Sacco, 1801.) (Author's document.)

In addition to his work on the true cowpox that confers protection from smallpox, Jenner also conducted research on the origin of cowpox. He had noticed that cowpox was a disease of milked cows, and was not seen in cows that were suckling their calves.

* The word "graft" was rarely employed when variolation started: smallpox was grafted to an individual. The more common expression was "to inoculate the smallpox". The word "to vaccinate" came into use in 1800, in Geneva and in London, and perhaps elsewhere (Bazin, 2000, p. 208).

7. Jenner, 1798, p. 3.

8. Husson, 1813, t. 7, p. 239.

Could cowpox have an external source? Jenner first eliminated a possible source related to the milking process since the epizootic disease of cowpox in Gloucestershire sometimes disappeared for several months or even years. The cleanest farms, where cows were milked only by women, were rarely infected.

He suspected the transmission of a disease called "*the grease*" that could be transmitted from the horse to the cow by people tending both animals. Moreover, Jenner observed that, among his clientele, blacksmiths and ferriers often presented resistance to variolous inoculation, even without having contracted the disease[9]. He even insisted on the necessity that the horse infection pass through the cow before infecting humans: "*It is curious also to observe that the virus which with respect to its effects is undetermined and uncertain previously to its passing from the horse through the medium of the cow, should then not only become more active, but should invariably and completely possess those specific properties which induce in the human constitution symptoms similar to those of the variolous fever, and effect in it that peculiar change which forever renders it unsusceptible of the variolous contagion.*"[10] He later abandoned this idea in the face of ample evidence to the contrary. Several authors, including Loy in England and Sacco in Milan among others, reported that they had used horsepox matter to successfully vaccinate humans[11].

The *grease* and horsepox are two infectious diseases of the horse, whose shared symptom is "*painful discharge in the heels*". But horsepox also presents as pustular naso-labial eruptions, and sometimes generalized lesions on the entire body. Tanner, a veterinary surgeon in nearby Rockhampton and Jenner's neighbour, was the first to obtain a cowpox vesicle in 1800 by inoculating *grease* matter on a cow teat. The lymph from this vesicle was transferred to a child, conferring cowpox (or at least a similar pustule!). Jenner was given a sample of this lymph; he in turn gave some of it to the *Small-pox Hospital*. "*He* (Mr. Tanner) *succeeded in communicating the disease to a cow by inserting some liquid matter taken from the heel of the horse. This produced on the teat of the cow a complete vaccine pustule.*" He observes: "*From handling the cow's teats, I became infected myself and had two pustules on my hand, which brought on inflammation and made me unwell for several days. The matter from the cow and from my own hand proved efficacious in infecting both human subjects and cattle.*"[12]

One year later, after many trials, Loy conferred to four cows the infection of a horse presenting a severe form of *grease* with generalized eruption, although he had always failed in the past when he used lymph from horses with *grease* only in the heels[13].

The supposed equine origin of the vaccine, not specifically demonstrated, gave rise to much criticism of Jenner's work. Pearson, Jenner's most notable adversary at that time, seized the opportunity to emphasize this questionable point. Since he had not succeeded in transmitting the *grease* from the horse to the cow, nor from the horse to humans, he attacked this aspect of Jenner's work. Woodville, Simmons and Coleman were as unsuccessful as Pearson[14]. It was clear that one factor was crucial in all attempts to transmit the horse infection to the cow: the stage of the disease when the sample was taken. If the sample was collected at the vesiculous stage, transfer was possible,

9. Moore, 1817, p. 14.
10. Jenner, 1798, p. 52.
11. Anonyme, 1812, p. 14.
12. Baron, 1838, t. 1, p. 249.
13. Loy, 1801 (1889), p. 275.
14. Husson, 1803a, p. 31; Baron, 1838, t. 1, p. 249.

but at the pustular or ulcerative stage, it most often failed[15]. Another crucial factor perturbing experiments at the time was the absence of sterility of the inoculating instruments. Lancets and needles were not always cleaned well enough between two inoculations, and virus from a previous procedure could contaminate the inoculum of the next procedure.

This problem, poorly understood given the state of knowledge at the time, kept recurring in experiments involving interspecies inoculation of sheeppox, swinepox, etc.

The First Vaccination, May 14, 1796

Jenner knew he had to go on from the stage of observation to the stage of experimentation. After all, Hunter had reacted to previous hypotheses that Jenner had sent him by saying: "*But why think, why not try the experiment?*"[16]

Cowpox cases directly inoculated from cows to humans have generally been described as benign, although this was often far from being true. Few descriptions exist, and Jenner's is that much more valuable since he cannot be suspected of wanting to detract from the vaccine: "*Inflamed spots now begin to appear on different parts of the hands of the domestics employed in milking, and sometimes on the wrists, which quickly run on to suppuration, first assuming the appearance of the small vesications produced by a burn. Most commonly they appear about the joints of the fingers, and at their extremities; but whatever parts are affected, if the situation will admit, these superficial suppurations put on a circular form, with their edges more elevated than their centre, and of a colour distantly approaching to blue. Absorption takes place, and tumours appear in each axilla. The system becomes affected - the pulse is quickened; and shivering, with general lassitude and pains about the loins and limbs, with vomiting, come on. The head is painful, and the patient is now and then even affected with delirium. These symptoms, varying in their degrees of violence, generally continue from one day to three or four, leaving ulcerated sores about the hands, which, from the sensibility of the parts, are probably very troublesome, and commonly heal slowly, frequently becoming phagedenic (a species of ulcer spreading very rapidly*[17]*), like those from whence they sprung. The lips, nostrils, eyelids, and other parts of the body, are sometimes affected with sores; but these evidently arise from their being needlessly rubbed or scratched with the patient's infected fingers. No eruptions on the skin have followed the decline of the feverish symptoms in any instance that has come under my inspection, one only excepted, and in this case a very few appeared on the arms: they were very minute, of a vivid red colour, and soon died away without advancing to maturation; so that I cannot determine whether they had any connection with the preceding symptoms*"[18]. Jenner's procedure of transmitting the disease from one human being to another involved some risk. But transposing the Sutton variolation technique to the cowpox inoculation no doubt reduced the severity of symptoms following cowpox inoculation, as well as those due to cowpox transmission from one person to another, producing a disease called vaccine (throughout Chapter 3 the word "*vaccination*" is used to refer to "*cowpox inoculation*", and "*vaccine*" or "*vaccine lymph*" to the cowpox inoculated to humans[19]).

15. Monteils, 1874, p. XXVII.
16. Baron, 1838, t. 1, p. 33.
17. Hooper, 1817, p. 613; Dorland's Medical Dictionary, 2000, p. 1364.
18. Jenner, 1798, p. 4.
19. Hooper, 1817, p. 842.

When Sarah Nelmes, a dairymaid from the Berkeley area, was infected with characteristic cowpox by one of the farmer's cows, Blossom, Jenner decided to seize this opportunity: "*I selected a healthy boy about eight years old, for the purpose of inoculation for the Cow Pox.*"[20] It is noteworthy that for his first transfer of cowpox/vaccine to man, Jenner chose the passing from human to human, rather than from cow to human, which is, *a priori*, a sign of caution.

The boy in question was the son of a farmhand who sometimes worked for the Jenners. On May 14, 1796 inoculum taken from Sarah Nelmes's hand was transferred to James Phipps's arm, on which Jenner had made two superficial scratches. "*On the seventh day he complained of uneasiness in the axilla, and on the ninth he became a little chilly, lost his appetite, and had a slight head-ache. During the whole of this day he was perceptibly indisposed and spent the night with some degree of restlessness, but on the day following he was perfectly well.*"[21] Jenner submitted him to a variolation test with variolous matter on July 1, and then to another a few months later. The boy's symptoms were negligible, demonstrating the success of Jenner's experiment. Thus, James Phipps was protected from smallpox thanks to inoculation with a cow disease, cowpox, which had given him a benign disease, vaccinia. Jenner inoculated James Phipps again with smallpox five years later, without producing an inflammatory reaction[22]. Variolation tests were commonly practiced to assess the immune status of patients, or of those who had had a pustulous disease not clearly identified or having occurred very long ago, as had been the case for the French king Louis XV, who was believed to be protected from smallpox following a pustulous disease, but who died of smallpox a few years later to everyone's surprise.

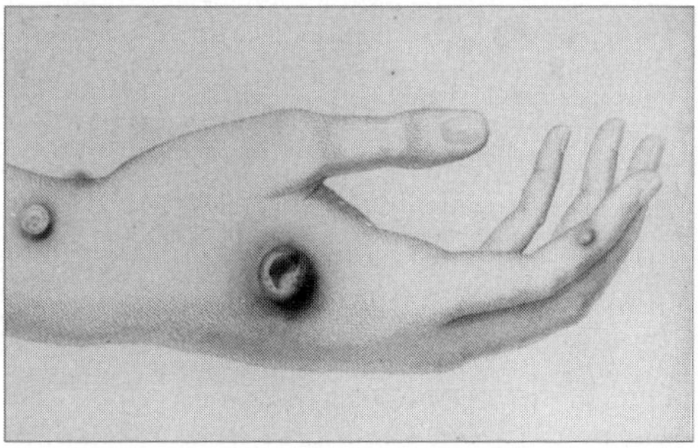

Figure 3. Illustration from Edward Jenner's first book, showing Sarah Nelmes's hand. Her cowpox pustules were the source for Jenner's smallpox vaccination. (Author's document.)

Certain moralists in the medical field find it fashionable to assert that Jenner, when he variolated James Phipps - the boy being vaccinated -, subjected his young patient to a great risk. These people only succeed in showing themselves ignorant on the subject! Jenner was a variolator and by variolating James Phipps, he was only performing a routine procedure of his medical practice. Michael Grodin, a professor of Medical Ethics at Boston University (1992) who, in a book entitled "*The Nazi Doctors and the Nuremberg Code*" wrote: "*Perhaps the earliest evidence of experimentation on children dates from 1776* (sic), *when Edward Jenner inoculated an 8-year-old boy with cow-pox material.*" [And the reference is E. Jenner... London: S. Low, 1789 (*sic*)]. Jenner knew of many cases of transmission of cowpox to humans and he variolated certain of his patients. Grodin

20. Jenner, 1798, p. 32.
21. Jenner, 1798, p. 33.
22. Royal Commission, 1889, p. 94.

continues: "*It should be noted that up to the nineteenth century, almost all medical practice may be considered uncontrolled, unstandardized experimental therapeutics or, quite simply, human experimentation of a purely empirical nature*."[23] It is obvious that all medical progress passes through a phase of experimentation. The example of variolation shows that this simplistic and morally flawed view is not borne out by reality. Examples of a relatively correct enquiry on the effects of variolation started very early, at the beginning of the 18th century, in particular in England under the influence of Jurin[24a].

Etienne Vermeersch (1994), in a book called "*The Ethics of Animal and Human Experimentation*"[24b], also gave a curious opinion: "*Being acquainted with some classical examples of research procedures that we now consider as utterly immoral, we are inclined to place all of them exclusively in the past. There are the vivisections on criminals by Alexandrian physicians of the third century BC; there are the well-known cases of Jenner's and Cotton Mather's vaccination experiments and Walter Reed's research on yellow fever*". This cutting opinion is based on a reference from Reich[24c]. The examples of Jenner and Cotton Mather are particularly badly chosen. They are two quite different methods of protection against the smallpox separated in time by 80 years. Cotton Mather introduced variolation into North America, and Jenner initiated world wide vaccination. Their cases are classed as "*well known*" and it is implied that these people ended up being pilloried by history. There is nothing to substantiate this opinion, which is not based on any historical reality. The variolation of Cotton Mather was a new practice but supported by much published work. Jenner's vaccination was a novelty but without any great risk and the variolation of James Phipps, a month later, was a medical practice current at the time and many members of the royal families of England, Russia, France made use of it.

In a similar vein, Robert Brines, editor of *Immunology Today*, an excellent immunological journal now *Trend in Immunology*, with a very large readership, wrote: "*With hindsight, Jenner's experiment appears to be the audacious and pioneering act of a visionary. However, at the time it was viewed with the skepticism and horror that would confront a modern-day attempt to inoculate a healthy child with HIV-infected tissue. If Jenner had been wrong, or if the actual inoculation had been carried out ineptly, James Phipps would have been exposed to the full force of the 'red death', the scourge from which Jenner is now credited with saving us*."[25] This accusation is totally baseless.

Rosalind Stanwell-Smith wrote in *The Journal of the Royal Society of Medicine*: "*The more accurately to observe the progress of the infection, I selected a healthy boy...*" *(Jenner, 1796). The boy was James Phipps, the 8-year-old son of a labourer. On 14 May 1796, Dr. Edward Jenner inoculated the boy's arm with cowpox. In July an excited Jenner wrote to his friend Edward Gardner: 'The boy has since been inoculated for the smallpox which as I ventured to predict produc'd no effect. I shall now pursue my experiments with redoubled ardor'... It was Jenner's remarkable - and today unthinkable - experiment on a young boy that earned him a unique place in vaccination's history*."[26]

Jenner used a test solely for the purpose of knowing the degree of protection against smallpox conferred on his patient, a classic test at the time. An example

23. Grodin, 1992, p. 121.
24a. Jurin, 1725; Jurin, 1756a & b; Dixon, 1962, p. 234.
24b. Vermeersch, 1994, p. 3.
24c. Reich, 1978, p. 684.
25. Brines, 1996, p. 203.
26. Stanwell-Smith, 1996, p. 509.

among many others: "*In these early days of the discovery, almost every case of vaccination was made a test of the alleged protection* (in England). *Dr. Jenner, writing in 1801, says, 'upwards of 6,000 persons have now been inoculated with the virus of cow-pox, and the far greater part of them have since been inoculated with that of small-pox, and exposed to its infection in every rational way that could be devised, without effect;' and Dr. Woodville (giving public evidence in 1802) said that, within two years (1799-1801) they were vaccinated at the Small-pox Hospital 7,500 persons, of whom about one half were subsequently inoculated with small-pox matter, and in none of them did small-pox produce any effect.*"[27]

In his first book, Jenner describes a few cases where the persons inoculated, or who had caught cowpox naturally, were subsequently variolated unsuccessfully. He also describes individuals resistant to cowpox after having had smallpox. Jenner writes about his work with caution and modesty. A first, rather elementary version of his treatise sent to the Royal Society in March or April 1797 was returned to him with the comment that it would be wiser not to promulgate this manuscript, that did not seem very serious, and did not study enough cases to convince anybody. On top of everything else, the book was based on common lore! A letter from Everard Home, John Hunter's brother-in-law, dated April, 22, 1797 and addressed to Sir Joseph Banks states: "*If 20 or 30 children were inoculated for the Cow pox and afterwards for the Small pox without taking it, I might be led to change my opinion, at present however I want faith.*"[28] In 1798, Jenner published his treatise with four beautiful colour illustrations, at his own expense.

Jenner was convinced that his procedure offers numerous advantages. First, cowpox is not naturally transmitted from one human being to another, and can only be transmitted through a minor surgical intervention (vaccination) or following inadvertent contamination by scratching and infection of the same person, or from one person to another. Jenner proved his argument by pointing out that James Phipps himself, when he was inoculated with cowpox, slept in a bed with two other children, a domestic arrangement very common at the time. These children were not contaminated, although they had had neither smallpox nor cowpox[29]. In addition, this method only gives the inoculated person a benign disease, not at all comparable to that contracted after variolation. Finally, he stated that the method provides protection equivalent to that of natural smallpox. This last point is debatable, if not mistaken, but Jenner firmly believed it to be true and did not change his opinion: "*Duly and efficiently performed, it* (the vaccination) *will protect the constitution from subsequent attacks of small-pox, as much as disease itself will. I never expected that it would do more, and it will not, I believe, do less.*"[30] In fact, Jenner believed in the unicity of the smallpox and cowpox.

Was Jenner the first to vaccinate? No. The use of vaccine, that is, of lymph from cowpox, appears to have been known for a long time, in England as well as on the Continent. Hufeland maintains that the protective properties of cowpox against smallpox were discovered in 1769, in Germany, but he gives no precise details[31]. In

27. General Board of Health, 1857, p. xiii.
28. Home quoted by Baxby, 1999, p. 108.
29. Jenner, 1798, p. 68.
30. Baron, 1838, t. 2, p. 135.
31. Hufeland, 1841, p. 449.

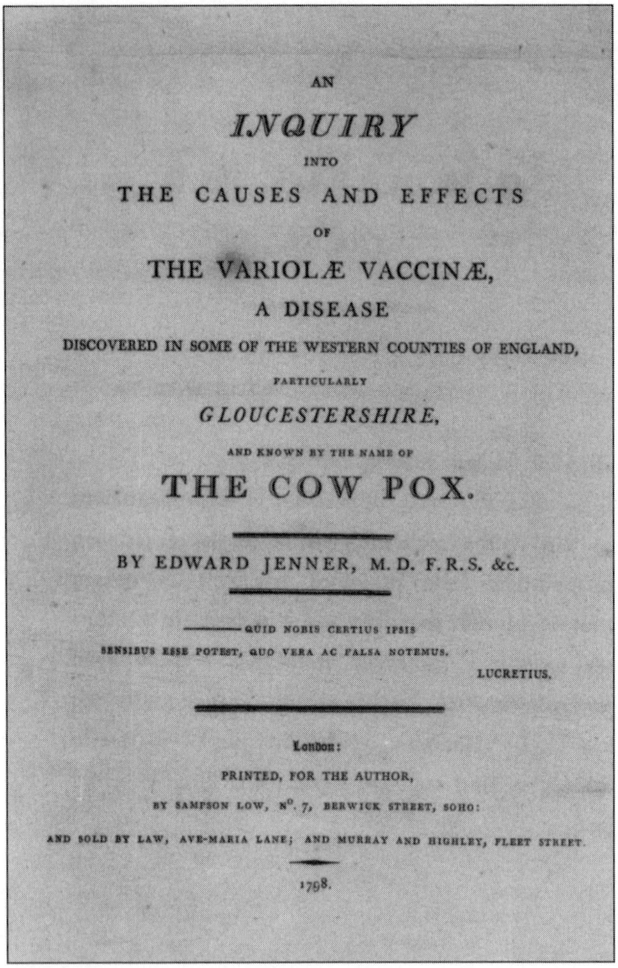

AN

INQUIRY

INTO

THE CAUSES AND EFFECTS

OF

THE VARIOLÆ VACCINÆ,

A DISEASE

DISCOVERED IN SOME OF THE WESTERN COUNTIES OF ENGLAND,

PARTICULARLY

GLOUCESTERSHIRE,

AND KNOWN BY THE NAME OF

THE COW POX.

BY EDWARD JENNER, M. D. F. R. S. &c.

——QUID NOBIS CERTIUS IPSIS
SENSIBUS ESSE POTEST, QUO VERA AC FALSA NOTEMUS.

LUCRETIUS.

London:

PRINTED, FOR THE AUTHOR,

BY SAMPSON LOW, Nº. 7, BERWICK STREET, SOHO:

AND SOLD BY LAW, AVE-MARIA LANE; AND MURRAY AND HIGHLEY, FLEET STREET.

1798.

Figure 4. Flyleaf of Edward Jenner's first book (1798). (Author's document.)

1784, in Montpellier (France), Mr. Rabaut, known as Pommier, a protestant minister, had occasion to see cows afflicted with an eruption that the people in the region called "Picotte" and which looked like smallpox. Mr. Rabaut suggested to Mr. Pugh, a British surgeon visiting the city at the time, in the presence of Mr. Ireland from Bristol, "*the idea that it might be possible to inoculate a man with matter from cow lesions...*"[32]. This actual conversation, not followed by any experiments, was widely invoked in the nineteenth century to attribute a French origin to smallpox vaccination. Husson's reference to the story is phrased in these terms: "*The following facts that leave no doubt whatsoever about the French origin of the vaccine...*"[33]. This supposed origin is obviously fictional.

The farmers of Gloucestershire were familiar with cowpox. Around 1788 or 89, when Jenner went to the Royal Society to present his study on the nesting habits

32. Husson, 1812, p. 116.
33. Husson, 1821, p. 362.

of the cuckoo[34], he took with him a drawing of a pustule on the hand of a milkmaid infected by cowpox. He showed the drawing to his friends. The pustule was quite ordinary. It was said that people who had cowpox were protected from smallpox, but this belief based on folk wisdom could hardly be trusted. Around 1760, the duchess of Cleveland was said to have boasted that she was safe from smallpox because she had had cowpox[35]. An English farmer named Benjamin Jesty had inoculated cowpox pus into his wife and two of his sons in 1774, to protect them from smallpox. But his wife had a strong reaction to this inoculation, and Jesty had to have her treated by a doctor. The experiment was not repeated. In fact, poor Jesty was called a brute and was harshly chastised for his initiative[36]. Mr. Nash, a Shaftsbury surgeon who died in 1795, left a manuscript whose latest observations seem to have been recorded in 1781; they state that cowpox (in humans) is not contagious, that it does not cause lesions, and that it provides reliable protection against smallpox...[37]. Another person who preceded Jenner was Peter Plett who, in 1791, is said to have inoculated cowpox into three children in his classroom in Husselburg (Holstein)[38]. When Fewster and Sutton observed that many peasants whom they had subjected to variolisation had no reaction to the procedure, "*they learned from these peasants that their resistance to smallpox was due to the fact that they had previously suffered from a pustulous disease contracted by milking cows with cowpox. They conducted further research to test this assertion, which appeared to be true; Mr. Fewster conveyed the information to a medical Society of which he was a member; but no one thought to put this valuable observation to good use*"[39]. In fact, Mr. Fewster of Thornbury, member of the Convivio-Medical Society like Jenner, is known to have discussed the possible use of cowpox as protection against smallpox. But he did not really believe in it, since in October 11, 1798, he wrote to Mr. Rolph, a Peckham surgeon: "*I think it* (naturally contracted cowpox) *is a much more severe disease in general than the inoculated small-pox. I do not see any great advantage from inoculation for the cow-pox: inoculation for the small-pox seems so well understood, that there is very little need of a substitute.*"[40] This letter is reproduced by Pearson in his book "*Inquiry concerning the History of the Cow Pox*". However, immunity against smallpox in all these "vaccinated" individuals had not been tested by variolation. The result was uncertain.

Finally, studies show that vaccination had long been known around the world. "*A passage in the Sancteya Grantham, a Sanskrit text attributed to d'Hauvantori, proves that vaccine inoculation was practised in India in very early times... Mr. William Bruce, consul in Bushire, wrote to Mr. W. Erskine of Bombay (Annals of chemistry and physics, t. x, March 1819) that the vaccine had been known for a long time in Persia... Mr. de Humbold (political essay on the kingdom of New Spain) proved that it had been years since the inhabitants of the Andes mountain chain had noticed the preventive effect of vaccine; A negro (loc.cit) unsuccessfully inoculated with variola, refused to be inoculated again, alleging that when he was milking the cows of the Andes mountain chain, he had contracted a sort of*

34. Jenner, 1788, p. 219.
35. Anonymous, 1914, p. 51.
36. Wallace, 1981.
37. Husson, 1803a, p. 17.
38. Anonyme, 1895c, p. 346.
39. Guersant, 1846, t. 30, p. 393.
40. Baron, 1838, t. 1, p. 49.

eruption similar to that seen on cow udders, and which gives life-long protection from small-pox to those who had taken that particular disease."[41]

It is difficult to assess the authenticity of these texts. We can, however, agree with Bousquet: "*From this point of view, Jenner suffered the fate of all inventors. When he announced the vaccine he was called a visionary, and when he proved its effectiveness he was reminded that it had been known in the East Indies since time immemorial.*"[42]

Jenner's great merit was to prove the reality of his own observations to doctors and to his contemporaries, much to their amazement. He succeeded in doing so through the use of variolation tests. Thanks to the clarity with which he described his observations, and to the relative simplicity of his experiments, he attracted the attention of his colleagues to the phenomenon. Woodville and Pearson conducted variolation tests on three cowherds on a farm in Marylebone, who had been contaminated with cowpox. All three inoculations were negative and confirmed Jenner's claims[43]. Mr. Cline, professor of surgery at the *St Thomas's Hospital* of London, first tried vaccination in June 1798. His patient was a child with an affection of the hip, who had never had smallpox. Cline believed that moderate inflammation of the hip following vaccine injection could be beneficial. Was he also considering possible protection against smallpox? There is no way of knowing. But the vaccination was as Jenner had described it and the subsequent variolation was negative[44]. Cline, who was Jenner's friend, hastened to reveal these events, which confirmed Jenner's claims. Because he had treated his young patient in collaboration with Dr. Lister, former physician at the Smallpox Hospital, his opinion carried additional weight.

In November 1798, Pearson, a British physician, published a booklet on cowpox inoculation. In it, he described cases of natural cowpox and subsequent immunity to smallpox[45]. In the early months of 1799, cowpox inoculations in humans were limited to those carried out by Jenner, Cline, Thornton de Strout who used "matter" from a Stonehouse cowherd, and Drake de Strout, who used inoculum sent by Jenner. All these inoculations caused the formation of more or less ulcerous wounds that had to be treated. This does not mean that they were necessarily very serious[46].

On January 1799, W. Woodville, director of the Smallpox and Inoculation Hospital in London, one of the most respected figures in the field, learned about a few cases of cowpox in a London dairy (in Gray's Inn Lane)[47].

For centuries cows starting lactation were brought to dairy farms located in cities or in their close surrounding areas, in order to provide fresh milk for the inhabitants. Once the lactation period ended, they were sent back to their farms, or sold. A veterinary student named Tanner, summoned for a consultation, diagnosed a case of true cowpox. What expertise did he possess? He was (perhaps) related to a veterinary surgeon named Tanner practicing in Rockhampton, near Berkeley, a region where numerous cases of cowpox had been reported. Out of the hundred cows in the London herd, fifty-four contracted the disease.

41. Guersant, 1846, t. 30, p. 393.
42. Bousquet, 1833, p. 1.
43. Creighton, 1889, p. 102.
44. Jenner, 1799, p. 54.
45. Pearson, reprinted in Crookshand, 1889.
46. Jenner, 1799, p. 33; Jenner 1800a, p. 104; Creighton, 1889, p. 103.
47. Aubert, 1801a, p. 7; Copeman, 1899, p. 68; Moore, 1817, p. 26; Woodville, 1799.

Three or four persons who milked these cows were also infected. Illustrious and less illustrious members of the medical profession in London were invited to examine these cases. Sir Joseph Banks, Lord Sommerville, Sir William Watson, Drs. Pearson and Willan, Mr. Coleman and others all gathered on the farm, and compared the illustrations in Jenner's book with the lesions found on the hands of three servants of the household, including a woman named Sarah Rice. Without a doubt, the pustules were identical. Six or seven patients at the Smallpox and Inoculation Hospital in London were vaccinated by Woodville with lymph from Sarah Rice; then, several other patients were vaccinated with "matter" collected from the first group inoculated, which was distributed to other vaccinists[48].

After a number of diversions, the effectiveness of the protection afforded by vaccine inoculation was generally admitted. But this victory was not won easily. One of the first to contest the Jennerian method was W. Woodville, head of the Smallpox and Inoculation Hospital in London. In May 1799, he published a report entitled "*Reports concerning a series of Inoculation…*", in which he declared that substituting the cowpox to the variola (smallpox) was not desirable: "*Now if it is admitted that, at an average, one of five hundred will die of the inoculated Cow Pox, I confess I should not be disposed to introduce this disease into the Inoculation Hospital, because out of the last five thousand cases of variolous inoculation the number of deaths has not exceeded the proportion of one in six hundred.*"[49] In reality, Woodville had probably mixed smallpox matter with cowpox matter on the premises of his hospital where the two were used for inoculations[50]. De Carro and de Laroque believed that Woodville himself transported the smallpox and contaminated his patients[51]. Woodville did not admit his error[52], but took the necessary precautions to avoid this mistake henceforth. In time, Woodville became a fervent supporter of the Jennerian method.

How available was the vaccine? Jenner himself remarked that from May 1796 until the spring of 1798 there was not a single case of cowpox among his clientele[53]. Jenner the vaccinist was very soon confronted by a lack of cowpox "matter"! Jenner the inoculator (the variolation practitioner) had never found himself in such a situation, because variolic "matter" was available everywhere, at that time! But cowpox was seasonal, erupting in the spring and only rarely. What could be done? "Variolous matter" could be preserved between glass slides away from the light, for a limited time. This method was tried for vaccine, with similar results. Jenner then opted for vaccine inoculation from person to person, or from arm to arm, as it was called at the time, to maintain a constantly available source of vaccinating "matter". But this arm-to-arm transfer of vaccine required great numbers of new subjects who had not had smallpox. An adequate system of donors called vaccinifers had to be organised and authorized. First, the children in orphanages were used as donors; then inoculated children of all social classes, but most often poor children, abandoned or with mothers receiving public assistance. Very quickly, centres where the poor received free vaccination were created; this in turn guaranteed the conservation of the vaccine strain and its production.

For example, according to Bryce (1802), England offered free vaccination: "*In order that the poorer classes of mankind might reap equal advantage from this important discovery,*

48. Woodville, 1799.
49. Woodville, 1799.
50. Ballhorm, 1801, p. XI; Bryce, 1802, p. 51; Copland, 1859, v. IX, p. 1419; Scofield, 1810, p. 21.
51. Ranque, 1801, p. 85; de Laroque, 1805, p. 174.
52. Woodville, 1800.
53. Jenner, 1798, p. 34.

as the more rich, and that all ranks might have an opportunity of co-operating for the general good of society in accelerating the extermination of smallpox, public institutions were soon established in most of the great cities of England, where gratuitous inoculation for cowpox was to be performed to all those who should apply."[54]

Jenner continued to vaccinate all his life; this allowed him to preserve his vaccine strain. According to Lettsom's account: "*For some time now, he* (Jenner) *told me, I have taken the habit of dedicating one morning a week to the inoculation of the poor… In the midst of these trees there is a small hut-like pavillion; it has only one room, and I only had it built to give this part of the garden a rustic look. I have converted it into a useful space, and the crowd I have to inoculate gathers there and waits for me to arrive. This is why I have called my little hut the vaccine Temple; and just like a zelous priest, he added smiling, I am always eager to find it filled with the faithful…*"[55]. This little hut was apparently built by the Reverend Ferryman, a friend of Jenner's, to serve as a locale for vaccination: one room, a chimney, a door surrounded by wood logs to create the appearance of a rustic cottage, no windows[56]. The hut still exists, in the garden of the Jenner Museum in Berkeley.

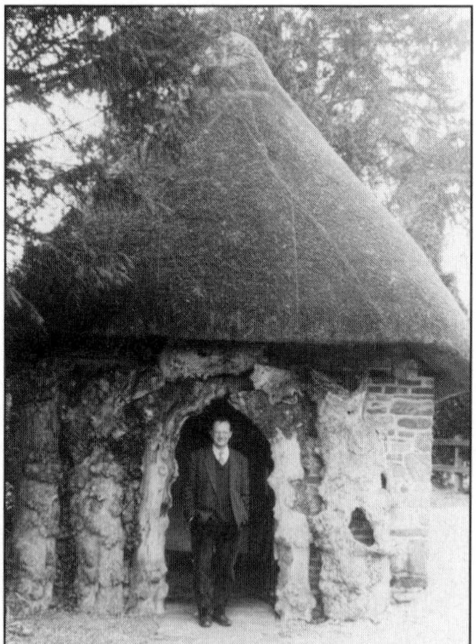

Figure 5. The "Vaccinia Temple" in the garden of the Chantry Cottage which must be very similar to how it appeared in Jenner's day because of its simplicity. (Author's photograph.)

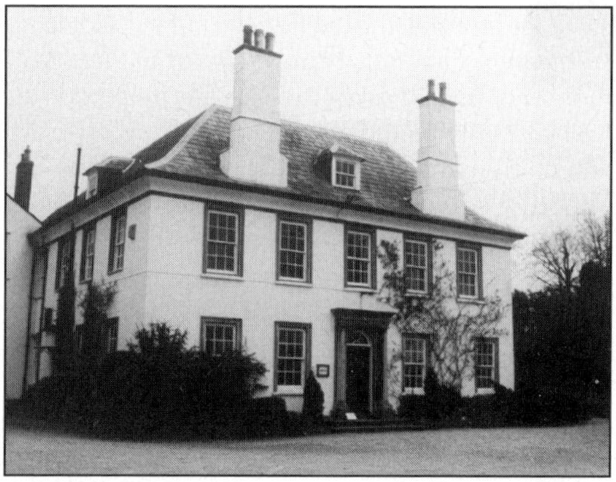

Figure 6. Chantry Cottage, Berkeley, Jenner's home, now the very interesting Jenner Museum. (Author's photograph.)

In 1799, in his second book on the vaccine, Jenner expressed his pleasure at Pearson's writings[57]. But this complicity proved to be short-lived. Acting rather unscrupulously, Pearson soon tried to claim merit for Jenner's discovery. On December 2, 1799, he

54. Bryce, 1802, p. 12.
55. Lettsom, 1811, p. 37.
56. Baron, 1838, t. 2, p. 297.
57. Jenner, 1799, p. 2.

founded an Institute for Vaccine Inoculation in London, under the patronage of the Duke of York and Lord Egremont[58]. Jenner's participation was requested, provided that the directors of the Institute accept him as an "*extra corresponding physician*" with the obligation of contributing one guinea per year as a subscriber with the right to send patients. Of course, Jenner politely declined, and informed the Duke of York and Lord Egremont of the situation. The latter was favourably inclined toward Jenner because of an earlier incident: Pearson had sent vaccine contaminated with smallpox virus to the surgeon of this gentleman. The inoculation of this virus to fourteen people had made them very sick, and they had contaminated two family members, one of whom died. Solicited by Lord Egremont, Jenner had explained the reasons for the accident so well that he gained Egremont's patronage. Very rapidly, Pearson's institution lost the support of these two high-ranking men. But after this incident, Pearson became a bitter adversary of Jenner's and tried in every way possible to discredit him.

However, Jenner's friends succeeded in founding a Society supported by voluntary subscription "*for the extermination of the small-pox*", following a "*very numerous and highly respectable meeting, holden at the London Tavern, on Wednesday, January 19, 1803, to consider of the best means to be adopted for the extermination of the Small-Pox*", and launched an "*Address to the public: the dreadful havock occasioned by that horrible pestilence, the Small-pox, which in the United Kingdom alone, annually sweeps away more than 40,000 persons, has long been a subject of deep regret to every humane and reflecting mind. The inoculation* (variolation) *of this disease has opposed an ineffectual resistance to its destructive career... A new species of inoculation has at length been providentially introduced by our countryman, Dr. Jenner, which, without being contagious, without occasioning any material indisposition, or leaving any blemish, proves an effectual preservative against the Small-pox. The house of Commons having investigated this subject with the most scrupulous attention, and being perfectly convinced of the superior advantages resulting from this discovery, have given the sanction to the practice... A motion having been made... That this meeting do form itself into a Society for the extermination of Small-pox... was then carried unanimously. Three gentlemen by appointed Trustees... a committee by now appointed for considering of and forming a Plan for the purpose of carrying into effect the important object of this Society... That the thanks of this Society be given to the Governors and Officers of the Small-pox Hospital, for their very liberal offer to co-operate in the purposes of this Society. Resolved unanimously, that all Bankers of London, Westminster and Southwark, and the Members of the Committee, be requested to receive subscriptions.*"[59] On February 3, 1803, Jenner became President of the "*Royal Jennerian Society*", whose patrons belonged to the highest spheres of society: Patron, the King; Patroness, the Queen; vice-patrons, a prince and five dukes; vice-patronesses, six princesses and a duchess, etc. The Medical Council had Edward Jenner for president, J.C. Lettsom for vice-president, and forty-seven members... as well as a secretary, John Walker. Thirteen vaccination stations were opened in the capital: one at the Central House on Salisbury Square, Fleet Street, and one in each of the twelve London districts defined by the statutes. At the central house, free vaccination was performed from 10 in the morning to 3 in the afternoon every day except Sunday. At all thirteen locations, people were vaccinated four days a week. Each vaccinator kept an

58. Anonymous, 1914, p. 73; Valentin, 1802, p. 3.
59. Jennerean (*sic*) Institution, 1803, p. 192; Address, 1803.

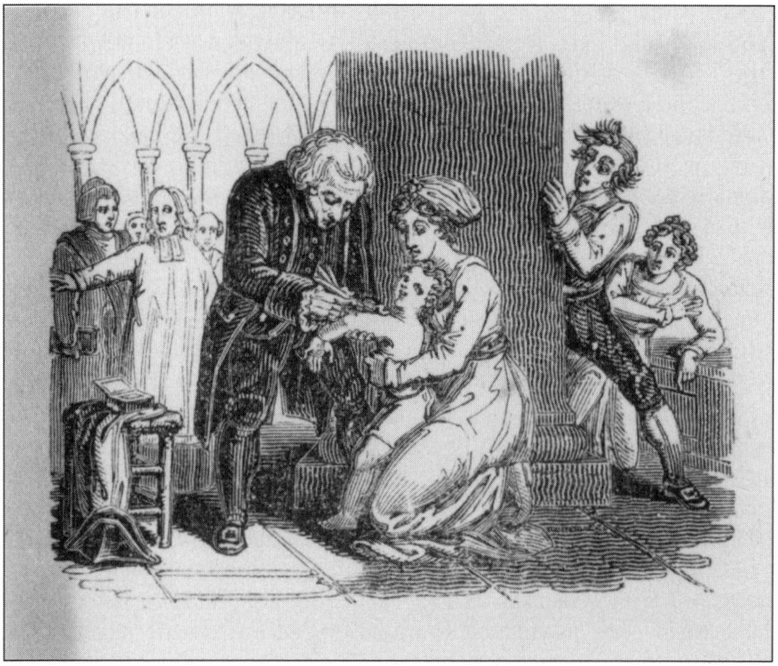

Figure 7. A curious anonymous representation of vaccination (Delavigne, 1826)[60], depicting this practice in a religious setting. The vaccinator could be Jenner, whose family was very religious.

inoculation register. In eighteen months, 12,288 vaccinations were performed, and 19,352 doses of vaccine were sent to cities throughout Great Britain and to other countries[61]. Unfortunately, this society only existed for a short period, because Jenner strongly disagreed with the ideas of the resident vaccinator, John Walker, which greatly differed from his own. As soon as 1805 he ended all contact with Walker. The members of the Institution had to proceed to several votes to remove Walker from his position.

A few months later, Mr. George Rose, treasurer of the Navy, was charged with creating a new institution, governmental this time. Rose asked Jenner to draw up a plan and establish a budget. Jenner's plan (modified to say the least, since some stipulations were certainly contrary to his view) was submitted to the House of Commons on June 9, 1808 under the title *National Vaccine Establishment*, administered by the College of Physicians and the College of Surgeons. Approved in October 1808, the new Establishment was governed by a Vaccine Board with eight members, and had as President Sir Lucas Pepys. Four members were from the College of Physicians, four from the College of Surgeons. A member's annual salary was a hundred pounds. The mission of the Board was to vaccinate London, and to send vaccine to anyone who asked, even when requests came from distant locations, "*but it had never possessed either apparatus or authority for any general system of vaccination*" in Great Britain[62]. Jenner was named Director, a position from which he soon resigned, as he could not promote his ideas,

60. Delavigne, 1826, p. 27.

61. Royal commission, 1889, p. 69; Royal Jennerian Society, 1803.

62. General Board of Health, 1857, p. lxviii.

caught between these two Colleges to which he could not belong because he did not have the necessary diplomas, to say nothing of the fact that his many enemies or those who were envious would bar the way.

"*Dr. Jenner, on account of his experience, his public merits, and his public rewards, which has seemed to engage him in the service of Vaccination; and also for the part he had taken in the constitution of the establishment, was Unanimously elected to fill the place of Director; though he afterwards declined to act in that capacity.*"[63] In reality, he was soon criticized for being at once the initiator of vaccination and, as Director, its official defender in litigious situations where he would have to evaluate the method[64]. Despite this problem, diffusion of the vaccine by the new institution was very effective, although the first reports are a little vague about the periods they cover[65]. On May 25, 1809, "*the numbers vaccinated have already amounted to 733* (in London)*; and 2,580 charges of Vaccine Fluid have been sent to various persons, many of them residing in distant parts of the country; and they have each been furnished, not only with several glasses, ivory points or lancets upon which it is conveyed, but likewise with printed instructions for the right use of it, and for ascertaining, as far as possible, the degree of security afforded*"[66]. The reports that followed indicate: January 22, 1810: 1,493 persons vaccinated in London and 16,749 charges of vaccine lymph distributed[67]; in the year 1812, 4,521 persons vaccinated in London and 23,219 charges of vaccine lymph distributed[68]; in the year 1816, 7,771 persons vaccinated in London and 44,376 charges of Vaccine Lymph distributed[69]; in the year 1820: "*6,933 persons were vaccinated in London, 48,105 charges have been given to the public and that 77,467 have been vaccinated in Great Britain and Ireland...*"[70]; in 1824, "*77,800 charges of lymph*"[71]. The last reports are brief but precise, and show vaccine shipments to destinations all over the world. The 1824 report ends with: "*We have sent Matter, since our last report, to almost every quarter of this country, and to most of the colonies; and also to Lisbon, to Madrid, to Cochin-China and to China; and it has been received every where with grateful acknowledgments: so that the name of Great Britain is associated throughout the world with acts of beneficence as well as power.*" [72] Vaccine distribution was free in England: "*The British government has made but one effort to diffuse the benefit of the cow-pox, by endowing an institution in the metropolis for the gratuitous vaccination of the poor, supplying lymph to applicants in all parts of the kingdom free of expense.*"[73] The clergy is mentioned several times in reference to the crucial role it played in convincing the people (lower classes as indicated in the text) of the benefits of vaccination[74], in Sweden[75], in Great Britain, in Spain, in Mexico and in Peru[76]. Starting in 1808, when the National Vaccine Institution was created, the Royal Jennerian Society lost its promince[77] but continued to exist.

63. Pepys, 1807.
64. Crookshank, 1889, t. 1, p. 228.
65. National Vaccine Establishment, 1810-1825.
66. Pepys, 1810.
67. Pepys, 1810.
68. Milman, 1813.
69. Latham, 1820.
70. Halford, 1821.
71. Halford, 1825.
72. Halford, 1824.
73. Cross, 1820, p. 235.
74. National Vaccine Establishment, 1810-1825.
75. Hedin, 1814.
76. Milman, 1813.
77. Baron, 1838, t. 1, p. 578.

Variolisation, with its risk of transmitting smallpox, soon became mistrusted in many countries, as it already was in New England between epidemics. In 1808, the Committee (probably of the House of Commons) recommended to the King that he prohibit variolation, at least "*three statute Miles within the distance of the utmost boundary of houses adjoining to each other, of any City, Town, Hamlet or Village of the United Kingdom in which there are ten houses adjoining to each other, under the penalty of forfeiting Fifty Pounds for every such Offence...*", the penalty to be shared equally between the denunciator and the poor, or those who might have caught smallpox from the inoculation. Finally, variolators had to inscribe in large letters on the house or houses where they inoculated "*Smallpox Hospital*" or "*Pesthouse*"[78]. However, the point that remained problematic was the respect for individual freedom: "*The work commences with a doubt, whether it would be consistent with British liberty, to restrain small-pox inoculation.*"[79] Variolisation was completely prohibited in England in 1842[80].

The Remarkable Speed of Dissemination of the Jennerian Vaccination

Edward Jenner met with extraordinary good fortune. The variolation test was the key to his success. He found himself in a situation rarely encountered by those who hope to develop a vaccine...

Variolators, like himself before 1796, could use the "Sutton" method on a subject, and then revariolate him a few weeks or months later to assess whether or not he was protected from smallpox, but within the limits of certain constraints. However, in the case of a test-variolation, these constraints were more administrative than medical in nature. The risk of more or less serious adverse effects, and the danger of contaminating those with whom the subject was in contact, were only real if the variolation had failed! Variolations as tests on already variolated persons were commonly done.

Using the "Sutton" technique (small scratches, small quantities of vaccine lymph...) and the "arm to arm" system, Jenner, the vaccinator, considerably reduced adverse side effects. Moreover, Jenner had an extraordinary advantage: the possibility of testing the results of his vaccination on the vaccinated individual himself, with the help of smallpox itself. At the time of his discovery, variolations were frequent, sometimes forbidden in certain places, but not totally forbidden, as they would become in the years that followed. Finally, Jenner provided a very good quality vaccine (with few side effects, producing very good and relatively lasting immunity, easy to make and inexpensive...) against a dread disease.

One of the major problems of vaccine development is demonstrating the value of the product. This value has to be shown based on data acquired as quickly as possible, for reasons of financial cost, and in terms of the immunity of those vaccinated. In addition, it is necessary to wait until those vaccinated, and a control group, are subjected to "natural" contamination, which takes a long time and is expensive. Using variolation, Jenner could test on the patient himself, and demonstrate the quality of smallpox protection conferred to him. There is no other example of a vaccine against an often deadly disease, tested on the inoculated subject himself.

78. Committee, 1808.
79. Adams, 1809, p. 3.
80. Hopkins, 1983, p. 86.

The most interesting aspect of this episode in the history of vaccination is without doubt the speed with which this empirical procedure, created by a relatively obscure country surgeon, spread through England and then throughout the world, spreading far and wide, out of Jenner's hands. The usual method was to vaccinate and then check the effectiveness of the vaccine by variolation, according to Ballhorn, the great vaccinator of Hanover. "*The number of vaccine inoculations performed in London was 15,000 in August 1800, and the number of variolic inoculations tried subsequently without the least effect was 5,000.*"[81]

How was vaccination introduced on the Continent? Great Britain and France were on bad terms. Most of the other countries were neutral and some tended to be anglophile. As early as 1799, in Hanover, a British Crown possession on the European continent, more or less successful vaccinations were performed[82]. In 1800, after Stromeyer spent some time in England at the request of the Duke of Hanover, he and Balhorn vaccinated successfully. On November 1, 1800, 1,000 people had been vaccinated by them or by their colleagues. Hanover became the first continental centre for vaccination[83], followed by Vienna, Berlin, Geneva, Turin, Paris, etc. In 1801, Jenner himself wrote that one hundred thousand people had already been vaccinated with cowpox, at minimum, as he modestly added. Jenner's first book was translated into numerous languages, first into Latin in Vienna (1799) by Careno, then in French in Lyon (1800), and many other languages, Pavia (1800)[84], Haarlem and Madrid (1801), Springfield (1800 or 1801), Lisbon (1803), Privas (1805), Modena (1853), Sydney and Baton Rouge (1884), London (1889, 896, 1966), New Orleans (1890), St. Petersburg (1896), Philadelphia (1909), New York (1910, 1939, 1996), Leipzig (1911), Milan (1923), Denver (1949), Birmingham (1978) and perhaps elsewhere...[85]. Numerous writings on the subject were published in "enlightened" circles, and very quickly at all levels of society.

The earliest information about vaccine inoculation arrived in Italy at the end of 1799. In the March 1802 issue of the *Philosophical Magazine*, Sacco recounted that in September 1800 he had had occasion to examine a number of cows from Switzerland which had been brought to the Lugano fair. Speaking with local farmers, he learned that in the area there were cows with pustules on their udders. Soon, he was taken to a farm where he found two cows in the early stage of the disease. The next morning, Sacco returned to see these animals which seemed to be suffering. The spots had changed into pustules and, with the help of the cowherds, he dipped wires into the pustule fluid. "*I proceeded to test the virus collected from the pustules of infected cows... Not having had small-pox myself, I was the first to have confidence in the vaccination, and the test inoculation with small-pox to which I submitted afterwards did not produce any effect.*"[86] Thanks to his powers of persuasion, Sacco convinced his family and friends to be inoculated with this matter! Three hundred people were soon inoculated. In a very short time, Sacco stopped smallpox epidemics in Guisarme and Sestos[87] and was named Director of vaccination of the

81. Balhorn, 1801, p. 47.
82. Bousquet, 1833, p. 109.
83. Balhorn, 1801.
84. Jenner, 1800b.
85. Balhorn, 1801; Bazin, 2000.
86. Sacco, 1801, p. 22.
87. Sacco, 1813, p. 3.

Cisalpine Republic and then of the Kingdom of Italy[88]. "*Orphans were placed at my disposal so that I could carry out public experiments and, at the Saint-Catherine Hospital for Found Children, a Commission of physicians and surgeons was created for this purpose.*"[89]

Numerous test inoculations (variolations) were performed as well; in Milan seventy-three people submitted to test inoculations before civic authorities; in Pavia they were performed by Pr. Scarpa, and they continued in Bologna, Brescia, Venice, Florence...[90]. When an epidemic broke out in Bologna, Sacco's foresight stopped its ravages and he was awarded a gold medal created for the occasion[91]. On November 5, 1802, a stipulation from the Minister of the Interior was aimed at providing for free vaccination of the poor and almost total suppression of the practice of inoculation (variolation)[92]. On March 9, 1804, the government of the Republic gave vaccination a new and concrete impetus[93]. Dr. Sacco inaugurated a prize of 50 sequins (500 francs of that era) for every vaccinated person who could prove that he had suffered a genuine smallpox infection following his vaccination[94]. Sacco sent his new strain of the Lombardy vaccine to de Carro, and to Pearson in London.

In Austria, on the 29th or 30th of April 1799, Ferro used the vaccine sent by Pearson to inoculate his three youngest children in the presence of several doctors, including de Carro and Peshier. De Carro, impressed by the success of the experiment, vaccinated his sons Charles and Peter[95]. A few months later, he variolated them. Soon, authorities prohibited vaccination, confusing it with variolation. Vaccination started again in March 1802. De Carro played a crucial role in the diffusion of vaccine in Europe, by sending it to many countries[96].

A short time later, the Prussian College of Medicine became convinced of the value of the procedure, and by the end of 1800 almost 2,000 Prussians were already vaccinated. "*Two of the children of the King of Prussia were inoculated with the vaccine at the end of March (1802), by Drs. Brown and Hufeland. It was the first example of this kind given by a sovereign.*"[97] In three years, 80,000 people were vaccinated, and in 1810, a further 600,000. In Bavaria, King Maximilian Joseph issued a decree stating that any person not artificially or naturally variolated, above a certain age, who neglects to be vaccinated, would be subject to an annual penalty that would increase year by year[98].

In a long letter to Dr. Ring, F.G. Friese informs him that he has received vaccine from De Carro, and that he has successfully vaccinated three people in Breslau on December 28, 1800. When he lost his vaccine strain, he obtained more vaccine from Berlin and started to vaccinate again; at the end of 1800, 10,000 people had been vaccinated in Breslau and Silesia[99].

---

88. Sacco, 1813, p. 4.
89. Sacco, 1813, p. 4.
90. Sacco, 1813, p. 122.
91. Sacco, 1813, p. 7.
92. Sacco, 1813, p. 6.
93. Sacco, 1813, p. 10.
94. Sacco, 1813, p. 130.
95. De Carro, 1799, p. 337; Sigerist, 1950, p. 3.
96. De Carro, 1799, p. 337; Sigerist, 1950, pp. 7 & 54.
97. Valentin, 1802, p. 15.
98. Cross, 1820, p. 242.
99. Friese, 1803, p. 128.

De Carro sent vaccine to Geneva. The first time he sent it, the vaccine was inactive on arrival; the second time, it produced more or less severe side effects in those who received it, and the trials were stopped. It would be Dr. Odier[100] who would introduce vaccination in Geneva.

On the fourth complementary day of year 8 (September 21, 1800), 600 children were successfully vaccinated[101]. By the end of 1801, 1,500 Geneva residents had been vaccinated. "*The combined efforts of the physicians and surgeons of the city* (Geneva) *to spread this practice greatly distinguish and honour them. We are aware of the notice to fathers and mothers, drawn up so that priests in the churches may be requested to distribute it to the father and Godfather of the child brought to them to be baptised*"[102].

In Belgium, on Thermidor 15th of year 9 (August 3, 1800), the commissioners of the Society of Medicine attested that 739 individuals had been vaccinated in Brussels, either in physician's offices or at the Saint-Pierre hospice, where twelve beds were reserved for the vaccination of the poor[103]. Elsewhere, Dr. Demaret of Gand received vaccine from England on September 7, 1800... and started to vaccinate immediately. Vrancken vaccinated on a large scale in Antwerp and received a gold medal from Napoleon[104].

In Denmark, vaccination was introduced in 1801. A committee was hastily constituted to evaluate the procedure. On December 5, 1801, it submitted a report to the king, who created a vaccination establishment in 1802, and made vaccination compulsory in 1810.

Friese sent vaccine to Moscow, where vaccinations had started in October 1801, in a home for orphans; the first vaccinated child was given the name "Vaccinoff" and was to be granted a pension for life[105]. Vaccination spread very quickly throughout the Russian Empire; Friese goes on to say: "*In consequence of this success, Her Majesty, the Empress Dowager, has graciously presented me with a valuable brilliant ring, accompanied with a very polite letter.*"

"*In July 1800, Dr. Marshall, supported by Dr. John Walker, informed the Committee of the House of Commons that he had introduced the vaccine on his Majesty's vessel Endymion; eleven crew members were vaccinated... He also vaccinated soldiers of the Gibraltar garrison... Vaccination met with the same success in Minorca, where it was performed... The practice was also introduced in Malta... In Sicily, where smallpox was even more devastating than in Malta, the introduction of the vaccine was greeted with enthusiasm... The benefits the vaccine brought to Palermo caused Naples to desire the vaccine for its own population.*"[106] Marshall wrote to Jenner from Palermo: "*It is not unusual to see in the mornings of the public inoculation at the Hospital a procession of men, women, and children, conducted through the streets by a priest carrying a cross, come to be inoculated.*"[107] Of course, the entire British Navy was vaccinated without delay.

In 1802, the vaccine imported into Greece by Dr. Scott was used in Athens, Argos and Corinth...

100. De Carro, *in* Sigerist, 1800 (1950), p. 42; Odier, 1800, p. 14.
101. Odier, 1800, p. 28.
102. Valentin, 1802, p. 10.
103. Société de Médecine de Bruxelles (Brussels Medical Society), 1800, p. 2.
104. Vrancken, 1851.
105. Friese, 1803, p. 128.
106. Thornton, 1808, p. 34.
107. Baron, 1838, t. 1, p. 403.

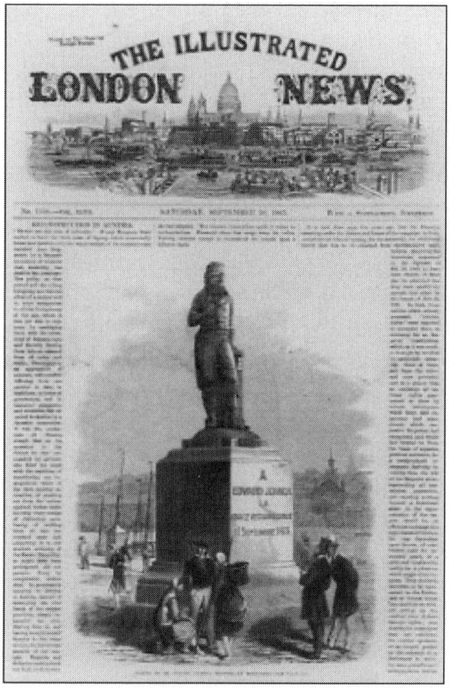

Figure 8. Saturday, September 30, 1865 *Illustrated London News* published on its cover the unveiling of Jenner's statue in Boulogne-sur-Mer (France). *"Statue of Dr. Jenner, lately erected at Boulogne-sur-Mer"*. The pedestal bears the inscription *"A Edward Jenner, La France reconnaissante, 11 septembre 1865"*. This illustration was also published in issue N° 593 of *L'Univers illustré*, of November 28, 1866, with this caption: *"Statue erected to the memory of Jenner, on the square of the sea resort at Boulogne, after a photograph."* Located in front of the fish market, Jenner's statue faced the port and the ships, which is not the case on the illustration. At the start of the 20th century, the statue was moved to the front of the Françoise Tower, on the edge of the boulevard encircling the city. On one of the sides of the pedestal, an inscription to the memory of William Woodville honours the man who made a long voyage from London, through Denmark, to come to Boulogne where French children were vaccinated and, above all, to make a reliable strain of vaccine available to French vaccinators.

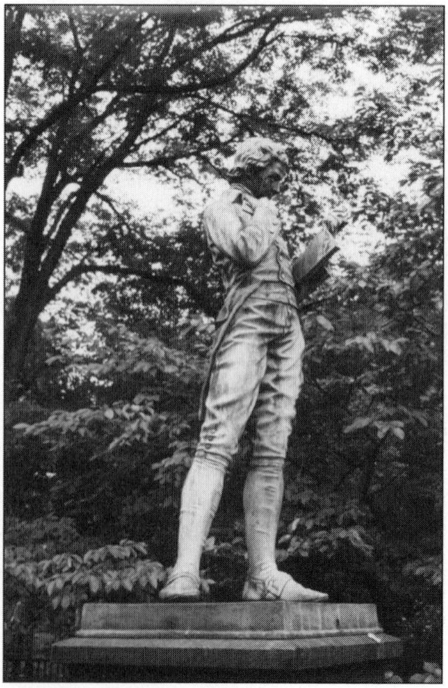

Figure 9. A Japanese foundation asked the University of Arts of Tokyo to sculpt a statue in honour of Jenner. The artist Unkai Yonehara was chosen to execute the work. Unveiled in 1904, this attractive statue represents Jenner as a young man, full of charm. It is located near the National Museum of Tokyo, in the Ueno Park. (Author's photograph.)

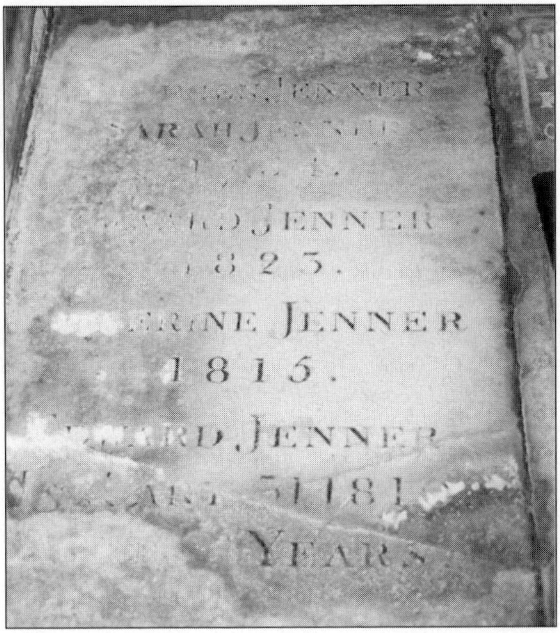

Figure 10. Edward Jenner's tomb, in the heart of the Berkeley church, is modest. Its simplicity reflects the man's character. From top to bottom, the names inscribed on the gravestone are: Stephen Jenner, Sarah Jenner, 1754 (Edward Jenner's parents); Edward Jenner, 1823; Catherine Jenner, 1815 (his wife); Edward Jenner, January 31, 1810 aged 21 years (their eldest son). (Author's photograph.)

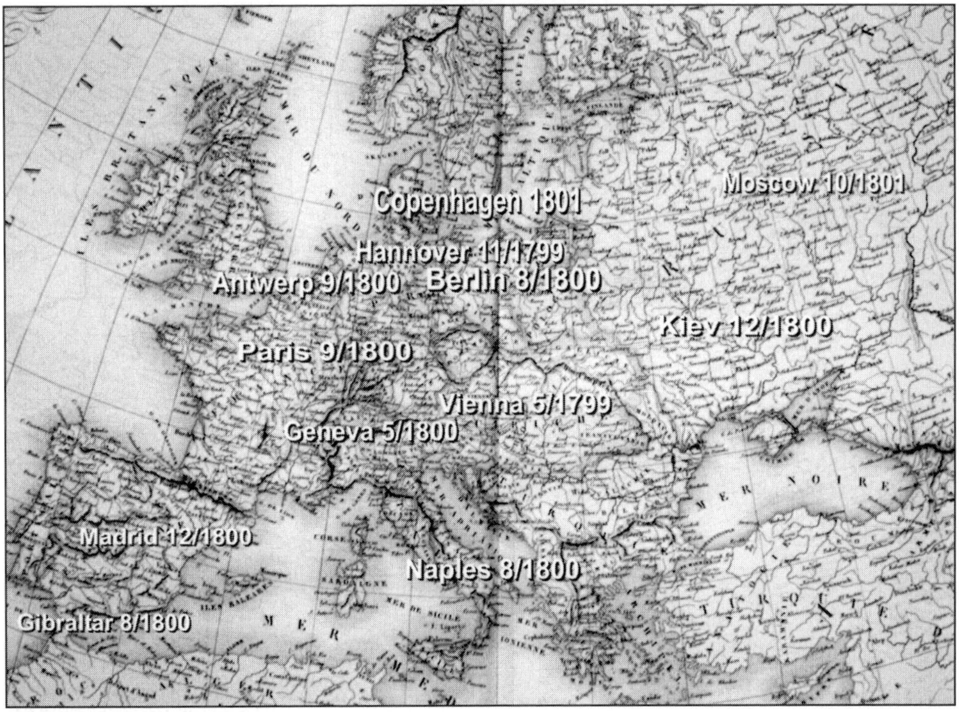

Figure 11. The remarkable speed of dissemination of the Jennerian Vaccination in Continental Europe. (Author's document.)

In 1803, Dr. Lafond, a French physician, brought it to Salonica, capital of Macedonia, and Dr. Moreschi, a Venetian, introduced it to the islands of Cythera and Ithaca[108].

Between 1799 and 1802, practically all major centres on the European continent acquired the vaccine. Jenner's procedure literally flooded Europe. "*No invention, no doctrine has been greeted with greater enthusiasm; no discovery has ever spread among civilized populations with greater speed.*"[109]

Of course, sending the vaccine out of Europe was more difficult. Jenner describes his attempts to send it to the East Indies: "*I made… my first attempt toward the end of 1799, by sending my works on the vaccine and a large quantity of cow-pox virus aboard the ship Queen East Indiaman; but unfortunately this vessel was lost at sea… I was summoned twice by the Secretary of State (Lord Hobart) who had received pressing requests for the cow-pox virus to stop the ravages wrought by small-pox in certain regions, particularly in the Island of Ceylan… This was my request: That aboard a vessel sailing to India, twenty recruits or other men from any State, who had never had small-pox, be chosen and that I would have them accompanied by a surgeon experienced in the practice of vaccination. That by this method I may assure the success of vaccination in all our establishments. After some deliberations, all my propositions were rejected…*"[110].

Fortunately, de Carro sent vaccine from Vienna to Constantinople, where it arrived in December 1800. Dr. Whyte inoculated the vaccine to the first child, whose father was Lord Elgin, the British ambassador. Soon, the vaccine crossed the desert, the Tiber and the Euphrates, and reached Baghdad and Bassora, then Bombay (now Mumbai) in India and finally Colombo in August or September 1802[111]. De Carro received a silver snuffbox from Jenner, containing a lock of Jenner's hair; it was his reward for enabling the vaccine to reach India[112].

Some vaccine virus was forwarded by George Pearson, of London, to Dr. David Hosack, of New York, in the year 1797[113]. In 1799, vaccine virus was exported by Pearson to Boston, but these trials were not conclusive. However, in December 1798, the *New York Medical Repository* reprinted in its columns a review of Jenner's book originally published in *The Analytical Review*[114]. Soon afterwards, Dr. Benjamin Waterhouse received Jenner's first book, then Pearson's book, which supported Jenner's conclusions. Waterhouse presented this information to Bostonians: "*Something curious in the medical line*", in the Colombian Sentinel, and later at the American Academy of the Sciences and the Arts, before President John Adams. Finally, on July 8, 1800, Waterhouse successfully vaccinated four of his children and three servants in Cambridge (Massachusetts) with vaccine received from Drs. Creaser and Haygard from Bath, to whom Jenner had sent it himself[115]. These vaccinations were the first on the American continent[116]. A little later, one of Waterhouse's children was variolated unsuccessfully, showing that he had immunity to smallpox. Vaccination was carried out at a steady pace in New England. But at the same time, a sort of vaccine black market developed

108. Auber, 1805, p. 5.
109. Valentin, 1802, p. 15.
110. Lettsom, 1811, p. 33.
111. Keyt, 1803, p. 391; Méglin, 1811, p. 52.
112. Munaret, 1860, p. 12.
113. Copland, 1859, p. 1415.
114. Blake, 1959, p. 177.
115. Waterhouse, 1809, p. 18.
116. Woodward, 1932, p. 23.

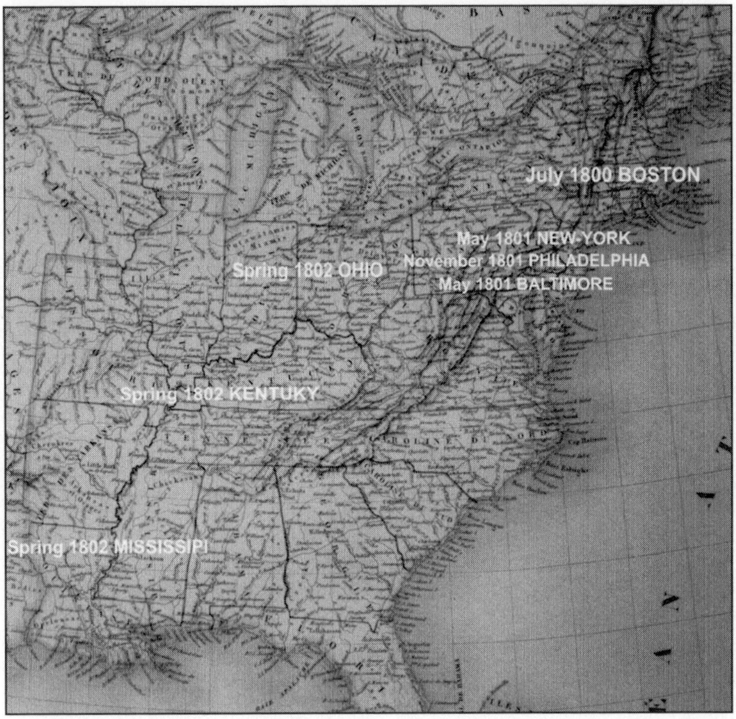

Figure 12. Diffusion of the vaccine in the USA. (Author's document.)

in Boston; fragments of shirts from vaccinated persons, presumably with vaccine absorbed into them, were being sold. At the end of 1800, in Marblehead, a village North of Boston, 58 people were infected with smallpox after using "vaccine" from a sailor arriving from England, who was presumed to have been vaccinated, but who in fact had had smallpox. Waterhouse played a major role in the diffusion of vaccine in North America. Unfortunately, in order to avoid a vaccine black market, he tried to control the vaccine financially by asking his colleagues for 150 dollars, or a quarter of their profits. Very soon, Waterhouse's "clients" were getting their supplies directly from England. Waterhouse himself lost his vaccine strain and had to wait until March 1801 to start vaccinating again. Waterhouse realised his error and abandoned his commercial ideas. In effect, he had only been imitating a great number of physicians who had made fortunes in Europe: Tronchin, Ingenhousz, Dimsdale, Gatti and even the Suttons, inoculators without diplomas. There were many others: de Carro, the Viennese physician, in a letter to his friend Marcet, dated June 26, 1799, tells him that he intends to advertise vaccination and to vaccinate whoever asks, and that he will gain great financial benefit by doing so[117]. In fact, famous inoculators gained their prestige and fortune from their competence at practicing a more or less dangerous technique that could have catastrophic consequences for their patients. The simplification and almost total elimination of danger linked to vaccination put an end to the need to seek out highly qualified inoculators.

In Boston, Waterhouse vaccinated a servant of New York Governor Sargeant, who brought the precious vaccine to New York, his own person serving as culture medium.

117. Siegerist, 1950, p. 33.

"For its introduction into the city, we are indebted to the persevering and philanthropic exertions of Dr. Valentine Seaman, who, on the 22nd of May, 1801, procured virus from the arm of Governor Sargeant's domestic... and fortunately arrived here at the proper period for procuring the virus. With this infection he inoculated several, and was happy enough to communicate the genuine affection. There had been virus received in this city during the preceding winter, but unfortunately, it gave rise to a spurious disease."[118] However, although vaccination was well-accepted by the medical profession in Boston, the population had reservations as to its value. In 1802, Waterhouse convinced the Board of Health of Boston to conduct a public experiment. A temporary hospital was established on Noddle's Island (now known as East Boston, around the airport side of the tunnels crossing the sea between Logan Airport and Boston downtown) and 16 young volunteers were vaccinated in August, then variolated in November, with special permission, two unvaccinated controls and a young man vaccinated two years earlier. The experiment was completely successful and produced the desired outcomes.

In 1801, the vaccine had already reached Georgia, the Carolinas and Kentucky...[119]. Dr. Coxe sent vaccine to New Orleans and to Martinique from Philadelphia.

Although Waterhouse's proposal of free vaccination for the poor in New York had originally been rejected: *"In January 1802, an institution was established in this city for the purpose of vaccinating the poor gratis, and of keeping up a constant supply of the genuine matter... This Institution has since been connected with the New-York City Dispensary, and a physician is appointed for the express purpose of vaccinating such as may apply for that purpose."*[120] In March 1802, the city of Baltimore created a similar institution[121]. In September 1802, the Board of Health of Boston accepted the idea of an institution for vaccinating the poor and conserving the vaccine by paying indigent mothers to convince them to vaccinate their children and to come back a few days later for vaccinal lymph to be taken. Vaccinations continued, with more or less interest shown by the population, depending on its fear of smallpox infection. In 1809, the city of Milton, frightened by numerous cases of smallpox, decided to set an example. It organised a town meeting on July 6 to consider the possibility of general vaccination. To pacify the population, a large survey was conducted and its results were read in public. In addition, the committee required a physician, Dr. Holbrook, to vaccinate for twenty-five cents, instead of the usual five dollars demanded in Boston. Three hundred and thirty-seven people, almost a quarter of the population of Milton, were vaccinated in a very short time. This example was important because it showed the effectiveness of general vaccination, which could be repeated at predetermined intervals[122].

Vaccinations continued, governed by various laws applied more or less strictly. Thus: *"An act was passed in Massachussetts, in 1810, providing that 'it shall be the duty of every town to choose persons to superintend the inoculation of the inhabitants with cow-pox.' This law was repealed in 1836, and the Revised Statutes provide 'that each town may make provisions for the inoculation of the inhabitants'. This change, as Mr. Shattuck*

118. Scofield, 1810, p. 24.
119. Valentin, 1802, p. 8.
120. Scofield, 1810, p. 25.
121. Blake, 1959, p. 180.
122. Milton, 1809; Blake, 1959, p. 183.

states, leaving it optional with the towns to do or not to do it, has probably caused the loss of many lives. Under the operation of the old law, many towns were accustomed, once in five or more years, to have a general vaccination of the inhabitants; but this custom, it is stated, has been generally discontinued, and the inhabitants are left liable to the disease from every fresh exposure. The same remark will apply to most of the States, and even large cities that have independent boards of health. Boston has provided that no child shall be admitted into the public schools without a certificate from some physician that it has been vaccinated. It also, as well as New-York and most of our cities, provided for the gratuitous vaccination of the poor; but the means provided are very inadequate to the end proposed. It is not yet safe exactly to presume on the intelligence of the lower classes in our large cities; as long as this is the case, compulsory measures will be necessary. Not only cities, but all towns and villages, however scattered the population, should have local boards of health, acting under a general State law, empowered, among other things, to provide for and enforce, if necessary, a general vaccination of the inhabitants as often, at least, as once in five years."[123]

Vaccine sent by Jenner even reached the parishioners of clergyman-physician John Clinch, who exercised his ministry in Newfoundland. In 1802, he wrote to his friend Jenner that he had vaccinated over 700 persons, who had proved to be perfectly resistant to variolation or contagion[124].

How did vaccination come to be known in Spain? "… *a Latin translation of Jenner's works was sent to Madrid. Several French books on the same subject followed; and the vaccine was favourably received and encouraged by the Government, beyond what could have been looked for. Vaccination was also gradually introduced into Cadiz, Seville, Barcelona, and the principal cities of Spain; and an enterprise was at length set on foot for extending the vaccine, which surpassed all that had been done by the most energetic European sovereigns. The merit is chiefly due to Dr. Francisco Xavier Balmis, Physician to His Catholic Majesty, a man of learning and talents, who, by persevering solicitations at court, obtained a commission for propagating the vaccine in the Spanish American and Asiatic domains; and, to defray the expense he obtained the rare and profitable permission of freighting a ship of a variety of good, and of trading at every port he touched.*

On the 30th of November 1803, he commenced his voyage from Corunna, accompanied by a number of medical gentlemen with subordinate commissions. Two-and-twenty healthy children were taken on board, that the vaccine might be continued in the most active state by successive vaccinations; and perhaps no ship was ever freighted with so precious a cargo. Balmis first pointed his fortunate course to the Canary Islands; where he vaccinated a number of children, and left instructions for perpetuating the practice. He next proceeded to Porto Rico and the Caraccas, leaving at both a preventive for some of those poisons which three centuries before had been carried thither by the Spaniards. At the Caraccas the medical officers divided, for the better accomplishing the object of their mission. Don Francis Salvani was dispatched to the south, and was shipwrecked at the mouth of the river of the Magdalena; the children and all however, got safe ashore, and reached Carthagena. After establishing Vaccination there, Salvani crossed the isthmus of Panama, carrying the Vaccine to the south-west coast of America, and diffused it among the interior provinces, and to Lima, Chili, and as far as Charcas. In the mean time, Balmis, the director, sailed to the Havannah, and then to Yucatan.

123. Copland, 1859, p. 1415.
124. Jenner, 1805 (1998), p. 163.

At this place the medical gentlemen divided again; Prof. Francis Pastor proceeded by land to Villahermosa in the province of Tobasco, propagating the Vaccine through the district of Cividad Real de Chiapa, and onwards to Guatemala. While Balmis sailed to Vera Cruz, then traversed the Vice-royalty of New-Spain, and the Interior provinces, and returned to Mexico, the point of reunion to Prof. Pastor. During the whole of these extended peregrinations, the vaccine was planted in every province; councils were instituted in the capital cities; professional men were charged with the preservation of the sacred deposit, and made responsible to the King. The director next prepared to convey the blessed lymph to the Spanish possessions in Asia. For which purpose he crossed the continent, and travelled to Acapulco on the western shore of America. He then embarked with six-and-twenty children, to secure by successive Vaccinations, the preservation of the lymph in a voyage across the Pacific Ocean. His arrival at the Philippine Iles was hailed with transports, and the captain-general gave every assistance in his power to extend the Vaccine to the furthest coast of Asia. The Archipelago of the Visuvian islands was then at war with Spain; but Balmis was a true disciple of Hippocrates, and distributing the Vaccine, as in every other exertion of his medical functions, he considered the enemies and friends of his country, equally as men. Having at length reached the extremity of that empire in which it is boasted the sun never sets, he shaped his course to Macao; and established the Vaccine both there and at Canton.

In returning to Europe, Balmis touched at St Helena; where, to his great surprise, he learned that the Vaccine had been positively rejected by the English settlers. But this Spanish physician, by relating his success, overcame their prejudices against the discovery made by their own countryman, and then returned to Spain.

Two years were nobly spent by this excellent man, in putting a vaccine girdle round the globe; and it is an additional pleasure to have learnt, that by trading during his circumnavigation, he acquired an easy fortune."[125] Pruen and Thorton indicate that Balmis came back on a Portuguese vessel, which must have considerably reduced his opportunities for personal commerce[126]. Moore does not specify the origin of the Spanish vaccine - after all, having a book on vaccine is not the same of having the vaccine! According to Husson, vaccine was sent from Paris by the central vaccine Committee to the Spanish Minister, Mr. Alonzo, in Madrid, who distributed it to the medical profession after having had himself vaccinated first[127].

Japan, at the time, was a very closed country, with commercial ties limited to the Netherlands and China. In 1803, Hendrick Doeff, head of the Dutch commercial mission in Nagasaki, informed a Japanese interpreter, Sajuro Baba, about Jennerian vaccination against smallpox. The first vaccination in Japan was performed in 1824 by Goroji Nakagawa, who was born in a small village in Northern Japan. In 1807 he was captured by the Russian navy and taken to Siberia as a prisoner. There, he worked for five and a half years as assistant to a Russian physician. Just before he was sent home, he learned about Jennerian vaccination and received one or two books on the subject. Liberated, he went south of Hokkaido island, to Matsumae, where he was immediately quarantined as were all Japanese returning from foreign countries. Because smallpox was endemic around him, he proceeded to vaccinate, successfully, and he even taught local physicians to do it. Sajuro Baba came into possession of the book on the vaccine brought back by Goroji Nakagawa, and translated it into Japanese. It

125. Moore, 1817, p. 266.
126. Pruen, 1807, p. 33; Thorton, 1808.
127. Husson, 1803b, p. 47.

was published in 1850. In 1837, an American physician and missionary, Peter Parker, vaccinated several people in the Ryukyu Islands. In 1846, it was a British missionary physician who propagated the method in the same islands. These trials seem not to have had concrete consequences. But on July 17,1849, a Dutch physician, Otto Mohnike, and a Japanese physician, Soken Nabeshima, succeeded in vaccinating one out of three children treated in Nagasaki by using variolous scabs sent from Djakarta. Mohnike started to send the vaccine away: on August 6 to Saga, on September 21 to Hiroshima, on September 22 to Kyoto, where a "house of vaccination" was created almost at once; on October 16 to Osaka, on November 11 to Edo (Tokyo), on November 25 to Fukui... Soon, Japan was completely open to vaccination. In 1857, a private foundation for vaccination was established in Edo (Tokyo), quickly becoming the "Government Vaccination House", itself transformed into the "Institute for Western Medicine" in 1863[128].

In 1875, a smallpox epidemic ravaged the Far East and killed the Emperor of China. But the Japanese Mikado and his wife, both vaccinated twice, escaped the contagion[129]. The "Compulsory Vaccination Act" came into effect in 1876[130]. In 1879, a Japanese mission visited European establishments producing animal vaccine, and soon Japan started its own production. Revaccination every five years was compulsory[131].

In 1892, coming back from Germany where he worked for 5 years with Koch, Behring, Kitasato obtained donations and founded in the Shiba Park in Tokyo an establishment for the study of infectious diseases, which quickly became an official Institution. Then, in 1905, an Imperial decree reorganised a number of institutions, including the one for vaccine and Kitasato's institution, bringing them together in a vast complex located on Shirokane Hill. Kitasato was named its first Director. Mr. Umeno, a veterinarian, prepared 1,700,000 vials of animal vaccine every year, enough to vaccinate 8 million people out of Japan's total population of 45 million[132].

The diffusion of Jennerian vaccination was extremely rapid in most parts of the world. However, populations submitted to it more or less readily depending on the fear of a near-by smallpox epidemic, on direct legal obligations, or on indirect obligations such as the need for a certificate for admission to schools, hospitals... or eligibility for financial assistance... Thus: "*Vaccination was introduced into Denmark in 1800... In a circular addressed in July 1916 to all magistrates and bishops, it was ordered that all should be vaccinated, without a compliance with which injunction no individual could be received at confirmation, admitted to any school or public institution, or bound apprentice to any trade. Priests were also forbidden to marry those who had not either the small-pox or the cow-pox.*"[133] Even in countries with high standards of hygiene, epidemics broke out periodically, when persons arriving from countries with smallpox had the disease in its incubation stage. There is no doubt that failure to apply a general policy led to the persistence of smallpox on all continents, until a decision was made by the World Health Organisation to implement a common program for the eradication of the disease.

128. Matsuki, 1998, p. 11.
129. Anonyme, 1875, p. 980.
130. Matsuki, 1998, p. 11.
131. Anonyme, 1898, p. 536.
132. Chaboseau Napias, 1909, p. 692.
133. Cross, 1820, p. 241.

Arrival of Jennerian Vaccination in Napoleonic France, from 1800 to 1815

*"Lightning rods are to houses what vaccine is to humanity."**
Mrs. Gaspard Monge.

It has often been said that in France the first mention of Jenner's work appeared in a note published in Dezoteux and Valentin's book *Traité historique et pratique de l'inoculation*, which refers to certain 1798 texts from the journal *Bibliothèque Britannique* published in Geneva[134], which, at the time, was the "prefecture" of the French department of Léman. In their book, Dezoteux and Valentin, two fervent inoculators, reveal their understanding of Jenner's texts with obvious scepticism: "*... as a result the pus of the horse-pox, passing through the cow udder, suffers a modification that augments its activity, and which renders the human body inaccessible to ordinary small-pox; that this matter is not a preservative without this intervention* (sic)*... It is in the spirit of caution suitable to the examination of new things, and particularly of the originality of such experiments, that we present this notification.*"[135] It is clear that the implication of horsepox complicated the presentation of Jenner's work. His readers were disconcerted by this point, which at the time was decidedly of secondary importance. It is true that the text in *Bibliothèque Britannique* insists strongly (and even repeatedly) on the role of the transmission of the virus from the horse to the cow, then to man: "*It is also highly remarkable that the virus of the horse, whose effects are precarious, uncertain and undeterminate before passing through the cow udder, then becomes not only more active, but also invariably endowed with this specific property of producing constantly in the human body symptoms similar to those of variolic fever, & of producing in it this change that makes it forever unsusceptible of the variolous contagion.*"[136] Some time was needed for this idea to dissipate.

Vaccination was first introduced in France in 1799, but early attempts were short-lived, for it was difficult to obtain cowpox virus, and even more difficult to conserve it, since no system had been devised to allow for this. Several unsuccessful attempts were carried out in Paris in 1799[137]. Elsewhere in the country, attempts were successful in Alsace (August 1799 and September 1800), and especially in Rochefort in March 1800, where Dr. Bobe-Moreau vaccinated successfully[138].

Paris started to take action as well: "*At the start of year VIII (1799), the Paris School of Medicine named commissioners to gather information and work with the members of a Commission created at the same time within the National Institute.*"[139] The intention was good, but produced few results. However, on the 21st of Floreal of year 8 (May 11, 1800), an influential man with strictly magnanimous intentions, and aware of the benefits of vaccination, the Duke de La Rochefoucault-Liancourt, recently back in France after

* Letter to her daughter Jeanne-Charlotte-Emilie and to her son-in-law Nicolas-Joseph Marey, dated 8th Prairial year XII (May 28, 1804), discussing the proper manner of installing a lightning rod on the Castle of Pommard (French department of Côte d'Or), about to be completed... (Marey-Monge family archives).

134. Anonyme, 1798, p. 258.

135. Dezoteux, 1799, p. 301.

136. Anonyme, 1798, p. 367.

137. Aubert, 1799, p. lviij; Aubert, 1801a, p. xxxij; Aubert, 1801b, p. V; Husson, 1800, p. 98; Husson, 1803b, p. 5; Portal, 1803, p. 212.

138. Darmon, 1986, p. 177; Hervieux, 1897, p. 180; Méglin, 1811, p. 5; Viaud, 1907, p. 681.

139. Duffour, 1808, p. XIV.

living abroad during the French Revolution, created a Society with some friends and acquaintances. These included Thouret, Director of the School of Medicine, and a subscription was started for the diffusion of this prevention method in France[140]. The first meeting of the Medical Committee of the Society of subscribers, composed of La Rochefoucault-Liancourt, Thouret, Delaroche, Chanseru and Parfait, took place at La Rochefoucault-Liancourt's residence "*near la Magdelaine*"[141]. A central committee composed of "*nine learned physicians*" was also created[142].

Because vaccination had still not begun, tired of waiting, at the start of year 8 (end of 1799 or start of 1800), a volunteer, the young Genevese Dr. Aubert, offered to go to London and learn the procedure from Jenner and Woodville. He was the envoy of the Institute Commission and of the School of Medicine, entrusted with bringing back answers to "*questions in regard to three main points: 1° pustulous eruption on the cow udder, which provides the inoculum; 2° selection of the matter to inoculate, and the means of preserving its effectiveness; 3° the effect produced by the Vaccine in humans*"[143]. The major aim of the Central Committee (of vaccination, in Paris) was to test the value of Jennerian vaccination before deciding to adopt it. "*The Committee first addressed itself to various members of the Public Administration, whose assistance could be helpful; and we* (the Committee) *must acknowledge here the willingness with which our efforts were supported in every instance. We needed subjects suitable for inoculations; the doors of the hospices were opened to us... Above all, the Committee had to obtain vaccine fluid for these operations. It turned confidently to the members of the Institute created in London for this inoculation, Mr. Pearson, Mr. Nihell, etc.; and for the relations it had to entertain with these learned men, it obtained, from the Minister of external Relations, citizen Talleyrand-Périgord, as well as from Sir Otto, Commissioner of the Republic in England, all the facilities it might have wished.*"[144]

A vaccination centre was established near Paris, in Vaugirard, in a house rent by Mr. Colon, for the purpose of conducting these tests. Forty subjects could be accommodated on the premises[145]. "*The Committee had chosen, for its experiments, a locale... Children from the La Pitié hospice were soon brought there in sufficient numbers; and the trials started...*"[146]. A new strain of vaccine arrived, on Prairial 7th, year 8 (May 27, 1800) in "*an ampule filled with hydrogen gas and perfectly sealed*"[147]. This trial seems different from those described previously. Results were probably negative, because after a few inoculations it became obvious that the cowpox virus had degenerated.

Fortunately, Aubert, accompanied by Dr. Woodville himself and by an English physician, Nowel, who had been practicing in Boulogne-sur-Mer before the beginning of hostilities between Great Britain and France, came back from England during the preliminary stages of the peace of Amiens. Talleyrand himself provided their passports! They had to pass through Denmark, in Altona, before reaching France on the ship of a neutral country. Nowel probably insisted that they land at Boulogne, for he had been practicing medicine there for several years. Having recovered his "old" clientele, Nowel

140. Husson, 1803b.
141. Parfait, 1804, p. 42.
142. Husson, 1803b, p. 7; Guersant, 1846, t. 30, p. 393.
143. Aubert, 1801b, p. V.
144. Husson, 1803b, p. 7.
145. Colon, 1800, p. 6.
146. Husson, 1803b, p. 8.
147. Barrey, 1800, p. 11.

vaccinated three little girls, Marie Spitalier, Sophie Hedouin and Beugny on June 19, 1800. By the time customs problems were solved a month later, the same lymph was inactive when it arrived in Paris on Thermidor 7th, year 8 (July 26, 1800). Nowel was called to the rescue; lymph, often called "*Boulogne matter*", was obtained in Boulogne and sent to Paris, where on Thermidor 20th, year 8 (August 8, 1800), Mr. Woodville inoculated it to François J.B. Eugène Colon, 11 months, 20 days old and "*breaking in his teeth*", son of the owner of the house in Vaugirard, the vaccine hospital[148]. Colon sent his vaccine generously all over France to many physicians, including Jadelot, Corvisart, Coladon, Valentin, Husson, Tessier, Voisin, Tarbès..., as well as overseas.

The value of the vaccine as protection against smallpox had to be demonstrated as well: "*On Fructidor 3rd, year 8* (August 21, 1800)*, having learned that at Madame Necker's hospice* (the present-day Necker Hospital)*, near the locale of its experiments* (Colon's house in Vaugirard, still being used)*, there were two children suffering from the small-pox, the Committee decided to take advantage of the occasion to start its counter-trials. Three of the children who had been vaccinated were taken there (Armand, Valois and Blondeau), two having received the vaccine on Prairial 13th* (June 2, 1800)*, and one vaccinated on the 20th* (June 9, 1800) *of the same month* (vaccinated children with dubious status prior to receiving the Boulogne matter)*, thus, all three vaccinated about three months earlier. Each child was given two inoculations of the fresh matter in each arm; in the case of one of the children, the procedure was performed by the most accredited inoculator in Paris, the citizen Goetz, whom the Committee, eager to prove its impartiality, had invited to follow its experiments.*"[149] Goetz was not convinced, and in 1802 he published a book entitled: "*De l'inutilité et des dangers de la vaccine, prouvées par les faits*" (Of the uselessness and the dangers of the vaccine, demonstrated by the facts.)

Until that point, the funds collected by the subscribers' Society had sufficed to cover the costs of the central committee's experiments, and the studies had advanced rapidly. On Pluviose 5th, year 9 (January 25, 1801), having run out of funds, the Committee turned to the Prefect of the Seine Department; it requested that a permanent establishment for free vaccine inoculation be created, serving as a place of instruction for inoculators: the premises, furniture and linens for this establishment, representing an annual budget of 4,000 to 5,000 francs. The committee wanted to sever relations with Colon, with whom it now found itself in conflict. There were also complaints about the roads (muddy in winter, dusty in summer) that linked Paris to Vaugirard. A new subscription was going to be made, but the committee did not hope to collect more than half of the required sun. It therefore solicited the "*citizen Prefect to consent to come to its rescue for the remaining amount, which could total about two thousand five hundred francs*"[150].

The vaccination centre was transferred out of the Vaugirard house, to "*a more comfortable, more central location... a spacious and permanent locale, where children of indigent families would receive free vaccination, and which could always supply an adequate quantity of vaccine... The Saint-Esprit house, near the City Hall... and as stipulated by an Order of Prefect* (Frochot) *on Pluviose 19th, year 9* (February 8, 1801)*... an inoculation hospice was created, for the use and under the supervision of the Committee... The hospice entrusted to the intelligent care of Mrs Dubois, sister of Charity.*"[151] Inoculation and treatment were to be free...

148. Colon, 1800, p. 27.
149. Husson, 1803b, p. 104.
150. Comité médical, 1801, p. 13.
151. Husson, 1803b, p. 17.

Shortly afterwards, in 1802, this establishment was classified as a civil hospice and was placed under the supervision of the Administrative Board of Paris Hospitals[152]. The budget consisted at first of subscriptions, supplemented by funds for hospices[153]. What is remarkable is the speed with which the Prefect responded to the request of the central committee, a private agency: less than two weeks! The Committee would meet twice a "decade" (the ten-day week of the French Revolutionary calendar). The vaccination hospice, at the corner of Hautefeuille Street and St. André-des-Arts Square (not far from Saint-Michel Square) was where the meetings of members of the central vaccine committee were held every Friday afternoon between three and five. Tuesdays and Saturdays, from noon to three, Mr. Husson vaccinated anyone who came[154]. Because the house looked rather stark, on March 13, 1810 Husson asked the Minister of the Interior for funds to plant two yew trees in front of the main entrance, and buy a hundred francs worth of lanterns to create a more pleasant atmosphere "*by placing an illuminated circle around the house*"[155]. A few days later, Husson ordered what he needed. The minister did not hesitate long: the success of the vaccine was assured!

The central vaccine committee was to serve the public, and particularly the Parisian population, by informing and inoculating. On October 20, 1800, over 150 children were vaccinated[156], and on February 21, 1801, over 1,000[157]. The committee encouraged research to validate the promise of the vaccine. Almost all its members had children in their charge: "*Citizen Pinel at Salpêtrière; citizen Mongenot at the Orphanage for girls, at the Sèvres limits; citizen Jadelet at La Pitié; and the Hospital for sick Children with citizen Marin; as well as the Prytanée* (military school) *all constituted additional hospices that could be regarded as annexes of the institution specifically entrusted to the Committee.*"[158] All these vaccinations were important, because the children involved could all be observed for a long enough period to validate the facts reported. The data had to be coherent: "*A model of uniform tables was printed for recording the details of individual observations. We took care to record the names of the children and of their families, their age, their place of residence, the date of the inoculation, the names of the donors of inoculated matter, the stage of pustule development when matter was taken, the principal characteristics of the procedure, and its termination. All these tables, carefully brought together at the meetings held at the Committee's hospice, provide an account of the vaccinations performed; they are the essential elements of the great experiment we have conducted.*"[159]

The central committee was looking for new sources of vaccine; it countered attacks against the vaccine by denouncing examples of bad faith and distortion of facts. The vaccination hospice became a teaching centre where demonstrations were carried out; it also maintained active correspondence with provincial doctors. Finally, the central committee met all requests for vaccine fluid. The charity work offices of the twelve Paris municipalities, and the Louvre Medical Society vaccinated free of charge or facilitated access to vaccination for all[160].

152. Husson, 1802, p. 3.
153. Frochot, 1801, p. 15.
154. Anonyme, 1801; Duffour, 1808, p. XXVIJ.
155. BANM, Ms 1611-739, letter n° 872.
156. Comité médical, 1800, p. 37.
157. Comité médical, 1801, p. 1.
158. Husson, 1803b, p. 20.
159. Husson, 1803b, p. 21.
160. Husson, 1800, p. 28; Portal, 1803, p. 212.

The Institute also named a Commission to supervise all work on the vaccine, but particularly the work of the central committee. But the Commission insisted on specifying: "*We are not, however, united by the bonds of association to this Committee, thus remaining unaffected by its success and its glory, and we have remained impartial witnesses...*"[161]. Numerous committees came into existence on their own in the provinces, and already existing medical societies propagated the vaccine, as was the case in Paris, Lyon, Marseille, Tours, Bordeaux, Nantes...[162]. Prefects were soon given the task of creating local committees and free vaccination establishments where none existed. Departmental administrative boards recommended that childbirth courses be supplemented with lessons on the vaccine, and health officers were charged with vaccinating in their sectors. Military authorities followed suit and strongly encouraged the vaccination of personnel under their command.

Throughout the entire period of its operations, the central committee worked with civil, military and religious authorities of the Napoleonic Empire, whose influence extended from Rome to Hamburg. It played a major role in the spread of the vaccine to foreign countries, thanks to its publications and the doses of vaccine it sent to Rotterdam, Geneva, Stockholm, Brunswick, Kiel, Raguse (Dubrovnik), Torino, Berlin, etc. An official letter was sent by the Minister of the Interior to departmental prefects, on Prairial 6th, year 11 (May 26, 1803). It described the benefits that could be expected from Jennerian vaccination, based on the first 1803 report of the central vaccine Committee, approved by the national Institute. Each prefect received two copies of the report, and was charged with introducing the vaccine in hospices for children, organising a vaccination service in subprefectures to allow poor families to have their children vaccinated, and recommending to Ministers of Culture, charity committees and public authority officials to use all their influence in favour of adopting vaccination[163].

It became urgent to obtain official status for the society of subscribers and its Central Committee, which had been government subsidized while having private status. The Society had to submit a request, and have the help of the national Institute, for a new society to be created by Chaptal, Minister of the Interior, on Germinal 14th, year 12 (April 2, 1804), bearing the name "*Société pour l'extinction de la petite vérole en France par la propagation de la vaccine*" (Society for the eradication of the small-pox in France by the propagation of vaccinia.) A medical committee was selected among the members, and a common secretariat for both bodies was appointed. The medical committee was to meet once a week and receive, for its services, "*a silver coin the size of an "écu": one side bearing the effigy of Emperor Napoleon. At the bottom, in exegesis: For the vaccine; on the other side, Asclepios and a woman representing Beauty; with the legend: Health and beauty, etc.*"[164]. This coin seems to resemble a smaller version of the "*Napoleon I - The vaccine*" medal coined by Bernard Andrieu (1804). Husson was named secretary of the Society and the Committee.

The thirty-four members of the Society, some individuals entrusted with political functions, physicians and the sixteen Committee members were named by an Order issued the same day and signed by Chaptal. This central organisation, under the auspices of

161. Portal, 1803, p. 212.
162. Emonnot, 1801; Capelle, 1801.
163. Coulomb, 1803, p. 183.
164. Parfait, 1804, p. 75.

the Minister of the Interior, was to work in collaboration with departmental agencies answering to prefects. Vaccination had become completely official under the Napoleonic Empire, in four years![165] There had, however been some resistance: "*Although most mayors showed so much zeal, we have to admit that their example was not followed everywhere...*"[166].

By issuing his decree of March 16, 1809, Napoleon showed his attachment to the fight against smallpox:

- attribution of an annual sum of a hundred thousand francs to cover costs,

- establishment of twenty-five depositories for the conservation of vaccine in the departments (with constant availability of four vaccinifer children) and an equal number of committees responsible for spreading the vaccine and for relations with the central vaccine Committee,

- obligation on the part of department prefects and local subprefects to attend general vaccination sessions,

- creation of a free vaccination room in hospices where vaccinations were to be performed on specific days such as Sundays or market days,

- obligation to vaccinate children raised as wards of the state in the first three months of life... all individuals admitted to an educational institution, a factory, a workshop... the poor receiving government assistance or public charity.

These stipulations were to take effect on January 1, 1810[167]. Nominations to the position of Director of vaccine depositories were carried out in hospices by the prefects, who often named their own protégés... The Central Committee received many requests for recommendation, and later complaints[168].

As for the Church's position, vaccination received practically unreserved support from the representatives of various religions. Some of them were very active, convinced that it was their duty to contribute to this effort. It is hard to say if this was true for all church officials. Pressure from imperial power must have been great, and attempts to resist were neutralised, at least in part. The annual reports of the central vaccine Committee show the names of the persons who worked most diligently to distribute the vaccine. According to the first report, for 1803, the Committee awarded medals of encouragement to an archbishop, a priest and two vicars, out of twenty persons quoted. Thankful acknowledgement is expressed to eight archbishops or bishops for having preached publically in favour of vaccine use[169]. On the occasion of Napoleon's coronation (December 2, 1804), Pope Pie VII came to Paris: "*Finally, the Committee took advantage of the sovereign pontiff's stay in Paris, to try to persuade him to recommend the new method to all the clergy in France... Our expectations were not deceived: the Pope accorded a kind reception to the delegation charged with this mission; and fully convinced of the benign nature and the immense benefits of the vaccine, he expressed in his answer that he applauded the work of the committee, and that he took the greatest interest in the success of a discovery both precious and useful to humanity, whose beneficial effects are confirmed by experience.*"[170] Archbishops

165. Chaptal, 1804.
166. Husson, 1818, p. 34.
167. Husson, 1809, p. 1.
168. BANM, Ms 1611-739, letter no. 878.
169. Husson, 1803b.
170. Husson, 1806, p. 27.

and bishops wrote pastoral letters[171]. "*Monsignor the Bishop ordered that a recommendation be made in each parish in favour of vaccination. Several ecclesiastics have given support to the mayors in the effort to spread it in their communities.*"[172]

The Bishop of Besançon, very favourable to the vaccine, informed the Central Committee of the obstacles he noted to the spread of the vaccine: the ignorance of country doctors, sordid interest in the gains to be made by treating smallpox sufferers, the small compensation given to vaccinators, the carelessness of parents who do not bring their children to vaccination appointments, and "*finally the terrible admission, thorn from them by misery, of a few parents who wish for small-pox to deliver them of their children*"[173]. The Catholic Church maintained this favourable position toward vaccination throughout the duration of the First Napoleonic Empire[174]. The Reformed Church took the same position, and certain vicars earned distinction. Marron, president of the Reformed Church Consistory, gave an address to his parishioners on September 29, 1811 in favour of the vaccine[175]. Mr. Benjamin Hussey, Nantucket Quaker (Massachusetts, Eastern United States), living in Dunkerque, received a gold medal on March 6, 1812 "*as a reward for the effort he deployed in the propagation of the vaccine*"[176]. "*Jews and Protestants were also partisans of the vaccine. We have noted that most Jews have had their children vaccinated.*"[177] A prospectus issued by the Central Israelite Consistory and addressed to the members of the various departmental consistories of the Empire, enjoined them to prevail upon all parents to vaccinate their children[178].

There were even individual initiatives, as innovative as they were original: "*Thus, Mr. Dupaquier, priest of Saint-Romain, department of the Côte d'Or, after having convinced his parishioners to use the vaccine, either through his exhortations, at church or privately, entered in agreement with the mayor of his village that the day of vaccination should be a festivity appealing to the inhabitants of the countryside. He had all the children in his village wear their best clothes, closed the school, so that vaccination day became a holiday. Not a single child was missing from the procedure.*"[179] Clearly, National Poliomyelitis Vaccination Days are not a new invention.

Cowpox vaccination also encountered pockets of resistance, or at least of indifference, as time went by: "*... We regret to announce that in some regions of France, specifically in the departments of Gironde, Orne, Sarre, Loire, de Marengo and the Two Nethes, the clergy did not support, as it should have done, the intentions of the Government regarding the propagation of the vaccine.*"[180] France annexed Piemont in 1799 (and held it until 1814-1815). Divided into departments, the territory sent reports, in French, to the Central Committee. They reveal a curious and apparently singular opposition to the vaccine. In 1802, on the occasion of the creation of the new Veterinary School in Turin, Giovanni Brugnone, its Director, opponent of vaccination, invokes, among

171. Husson, 1805, p. 20; Latour, 1804, p. 11.
172. Serriere, 1807, p. 12.
173. BANM, Ms1602-730, p. 21.
174. Husson, 1814.
175. Marron, 1811, p. 5.
176. Kenny, 1812, p. 11.
177. Serriere, 1807, p. 12.
178. Sasportas, 1811, p. 11.
179. Husson, 1812, p. 37.
180. Husson, 1809, p. 26.

other objections: "*The fear of making cow-pox indigenous in cows of a region where it had not existed is one of the strongest motives that have opposed until now the general adoption of the vaccination...*" Huzard responded to this concern by emphasizing that cowpox is not an anthrax-type disease, adding that he had had his four children vaccinated[181]. Moreover, not far from Turin, in Lombardy, Sacco had found a local strain of cowpox.

The Vaccination Technique

How was Jennerian vaccination, also called "*arm to arm*" or "*human*", practiced? Many descriptions exist. They all derive from the techniques of variolation, sometimes improved to increase the speed of the operation[182]. Using small lancets or needles, the skin of the person to be vaccinated was scratched lightly (so that bleeding was avoided), or the skin was punctured lightly, then the dermis was rubbed, to introduce on very small areas vaccine lymph taken from a person vaccinated a few days earlier, or lymph that had been conserved. The procedure itself could take various forms: puncture: "... *I made three punctures on each arm of Adrien de Laroque, my third child, eleven months old at the time. No blood appeared, and the punctures were so lightly made that the child*

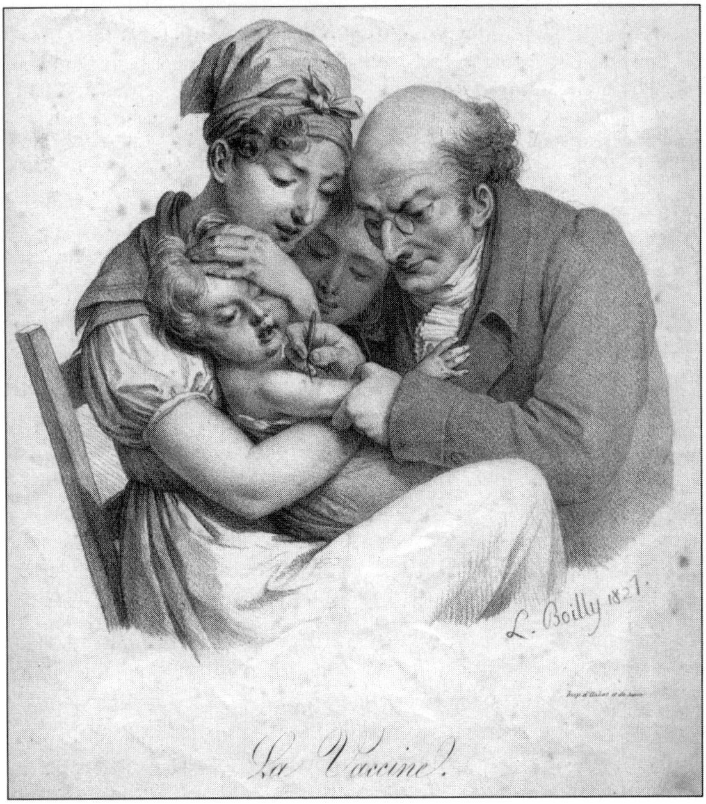

Figure 13. Example of Jennerian vaccine. "*The Vaccine*" by L. Boilly, 1827.

181. Carpanetto, 2004, p. 135.
182. Redman Coxe, 1802, p. 91; Ring, 1803, p. 296.

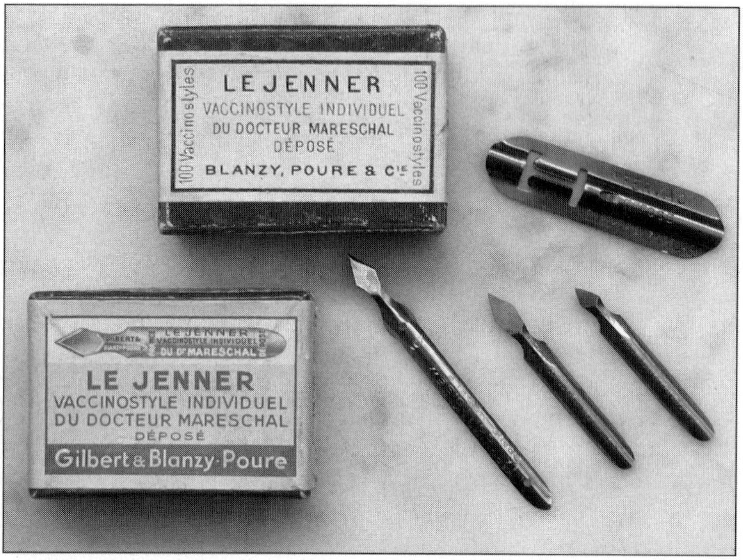

Figure 14. To improve vaccination hygiene, in 1890 Dr. Mareschal had the idea of using writing quills instead of lancets. They were quickly transformed into vaccine-pens that were sold in boxes of one hundred. The manufacturers were the same. This was one of the first single-use medical instruments, or at least easily reusable after sterilisation. Vaccine-pen holders were also available. It is quite possible that this type of vaccine-pens had been invented elsewhere. (Author's document.)

continued to play and to laugh during the entire operation."[183] In a letter dated Prairial 5th, year 13 (May 25, 1805), Husson describes Sacco's method: "*The parishioners are advised at the previous sermon, the bells ring when Sacco arrives, and crowds hasten to the sacristy, located within the church, to be vaccinated...*" Husson is very impressed and recounts (in the third person, in the annual report of the Central Committee): "*A short time later, one* (Husson) *of us had occasion to see doctor Sacco in Italy, and to appreciate the excellence of his method: he uses a hollow needle with a groove on one face, enclosed in a double-arm casing, like a lancet; it is with this instrument that he loads the vaccine first, so that the groove fills up, then vaccinates in less than a quarter of an hour over a hundred children, although he practices at least four punctures on each of them... This is the same method he* (Husson) *has used for the past six months to carry out vaccinations at the vaccine hospice.*" With his grooved needle, Sacco could give fifteen children four inoculations each in less than two minutes, before refilling his needle... Husson enthuses: "*He vaccinates like women knit.*"[184]

A Jennerian vaccination was not very painful. The procedure itself was followed by three distinct stages. The first was a stage of inertia lasting three or four days; the vaccinated area showed no reaction. This was followed by a period of inflammation, until the twelfth day. The rising of a pustule at the point of vaccination, its development and maturation, are described carefully, because their observation makes it possible to distinguish the true vaccine, also called "genuine", which confers protection, from the false (spurious) vaccine, which does not. General signs can appear during this

183. de Laroque, 1805, p. XXV.
184. Husson, 1806, p. 79; BANM, Vaccine 2, file 2 (A), no. 6.

period. They were often taken to indicate successful vaccination. The dessication period follows, with the forming of a scab which dries and falls off, usually leaving a deep and permanent scar[185].

A major element of the vaccination process was examination of the point of inoculation by the vaccinator, about one week after the operation: either the patient had a vaccinal pustule and the vaccine had taken, or there was almost no trace left of the vaccination, particularly no pustule, which meant that the vaccination had failed for some reason, or that the subject was still immunised by an old vaccination or a previous attack of smallpox. The vaccinator had to interpret the result and deliver the precious vaccination certificate accordingly, either after a successful vaccination (a vaccinal pustule at the site of inoculation), or after three negative vaccination trials (no vaccinal pustule following vaccination).

Great numbers of counter-experiments (variolation tests) were performed. The most important were reported not only locally, but throughout the country and even on other continents. This was the case for an experiment conducted by the Paris central vaccine Committee, published in *Le Journal du Commerce* on November 24, 1801, and translated into English in Redman Coxe's book published in Philadelphia in 1802: "*It has been satisfactorily proved that during the whole time no febrile affection has been experienced* (by the person submitted to the counter-experiment), *and there was not on any of these individuals the least sign of general disease, or the smallest appearance of eruption.*"[186] In the hope of impressing hostile and indifferent populations, counter-experiments were sometimes practiced in spectacular ways: "*Marthe Agert had a daughter who was monstrously covered with small-pox: one day when I went to see her I found a crowd of people in her house, especially children, some vaccinated and some not; I took a few of each group and rubbed their hands against those of the sick girl, and it followed that those who had been vaccinated did not contract the disease, while the contrary happened to the others.*"[187] A hasty demonstration! "*Mr. Bonetty, health officer at Chibiers (Hautes Alpes department), took off the shirts of two small-pox sufferers and dressed in them two children he had vaccinated himself. Eight days later, when no small-pox symptoms had appeared, he had them take off the infected shirts before the inhabitants of the village, astounded by the success of this experiment.*"[188] The washerwomen of this village must not have been overworked!

Some counter-experiments were altogether scandalous: "*Six little Negros, the first to be vaccinated on Reunion Island, were put on a ship returning from slave trade, and infected with variola: the ship was placed in quarantine. These six children stayed on the ship three months, remaining constantly at the centre of infection; they lived, ate and slept with small-pox sufferers, some of whom died. Small-pox was inoculated twice to these children, in ample doses. They were not contaminated and stayed in perfect health. These six vaccinated children lived for fifteen days in the midst of twenty Negros with confluent small-pox, six of whom died; and with 25 other Negros with scabs, in dessication, who had survived while seven infected individuals died during the crossing of the trade ship. All of them were housed on the tween deck of the ship, in a space measuring 8 by 12 feet* (2.56 by 3.84 meters, that is, about 10 square meters). *This counter-experiment deserves a place among*

185. Husson, 1800, p. 36.
186. Redman Coxe, 1802, p. 62.
187. Latour, 1804, p. 18.
188. Moreau, 1824, p. 11.

the immense number of experiments conducted in Europe."[189] A place, yes, but not a place of honour! This episode of the ship *La Jeune Caroline* is also recounted by Husson, Secretary of the Society for the Extinction of Small-pox[190]. No one seems to have been shocked at the time, not even prefects, archbishops and bishops, to say nothing of Guillotin, Corvisart, Pinel, Huzard... who attended the general meeting of the Society where this very peculiar test was described. Of course, at the time, this kind of ferocity did not shock these French notables (nor, very probably, those of other countries)...

For years, in the beginning, vaccine matter travelled most often by mail, at the speed of horses or of wind in the sails, but arrived at its destination. It was dry when it arrived. To thin it, it was dissolved in water or... in saliva[191]. This lack of asepsis had, sometimes, very serious infectious consequences, but germ theory was not yet known at the time.

Arm-to-arm Jennerian Vaccination, 1815 to 1864... or until the End of the Century!

In France, the fall of the first Empire (1815) and the advent of the Restauration did not change the attitude of French civil and religious authorities toward vaccination. Churches continued to praise its merits, but only after a period of adjustment to the new regime: "*The Central Committee cannot cite, for 1817, any Archbishop or Bishop who published new pastoral letters in favour of the vaccine.*"[192] The Catholic hierarchy was perhaps confusing the vaccine with the Empire's political regime, and preferred to show itself prudent on the subject. But its position evolved rapidly. In time, the vaccine was no longer considered "imperialist", and the Catholic church took up, once again, its efforts for the spread of the vaccine, to the great benefit of the authorities, and of their constituents.

The December 20, 1820 ordinance which created the Royal Academy of Medicine in France, assigned the institution a number of responsibilities, including vaccination. The problems related to the establishment of this Academy, such as its lack of headquarters, prevented it from carrying out this function immediately. The Academy officially received the attributions of the Central Vaccine Committee through an Order issued by the Minister of the Interior on July 17, 1823. The Central Vaccine Committee and the Society remained active until this date.

The Academy named a Commission immediately, to supervise vaccine quality and distribution, and to carry out free vaccination sessions. Bousquet was the first physician to assume the role of vaccinator for the Academy, almost invariably on Tuesdays and Saturdays. "*In addition to children living in the city, I see the children in hospitals who, by this exchange without which society could not survive, conserve and perpetuate the vaccine fluid indefinitely.*"[193] The vaccine maintenance and free vaccination service followed the Academy in its transfers, from Poitiers Street to rue des Saints-Pères, then to Bonaparte Street, where it established its headquarters until it was dissolved.

189. Parfait, 1804, p. 61.
190. Husson, 1805, p. 27.
191. Balhorn, 1801, p. 73; Sacco, 1813, p. 216; Valleix, 1860, t. 1, p. 175.
192. Husson, 1819, p. 35.
193. Bousquet, 1833, p. VJ.

Dr. Crouigneau, Vaccine Director at the Dijon prefecture, describes the beginnings of vaccination in the Côte d'Or department until 1861, in a long report (probably the only document covering this period, in the possession of the BANM*). Vaccination started as early as 1801, but Crouigneau is not aware of any written records until 1805. Another source indicates May 1801 to be the start of vaccinations, and reports that 52 vaccinations were already performed in June 1802[194]. Crouigneau himself speaks of 77 in 1806, and 300 in 1807. On May 1rst 1808, the city of Dijon established "*a vaccine room in the locale known as la Miséricorde... open every day, for the children of the poor of this city, and even of neighbouring villages, between eleven in the morning until noon*". All vaccinations were free, but vaccination certificates were required for admission to schools or hospices[195]. The 1809 imperial decree led to the establishment of a vaccine depository in Dijon, and to the appointment of its vaccine committee, whose first meeting took place in July 1810. This was followed by a letter from the Bishop of Dijon to his priests, and by letters from prefects to mayors and to health officers. On October 4, 1810, the prefect wrote to the mayor of Dijon to ask that prison inmates be vaccinated, and that families whose children were not vaccinated be denied the assistance of Charity Offices. Three other vaccine depositories were created in Beaune, Semur and Chatillon, regional county seats (subprefectures).

There were two vaccination seasons, one in the spring and one in the autumn, with additional sessions organised in case of a perceived risk of an epidemic. County vaccinators warned mayors, as well as urban and rural priests, of their visits; on vaccination days, they were helped by local teachers, who acted as secretaries. The town paid the vaccinator one franc for each person vaccinated. If their budget was insufficient, the department contributed to the vaccinator's remuneration. No figures have been found for the period between 1808 and 1811. Between 1811 and 1818, 23,648 vaccinations were performed free of charge. Between 1820 and 1859, for a population of 368,000 to 393,000 inhabitants and 402,187 births, there were 340,930 vaccinations. According to Crouigneau, children were vaccinated at about the age of 6 months, an age by which ten percent of them would have already died, which indicates that the great majority of children were vaccinated, although the statistics include some adults. The author of the report prepared by the Academy's vaccine Commission adds: "*The care with which vaccine services are performed there* (the Côte d'Or) *certainly contributes to this satisfactory result.*"[196] In this "well-vaccinated" department, over the same period (about fifty years) there were still 6,405 cases of smallpox, 788 disfigured or maimed individuals, and 796 deaths revealed by census[197].

Vaccination and its (Major) Problems

In 1838, the Paris Academy of Sciences formulated a series of questions, for a contest offering the substantial Prize of 10,000 francs (about 30 to 35,000 euros) to be awarded in 1842. The questions can be summarized as follows:

- Is the preventive virtue of the vaccine temporary or permanent?

* BANM: *Bibliothèque de l'Académie nationale de Médecine.*

194. Dumay, 1848, p. 6.

195. Degroise, 1808 (1990).

196. Blot, 1876, p. 18.

197. Crouigneau, 1861.

- Does cow-pox offer more persistent protection than vaccine passed numerous times to humans?

- Assuming that the vaccine becomes weaker with time, should it be renewed and how?

- Is the intensity of local responses to the vaccine correlated with the effectiveness of protection against small-pox?

- Is it necessary to vaccinate the same person several times, and if yes, after how many years?[198]

The Academy of Sciences received thirty-five dissertations, most of them voluminous. Two were written in German, another in Latin, yet another was a large volume *in folio* of 769 pages accompanied by an atlas, a fifth was comprised of three volumes *in-quarto*, etc. The Commission, composed of Mr. Magendie, Mr. Brescht, Mr. Duméril, Mr. Roux and Mr. Serres (author of the report), apparently took five years to read and assess these dissertations. In 1845, the Commission submitted its report and on March 10, 1845 the Academy divided the prize between Mr. Bousquet, Mr. Fiard and Mr. Steinbrenner, giving half to the first and dividing the other half between the other two[199]. Mr. Fiard did not publish his work, probably because of his early demise[200]. Bousquet's report, as well as Steinbrenner's, are both of excellent quality. They reveal clearly the concerns of French vaccinators and the problems they faced, but we can now see that these five questions illustrated only some of the difficulties to overcome! It is very likely that problems were very similar in every country, especially in the Western World.

Are Cowpox, Horsepox, Sheeppox, Vaccinia and Smallpox the Same Disease due to a Single Agent?

The possible relatedness of the smallpox virus, the variolovaccine, cowpox/vaccinia and, to a lesser extent, horsepox and sheeppox has been the subject of many studies which have given rise to numerous hypotheses.

• **Smallpox and cowpox/vaccine; variolovaccine.** According to Baron, Jenner really considered the vaccine a mild form of smallpox, protecting against smallpox based on the accepted principle that a person can only have smallpox once[201]. Most vaccinators after Jenner were of the same opinion, but the principle had to be proven... and this was hard to do given the state of knowledge of that era. In order to resolve the debate as to the unicity or duality of smallpox and cowpox, attempts were made to transmit smallpox to cows so as to obtain cowpox that would become vaccine when retransmitted to humans; this virus was named "variolovaccine". The possibility of infecting a bovine with the smallpox virus was described in a letter from Waterhouse to Jenner, dated April 24, 1801[202].

Apparently, in 1801 Gassner had succeeded in transmitting smallpox to a cow, and from this animal to children[203]. Sacco, on the other hand, tried to inoculate smallpox into cows, horses, dogs, calves, oxen, sheep, pigs, etc. without any convincing results[204].

198. Serres, 1845, p. 624.
199. Serres, 1845, p. 662.
200. Bousquet, 1858, p. 18.
201. Baron, 1838, t. 1, p. 241.
202. Ashworth-Underwood, 1949, p. 823.
203. Seaton, 1868, p. 57.
204. Sacco, 1813.

A sensational article was published in the November 1831 issue of the *Archives générales de médecine*. A certain Sunderland, physician in Bremen, had covered a cow "*in the blanket of a small-pox patient. The animal caught the disease which, when given back to humans, changed, he says, into vaccine. If all this is true, the demonstration has succeeded and the nature of the vaccine virus is known; but I must admit that I still have some doubts*"[205]. The French Academy of Medicine asked the Minister of Commerce (in charge of health, at that time) for means to confirm Sunderland's discovery. The experiment was reproduced by Delafond, Director of the Alfort Veterinary School, with three cows that were covered with blankets and shirts from smallpox patients at the Hôtel-Dieu Hospital. The attempt failed; it was tried again with a dog and a pig, but these animals, not inclined to wear this apparel, quickly threw it off: the pig in two hours, the dog in twenty-four[206]. The experiment ended there. Several similar studies were carried out, in different countries, without success. However, these trials focused attention, once again, on the idea of variolation for cows. Ceeley of Aylesbury was able to induce pustules by inoculating cows with the smallpox virus, not on the udder but on the mucous membrane of the vulva[207]. He is said to have successfully performed at least 60 passages from animal to animal, and over 2,000 vaccinations with the variolovaccine that he obtained. However, Ceely's assistant, Taylor, who had been vaccinated as a child, and who accidently injected himself with the variolovaccine, had a benign case of smallpox, a modified form, but quite real. Worse still, Ceely admitted that he had had great difficulty convincing the families, friends and neighbours of those "vaccinated" that their symptoms were not those of smallpox[208]. In 1860, Martin of Boston vaccinated fifty people with lymph from the vesicles on the teat of a cow which had been inoculated with pustule contents taken from a man who died of smallpox. Almost all those who were inoculated developed smallpox, which is not surprising, and three of them very regrettably died[209]. However, several strains of variolovaccine, obtained by Fischer or by Voigt in Germany, Haccius in Switzerland, Thiele in Russia and King in India by inoculating smallpox virus to calves were widely used, apparently with the desired results[210].

The technical possibilities for determining the unicity or duality of the "viruses" (in the sense this term was used at the time) of smallpox or cowpox were too limited to provide an answer. One of the most rigorously conducted experiments, carried out by Chauveau and the Lyon commission, between 1863 and 1865, concluded that the two viruses were not identical[211].

• ***Grease*, horsepox and cowpox.** The *grease* and horsepox are two infectious diseases of the horse, whose common symptom is painful discharge in the heels. About 1800, Loy, a surgeon in Pickering, York county, was successful, after many attempts, in communicating to four cows an infection from a horse suffering of *the grease*, who was severely ill and had generalised eruption; Loy had always failed previously, when he took lymph from horses with *grease* localised in the heels: "*This fact made me suspect that there are two kinds of Grease, different from one another in their capacity to transmit*

205. Bousquet, 1833, p. 334; Emery, 1832, p. 23.
206. Gérardin, 1835, p. 37.
207. Anonymous, 1902a, vol. VIII, p. 6119.
208. Dupuy, 1894, p. 19.
209. Copeman, 1899, p. 49; Anonymous, 1902a, vol. VIII, p. 6119.
210. Conklin, 1886, p. 318; Copeman, 1899, p. 67; Anonymous, 1902a, vol. VIII, p. 6119.
211. Chauveau, 1865, pp. 417 & 513.

the disease to humans or animals... The most curious fact revealed by these experiments is the attribute possessed by Grease matter, of communicating to humans a disease that will prevent small-pox infection, whether this matter is used directly from the original source, or after having passed through a more complex circuit..."[212]. Other examples, similar in nature, have been published. They shed no particular light on this problem, other than the fact that the difference between constitutional *grease* and local *grease* was identified very early. Many people were vaccinated with virus of equine origin, for example, with Sacco's strain (*see below*), with no particular problem.

• **Cowpox, vaccine and sheeppox.** The resemblance between these diseases of cows and sheep gave rise to attempts at crossed inoculation. In a treatise entitled "*Mémoire sur la vaccination des bêtes à laine*" ("Dissertation on the vaccination of wool-covered ruminants"), in 1804, Voisin, Assistant Chief Surgeon of the civil and military hospice of Versailles, reports: "*1°. That wool-covered animals have the capacity to receive human vaccine, and to transmit it unaltered to the cow. 2°. That cow-pox in cows, induced by vaccine matter from wool-covered animals transmits the vaccine to humans without alteration...*"[213]. Sacco also attempted to transmit sheeppox to humans, a technique called "clavelisation"[214]. "*... The disease was the true small-pox of sheep... I collected at this place* (Capoue, in 1804)*, with the greatest care, matter from the ripest pustules, in small tubes, with the intention of testing it at the earliest occasion... I went to see doctor Legni, physician-surgeon of the army; I informed him of my plan, and my desire to attempt experiments with the sheep matter collected in Capoue. He lent me his help with the greatest sincerity; he found me six children who were all inoculated with this lymph that was still fluid; and I also injected two other young children with true vaccine, so as to compare the effect.*"[215] The children were examined by the same physician, who concluded that this matter (sheeppox) was identical to that of vaccine. In the course of the following months, Legni inoculated sheeppox matter into about three hundred children. Carried away by his enthusiasm, Sacco seemed to think that many, if not all, animal diseases presenting pustules could serve as vaccines for each-other, and particularly that cow-pox inoculated to sheep protects them from sheeppox, and that the sheeppox matter inoculated into humans protects them from smallpox[216]. These experiments could not be repeated. Sacco and Legni's material was probably contaminated with vaccine. But, once again, this illustrates the care free way with which almost anything was inoculated to patients who were unaware of the danger to which they might be exposed.

In conclusion, cowpox and horsepox were used as vaccines in humans with apparently similar results, but the identity or even the degree of relatedness of these "viruses" was unknown. Cowpox or horsepox strains were exchanged between production centres many times, so that the origin of vaccine strains was difficult to determine.

Does Vaccination Confer Permanent Protection? Is Revaccination Necessary?

This essential problem was the subject of endless discussion between 1810 and 1850. Jenner, like his associates, firmly believed that vaccination protected for life, based on

212. Loy, 1801, p. 283.
213. Voisin, 1804, p. 17.
214. Dorland, 1945, p. 338.
215. Sacco, 1813, p. 318.
216. Sacco, 1813, p. 340.

his observations of variolation tests in those who had had smallpox or those who had had previous variolation. However, from the earliest days of vaccination, smallpox cases contracted after vaccination troubled the minds of even those best-disposed toward vaccination, and excited the anti-vaccinists. Two explanations were possible: either the vaccine lost its virtues over time by regular transmission from arm to arm every eight to ten days, or the vaccination had simply been incorrectly performed. Jenner was convinced that incorrect vaccination, which did not allow the virus to "do its work", was the explanation.

Goldson, a Portsmouth physician, brought into question indefinite vaccinal protection as early as 1804. He suggested a three to four-year period of efficacy[217]. On July 15, 1806, Pearson made a declaration regarding the non infinite effectiveness of the vaccine, based on two smallpox cases after vaccination, observed in his institution[218]. Robert Grosvenor's smallpox created a big stir. This young man fell ill on May 6, 1811, after having been vaccinated about ten years earlier by Jenner himself; his arm bore the vaccination scar. He had a very bad case of smallpox, which fortunately ended quite quickly (varioloid?). Only a few weeks after this incident, the son of Sir Henri Martin, who had also been vaccinated a few years earlier, contracted a mild form of smallpox. It was Thomson who, in 1820, invented the word "varioloid" to designate certain classic forms, or more or less aborted forms, of smallpox and of varicella[219]. At the time, certain individuals who had been vaccinated or those individuals who had had smallpox, more or less immunised against smallpox, could have attenuated signs of the disease. Even the most ill only had an altered form of smallpox called varioloid, whose prodromes and symptoms, in the incubation and suppuration stages, were the same as those of smallpox. "*On the seventh or eight day, the eruption ends abruptly and dessication begins. Between the tenth and twelfth day, all symptoms disappear. Based on the comparison of the two eruption stages, if nothing else, varioloid appears to be merely an aborted form of small-pox.*"[220] It is more likely that the varioloid was a case of smallpox whose evolution was arrested by the somewhat delayed onset of a secondary immune reaction. These cases were not always benign, since some of them caused the death of the patient.

In France, belief in indefinite immunity conferred by vaccination persisted. In 1812, the *Institut de France* asked Berthelot, Percy and Hallé to conduct a study on vaccination; Hallé prepared the report. Its conclusions review the seven observations made by the Central Committee, and confront them to 2,671,662 vaccinations performed: 1 failure out of 381,666 vaccinations, which requires no further comment, as the authors of the report rightly assert[221].

After several years had elapsed from the date of the introduction of vaccination, it was observed that cases of smallpox occasionally occurred in the persons who had been vaccinated. It was emphasized that the protective power of vaccination was only temporary, gradually becoming weaker as the individual grew older. Early observations in support of this belief were made in Copenhagen and in London. The number of persons attacked by modified small-pox increased in Copenhagen between 1809 and 1823, and

217. Copland, 1859, p. 1425; Creighton, 1889, p. 317.
218. Steinbrenner, 1846, p. 33.
219. Thomson, 1820, p. 19.
220. Bousquet., 1833, p. 189.
221. Hallé, 1812, p. 47.

in 1824, 412 cases were admitted to hospitals, of whom 257 had been vaccinated and in 1825, 623 cases, of whom 438 had been vaccinated. The mortality among those vaccinated was much lower than among the unvaccinated. By far the greater number of smallpox cases which occurred after vaccination were in persons who had not been vaccinated within a period of 15 years[222]. In 1823, Gregory, a physician at the Hospital for Smallpox and Vaccination in St. Pancras (London) once again raised the question of the number of cases of smallpox occurring in vaccinated individuals. "*Cases of smallpox after vaccination are, without any doubt, more frequent than relapsing cases of smallpox.*"[223] The article is based on the comparison of data collected between 1810 and 1822. However, the author does not bring into question the duration of vaccine immunity, but only faulty vaccination due to the defective vaccine employed in the countryside (in the author's exact words). The concept of revaccination evolved with some difficulty, because it implied an imperfection of vaccination - the perfect example of an iconoclastic idea. Moreover, it could suggest a lack of care at the time of the initial vaccination, which was quite possible, as Dr. Titeca demonstrated at the Belgium Academy of Medicine (1885)[224].

The French vaccine Commission and the Academy were very reluctant to accept this concept. But elsewhere revaccination was already practiced in 1823: in Malta, Geneva and Northern Europe[225]. In 1829, in Wurtemberg, the practice of re-vaccinating the troops of that kingdom had already started[226]. There are numerous reports on the results of revaccinations in armies, and in populations, giving the rates of revaccination that took place in the populations involved.

Often, at least a third of those who were revaccinated "took" the vaccine: that is, developed a vaccine pustule, which did not happen with immunized subjects. This provided exact information on the immunity of a person or of a group of people. In 1845, cases of smallpox were so numerous at Hôtel-Dieu that Magendie, member of the vaccine Commission of the Academy of Sciences, had all his patients revaccinated, and none of them contracted smallpox[227]. Magendie's prestige, or the results obtained with revaccination in neighbouring countries, led to a change of opinion. Around 1850, revaccination became strongly recommended in France. It was the army that took the initiative of recommending it in 1858, but its application was difficult to accomplish. Revaccination of the whole population was made compulsory in Denmark in 1871 and in Rumania in 1874; in Holland it was made mandatory for all school children in 1872[228].

The Search for Cowpox or Horsepox to Regenerate Vaccine Strains

The accumulation of smallpox cases after vaccination, varioloid or not, led the medical profession to ask themselves if the vaccine itself did not degenerate with time. New sources of vaccine, that is, of cowpox had to be found. In France, this was a constant concern of the Central Vaccine Committee, and later of the Academy of Medicine.

222. Abbott, 1889, vol. VII, p. 509.
223. Gregory, 1823-4, p. 806.
224. Abbott, 1889, vol. VII, p. 509.
225. Bousquet, 1857, p. 17.
226. General Board of Health, 1857, p. XXXIV.
227. Camus, 1921, p. 239; Serres, 1845, p. 624.
228. Anonymous, 1902a, vol. VIII, p. 6119.

But this opinion was not shared by everyone. Thus, the 1854 report of the British National Vaccine Board states: "*We feel it our duty, in order to dispel any doubts which may still affect the public mind, to repeat what we have so frequently stated with unabated confidence, that the vaccine lymph does not lose any of its prophylactic power by a continued transit through successive subjects, and that is a fallacy to predicate the necessity of resorting to the original source of the cow for a renewed supply.*"[229]

• **The Search for Cowpox.** Cowpox* was a well-known disease in Great Britain, in the Holstein region (northern area of present-day Germany) and in Lombardy, but how frequently did it occur? In France, the disease was unknown at the end of the 18th century. Valentin wrote that when he returned from America at the start of 1798, he had occasion to speak with highly competent veterinarian Jean-Baptiste Huzard about the presence of cowpox in cows, and horsepox in horses, and the transmission of that disease to cows. Huzard assured him that he had neither seen nor heard talk of any such disease[230].

The first confirmed case of cowpox on French territory occurred in Passy. "*On March 21, 1836, a dame Fleury, dairy woman in Passy, Longchamp Street, n° 21, arrived to consult doctor Perdrau at his medical residence in Chaillot; she had 3 pustules on her right hand...*". She was sent to Bousquet, official vaccinator of the French Academy of Medicine, who inoculated lymph from one of dame Fleury's pustules to nine children, by performing three injections of the old vaccine in one arm, and three in the other arm using the new "Passy vaccine"[231], thus mixing the two strains...

Thirty years later, on May 1, 1866, Depaul, Bousquet's successor, had reason to be greatly delighted. He had "*had the good fortune of discovering a source of cowpox*", and he hastened to tell his colleagues at the Academy about it. "*I hope that no one will be able to say any more that our cowpox is only human vaccine transmitted to the heifer.*"[232] This case of cowpox detected in Beaugency is interesting because this strain of "matter" was distributed to many centres, including that of H.G. Martin in the United States.

While cowpox was frequent in Europe (at least in Great Britain, France, Germany, Holland, Italy, Switzerland)[233], it was rare elsewhere, but detected in Bengal, Mexico, South America, New England, Pennsylvania, California...)[234], or existing but not identified.

In the United States, cowpox (often called Kine-pox as Waterhouse proposed) was observed for the first time in 1844, in Torringford (Conn.) by Dr. John Yale, then by Dr. Currier in Lexington (Mass.) in 1850, then by Drs. E. Cutter, H. Darlington, McMillan and Trask, Jonathan Brown, and finally by H.A. Martin in Cohasset[235]. Most of these observations led to the inoculation of children, as was the practice at the time. According to Conklin, "*previous to the discovery of the Cohasset stock in 1881, no perfectly authenticated case of natural cow-pox had ever occurred in America*"[236].

* Not to be confused with the pseudo-cowpox, a parapoxvirus having no cross-immunity with smallpox.

229. General Board of Health, 1857, p. XXXVI.

230. Valentin, 1802, p. 8.

231. Emery, 1837, p. 17.

232. Depaul, 1866, p. 590.

233. Abbott, 1889, vol. VII, p. 509.

234. Abbott, 1889, vol. VII, p. 509.

235. Abbott, 1889, tome VII, p. 509.

236. Conklin, 1886, p. 318.

One point remains doubtful: that of the origin of these cases of cowpox, part or all of which could have been caused by contamination spread by freshly vaccinated persons... in the United States and elsewhere.

Why were cowpox cases so rare, particularly at the start of the nineteenth century? Probably because they were not reported: "*In all likelihood, cowpox is often present on the farms of several other countries, but farmers do not speak of it for fear of finding it more difficult to sell their milk and butter.*"[237]

Cowpox is found mainly in Western Eurasia. Despite its name, cowpox virus circulates mainly in wild rodents such as bank voles (*Clethrionomys glareolus*), field voles (*Microtus agrestis*) and woodmice (*Apodemus sylvaticus*). Domestic cats are presently the species in which clinical disease is most often diagnosed. Human infection, although uncommon, can often be traced to contact with an infected cat, or sometimes direct contact with rodents. Cats probably become infected by direct contact with infected wild rodents, perhaps when hunting.

• **The Search for Grease/Horsepox as a Vaccine Source.** At the start of 1802, a coachman who looked after three horses with horsepox (*giavardo*), saw a vesicular eruption appear on his hands, accompanied by high fever and diarrhea. He was sent to see Sacco and "matter" taken from him was used to inoculate three small children and a cow. Two children developed a clearly identifiable pustule. Sacco described *giavardo* "*which attacks the pastern and sometimes the heel bulb of horses; it causes an inflammatory tumor that suppurates, and contains a sort of virus which, when inoculated to humans or to cows, produces a local pustule, circumscribed and regular... This pustule induces in humans the beneficial alteration that protects against small-pox...*"[238]. These phenomena were described to Jenner by Sacco in a letter written in French, whose content was reproduced by Copeman[239].

Having read Mr. Loy's book, which speaks of a generalised eruption, Sacco specified that he had not seen anything like this. He sent *giavardo* matter to Dr. de Carro in Vienna, and to Dr. Friese, Director of vaccinations in Silesia. De Carro was very happy with this "*giardonic matter*" (*sic*), as he testifies in a letter to Dr. Marcet: "*For almost 8 months I have been vaccinating in Vienna solely with the giardonic matter that Dr. Sacco sent me, and that he took directly from a horse's heel...*"[240].

In the period between 1860 and 1870, France experienced several epizootics of horsepox, and great numbers of children were "vaccinated" with this matter.

Transport and Conservation of the Vaccine

Because of its simplicity, *in vivo* transport, from person to person, was widely used. In the report dated Germinal 9th, year 9 (March 30, 1801) of the French vaccine Committee, we can read: "*It is by making vaccinated children travel that I spread this beneficial germ* (the vaccine) *through the villages...*"[241]. Transporting the vaccine to Central America and the Far East was accomplished exclusively with the help of orphans vaccinated one after the other. Later, animals were also used. The *Nouveau Monde*, a beautiful ocean liner belonging to the Compagnie transatlantique (Transatlantic

237. Balhorn, 1801, p. 35.
238. Sacco, 1813, p. 286.
239. Copeman, 1899, p. 33.
240. De Carro *in* Sigerist, 1804 (1950), p. 57.
241. Latour, 1804, p. 12.

Company) from Saint-Nazaire (France) was about to sail to Mexico, where a smallpox epidemic was at its peak. What could be done? Everyone had to be revaccinated. Lanoix (*see below*) could not provide so much vaccine in such a short time. He decided to inoculate a heifer and send it to Saint-Nazaire. Everyone was vaccinated on the ship and there were no fatalities[242].

Jenner made his first shipment of vaccine from Berkeley to London by using the shaft of a bird feather, sealed with wax[243]. Very quickly, Jenner began to use glass slides: "*Jenner would take a plate of polished crystal with a small indentation in its centre... he filled it so that the fluid created a slight swell; he then moistened another crystal plate with vaccinal fluid by placing it over an open vesicle, and applied the second plate over the first.*"[244] All methods tended to seal the lymph away from air, between two plates of glass or ivory, or inside a tube, away from light and, if possible, from heat.

Animal Vaccine: Solution to Vaccinal Syphilis?

Could Jennerian vaccine (also called human) be dangerous for the person receiving it? Jenner always considered the vaccine safe. Starting with its very first report, the 1803 French Central Committee denied any danger associated with the vaccine itself, or with any cow disease. The Central Vaccine Committee always maintained this position. In a letter dated July 7, 1809, Husson wrote, in the name of the Central Committee, to Mr. Moutillard, physician in Commercy: "*As to the successive weakening of the vaccine virus, and the susceptibility you attribute to it of becoming attached to other viruses or morbid humors that can pre-exist in the system of the vaccinated person, the Committee does not entirely agree with this opinion... Nor does it share the concept of foreign viruses that could complicate the vaccine, mix with its matter and produce, in the inoculated subject, diseases in accordance with his nature...*"[245]. This official position remained unshakable for a long time. The "*Instructions sur la vaccination*" (Instructions on Vaccination), sent to all vaccinators in 1830, expressed the same viewpoint[246].

This opinion was commonly accepted for a long time in most countries, although problems developed after some time: more or less serious cases of erysipelas, of pemphigoid bullae[247], epidemics of jaundice were reported, such as the one in Bremen, Germany, between 1883 and 1884, where the personnel of the "Weser" firm was vaccinated *en masse* through fear of the smallpox. Out of 1,349 vaccinated people, 191 became jaundiced, which was probably due, *a priori*, to a hepatitis virus[248]. Nevertheless, the Jennerian or human vaccine became the object of growing suspicion, essentially regarding syphilis contamination. According to Jeanselme, the first cases of syphilis transmission by vaccine were allegedly detected in 1814[249]. Examples of syphilis transmitted by vaccination accumulated... Some of them gave rise to much commentary. On June 16, 1852, Dr. Hübener, a homeopath, health official in Hollfeld (Bavaria), vaccinated eight children from Freimfeld. He used lymph taken from the arm of the child of Marguerite Keller, an unmarried, 29-year old woman. The vaccinated children

242. Marchal, 1869, p. 869.
243. Baron, 1838, t. 1, p. 151.
244. Valleix, 1860, t. 1, p. 171.
245. BANM, Ms 1611-739, n° 754.
246. Camus, 1921, p. 239.
247. Anonymous, 1902a, vol. VIII, p. 6119.
248. Stienon, 1885, p. 123.
249. Jeanselme, 1931, p. 523.

showed signs of syphilis. Their parents brought charges against Dr. Hübener. The Bamberg tribunal condemned him to two years imprisonment in a fortress. At his appeal, two experts presented opposing testimony, and the final verdict was 6 weeks in prison for having taken the vaccine from a sickly, stunted child, contrary to the instructions received by county physicians[250]. The medical profession felt under attack.

In 1864, Depaul, who had been named director of the vaccination Services of the Academy of Medicine (Paris), wanted to take precautions to avoid possible vaccine-related accidents, particularly vaccinal syphilis. Many physicians still doubt the reality of this occurrence. Over 2,000 vaccinations were performed at the Children's Hospital by Mr. Taupin with "*vaccine taken from children with all sorts of affections including syphilis, and he never observed a case of syphilis among the vaccinated children...*" Blot described the collection of vaccine at the Academy of Medicine: "*How do you think that a great portion of the vaccine used at the Academy is collected? What is the source from which we take it? Who makes this essential harvest? I will tell you. Until recently, things were done in the following way. We vaccinated here two, three, four or five children sent by the supervisor of services of the Maternity Clinic, and they returned to the Clinic afterwards. After eight days we went to the hospital to collect the vaccinal fluid each of these children might have produced. But who do you think, gentlemen, was sent to make this harvest, which was to serve to inoculate other children, at the Academy, in Paris or in the provinces? The Director of vaccinations, perhaps? Never. If not him, the assistant director? No again. In that case, you say, one of the members of the permanent vaccine Committee? Not at all. Well then, a young doctor who has distinguished himself, or at least an intern? Wrong again. It was... a simple office clerk of the Academy, an old and sickly man having no medical knowledge whatever, and agitated by senile tremors. I need not ask you to guess whether this poor man knew how to choose subjects, examine them or obtain information from the mothers. Even if he had been capable of this, it was the least of his worries. In any case, this is how our faithful employee arrived each week, all atremble, to perform his vaccinal harvest. Holding an ordinary lancet in his shaking hand, he plunged it parallel to the skin under the protrusion of each pustule; then, turning over the instrument abruptly, he removed, in one motion, the top portion of each vesicle. From the wound inflicted in this way, a more or less impure vaccine mixed with blood flowed out; tubes and glass plates were loaded with this fluid and brought back to the Academy, where, believe me, Mr. Robin's microscope was altogether useless for identifying the bloody fluid. I hope, gentlemen, that these details definitively edify you as to the value of the great care taken at the Academy, and that others are wrong not to take elsewhere.*"[251]

This text is reproduced *in extenso*, in a note, in Seaton's book[252] which intends to indicate to Anglophone readers the limits of the confidence that can be placed in French medicine. This procedure of vaccine collection is a little worrying, but there was no protest from the audience that day, nor during the meetings that followed... as Seaton points out. The text was published in the *Bulletin de l'Académie*... The Director to whom the text alludes was Bousquet, appointed head of the vaccine Service in 1823, and later Director of the same Service (between 1850 and 1864). He did address this question eventually in the course of what became an epic battle, but he did not contest Blot's description... which must have been exact! Blot went on to say that it

250. Tardieu, 1864, p. 366; Sée, 1855, p. 176.
251. Blot *in* Depaul, 1865, p. 285.
252. Seaton, 1868, p. 206.

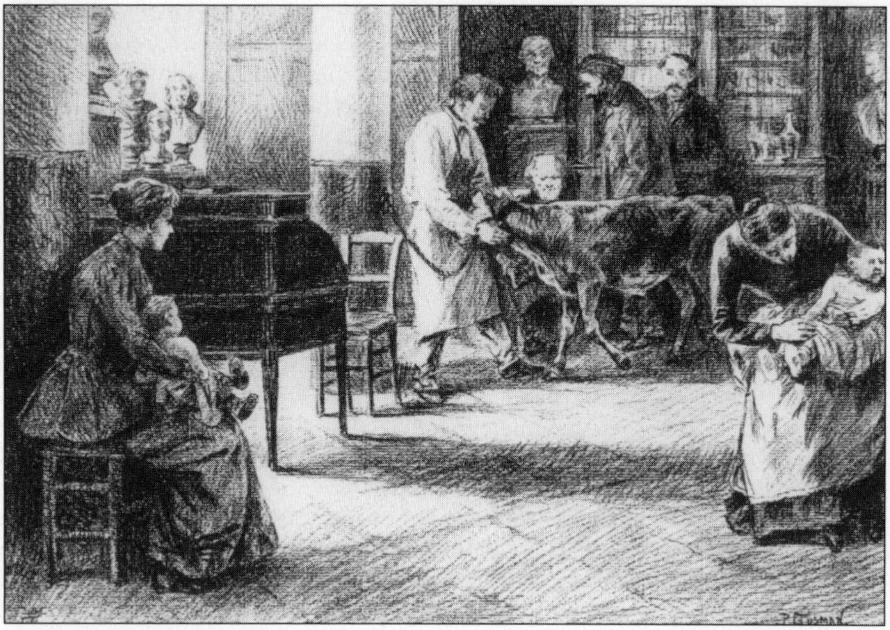

Figure 15. "*The public vaccination Service of the Académie de Médecine*." (Strauss, 1892)[253]. The Academy of Medicine was located on *rue des Saints-Pères*, in Paris, from 1850 until 1902. The premises were inadequate in size, particularly since the Academy was responsible for conserving the vaccine: maintaining the strain, finding new strains if needed, vaccinating children or adults who came there, sending tubes of vaccine to those entitled to receive them... A great deal of work and responsibility, little help from the State... The nave of the disused *Hôpital de la Charité* chapel was divided: near the front porch, a stable for the heifers off to the side, and the vaccination room in a section of the nave. The rest of the space was used as a conference room. (Author's document.)

was impossible to conduct a complete exam of the mother, to say nothing of the father... This is how things were: insufficient government funds, inadequate premises, no certainty concerning the reality of vaccinal syphilis... Who would be the first to attribute blame?

The meetings of the Academy of Medicine resonated with passionate discourse. On one side, the defenders of the vaccine who do not believe, at first, that it could have harmful effects, then admit it but do not tolerate that it should be said, invoking the disaster that would ensue from loss of confidence in the vaccine. On the other side, the partisans of the truth and, very quickly, of producing vaccine by using heifers, even if this meant a greater financial contribution by the State. The Academy of Medicine itself was caught in the controversy surrounding vaccinal syphilis... On August 19, 1865, a 27-year old man came to the Academy to be vaccinated. He was inoculated on both arms with vaccine taken from a 6-month old child, "pale and frail looking". A few weeks later, Dr. Millard diagnosed the young man with vaccinal syphilis. In Paris, it was the talk of the town... he was vaccinated at the Academy of Medicine! The Institution was morally responsible[254]. Depaul only learned of the contamination

253. Strauss, 1892, p. 147.

254. Depaul, called away by his professional obligations, had attributed the task of inoculations to an Academy employee who had been performing this function occasionally for many years.

in November. He immediately tried to find the other people vaccinated on the same day at the Academy, who might have been infected: nine children, thirty-three employees of a military Department, and the two vaccinifer children. Two children had already died, apparently from syphilis, and the other seven were infected with the disease. Three military personnel members were found at the Val-de-Grâce Hospital, their admission papers reading: "*Syphilitic intoxication determined by a vaccination performed at the Academy*".

One of the vaccinifers was still in good health, but the other died the next day... and his mother greeted Lanoix and Depaul with the words: "*Did he give the infection to others?*"[255] Of course, the Academy was very concerned, but the human vaccine was not forbidden because there were still no funds to improve the Vaccine Service.

Vaccinal syphilis was due to the transmission of syphilis Treponema along with the vaccine virus. How could the vaccine become contaminated? The easiest, most obvious culprit to designate was the vaccinifer. When a physician in private practice had to select a vaccinifer, knowing the family made it easier to make the right choice. But recourse to tubes of vaccine by the Academy or by provincial Centres must have been frequent, because arm-to-arm vaccination was very constraining for private practitioners. And collection methods in public Centres were... as good as their means allowed: "*As for the age and choice of vaccinifer subjects also specified in the pamphlet, they are based on well-known rules applied everywhere except perhaps at the Academy... But here there is an imperative that outweighs all others, that of never letting the source of vaccinal fluid run dry; and because the Academy often only disposes of hospice children or newborns, it cannot always show itself as scrupulous as private vaccinators... but I will continue to doubt the possibility of taking the syphilitic virus from a vaccinal vesicle.*"[256] Most cases of vaccinal syphilis described in the literature resulted from the inoculation of lymph taken from found children or from unmarried mothers, and this was the most common source of vaccinal lymph... The work of the Vaccine Service of the Academy was far from negligible. In 1866, as in many other years this institution sent to Paris, to the provinces or to the colonies 28,397 plates, tubes or lancets loaded with vaccine. Most of them, about 80%, contained vaccine collected from human beings[257]. The rest was vaccine produced in heifers; this was most often used locally. Vaccinations were performed in poor conditions.

There were also local centres of vaccine production and distribution which, around 1865, were also operating in difficult conditions. Vaccinators were required to work in deplorable conditions in city and town halls: "*This is in fact how vaccinations were generally carried out: children vaccinated on the corresponding day of the previous week, and those to be vaccinated, are assembled together in an often overcrowded room, especially in May and June, the months when mothers preferred to bring their children. The vaccinator has to assess quickly the results of his vaccinations of the preceding week, and at the same time choose vaccinifers for the inoculations he is going to practice. All this is done in public, before the impatient crowd of mothers and women accompanying children, in the midst of a deafening hubbub of screams and chatter. In these conditions, how could the doctor make a complete enough exam of the young subjects from whom he was going to harvest vaccine? In addition, the examinations should ideally extend to the mothers as*

255. Depaul, 1867, p. 1024; Fournier, 1889, p. 7.
256. Gilbert *in* Bousquet, 1865, p. 499.
257. Depaul, 1868, p. 70.

well. Once the choices are made for better or worse, and the vaccinations are being performed, some women raise objections: 'I don't mind you taking vaccine from my child, but only for two or three people, not for a large number. Why don't you take some from this woman's child, like from mine?' And a hundred more things of this kind. On the other hand, the decision to refuse some children as vaccinifers, pronounced in public, places, and will continue to place, suspicion in the minds of those present regarding the parents of the children not chosen, and creating such suspicion, whether it be grounded or not, is undesirable."[258]

Pellarin suggested that the children and their mothers be examined in a separate room if possible, and that the mothers of vaccinifers receive double remuneration. As to a thorough exam of mothers or fathers of the vaccinifers, that possibility would have seemed completely illusory. There are accounts of gynaecological exams, presented at enquiries following accidents, but in current practice it would have been impossible to perform them! Good intentions abounded, but reality prevailed.

This description of the difficulties in the functioning of the official French Vaccination Service is well-written and probably close to the real situation. It is more than likely that the same situation existed in many countries. Not surprisingly, the decrease of smallpox prevalence was very slow in the Western World. Production of vaccine in heifers was to allow considerable progress.

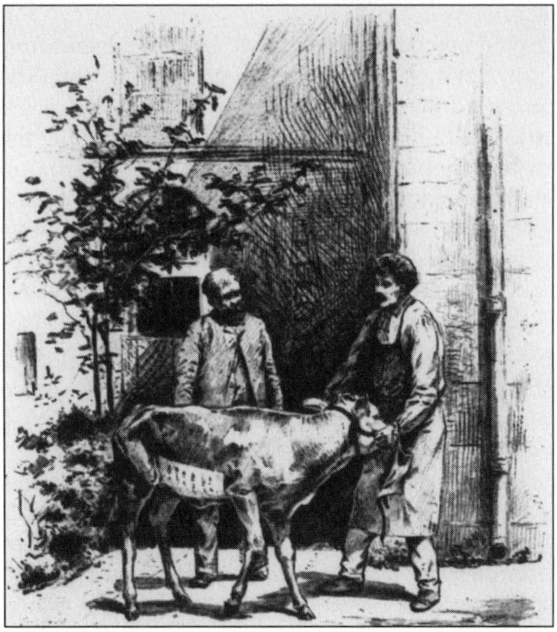

Figure 16. "*One of the heifers inoculated for vaccination.*" (Strauss, 1892)[259]. (Author's document.)

In September 1864, at the Lyon Medical Conference, Dr. Viennois presented studies on vaccinal syphilis. Dr. Palasciano, hospital surgeon in Naples, informed those present that animal vaccine was commonly used in Naples since the beginning of the century.

258. Pellarin, 1865, p. 505.
259. Strauss, 1892, p. 388.

Chambon, still a medical student at the time, was impressed with the Napolitan technique and succeeded in convincing one of his friends, Lanoix, to try it. On November 24, 1864, Lanoix left for Naples to learn Negri's technique. He came back with an inoculated heifer. Chambon was to house the heifer in Saint-Mandé, a Parisian suburb, where he created a private Institute of Animal Vaccine, one of the first private pharmaceutical establishments, at least in biotechnology!

Lanoix and Chambon were finally achieving out the dream, or nightmare, of certain vaccinators. "*Finally, there are vaccinators who, more scrupulous still, in order to remove any chance of wrong doing, wish to see an institution created where the cow-pox would be preserved continually, like vaccine is preserved in certain centres. This desire is certainly very philanthropic, but extremely difficult to put into practice. How would it be possible to have enough cows to allow for uninterrupted inoculations?... And dare I speak of the cost of such an enterprise? A spacious locale is needed to house the cows, men are needed to look after them, installations to contain them, etc. Finally, the costs are such that only the government could assume them. If a capitalist enterprise was involved, it would work for its own benefit, and the benefit for mankind would be forgotten.*"[260] Budding capitalism was already seen with disapproval by part of the medical profession! Dr. Vicherat from Nemours said of animal vaccine: "*If commerce, always shameful in the public health domain, has taken hold of this novelty, we have only ourselves and our era to blame.*"[261] And yet, it was private industry that played a major role in the development and production of vaccines in the world...

Quite rapidly, animal vaccine was adopted everywhere. But, at least in the beginning, it was accused, probably rightly, of not "taking" in humans. A crisis arose with the advent of the major smallpox epidemic that swept all of Europe in 1870 and 1871. Within the medical profession, at the 1870 Paris Medical Conference, while the smallpox epidemic was raging, great opposition was expressed to animal vaccine, in the presence of Lanoix himself... It was claimed that inoculation with animal vaccine was very inferior to human vaccine inoculation. Lanoix was overwhelmed with criticism: "*... countless cases of smallpox were observed in individuals vaccinated unsuccessfully by Mr. Lanoix's heifers, who believed they were protected from the plague... It is clear that we must return to the human vaccine...*"[262]. Lanoix and Chambon were used as scapegoats and attacked by qualified physicians who were renowned and influential, like Just-Lucas Championnières and Eugène Bouchut.

A few years later, when the problems associated with animal vaccine had been solved, the Academy of Medicine was still begging for a stable to house the heifers that produced the animal vaccine... In 1902, when some progress had been made, Academy president, Riche, declared: "*Our premises will be very suitable; the public will be seen in spacious rooms and in good conditions of hygiene; the stables will house twelve heifers, sixteen if need be.*"[263] He was describing the Academy's future premises on Bonaparte Street. At the military Val-de-Grâce Hospital, a vaccine centre was created in 1883; others opened in Lyon, Montpellier, Bordeaux...

However, opinions were still divided concerning the possibility of inoculating syphilis by vaccinating against smallpox, using the arm-to-arm method. The two reports of the

260. Bousquet, 1833, p. 252.
261. Vicherat *in* Blot, 1875, p. 165.
262. Gallard *in* Caffe, 1872, p. 92.
263. Riche, 1906, p. 31.

British Royal Commission appointed to inquire into the subject of vaccination are not clear on this point and advance many arguments against the existence of vaccinal syphilis, particularly the occurrence of congenital syphilis[264].

Elsewhere in Europe, animal vaccine was adopted by practitioners between 1865 and 1885. A vaccine Institute was created by Warlomont in Belgium, in 1865; its mission was to produce animal vaccine and distribute it free of charge. The operation of the Institute was taken over by the Government in 1868, and the name was changed to State Vaccine Institute, and later to Central Vaccine Office[265]. In 1882, Charles Haccius founded a Swiss Vaccine Institute in Lancy, near Geneva. He received government grants and sent his products to most Swiss cantons free of charge. His facilities were modern; 3 or 4-month old calves were bought from neighbouring farmers, kept under observation for four or five days, and then used to produce vaccine. The fact that they

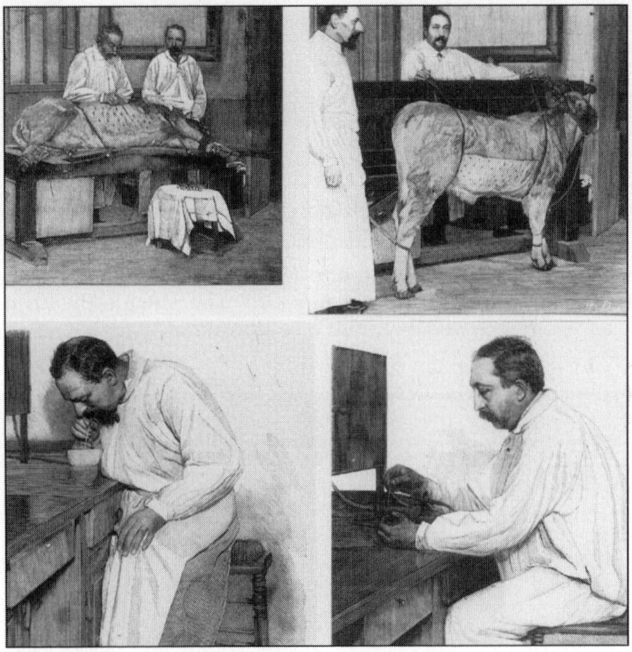

Figure 17. Animal vaccine. At the 1864 Lyon medical Conference, Dr. Palasciano revealed that in Naples vaccine production was accomplished with heifers, and no longer by Jenner's arm-to-arm method. After much discussion, this procedure was adopted everywhere, because it avoided contaminating subjects with the infectious germs of vaccinifers, and it preserved the original properties of the vaccine strain. The Academy of Medicine produced 40,000 tubes of vaccine in 1892, a considerable achievement. Top right: heifer inoculated a few days earlier and attached to a tilting table (*Le Monde illustré*, December 17, 1892); top left: "*Vaccine harvest*"; bottom left: "*Filling of vaccine tubes… Introduction by suction of the product.*" This product was composed of derm particles from the heifer, seeded with lymph and triturated with glycerin. Pipetting by mouth, even with a cotton wad in the opening of the pipette, was a dangerous practice which disappeared when techniques improved; bottom right: use of a blowpipe for closure of tubes. (*La Petite Revue*, January 14, 1893.)

264. Royal Commission, 1889, p. 130; Royal Commission, 1890, p. 310.
265. Warlomont, 1883, p. 186.

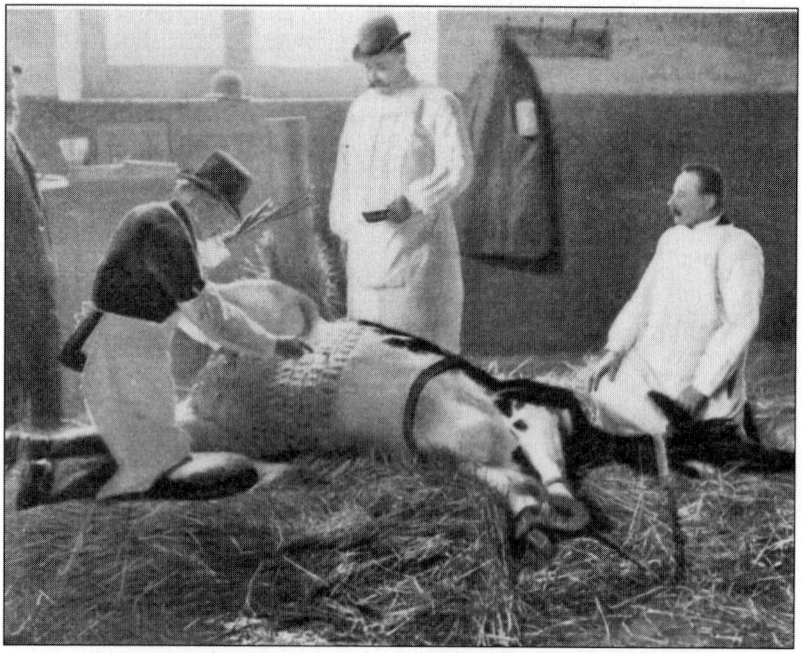

Figure 18. "*At the Cureghem vaccine Institute (Belgium). Mr. Degive, Director of the State Veterinary Medicine School, makes a vaccine harvest.*" The tilting table was not yet in use. *Le National illustré*, 12th year, n° 9, March 1, 1903; or *Illustration européenne*, 33rd year, n° 7, February 15, 1903.

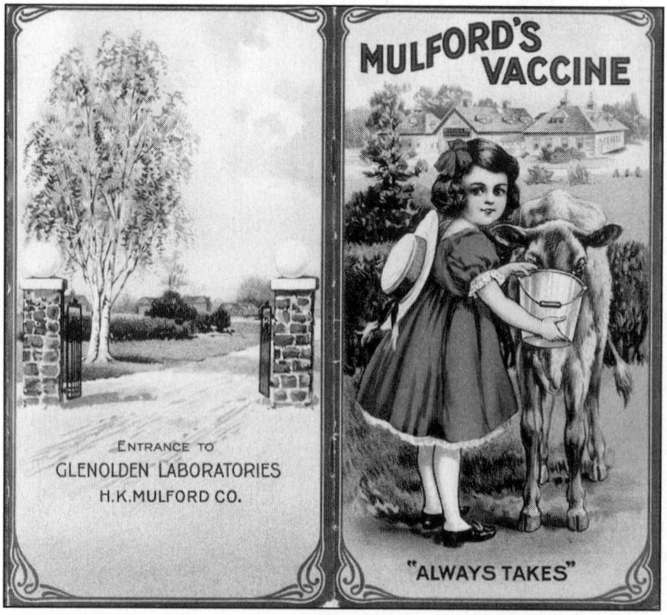

Figure 19. A polished presentation by an American vaccine firm. This is a prospectus for Mulford's Vaccine from the Glenolden Laboratories of the H.K. Mulford Company, whose motto was "*Always Takes*", which relates to the quality of the animal vaccine. (Author's document.)

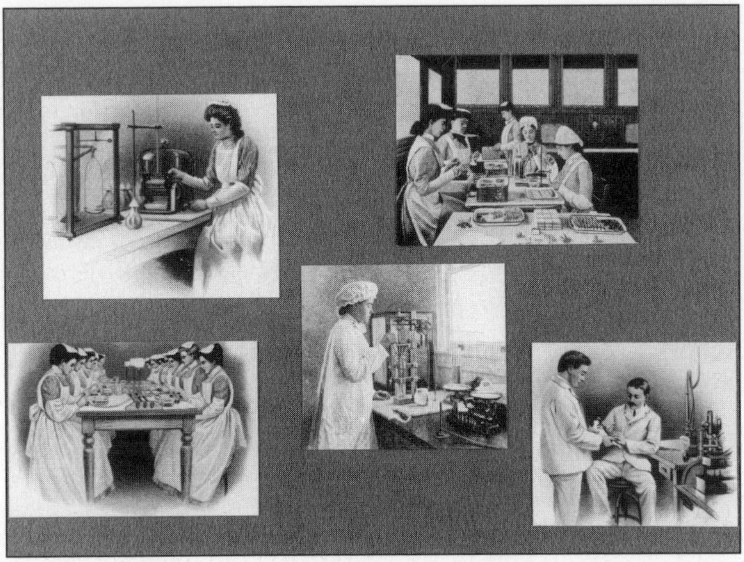

Figure 20. Mulford's Vaccine. The work in the laboratories. Top left: "*Trituration of the virus ensures uniform potency*". Top right: "*Filling tubes with lymph*". Centre: "*Glycerinisation of virus*". Bottom left: "*Filling tubes with glycerinised lymph*". Bottom right: "*Testing vaccine on guinea pig to ensure purity and potency*". (Author's document.)

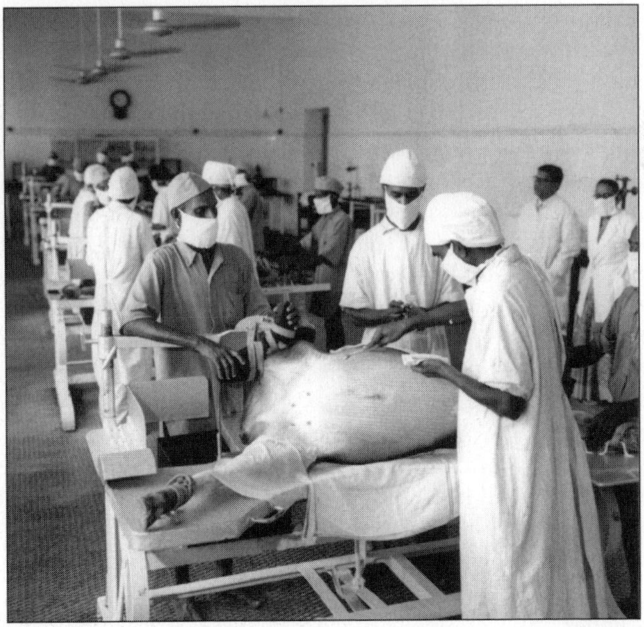

Figure 21. At the end of 1962, India launched a major vaccination campaign against smallpox. Massive quantities of lyophilised vaccine were needed for use in tropical conditions. At the Royal Institute of Preventive Medicine in Madras, with the help of the WHO and of UNICEF, vaccine was prepared, as everywhere else at the time, using the old method of virus culture on heifer skin. Of course, although the technique was a century old, hygiene conditions for harvesting had been much improved. (Photograph P.N. Sharma, reproduced courtesy of the WHO.)

were resold to butchers made it possible for them to be inspected once they had been slain, and to obtain a certificate from a veterinarian attesting that they had been in good health. The vaccine harvest was processed and placed in coloured glass tubes. The Swiss installation was remarkably clean. But Mr. Haccius complained of being unable to obtain from official vaccinators permanent written records of the vaccinations performed using his vaccine[266]. England continued to resist this method of production until the turn of the century.

The animal vaccine finally won the battle. Presenting no risk of transmitting syphilis, and allowing massive production, it was the only one to survive. Jennerian vaccine disappeared completely.

How to Encourage the Population to Be Vaccinated?

"*One cannot imagine the effect that example and a little money can produce on the poor*." Buchan, 1799[267].

Having a vaccine supply was obviously important, but vaccination candidates were also necessary. In the 18th century, smallpox concerned all segments of society, from the richest to the poorest. However, inoculation was essentially practiced among the rich, who were concerned with avoiding future risks. This was not the case among the poor, who were preoccupied with daily survival. In the 19th century, thanks to improved conditions of hygiene and more efficient isolation of smallpox sufferers, a new phenomenon emerged: epidemics started among the poor and then spread to the rest of the population. This caused "the rich" to become aware of their obligation to protect "the poor", at least to some extent, for the sake of protecting themselves. However, well-meaning men took an interest, very early, in organising vaccination for all.

The educated classes learned about vaccination by reading newspapers, and the information travelled by word of mouth or in correspondence. In addition, fear of contagion during epidemics influenced behaviour. In a short time, free vaccination for the poor was organised, and social assistance was denied them if they refused. Yet it is obvious that vaccination did not extend to the entire European population. Making the trip was difficult and, if vaccinators did not meet candidates where they lived, poor people could not afford to travel, especially with babies and small children. It was not until the end of the 19th century that a more or less universal vaccination system covering the entire territory became a reality.

Very different positions on the question were adopted in different countries, depending on their views on individual freedom or, inversely, on individual responsibility to society. Countries used to legal decisions passed vaccination laws very quickly: Bavaria made vaccination of all children compulsory in 1807, Denmark in 1810, Sweden in 1814, Wurtemberg and Hesse in 1818, Rumania in 1874, Hungary in 1876, Serbia in 1881[268].

In Prussia, a law passed in 1835 required vaccination, and families in which unvaccinated children under one were infected with smallpox were punished. In 1864, a law applying to all States of the German Empire came into effect: all children not yet

266. Copeman, 1899, p. 232.
267. Buchan, 1799, p. 179.
268. Anonymous, 1902, vol. VIII, p. 6119.

inoculated had to be vaccinated before the age of two; breaking of this law was punishable by imprisonment and other penalties. In Switzerland, vaccination was compulsory in all cantons except Uri, Glaris and Geneva[269]. Only a few States or cities of the United States had vaccination statutes; in Lower Canada, vaccination was not compulsory. It was compulsory in South Australia (1872), Victoria (1874), Western Australia (1878), Tasmania (1882), Calcutta (1880)... In the countries listed below there was no legal compulsion but governmental facilities and pressure on various classes of the population more or less directly under government control, such as soldiers, state employees, apprentices, school children, was evident: France, Italy, Spain, Portugal, Belgium, Norway, Austria, Turkey[270].

The example of Great Britain, country of origin of inoculation and vaccination in Europe, is interesting. The question of obligatory vaccination was first brought before the House of Lords in 1840, in answer to a petition submitted by the *Medical Society of London*[271]. A bill was introduced, requesting the organisation of vaccination sessions for the poor under the authority of the Boards of Guardians. The House of Commons ratified it. All children born after August 1st of that year had to be vaccinated free of charge; parents of unvaccinated children were liable to fines equivalent to between 80 and 400 euros[272].

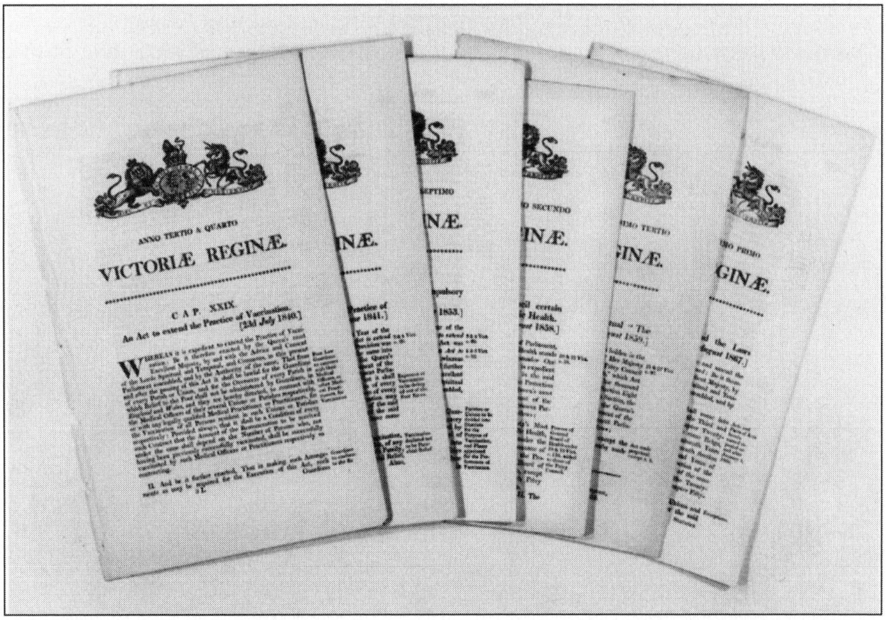

Figure 22. Queen Victoria and her government were very active in promoting smallpox vaccination in Great Britain. Six Acts of Parliament were needed to legalise compulsory vaccination, in 1840, 1841, 1853, 1858, 1859 and 1867. However, this did not last long, because these laws were weakened by a further act of 1898 recognizing conscientious objectors. (Author's document.)

269. Larousse du XIXe siècle, 2nd suppl., 1888, p. 1965.
270. Anonymous, 1902, vol. VIII, p. 6119.
271. Creighton, 1889, p. 302.
272. Anonyme, 1853, p. 64.

No less than six Acts of Parliament, in 1840, 1841, 1853, 1858, 1859 and 1867, were necessary to encourage, and then make vaccination mandatory, under pain of fines and even imprisonment. But, as McVail points out, resistance could lead to prison but not to forced vaccination[273]. Obligatory vaccination also produced reactions of revolt and much controversy, for example, in Leicester (1869)[274] or in Montreal (1885)[275]. Starting in 1898, a conscience clause amending the law in Great Britain made it easy to obtain exemptions. After that, the laws quickly lost their effectiveness.

After the stick, the carrot. It was clear that most people were indifferent to a vague threat; the only thing left was persuasion, an excellent method when it can be implemented. Positive encouragement was used widely, with generally favourable results. To combat the parents' inertia, novel ways of attracting them were devised. Each prefect had his own ideas: "*We saw poor families come for vaccination and receive not only protection from small-pox, but also suitable help with their difficulties… The mayor of Amiens… delivered a kilogram of meat to the parents of each poor child who was vaccinated. During the first month following this municipal order, over four hundred subjects were vaccinated.*"[276a]

Elsewhere, similar procedures were employed: "*In 1812 an alarm arose from the introduction of the variolous contagion, and the poor being backward in embracing vaccination, Dr. Rigby suggested to the court of Guardians that the additional inducement of a reward would more effectually bring them to submit to so desirable a measure than any other plan that could be devised. He urged his opinion with the same zeal and earnestness as he had done on many other occasions with the view to the obtening of public good, and in the end*

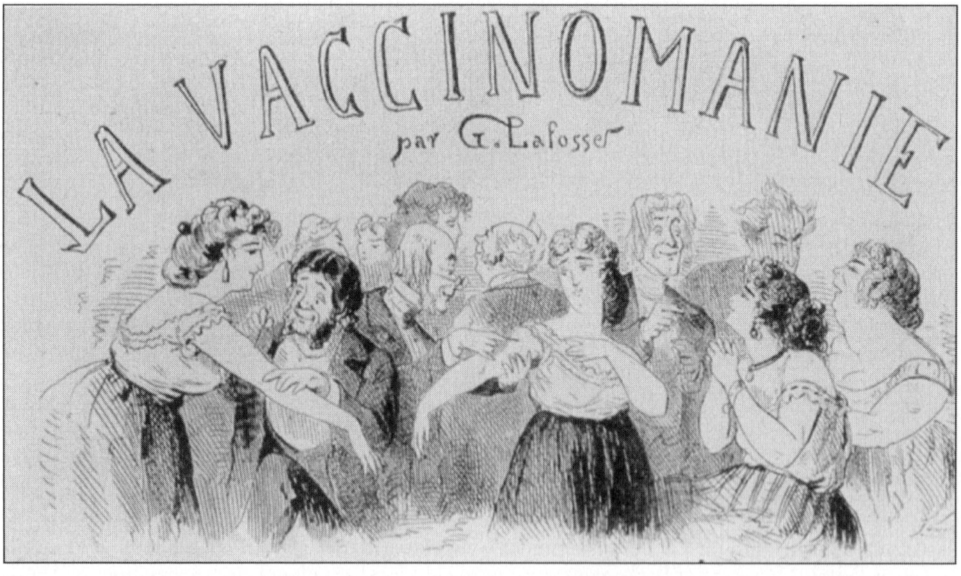

Figure 23. Vaccinomania. "*These doctors, these doctors! They see pretty arms, pretty shoulders, pretty…*". Song by G. Lafosse. (Anonyme, 1914)[276b].

273. McVail, 1919, p. 27.
274. Bazin, 2000, p. 130.
275. Bazin, 2000, p. 132.
276a. Husson, 1811, p. 17.
276b. Anonymous, 1914, p. 80.

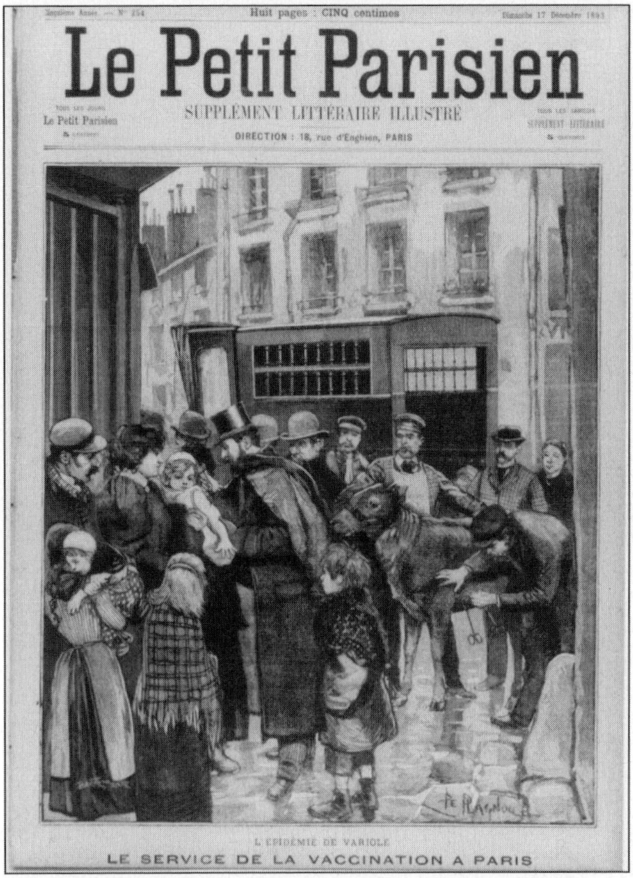

Figure 24. A smallpox vaccine session. The heifer, source of the vaccine, is brought to the location where the vaccinations are to be performed. Potential candidates admire the animal's good health, and are thus encouraged to present their arm to the vaccinator's lancet. The Chambon Institute had a contract with the city of Paris to vaccinate or revaccinate populations in the proximity of declared smallpox cases. Indigent mothers received two francs for each child they brought. As a scale of reference, the supplement of the *Petit Parisien* cost five centimes. (Reproduced from the *Petit Parisien*, illustrated literary supplement, n° 254, December 17, 1893.)

prevailed on the court of Guardians to allow half a crown to every poor person, who should bring a certificate from a surgeon of having satisfactorily through the cow-pox... The good effect of it (the half-crown donation) *was soon evident...*"[277].

In France, the Central Committee, and later the Academy's vaccine commission, took a strong position in favour of persuasion. In a letter dated August 16, 1810, Husson wrote to Mr. Forestier, surgeon in Avallon (Yonne): "*The government is loath to employ coercive measures. It thinks that in a matter it considers dependent on public opinion, persuasion should achieve everything, and constraint will achieve nothing.*"[278] In 1847, the idea of a legal obligation regarding vaccination was beginning to be promoted. Every report

277. Cross, 1820, p. 21.
278. BANM, Ms 1611-962, letter n° 962.

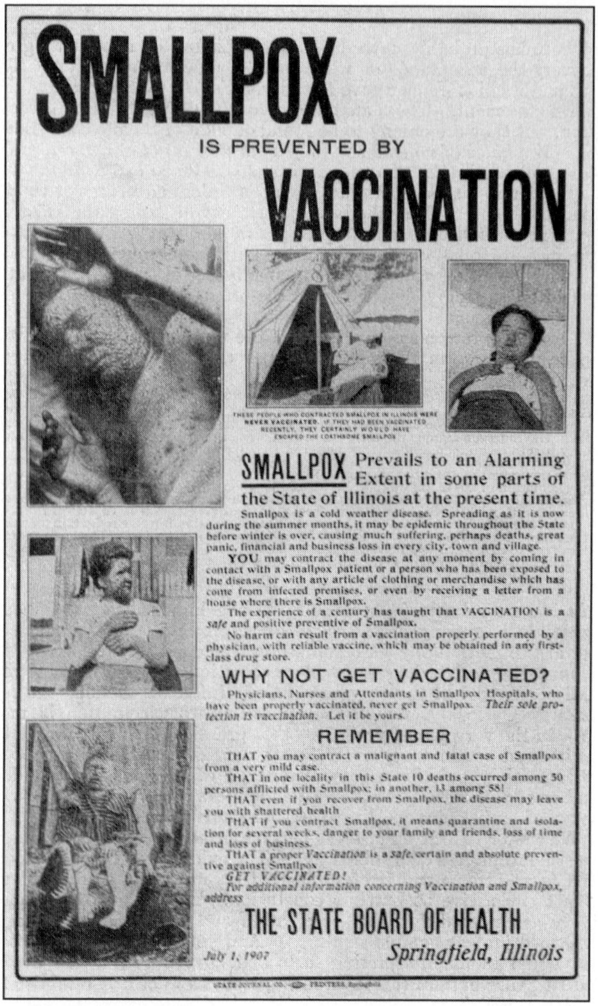

Figure 25. Public advertisement about smallpox vaccination. The State Board of Health, Springfield, Illinois, 1st July 1907. (Author's document.)

of the Academy of Medicine recommended compulsory vaccination, revaccination whenever possible and isolation of smallpox sufferers, particularly in hospitals: all measures in the public good.

One of the curious arguments used to promote compulsory vaccination was the benefit it had brought to the colonies of France, which extended its well-meaning protection to them. But French deputies remained deaf to this argument. In 1901, the Senate finally took an interest in the obligation bill. The law was passed on February 15, 1902: compulsory vaccination during the first year of life, compulsory revaccination at age 11 and 21. It took five years for the law to be applied; although the statute was never strictly enforced, mortality due to smallpox in France dropped drastically. Improved public hygiene, isolation of infected persons and vaccination of those who had been in contact with them probably did the rest.

For instance, Chambon and Ménard (Directors of the private Vaccine Animal Institute) signed an agreement with the city of Paris to vaccinate individuals who had had contact with smallpox sufferers or with their families. Posters announced the arrival of the vaccination Service. The heifer was transported to the site at the appointed time, and vaccinators went from door to door inviting people to be vaccinated or revaccinated free of charge. Seeing the healthy heifer on the street reassured people and gave them confidence, so that they could be persuaded more easily to be vaccinated[279]. Mothers who brought their children were given a small sum of money to compensate for lost wages.

The behaviour of royal families had had considerable impact from the start of variolation; the same was true from the beginning of vaccinations. "*We know that Leopold II, to set a good example for his loyal subjects, was vaccinated last week at the same time as Princess Clémentine. Since then, a veritable vaccination furor rages in Brussels...*"[280]. The influence of the media, which diffused unfounded rumours as well as well-established facts, was always considerable.

The Medical Professions and Vaccination

The medical profession in the Western World, as a whole, was very receptive to Jennerian vaccination. In France, in addition to physicians belonging to vaccine committees, be it the Central Committee of which Pinel, Bourdois, Husson, etc. were members, or Departmental Committees, numerous members of the profession took an active part in the spread of vaccination. Their names often appear in official reports: Voisin de Versailles, Valentin de Nancy, Levieux de Bordeaux, Barrey de Besançon, Pagès d'Alais (Alès), Guyétand de Lons-le-Saunier, Lalagarde d'Albi, Bounder de Dijon, Bretonneau de Tours... The Academy of Medicine and medical societies awarded prizes, medals, books, etc. to the best vaccinators, whose names were made known in official reports.

Here and there, the voice of discontent could be heard regretting the loss of medical visits by physicians to treat smallpox: "... *As things stand now, vaccination is so unprofitable for those who practice it that it would be better for them to see parents give up the vaccine in favour of small-pox, which at one time made physicians wealthy.*"[281] But such remarks were exceptional.

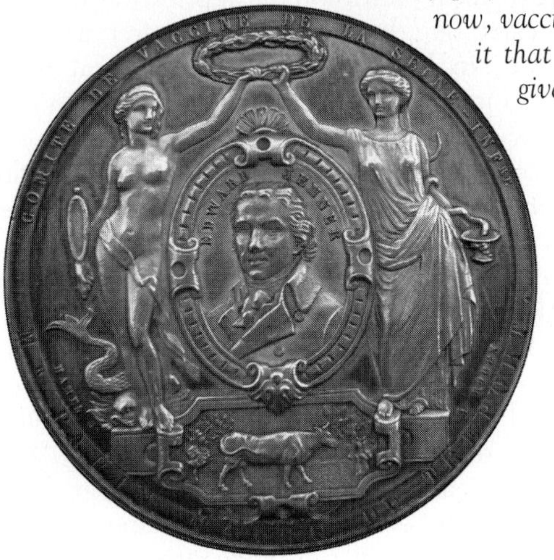

Figure 26. Silver medal bearing the portrait of Edward Jenner, coined by the Seine-Inférieure vaccine committee and awarded to Mr. Papin, mayor of Le Tréport. Obverse: Napoleon III (French Emperor: 1852-1870); verso: Edward Jenner. Signed Barre, Hamel at Rouen. Diameter 40 mm. The most dedicated vaccinators received medals (gold, silver or bronze) from the Central Committee or from departmental vaccine committees. (Author's document.)

279. Copeman, 1899, p. 203.
280. Anonyme, 1903, p. 110.
281. Anonyme, 1828-1830, t. 13, p. 308.

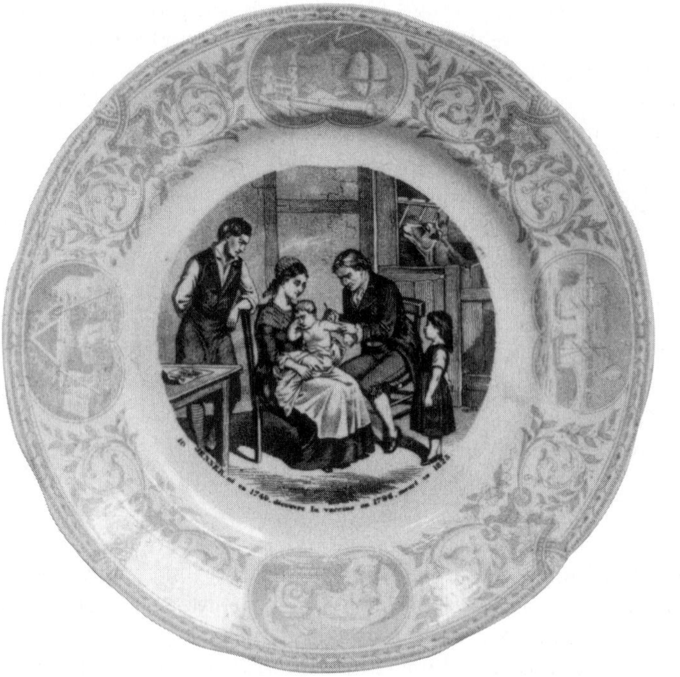

Figure 27. Jenner was classified as one of the great benefactors of humanity. This China plate from Sarreguemines (France) bears the inscription "*Jenner, born in 1749, discovered the vaccine in 1796, died in 1823*". The engraving shows a physician (most probably Jenner) vaccinating a child who is crying a little, under the gaze of his parents and a little girl. A cow in the nearby stable reminds us of the origin of the vaccine. (Author's document.)

Although vaccination was welcomed by the medical profession, its application was less well received, because it was difficult to carry out. In 1860, Dr. Munaret wrote a revealing description of vaccination rounds, in his department. Prefectoral rules required mayors to keep a list of children born in the current year, and of children not vaccinated the previous year. The date of vaccinations was officially posted. The mayor was supposed to be present during the visit of the physician-vaccinator. The physician chose one or more vaccinifer children, which was something mothers disliked, whether their child was chosen or not. A way to avoid this was to hide until the visit was over, not a difficult thing to do in a village. Parents did not like to have lymph taken from their children, and for this reason they did not come to the vaccine harvesting visit, or only came two weeks later, or even later than that...[282]. A second trip was made for the general vaccination session. Mothers expressed their fear of transmission of diseases other than the one related to the vaccine, and brought to bear problems that had come about in the family of the vaccinifer. The atmosphere became tense! Finally, the vaccinations were performed, thanks to much reassurance and to barley sugar (*sic*). Eight days later, a third visit was made to check the development of vaccine pustules and, perhaps, to vaccinate a few more children, so that yet another visit would have to be made a week later. The physician would also have to waste (*sic*) hours: "*writing*

282. Depaul, 1868, pp. 62 & 140.

in duplicate, biannual reports, their official registration, correspondence..."[283]. Dr. Munaret, a dedicated vaccinator, was not happy with government attitudes. He was not the only one. Financial benefit for the vaccinator was minimal, not to say non-existent. The stinginess of successive governments and their scant subsidies were mentioned even in the reports of the Central Committee or of the Academy of Medicine.

Unfortunately, it was difficult to form a definite opinion on the effectiveness of the smallpox vaccination, even in the countries where it was compulsory but not practiced rigorously, or where contamination from outside could occur. Statistics show that the British army and navy, rigorously vaccinated, had no cases of smallpox, while in the civil population cases of smallpox among "vaccinated" individuals were numerous. As to mortality rates due to smallpox among vaccinated and unvaccinated subjects, they seem about the same[284]. These rather unsatisfactory statistics show that vaccinations as well as revaccinations were never correctly performed in the 19th century in Western countries. The eradication of smallpox in countries with very poor levels of private and public hygiene had shown that vaccination was effective when it was scrupulously applied.

In conclusion, variolation and vaccination represent an important stage in active protection against infectious diseases. But the two procedures protected against one and the same disease: smallpox, a horrible disease, but not the only one. Protection against other diseases remained to be discovered. Attempts were made to find the cowpox/vaccinia of each disease, but in vain.

There are no other examples of human vaccine of the "vaccine" type. Veterinary medicine has a small number of vaccines of the "vaccinia type". Viruses without danger for their source species, as well as for the species receiving them as vaccine, are used. Protection is conferred by cross-immune reaction. The so-called heterologous vaccine induces immunity against the virus in question, as well as the other, related, virus which it has to combat.

A classic example is the use of the turkey herpes virus, for which the turkey is a source species in which it induces no pathology. It is used to inoculate and protect poultry from Marek's disease. Other examples exist, such as the Shope fibroma virus, used to protect rabbits from myxomatosis; the vaccine of rinderpest (cattle plague) against the peste des petits ruminants; the vaccine of sheeppox against lumpy skin disease. Measles vaccine has also been used to protect against rinderpest in cattle or distemper in dogs. These rare examples were not known in the 19th century and their relevance is limited to a small number of infectious diseases. Therefore, the "variolation" method was relied upon once again, that is, the "virus" or natural pathogenic agent was used, taking care to avoid serious accidents. It was a heroic era, not always medically irreproachable, and even less ethically so...

283. Munaret, 1860, p. 47.
284. Anonymous, 1902, vol. VIII, p. 6119.

4
Inoculation (Variolation) Reaches an Impasse

When did people realize that it could be useful to inoculate a disease artificially to avoid having it later? The exact moment in history is unknown, but it came in the wake of the discovery that many infectious diseases do not recur in the same subject. This observation, along with the awareness that infectious diseases are often less dangerous in children than in adults, was what impelled mothers to let their children play with other children who were obviously infected, so that they would all have chickenpox or rubella at the same time? What herd owner has not wished for all his livestock to become contaminated at the same time, to avoid drawn-out deterioration of his means of subsistence? The need to be protected against infectious diseases has long been obvious. As far as animals were concerned, the first methods of protection were probably confinement, isolation, slaughter and natural contamination. The example of variolation, widely known from the second half of the eighteenth century on, inspired adaptations of this technique to other diseases. Veterinary medicine, subject to few moral constraints, became an ideal field of action for some of these experiments. Many physicians, and later veterinary surgeons, took an interest in human or animal variolation, particularly in clavelisation, which was the subject of interminable discussions in medical (human as well as veterinary) or scientific academies and societies. Another path appeared gradually, thanks to Pasteur: that of viruses with attenuated virulence.

The Cattle Plague: 1744...

Cattle plague was certainly one of the most terrible disasters of world animal husbandry. "*The name cattle plague is given to an epizootic disease, not present in our country* (France in 1889), *producing fever, diarrhoea, extreme thinness, rapid walk and finally, in most cases, death.*"[1] This affection is also called contagious horned cattle typhus or typhus of big cattle. Cattle plague was endemic on the Steppes of Southern Russia. In Europe there were numerous epizootics of cattle plague, between 1710 and 1871[2]. This disease has disappeared from Western Europe after this last epizootic, and is about to be eradicated world-wide.

Epizootics followed one another, most often spreading from East to West, but sometimes the other way round, as cattle arriving by sea were being imported. In the Netherlands, Belgium and France serious cattle plague outbreaks raged throughout the eighteenth century, killing about 10 million bovines[3]. In an in-depth study on the cattle plague epizootic in Flanders, Ardresis, Calaisis, Boulonnais and Artois between 1774 and 1776, Mr. de Berg, of the city of Brussels, specifies: "*We must expect, in all places*

1. Peuch *in* Bouley, 1889, t. 17, p. 1.
2. Blancou, 2003; Vallat, 2009, p. 51.
3. Dunlop, 1996, p. 320.

where this disease exists & where it will exist, to lose two thirds of the animals infected in a canton composed of several villages." Actual figures are hard to find. In one Flanders canton, this cattle plague epizootic killed about a fifth of the cattle in three months[4].

As a result, systematic slaughter of sick cattle and of the animals with which they had been in contact was introduced at the start of an epizootic, following the precepts of Thomas Bates or Lancisi[5]. But when it was realized that this disease only attacked individual animals once, in Holland and in German cantons where the disease had become endemic, inoculation was attempted[6]. Dodson (actually Dobson), Layard and Bewley in England, Grashuis, Sandifort and Noseman, Kool and Tack in Holland and many others in Switzerland, in the German territories, almost all medical doctors, started to inoculate bovines and to look for inoculums from animals with "benign" plague, while avoiding those from more serious forms of the disease. Overall results were not impressive, mortality among the inoculated animals remaining about the same as that seen in bovines with natural contamination[7]. However, the favorable results obtained by Camper, van Doevren and Munnicks became known all over Europe. Inoculations were performed with "*a thick double thread soaked in the suppuration that runs from the nostrils of a sick animal, when the disease has not yet reached its peak...*"[8]. These observations were collected concerning 1100 horned cattle that were inoculated in Mr. Munnicks's presence, and surveyed afterwards. Results were not very satisfactory: at most, half of the inoculated cattle resisted infection, which was not sufficient for recommending the practice. In 1776 and 1777, Vicq-d'Azyr himself carried out some experiments on cattle, with similar results. Having read in the *Journal de Physique*, published by the Reverend Father Rozier (author of a 10-volume Dictionary of Agriculture), a dissertation by Mr. Mauduyt advising "*to test if the pestilent virus cannot be denatured by some process, I directed my attempts according to these observations, & I soaked the contagious strips in different acids, stable & volatile alkali, spirits and aromatics: none of these procedures hindered the progress of the inoculation...*"[7] The idea is interesting, because it predates that of Pasteur (or Toussaint) concerning vaccines with attenuated virulence. Vicq-d'Azyr continues his study by reporting the results obtained by Mr. Geert-Reinders, a Dutch cattle farmer, who inoculated using Camper's technique, with very poor results. "*Mr. Geert-Reinders observed, in a large number of calves he was feeding, that when the epizootic broke out among them, all those who were born of cows previously attacked by & healed of the epizootic, were very lightly infected & all survived, while almost all the others died.*"[7] Camper and Munnicks took this to be a hopeful sign, and after lengthy experiments made the following deductions:

"*1°. That calves born of cows previously infected & healed of the epizootic are disposed to resist a certain time the contagion of the disease, or that they heal of it very easily, if they contract it.*

2°. That the time during which they enjoy this favourable disposition being elapsed, these animals contract the epizootic in as dangerous a manner as the others.

4. De Berg, 1780, p. 616.
5. Pastoret, 2006, p. 86; Vallat, 2006, p. 40; Vallat, 2009, p. 271; Wilkinson, 1992, p. 51.
6. Vicq-d'Azyr, 1780, p. 163.
7. Vicq-d'Azyr, 1780, p. 163.
8. Camper, 1779, p. 321; Vicq-d'Azyr, 1780, p. 163; Vicq-d'Azyr, 1795, p. 233.

3°. That the period during which the calves possess this disposition is always close to their birth...

4°. Finally, that the calves with this disposition, & which in this interval contract the disease, either through natural contagion or through inoculation, are often infected in such a light manner, that it would be tempting to believe that their health is almost unaltered... we decided to inoculate the calves born of healed cows, at the age of one month or six weeks... By using this procedure, out of twenty inoculated animals, we only lost one... this year, the inoculation has been successful in over two thousand..."[7].

The conclusion of this report recommends slaughter in case of an emerging epizootic, and inoculation by the Camper/Reinders method in the troublesome event that the contagion has not been contained right from the start[7]. These remarkable data are among the first to be collected in immunology.

In 1853, Jenssen, physician and director of the Imperial Veterinary School of Dorpat (Russia), tried to use cattle plague inoculation on a large scale. He searched for a mitigated virus (a strain with attenuated virulence, as we would say now) by successive passages of the infectious agent to the animals. Losses showed fifty per cent at the first inoculation, and stabilised at more acceptable ratios. The preferred fluid for inoculation was tears from cattle inoculated with virus having already been "passed" several times to bovines. Two establishments for the inoculation of cattle plague were opened in 1860, one in Orenbourg, the other in Bondavevka; their mission was to study the value of this practice[9]. In 1864, the commission in charge of this work judged the results to be negative and had both centres closed.

Ramazzini and Lancisi are said to have connected cattle plague with smallpox as early as 1711. This idea was accepted by many others. To elucidate the question, "*in 1865, eight cows that had provided, for several days, virus for (smallpox) vaccinations performed by Dr. Lanoix, and that came from a Service he had created for this purpose, were sent by* Mr. M.H. *Bouley to England, where a cattle plague outbreak was then at its peak. Placed in contact with the infected animals, they all contracted the contagious typhus* (cattle plague), *either through simple cohabitation, or by inoculation*"[10]. Cattle plague and smallpox (more precisely, cowpox/vaccine) were two different infections.

In 1881, Piot, former lecturer at the Alfort veterinary school, was named Chief veterinary surgeon of Egyptian territories, in Cairo. Piot was aware of Toussaint and Pasteur's work on anthrax vaccination. He organised vaccination against the cattle plague or "*contagious typhus of horned cattle*" in Egypt and then in the State of Great Lebanon, apparently with successful results. Piot made his vaccine by heating virulent blood (source of virus), as Toussaint recommended (*see Toussaint's texts*).

Cattle plague has been eradicated in most countries by the slaughter of sick animals and those that might have had contact with them, with compensation provided to owners, or by use of vaccination in the twentieth century. Only one pocket of the disease remains, in Somalia, but it too will no doubt disappear in the near future.

---

9. Jessen, 1859, p. 652; Reynal, 1873, p. 369; Hurtrel d'Arboval, 1877, v. 3, p. 149; Peuch *in* Bouley, 1889, t. 17, p. 1.
10. Reynal, 1873, p. 369.

Inoculation against cattle plague was sometimes compulsory in infected French departments, upon prefectorial Order and with compensation to owners of cattle that died as a result of the operation[11].

Clavelisation, about 1800

Sheeppox, a disease dreaded by sheep-farmers, can be compared to smallpox in humans. Both have four distinct stages: inflammation, eruption, suppuration and desiccation. Sheeppox, like smallpox, can be discrete and benign, or confluent and malignant*. In about 1800, its contagious nature was well-known; the disease constituted a real economic problem: "*Its ravages* (of sheeppox), *he says* (Tessier), *taken all together, are more considerable than those wrought by the rot* (foot rot?) *and by the blood disease* (anthrax?). *Sheeppox sometimes kills half a flock...*"[12]. Recurrence of sheeppox is very rare. Therefore, it must have been tempting to use an ovine form of variolation. It is said that as early as the fifteenth and the sixteenth century respectively, the Serbs and the Swiss used clavelisation[13]. The example of the "Lady Montagu" variolation probably gave the method new impetus. In France, practically at the same period, the procedure was proposed by Chalette (1762-63), and then by the famous director of the Lyon Veterinary School (and Royal Rider) Bourgelat (1765)[14]. It actually started to be used at the turn of the century. Tessier predicted great benefits if clavelisation was adopted: "*Inoculation practiced everywhere on lambs strong enough to withstand it, will prevent treatment and concern. Flocks will travel safety, they will be led from market to market, without fear that they take or give an often deadly disease.*"[15]

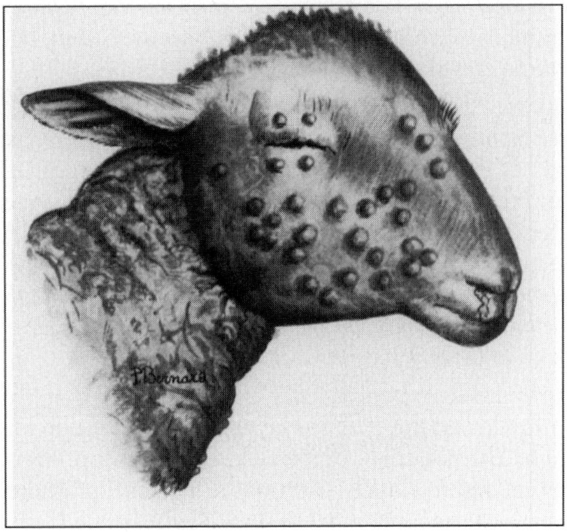

Figure 1. "*Sheeppox. Confluent eruption of the face.*" (Moussu, 1923)[16].

* But it can also affect internal organs.

11. Reynal, 1873, p. 369; Conte, 1895, p. 203.
12. Voisin, 1805a, p. 4.
13. Blancou, 2003, p. 40.
14. Hurtrel d'Arboval, 1826, v. 1, p. 281; Reynal, 1873, p. 526.
15. Tessier, 1790, p. 379.
16. Moussu, 1923, p. 247.

The arrival of the vaccine introduced the question: was it possible to protect sheep from sheeppox by a vaccine inoculation? Numerous experiments were conducted. The first experiments were inconclusive, probably due to the mixing of viruses. Godine le jeune reports: "*the variolous virus, inoculated to sheep, produces sheep-pox... the vaccine protects sheep from sheep-pox...*"[17], which is certainly not true... These results are surprising, since this work was closely followed by the Central Vaccine Committee, and financed by the Minister of the Interior. In fact, Godine specifies that during one of their visits to Alfort, Husson and his colleagues would be given "*a country dinner*"[18], which might explain certain things...

Voisin and his colleagues from the Agriculture Society of the Seine-et-Oise Department, who participated actively in this work, presented an experimental plan to improve the prevention of sheeppox, on March 8, 1805[19]. It is clear that the disease constituted a major concern at the time. Everyone took part in the effort: the Agriculture Society provided a flock of sheep, the mayor of Versailles authorised the avenues of the city to serve as pasture for the flock for the duration of the experiment, the Inspector of Taxes and Duties did not demand taxes on the entry of the animals into the city of Versailles, and the school principal allowed certain parts of the building (the new "lycée") and the vast courtyards of the establishment not yet in use to be occupied temporarily by the sheep. These had to be separated from the rest of the flock in order to be subjected to counter-experiments. The number of observers and witnesses, all very competent, indicates the significance of the study: the Central Vaccine Committee, the Medical Society, the Seine Departement Agricultural Society, the College of Arts, the *Société galvanique* (Galvinist Society)... The animals were identified: "*... They were vaccinated, then a wire necklace was placed around their neck; it was attached to a tin plate with an identification number.*" Forty woolly animals were inoculated (with vaccine); they had light symptoms but remained receptive to clavelisation.

The Central Vaccine Committee reports: "*But the important objective of our work was to apply the vaccine to sheep, to protect them from sheep-pox... Experiments aimed at this were numerous and tiring, repeated trips to the site were needed, the research was difficult and the results are still hard to evaluate; because the objective was important, no effort was spared to reach it.*"[20] Unfortunately, these efforts were unsuccessful and it was necessary to return to the inoculation of the sheeppox: "*It* (sheeppox inoculation to sheep) *seemed to us to be to sheep-pox what variolous inoculation is to small-pox... and that this operation* (clavelisation) *performed by a skilled veterinarian, and followed by three or four visits during the evolution of the inoculation, is enough to carry it out well...*"[21].

In 1808, Cuvier's report on "*les progrès des sciences naturelles*" already states that the clavelisation method is widely used in rural economy[22]. The clavelisation technique was promoted in articles, often in the form of instructions[23], or in books on rural economy or animal husbandry. The major problem related to clavelisation was a "normal" mortality rate of 4% after clavelisation[24]. The method probably improved with time, since Henry

17. Godine, 1803a, p. 29; Godine, 1803b, p. 226.
18. BANM, Vac 2, D4.
19. Voisin, 1805a.
20. Husson, 1806, p. 97.
21. Voisin, 1805b, p. 84.
22. Cuvier, 1810, p. 365.
23. Bouriat, 1811, p. 173.
24. Hurtrel d'Arboval, 1838, v. 1, p. 482.

Bouley reported it to be 1% in 1882[25]. Unfortunately, the mortality rate could also rise to 8% and even 25%[26]! Finally, as was the case with variolation, clavelisation was blamed above all for spreading the disease by contagion. In France, clavelisation became the subject of lengthy scientific and even political debates, in the Chamber of Deputies. It was submitted to the authority of prefects... Normally forbidden due to the risk of spreading the disease, it could become compulsory during epizootics, and had to be practiced by licensed veterinarians, with official (prefectorial) authorisation[27].

"*Sheeppox virus culture*" became a favoured technique, particularly in Germanic countries, under the influence of Pessina's work: "*ten young, perfectly healthy sheep are chosen, and inoculated with virus from a benign sheep-pox pustule. From among them, one is chosen: the one with the fewest, the most beautiful, the ripest pustules, and the product of their secretion is used to inoculate ten other sheep. Once again, the one with the most optimally developed pustule is chosen, and its virus is used to inoculate ten more animals... According to Pessina and other veterinary authors, this characteristic indicates that the virus has reached the stage where its inoculation will always produce a benign form of sheep-pox.*"[28] The technique consisted of inoculating sheeppox virus into ovines and of choosing, passage after passage, "*the strain*" that produced "*a single, beautiful pustule*". At the Vienna Veterinary School, where Pessina worked, one strain of sheeppox virus was transmitted for nine years (1836-1845), with thirty-three passages per year, without loss of virulence or preventive properties.

In 1923, clavelisation was still considered a valid method, but it was practiced in combination with convalescent animal serum. Conte recommended this sero-clavelisation procedure as early as 1906[29] (*see "sero-vaccination" later in this book*). Clavelisation is still used in animal-farming regions of Asia and Africa (particularly in the Maghreb). Today, there are vaccines made of modified viral strains preserved *in vitro* on cell cultures.

Louis Willems and Bovine Pleuropneumonia: 1852...

"... *Being a true citizen and friend of humanity, I felt obliged in good conscience to reveal my secret and thus share with all those whose animals are subject to the plague* (epizootic pleuropneumonia) *the fruits of my studies and my sacrifices.*" Willems, 1853[30].

Another disease, contagious pleuropneumonia of bovines, was also fought using inoculation of the wild "virus". This disease of cattle, one of the deadliest of the era, was endemic in many European countries, and particularly in Belgium. Many other countries such as the United States, parts of Australia and South Africa, and some regions of Asia were also infected[31]. Its contagious nature continued to be the subject of bitter controversies, as it had been for a long time. It was obviously an important subject.

Louis Willems, a Belgian physician having just obtained his diploma from the Faculty of Medicine of the University of Louvain, found himself confronted with this disease that

25. Bouley, 1882a, p. 311.
26. Peuch, 1882, p. 648.
27. Conte, 1895, p. 239; Viseur, 1873, p. 662.
28. Reynal *in* Bouley, 1857, t. 3, p. 729.
29. Conte, 1906, p. 356.
30. Willems, 1853, p. 36.
31. Salmon, 1896, p. 371.

was decimating his father's stables. The latter, a Hasselt distiller, bought young cattle that he fattened with by-products from his factory, to resell as beef cattle in the markets of neighbouring cities. Willems noted the contagious nature of the disease, and its transmission by the inoculation of pulmonary exudates. The idea of using inoculation came to him naturally, because "*in human medicine, epidemic and contagious diseases are often inoculated, and as a result become benign*"[32]. The classic inoculation into the base of the neck (imitating clavelisation) of pulmonary serosity from animals killed by pleuropneumonia transmitted the disease well, but in most cases killed the inoculated animals. Willems had the idea of inoculating not in the fetlock area, but at the end of the tail. The animal developed a much less serious disease. At times, problems developed at the point of virus insertion, be it gangrene or another problem, but the fact that an animal was missing the end of its tail did not diminish its value on the meat livestock market. But was "Willems's inoculation" profitable? This question was the subject of hundreds of hours of committee discussions, and filled thousands of report pages, ending in somewhat divergent conclusions. The inoculated animals were well protected from a subsequent attack of the disease, but the effects of the inoculation were not benign. In some cases, the cumulated losses in an inoculated herd were equal to those associated with normal epizootic risk. Official experiments were conducted in Belgium, France, Holland, England, Italy and perhaps elsewhere... on entire herds. The problem will never be entirely solved. In Belgium, the question even became political and protectionist, through the implicit refusal of veterinarians to accept a method invented by a... physician[33].

Willems was subject to attacks, and was glorified at the same time! To illustrate, in France, there was no winner of a contest comparing proposals for preventive and curative methods for "big cattle pleuropneumonia" in 1853, due to a lack of suitable submissions. *Le Journal Agricole* of Verviers, reprinted in *Annales de Médecine Vétérinaire* (Brussels), comments ironically: "*As we can see, all the noise made by sensationalist journalists interested in Mr. Willems's cause, as well as all the demonstrations made in good faith by very honourable persons misled by appearances, in favour of this inoculator; no less than the singular comedy these excellent cattle breeders played for his benefit, by promenading him through the streets of Hasselt, in a triumphal carriage with six richly attired oxen, all this did not suffice for the France of agriculture and veterinary medicine to leave him alone, while at the same time proclaiming him the Jenner of the bovine species.*"[34] All of which is neither kind nor true.

Willems was granted flattering awards such as that of Knight of the Order the Netherlands Lion[35], yet he received no honours in Belgium. Belgian newspapers did not speak kindly of him in their editorials. In the report on the work of the Royal Academy of Belgium, its Secretary wrote: "*In 1852, the honourable Dr. Willems had the idea of trying to prevent exudative pleuropneumonia by inoculating, in the stables belonging to his father, a Hasselt distiller, beef cattle with lung serosity taken from animals suffering from this disease. Mr. Willems believed that he had found the remedy he was seeking, and asked the Academy to evaluate his discovery. The commissioners chosen by our company to follow the experiments conducted at the Veterinary School by a Commission charged by the Minister of the Interior with observing the effects of the inoculation proposed by the Hasselt physician have expressed the opinion that, in the present circumstances, time and experience alone can*

32. Willems, 1852, p. 7.
33. Commission, 1854, p. 33 and many others; Husson, 1857, p. 166 and many others; Willems, 1853.
34. Anonyme, 1854, p. 586.
35. Willems, 1857, p. 107.

indicate the effects of the inoculation, in terms of prevention of epizootic pleuropneumonia, and that these inoculations do not have a sufficient basis in science."[36]

The report conclusions maintain a polite attitude toward Willems. But to say that his inoculations "*do not have a sufficient basis in science*" to be used, while the smallpox vaccination (cowpox/vaccine), which did not have any greater scientific basis, was commonly used... was unexpected. The conflict continued. Willem's method was never entirely accepted in his own country, any more than anywhere else. As the saying went: "*A pneumonia of the tail, what a paradox for science!*"[37]

Willem's efforts were admirable and worthy of interest. Were they rewarded? In the dissertation in which he reveals his secret to the Belgian Minister of the Interior, in 1852, Willems asks that his work be recognized: "*You see, Mister Minister, I have spoken openly and straightforwardly; I have revealed my secret to you and I count on your loyalty. If you should recognize the new method I discovered to be good and efficatious, I hope that you will see fit to reward my efforts and sacrifices appropriately.*"[38] Was the Minister generous? We will never know...

Cruzel wrote an excellent review of Willems's work[39].

In fact, it is probable, if not certain, that the inoculation of bovines against pleuroneumonia is a very old practice. In 1917, Tettaz wrote that it has long existed in West Africa[40]. An interesting episode related to the inoculation of this disease of cattle took place at the end of the nineteenth century. In 1880, de Rochebrune presented an original discovery to the Academy of Sciences (Paris). "*Naturalists and travellers of all eras, for reasons unknown, have kept absolutely silent about a race of domestic Cattle indigenous to Senegambia... This bovine race has a very exceptional characteristic that distinguishes it from other races: this characteristic is the presence on the nasal area of a veritable horn... this horn, sometimes conical, more often in the form of a quadrangular truncated pyramid reaches an average height of 0 m.060 to 0 m.075, a width of 0 m.55 and a thickness of 0 m.040; ... in a herd of a hundred heads, for example, there will always be fifty-five to sixty individuals with a perfectly developed nasal horn... It is therefore manifest that we are in the presence of a hereditary trait.*"[41] The "species" came to be called *Bos triceros*.

Five years later, de Rochebrune sent another communication to the same Academy, in which he made matters worse. He refuted detractors who suggested that the third horn of these bovines could have originated in "*a habit born in ancestral times* (which) *consists, among the Maures and the Pouls* (sic) *of Senegambia, of inoculating to their herds of cattle the epizootic pleuropneumonia virus (pneumosarcia, peripneumonic phthisis), a contagious disease frequently seen in their regions. The point of a primitive-shape knife, or the point of a dagger, is plunged in the lung of a subject killed by the disease, and an incision allowing penetration of the virus under the skin of healthy animals is made in the subnasal area. Experience has shown all the benefits of this preventive operation. The inoculation procedure used by English and Belgian cattle breeders, according to Wilhem* (sic) *(in Hasselt) and based on... seems to copy the method used by the Maures and the Pouls, a method that had remained unknown until now. Neither repeated blows on the subnasal area, nor the inoculation of the pleuropneumonia virus can be invoked as the origin of subnasal osteoporosis and of their characteristic horn, despite*

36. Sauveur, 1857, p. 79.
37. Quoted by Jonas, 1960, p. 15.
38. Willems, 1852, p. 33.
39. Cruzel, 1869, p. 248; Cruzel reviewed by Peuch, 1892, p. 542.
40. Fontaine, 1924, v. 2, p. 566.
41. de Rochebrune, 1880, p. 304.

what the Maures and the Pouls affirm. In effect, this inoculation is used for other races of cattle, with no phenomenon observed other than immunity to disease. The origin of Bos triceros *will no doubt remain an enigma for some time to come.*"[42]

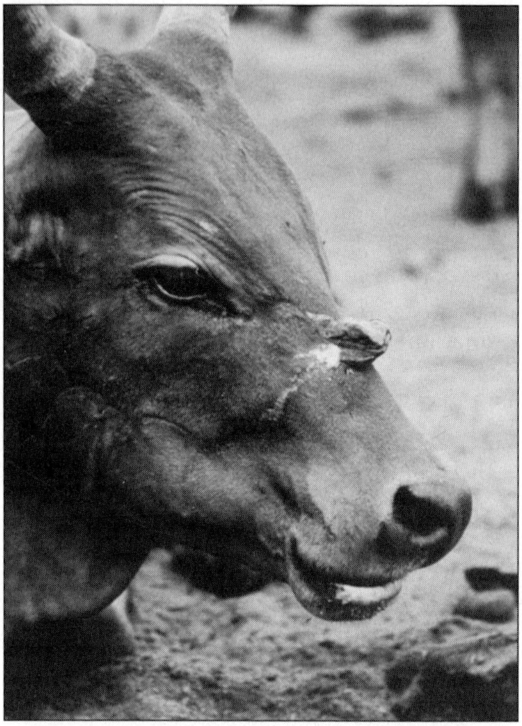

Figure 2. Photograph taken in 1986 in Ethiopia, showing on the nose of the zebu a mark of "variolation" against bovine pleuropneumonia, a technique still used in certain countries of the Sahel region. (Photo provided courtesy of F. Thiaucourt.)

In 1894, Willems himself spoke of the supposed use of this immunisation technique by the indigenous populations of the banks on the Zambezi River, for the protection of their cattle. But he denied the existence of this custom: "*As to the inoculation of Senegambia, it appears to be mere legend, for if Senegambians inoculated, as they were said to do, the pleuropneumonia virus into the subnasal area, with a knife dipped in the lung of an animal killed that died of the disease, 80 percent of the inoculated animals would be killed (Willems).*"[43]

In 1898, a Pasteurian team composed of Roux, Nocard, Borrel, Salimbeni and Dujardin-Beaumetz identified the pathogenic agent of contagious bovine pleuropneumonia. Pure cultures of this mycoplasma were produced at the *Institut Pasteur* and could be used to inoculate bovines[44].

Unfortunately, the method had the disadvantage of all "variolations", as Salmon explains: "*Inoculation has been adopted in many countries, and has undoubtedly lessened the death rate, but the disease is kept up and spreads where his practice is allowed. For this reason it should be prohibited wherever there is a possibility and disposition to eradicate the contagion... This disease has been eradicated from the United States, Norway, Sweden,*

42. de Rochebrune, 1885, p. 658.
43. Galtier, 1891, p. 574.
44. Nocard, 1898, p. 240; Metchnikoff, 1901, p. 499.

Denmark, Holland... Other countries long infected, and in which the contagion was thoroughly established, like Australia... have laboured long, in some cases making no progress, and in others being only partially successful... Neither treatment nor inoculation is permitted in European countries."[45] The only possibility of eradicating the disease is to kill diseased or exposed animals, and to use disinfection.

The traditional inoculation method, by insertion of small fragments of infected lung under the skin of the nose, is still used on a small scale. In Rwanda and in the area which includes Senegal and Ethiopia, that is, the Sahelian strip, bovines of the pseudo-species "*Bos triceros*" can still be found[46].

Syphilisation or Vaccination against Syphilis: 1844...

Syphilis was the object of some very curious and disquieting... attempts at preventive or curative vaccination. These were the first actual attempts at human vaccination (or variolation?), after Jenner's and before Ferran's or Pasteur's; as such, they merit discussion. They also help to explain why a segment of medical opinion, in Pasteur's time, had reservations about any new "vaccine".

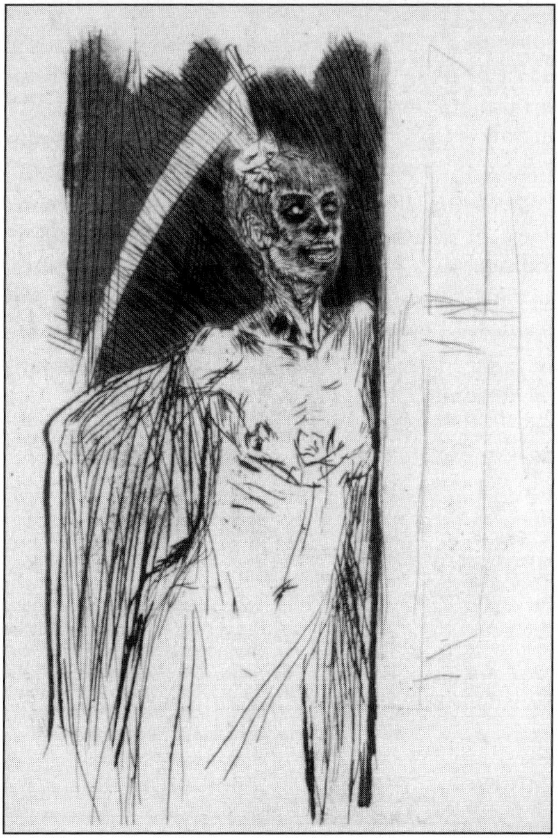

Figure 3. Mors siphilitica. Engraving by Félicien Rops, a Belgian engraver (1833-1898). (Author's document.)

45. Salmon, 1896, p. 371.
46. Thiaucourt, 2000; Blancou, 2003, p. 146.

Venereal diseases are classified as local or systemic. The first category includes several affections such as gonorrhoea or "the clap" and chancroid diseases (also called soft chancres); the second category includes syphilis and AIDS (acquired-immune deficiency syndrome). When syphilis first appeared in Europe around 1495, it was a particularly dreaded disease that caused thousands of deaths and infirmities. It was, rightly, distinguished from gonorrhoea. Later, due to certain unfortunate experiments, the two became confused.

Syphilis is a contagious disease caused by *Treponema pallidium*. Usually sexually transmitted, it develops in three stages. The first, called the primary stage, starts with a small, firm lesion called chancre (or hard chancre, hard sore) associated with chronic inflammation of draining lymph nodes. Primary syphilis heals spontaneously in a few weeks. Secondary manifestations occur, in the weeks or months following the first stage, and take the form of a skin rash or mucosal lesions such as roseola and mucous patches. Tertiary syphilis occurs months or years after the initial infection. It is characterised by general cutaneous, bone, vascular and even nervous symptoms, with paralysis and dementia. "Primary syphilis", the chancroid form, has often been distinguished from "constitutional syphilis", where the virus has infected the whole system and produced general symptoms of various types and in different parts of the body.

Gonorrhoea (also called "the clap" in popular language) is an infectious disease caused by *Neisseria gonorrhoea* and more rarely by other organisms such as Chlamydiae, mycoplasmas, trichomonas, etc. The disease usually takes the form of vulvitis, vaginitis or metritis in women, and urethritis in men. It is essentially local and much less dangerous than syphilis. If left untreated, it can have damaging effects.

Chancroid disease is a specific, local affection consisting of an ulcer called soft sore, soft chancre or soft ulcer. It is caused by the Ducrey's bacillus or *Haemophilus ducreyi*. Chancroid is an inoculable disease, and relatively benign. At one time it was common in Europe, but has now almost disappeared. Confusing it with syphilitic chancroids could lead to unfortunate errors in diagnosis, prognosis and, above all, treatment.

At the end of the eighteenth century, gonorrhoea, chancroid and syphilis were generally not clearly distinguished from each-other[47].

Attempts were made to differentiate between them by auto-inoculation, that is, testing on the same patient, but sometimes also on other persons who, if they did not have syphilis, were exposed to a real danger of contracting it.

"*I do not believe that patients always had reason to rejoice, to the same extent as we* (physicians) *did, in the marvellous discoveries that have marked the past twenty years.*"[48] Unfortunately, this comment is well-founded. These were some of the darkest pages of the history of preventive medicine. The success of the smallpox vaccination and of clavelisation opened new perspectives that attracted adventurous spirits. Using the smallpox-vaccine couple as a model physicians looked for the "cowpox-vaccine of syphilis" to vaccinate (as they very often wrote) against this disease. At least two major attempts were made, on slightly different scientific bases, to prevent the disease or to treat syphilitic patients, who were very difficult to cure.

47. Swediaur or Svédiaur, 1790, p. 1.
48. Dubois-Havenith, 1891, p. 604.

The first and by far the most active school of "syphilisation" was that of Auzias-Turenne. It began with a letter written by Auzias-Turenne on October 28, 1844 to the Academy of Sciences (Paris). "*The enlightened administration of the Natural History Museum, so well-meaning as far as encouraging useful efforts is concerned, having placed several monkeys at my disposal, I was able to ascertain through a number of experiments the possibility of inoculating the syphilis to these mammals...*"[49].

As Charles A. Lee recounts: "*This young physician* (Auzias-Turenne) *commenced, about 1844, a series of experiments with the view of testing John Hunter's doctrine of the non-communicability of syphilis to the lower animals. After many experiments and some failure, he succeeded in producing in monkeys, inoculated with chancre-matter, a true chancre, and the disease thus communicated to them was transferred to rabbits, cats, and horses. The malady was again returned by inoculation from these to the human species, the first trials in this regard having been made by Dr. Robert Weltz, of Würtzburg, on his own person. On four separate occasions Dr. Weltz succeeded in producing an unmistakable chancre on his own person, by inoculation from animals, and this was acknowledged even by Ricord* (a respected French Syphilis specialist of that period)."[50]

A few years later, in 1850, Auzias-Turenne went on to write: "*When successive chancres are transmitted to an animal by inoculation, whatever the interval of their succession, or however they are combined, the first chancre occurs more rapidly, becomes bigger, produces more pus and is accompanied by greater inflammation than the second; the latter is to the third what the first is to the second, and so on, until the animal cannot contract any more. This animal is thus vaccinated against syphilis, that is, his state of health relative to syphilis is analogous to that in which we find ourselves relative to small-pox, after having been inoculated with the vaccine or having had the small-pox. I designate this state by the word syphilisation or the term syphilitic vaccination.*"[51] This was the start of the stormy history of syphilisation.

In a letter dated August 22, 1851, sent to the *Union médicale*, a medical newspaper well-known at the time, Auzias-Turenne explains: "*To describe what syphilisation is, I think of a hiker who covers the two sides of a mountain, first from the base to the summit, then from the summit to the base. He represents the person who is undergoing syphilisation. The chancres correspond to the different portions of the road travelled. Thus, the primary syphilitic sore, sign of constitutional syphilis, represents the top of the mountain, and syphilisation represents the end of the voyage. This traveller approaches constitutional syphilis when he has his first chancres. Once he has reached constitutional syphilis, he goes beyond it by having other chancres that take him to syphilisation. Therefore, in order to avoid constitutional syphilis, he must not stop half way.*"[52] This metaphor is very poetic, but unfortunately very far from reality. Auzias-Turenne even adds, in the same letter: "*The first chancres are the hardest.*" It would be tempting to add "*... and the most costly*".

In truth, the method was traumatic. It must have been hard to bear all those lesions. Nevertheless, a number of people, physicians among them, were willing to serve as guinea pigs. In his presentation before the French Academy of Medicine on August 10, 1852, Baron Hippolyte Larrey specifies: "*A commission has been named to learn the story of* M.L. *and understand all the consequences of his regrettable syphilomania...* M.L.'s

49. Auzias-Turenne, 1844, p. 916.
50. Lee *in* Copland, 1859, vol. IX, p. 1489.
51. Auzias-Turenne, 1850, p. 719.
52. Auzias-Turenne, 1851 (1856), p. 363.

appearence, all covered with voluntary ulcerations and provoked pustules, was a distressing sight. There (at the Society of Surgery), *as here, the state of this unfortunate colleague, excessive partisan, voluntary victim of syphilisation, was an example of this blind belief that transformed insane devotion into veritable suicide by the slow poison of syphilis.*"[53]

Because the duration of protection was unknown to him, Auzias-Turenne added: "*Who would want to oppose syphilitic revaccination, if it should prove necessary? These revaccinations would only require a few inoculations since their sole purpose would be to prolong a previously acquired immunity that should not be completely exhausted!*"[54] To which Ricord answered a little unkindly: "*If you have syphilis, it means you were not given enough!!!*"[55] But Auzias remained true to his humanitarian principles: "... *I do not intend to practice syphilisation if there are those who are forever safe from the contagion.*"[56]

Using pus from chancroid as "vaccine", because it is the only chancre reinoculable to the same person, "syphilisators" like Auzias-Turenne only created immunity (if indeed they were creating immunity) that was inadequate for syphilis. Auzias-Turenne started his experiments on animals, and with them he quickly reached the limit beyond which the chancres were no longer reinoculable. He "*thought that chancroids were a form of weak virulence syphilis*"[57]. It is true that some inoculated subjects showed a real resistance to subsequent inoculations, but this was not always the case and, in addition, it was a transient state. Finally, the most serious problem was that by inoculating from person to person "matter" not simply from chancres, but from mixed chancres (chancroid and primary syphilitic sore), or outright from syphilitic wounds, syphilis was transmitted to patients who only had chancroid disease, not syphilis.

Auzias-Turenne only performed a limited number of "syphilisations" in humans. On several occasions he tried to have access to hospital patients or to the prostitutes of Saint Lazare (Parisian prison for women serving short sentences), without success. But his confidence in his method was unshakable: "*All those who have any form of syphilis should be given syphilisation, he says: all prostitutes, all military and navy men, all those who spend their lives together in large numbers in jails, prisons, factories* (sic), *in short, all those who can be exposed o the contagion. Syphilis could be eliminated in the whole world through universal syphilisation...*"[58]. He was able to practice "syphilisation" on a small number of patients, including one described by Rollet: this patient had received pus from mucous patches (a true syphilitic lesion) and found himself, in a very bad way, in Ricord's Service. The latter had to employ great diplomacy to dissuade the victim from bringing Auzias-Turenne to justice[59].

Curative "syphilisation" was practiced mainly by two "syphiligraphs": Sperino and Boeck. Sperino, chief physician and surgeon at the Torino Syphilicome (Italy), inoculated a patient suffering from osteocopic pain, mucous patches and syphilids, with between sixty and eighty chancres in one session. A few cases of cure (?) encouraged Sperino to have great expectations. His book presents ninety-six observations made over a period of about two years. Sperino did not practice "syphilisation" on any

53. Larrey, 1852, p. 967.
54. Auzias-Turenne, 1851 (1856), p. 363.
55. Ricord, 1856, p. 372.
56. Auzias-Turenne, 1851 (1856), p. 363.
57. Jeanselme, 1931, p. 335.
58. Auzias-Turenne, 1867 (1884), p. 682.
59. Rollet *in* Dechambre, 1884, 3rd series, t. 14, p. 684.

healthy person. As to what he foresaw for the future, in his own words: "*The prostitutes who have already had syphilisation, and who will return to the hospital with a new venereal disease, will be given the syphilisation treatment again, that is, they will be revaccinated.*"[60] Unfortunately, these women subjected to "syphilisation" quickly suffered recurrences.

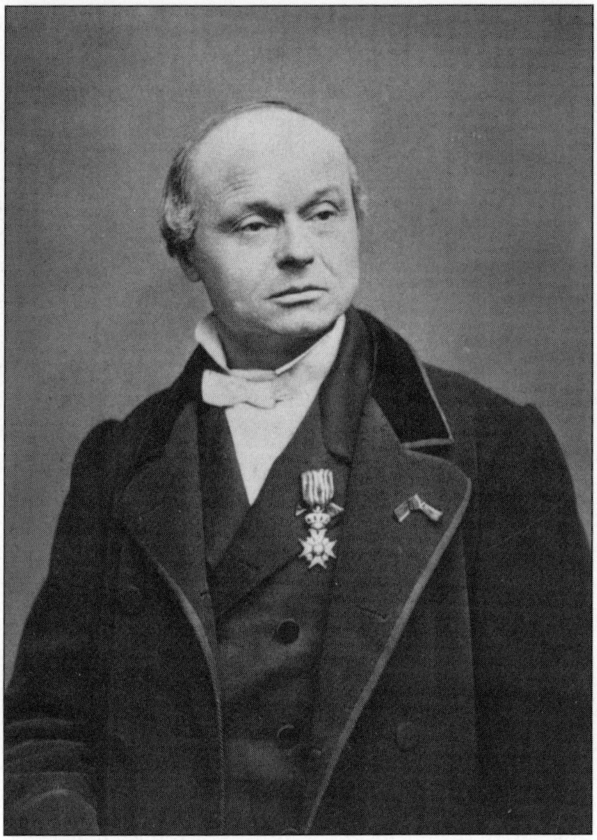

Figure 4. Portrait of Dr. Auzias-Turenne (1812-1870). Photo Goupil & Cie Editeurs à Paris, in *La Syphilisation*, Auzias's œuvre published thanks to his friends. Auzias-Turenne proudly wears "*the cross of the order of the polar star, awarded to him by the Norwegian government*", a decoration reserved to a very small number of dignitaries, since nominations were only made upon the demise of a bearer of the title. A drawing of this medal is etched in the tombstone of his grave at the Montparnasse cemetery in Paris. (Author's document.)

Carl Wilhelm Boeck, from Christiana (present-day Oslo, Norway), used the same curative syphilisation technique[61], and inoculated each of his patients between 96 and 700 times. Fournier quotes from Boeck's writings: "*To treat syphilis with syphilisation, I inoculated into the chest, the belly, the thighs and the arms. The smallest ulcers, in depth as well as in width, are obtained on the chest and the belly; (on the cheeks, where I inoculated to experiment, the effect is even weaker than on the chest); ulcers are larger on the arms; the biggest are on the thighs.*"[62] A similar text was published in *l'Union médicale*[63]. Ulcer induction experiments on the cheeks! Between October 1852 and July 1865, he performed syphilisation on 441 patients in Christiana, and at least 250 patients from his private practice.

60. Sperino, 1851, *in* Ricord, 1853a, p. 205; Sperino, 1853, p. 663.
61. Richelot, 1859, p. 731.
62. Boeck, 1874, p. 109.
63. Boeck, 1861a, p. 78.

Out of the 441 syphilisations performed before witnesses, 47 returned due to recurrence[64]. These data only cover a relatively short time, allowing no real perspective.

Boeck also established contact with the Anglo-Saxon world. He made at least one visit to England, where he treated twenty-one cases in four months[65]. The reports made by the physicians who witnessed Boeck's treatments are guarded. Henry Lee wrote, in 1866: "*There is little justification for repeating the dangerous experiment of inoculating a healthy individual with fluid from a pustule…*"[66]. "*We conclude… that the time needed to treat syphilis using this method* (syphilisation) *is so long, and the inconvenience associated with it are so great, that it should not be adopted, to any degree, in private practice in England.*"[67] However, Lane considered the method worthy of interest[68]. On the occasion of Auzias-Turenne's death, reference was made to "*Prof. Boeck who, at this very moment is travelling in America for the triumph of the idea Auzias-Turenne has brought to humanity*"[69]. What were the results of Boeck's voyage to America? In the work entitled A *Reference Handbook of the Medical Sciences*, published in New York, in 1888, syphilisation is described in these terms: "*The so-called process of 'syphilization' has not survived its brief period of notoriety. It was based upon a confusion respecting the nature of the syphilitic and the non-syphilitic sore, and is now not more than a curiosity in the literature of syphilis.*"[70]

Boeck was convinced that chancroids (soft sore) and primary syphilitic sores were identical, and that both were due to the same virus, with different strength (virulence): "*Chancroids, like primary sores, are the products of the same virus, but the different strengths of this virus produce the two forms. Chancroids are produced by the more energetic virus which, through its strength, develops an inflammation in its circumference, hindering absorption. Primary sores are produced by a less intense virus which does not develop an inflammation strong enough to stop absorption.*"[71] The other syphilisators held similar beliefs. This error was very regrettable, so much more so since Bassereau had distinguished the two diseases much earlier, in 1852.

It is difficult not to believe in a certain effectiveness of the treatment, given the very persuasive commentary circulating at the time, but the credulity of those who want to believe is sometimes limitless: "*The conclusions drawn by Dr. Boeck from eighty-four cases of syphilization, which he has treated up to March, 1856, are : 1st, that in all cases, without exception, immunity to the venereal virus is obtained, sooner or later, by inoculation of the poison; 2d, that the symptoms of syphilis present at the commencement of syphilization disappear during the employment of this mode of treatment; 3d, that the general health does not suffer in the least from syphilization; on the contrary, if the patient has been in weak health before inoculation, he most materially improves in strength and appearance during the process. These propositions are conceded as undoubted facts by Dr. Boeck's collegues, by Dr. Sperino, by M. A Turenne, by Danielsen, by Dr. Carlsson, and by Dr. Stenberg of Stockohm.*"[72] It must be stressed that the syphilis treatments of that era were dangerous, and their effectiveness uncertain.

64. Boeck, 1866, p. 212.
65. Lane, 1866, p. 171.
66. Lee, 1866a, p. 160.
67. Lee, 1866b, p. 165.
68. Lane, 1866, p. 171.
69. d'Anceny, 1878, p. XXI.
70. Hyde, 1888, p. 709.
71. Anonyme, 1864, p. 22.
72. Lee *in* Copland, 1859, vol. IX, p. 1489.

Several physicians, most of them French and Italian, also tried the method on themselves or on a small number of patients: Melchior Robert, Sirus-Pirondi, Simpson, Rodet, Turenne, Fouquet, Thirry, Gamberini from Bologna, Gulligo in Florence, Mottini (from Genoa), C. Riva, Caire (from Novara), Arena (from Torino), Flarer (from Pavia), Sigmund (from Vienna), as well as Scandinavian physicians: Boeck, Faye, Danielsen in Bergen, Bidenkap in Norway, Hjort, Wildhagen, Sternberg and Carlsson in Stockholm, Kalischer (Berlin)...[73] but their results were no better. And yet there was no lack of attempts... "*... The famous example of the courageous experimentator Lindmann, who inoculated himself with over 2700 chancroids...*"[74]. A German physician, suffering from a persistent case of syphilis, inoculated himself with over two thousand two hundred chancres, but without any tangible result[75]. Perhaps the two are one and the same man. Of course, no immunity was transferred to any of these inoculated subjects. Danielsen successfully inoculated syphilis to a patient using 287 chancres of chancroid pus. Five months later, the time required for all the chancres to evolve and scar, the same person received two inoculations of syphilitic chancre material (wound?) and developed constitutional syphilis in four weeks[76].

In France, Marchal (from Calvi) took up (and then was forbidden to practice) this treatment at Val-de-Grâce. In his presentation to the Academy of Medicine (Paris) on August 10, 1852, Larrey expressed his opposition to medical experimentation in military hospitals, without the authorisation of the Minister of War, and only if a proposal was made by the Board of Health[77]. On the other hand, Seutin, who was consulted by the Prefect of Police, expressed a favourable opinion.

Syphilisation continued to have advocates for many years: "*A remarkable thesis on syphilisation has just been defended before the Paris Faculty of Medicine, under the presidency of professor Nélaton, by Mr. Henri Guérault... yesterday's absurdity has become a scientific truth that was demonstrated today; and this result is due, above all, to the research conducted by Mr. Sperino, from Torino, and by Prof. W. Boeck, from the University of Christiania. Prince Napoleon, witness to the successes obtained by Mr. Boeck, awarded him the* Légion d'Honneur... *The judges were unanimous to congratulate the candidate for his courage to examine such a controversial subject, and for the talent he has shown in the accomplishment of his task. The honourable professors, and particularly Mr. Depaul and Mr. Nétalon, showed themselves favourable to syphilisation...*"[78]. Not to be outdone, the Norwegian government awarded the "polar Star", a decoration of great distinction, to Dr. Auzias-Turenne[79]. These gestures of courtesy, in a context such as this, show the limits of political attitudes in medical matters.

In contrast, opponents of this doubtful practice, from the very beginning, were many. On August 10, 1852, Begin concluded his presentation to the Academy of Medicine by saying: "*Considering all that is hideous, compromising, dangerous about syphilisation for the present and the future of individuals and their descendants, it is difficult to understand that this operation could have found a mind to conceive it, fanatics to submit to it, physicians*

73. Copland, 1859, vol. IX, p. 1489; Belhomme, 1864, p. 86; Boeck, 1861b, p. 330; Rollet *in* Dechambre, 1884, 3rd series, t. 14, p. 688; Sperino, 1853a & b.
74. Fournier, 1874, p. 118.
75. Belhomme, 1864, p. 85.
76. Rollet *in* Dechambre, 1884, 3rd series, t. 14, p. 685.
77. Larrey, 1852, p. 967.
78. Rambosson, 1857, p. 327.
79. d'Anceny, 1878, p. XI.

to perform it."[80] Ricord was probably the most determined. Dubois-Havenith concluded his review of syphilisation by saying: "*We should be grateful to Ricord for putting an end to the zeal of the Italian syphilisator* (Sperino) *and his followers. For at the rate things were going, the whole of Europe would soon have been infected with syphilis.*"[81]

Auzias-Turenne was no doubt a well-meaning man. He believed in his method. He asked to be autopsied after his death. The anterosuperior and lateral portions of his thighs bore numerous scars from the chancre inoculations he had given himself. Broca and Verneuil were present at his autopsy[82]. Auzias-Turenne's followers were most probably sincere, but thoughtless and careless. To make a judgement concerning syphilisators, one must read at least a portion of the enormous amount of literature written for or against them. In one of his syphilisation lessons, Auzias-Turenne provides a glimpse of the attributes that were used to describe him. He is speaking of a physician, opposed to his work but respectful of a colleague: "*He did not threaten, denounce or accuse me. He did not ignore, disdain, repulse, condemn, prohibit, humiliate, banish, shame, insult, blacken, hoot, boo, flout, decry, denigrate, abuse, defame, execrate, tear apart, offend, abase, curse, calumniate, vilify, abominate, exorcise, damn, despise, poison, embitter, debase, dishonour, stigmatise my name. He did not call me a foolish, stupid, ridiculous, absurd, visionary, temperamental, obsessed, impertinent, ignorant, deceptive, lying, bragging, fraudulent, phony, insane, mad, extravagant, rambling, careless, immoral, deceitful, swindling, hypocritical, mischievous man or (historical) thief*"[83]. Language is resourceful.

At least three commissions were named to study syphilisation: one by the medico-surgical Academy of Torino, on May 23, 1851; another by the Paris Academy of Medicine; and a third by the Prefect of Police of the Seine Department. On August 21, 1852, the Academy of Medicine accepted unanimously, with two abstentions (Depaul and Malgaigne) the conclusions of the commission's report, which were opposed to syphilisation. According to Dr. Richelot, French translator of John Hunter's work, the conclusions of the Torino commission were unfavourable to syphilisation as well.

The theory that defended this treatment method was erroneous: it confused chancroid, which was easily inoculable, with primary syphilitic sores, which could not be inoculated to the same subject. Around this time, the confusion ended. Syphilisators found it hard to admit their mistake. On the other hand, the transfer of syphilitic matter to healthy individuals was very likely, and clearly occurred several times, with disastrous consequences.

All these efforts came to an end rather quickly. By 1852, Auzias-Turenne himself changed his mind, so it seems, about the advisability of subjecting all persons living in a community to syphilisation[84]. In the 1870s and 1880s, no one believed in it any more. Fournier speaks of "*monstruous practices of syphilisation… Let us condemn the culpable experiments in which, for the sake of speculative research, syphilis was needlessly and with no excuse transmitted to healthy subjects… Hetero-inoculation should be forbidden in the name of the simplest, most elementary morality.*"[85]

80. Begin *in* Ricord, 1853, p. 110.
81. Dubois-Havenith, 1891, p. 604.
82. Jeanselme, 1931, p. 337.
83. Auzias-Turenne, 1852, p. 401
84. Auzias-Turenne, 1853, p. 35.
85. Fournier, 1874, pp. 118, 119 & 131.

What is somewhat surprising for physicians of this stature, is that judgement about syphilisation was strongly determined, or at least influenced, by philosophical principles rather than scientific facts. Two positivists, Littré and Robin, quoted in the 1855 edition of Nysten's Medical Dictionary (Nysten died in 1817, but his name stayed on a few subsequent editions) had this to say: "*Until now, the practice of syphilisation as a treatment method has been rejected as being more dangerous than useful considering the syphilis treatment methods offered by current medical practice. But from a scientific perspective, it should be noted that immunity against new chancres, despite an impure coitus or inoculation, seems entirely proven by Boeck and Sperino's confirming experiments... Syphilisation corresponds to the state of a person following vaccinal eruption or smallpox eruption.*"[86] However, they believe that, despite everything, it should be rejected as a preventive method, but studied more closely as a curative method. In 1866, in the 12th edition of the Dictionary, the entry on "Syphilisation" is twice as long, stating specifically: "*In Sweden and Norway, syphilisation has become a common practice in hospitals and private offices*"; the authors even present the good results (*sic*) obtained. From 1873 (13th edition) to 1886 (16th edition), these authors repeat the same message, while making some changes to the text. In the meantime, Littré and Robin both died and their Medical Dictionary was taken over by others. In 1893 (17th edition) the entry on syphilisation is considerably shorter. The method is said to have limited application, but is still considered useful. When Gilbert became editor of the Capuron-Nysten-Littré Medical Dictionary in 1908, the entry disappeared. He mentioned the method, but prohibited its use in humans.

An entire body of literature exists as well on the subject of the moral problems posed by protection against syphilis. For example, on syphilis prevention: "*We shall do it without regard for the scruples of certain persons who, for lack of knowledge, and no doubt based on observation, believe that fear of syphilis stops libertine behaviour, and as a result consider immoral any attempt to protect against this disease. They would be well advised to think of the women, children and other innocent persons who fall victim to the faults of others every day.*"[87] But absolute protection was considered even worse: "*In our opinion, syphilisation* (preventive) *is immoral! To give it to a child, a young man or an adult, is an invitation to debauchery, it is to make him invulnerable, provide him with a talisman that allows him to succumb without fear to all the ignominious behaviour and degradation of those who surrender to the pleasures of the flesh... Finally, should girls be given syphilisation? This unprovoked insult to their future conduct and to the morality of their husbands is profoundly revolting. Proper conduct is the best syphilisation.*"[88] Today, the same opinions are being expressed about AIDS.

Obviously, syphilisation gave rise to very serious hopes that are hard to understand today. In the Copland's Medical Dictionary, Charles A. Lee wrote, in 1859: "*I have given this account of syphilization as it is hardly known in this country* (United States). *It is manifest that it could not be rationally submitted to, but as a cure of the distemper, and not by a healthy person to prevent the infection of it. If, however, it be found to be by farther experience, not only a permanent cure, but also a permanent preventive, it will establish for itself a reputation not possessed by any other means...*"[89].

86. Nysten 1855, p. 1227.
87. Cullerier, 1843, p. 64.
88. Valleix, 1860, t. 1, p. 414.
89. Lee *in* Copland, 1859, vol. IX, p. 1492.

The second antisyphilitic vaccination campaign, much more modest, originated from the ideas of Diday, chief physician at the Antiquaille hospice in Lyon. As far as we know, Diday was the first to use the word "vaccination" in 1849 for an inoculation other than the cowpox-vaccine.

Diday had many patients to treat. Knowing that "constitutional" syphilis does not infect the same patient twice, and that it is enough to have "*a slight lesion, a few sheeppox pustules, a single vaccinal button, to prevent forever the onset of disease in an individual*"[90], Diday chose the blood of syphilitics in the tertiary stage, using them as donors to prevent infection in other patients. On June 26, 1848, he chose, rather than healthy men, "*for in that case validation of my trial would have to wait for a chance event that might be long in coming or might never come*"[91], sixteen patients with primary chancres (fifteen chancroids and one syphilitic sore). "*I made the tertiary patient lie down in an office separate from the rooms. With a scalpel, I made an incision about one centimetre long... The blood seemed red and pure. Immediately, I brought the donor into the next room where I had gathered the patients, with their arms already uncovered. As each one approached, I dipped a lancet into the bleeding wound of the tertiary, and I inoculated this blood into the same part of the left arm, and in the same manner, as for ordinary vaccine... The operation, whose aim I explained to them briefly, was accepted by them all with confidence, with the exception of one, whose resistance I could only overcome by first inoculating myself, before him, with an injection in the left hand.*"[92] Locally, the effects of these inoculations were "*just about insignificant*"[93]. Chancres and bubos (adenopathy, that is, inflammation of the corresponding lymph node) resolved normally. "*I noted carefully the name and address of my inoculated patients before letting them leave the hospital; then I gave them a signed promise to pay a small sum, six weeks later, if they came back at that time to be examined, and brought it back to me. Finally, to be sure they would come back themselves, I noted for each of them a small personal trait... such as a sign, a scar, a tatoo on the arm...*"[94]. "*Vaccination results*" after eight months were perfect, none of the patients developed syphilis, except one who had a primary syphilitic sore at the time of inoculation; he developed constitutional syphilis. It is not certain that mercury treatment could have changed the course of the disease. "*Despite the obvious impropriety of the expression, from an etymological point of view, I called my operation antisyphilitic vaccination.*"[95]

Diday was somewhat carried away by his success (?): "*As, on the one hand, a single syphilitic can serve to vaccinate thousands of bearers of syphilitic chancre, and as it is never indispensable to vaccinate them right away, we could and we should imitate the method used for vaccination against small-pox, and proceed by batches... Only, to be truly honest, I believe that certain tertiaries would willingly use their disease for profit. Like the beggars who refuse to let their disgusting infirmities heal, so that they can exhibit them to us, they would no doubt prefer to conserve the valuable remnants of a poison for whose every drop science, love of health and the philanthropic concern of hospital administrators are apparently eager to pay the highest price.*"[96]

---

90. Diday, 1849, p. 5.
91. Diday, 1849, p. 15.
92. Diday, 1849, p. 17.
93. Diday, 1849, p. 18.
94. Diday, 1849, p. 19.
95. Diday, 1849, p. 26.
96. Diday, 1849, p. 38.

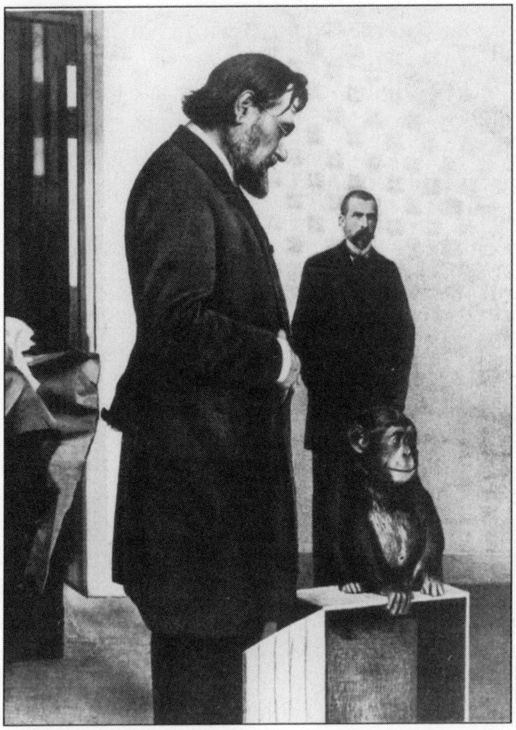

Figure 5. Drs. Roux and Metchnikoff at the Academy of Medicine, presenting the little monkey to which they succeeded in transmitting syphilis; the Beris Prize was awarded to them for this work. The little monkey presents a "beautiful lesion" *(une belle avarie)*, as was said at the time. This transmission of syphilis to an animal model raised hopes of treatment or prevention. Metchnikoff seems puzzled, Roux seems a little distant, reserved. Only the little monkey seems at ease. (*La Vie Illustrée*, no. 251, August 7, 1903.) (Author's document.)

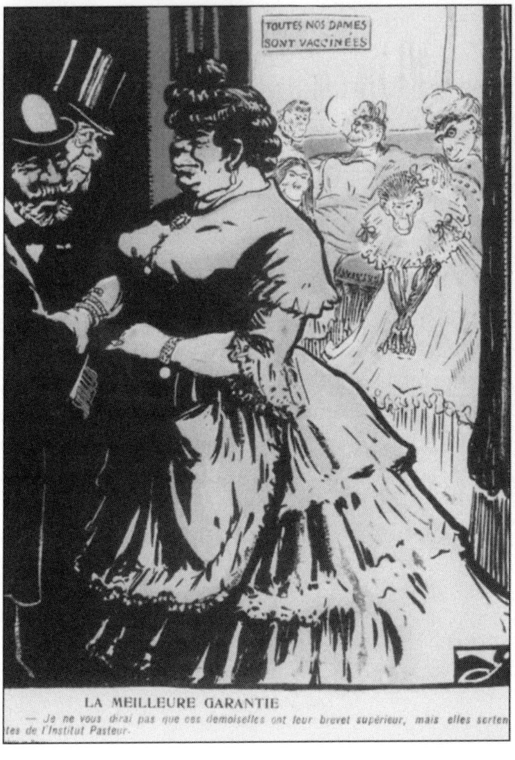

LA MEILLEURE GARANTIE

— Je ne vous dirai pas que ces demoiselles ont leur brevet supérieur, mais elles sortent de l'Institut Pasteur.

Figure 6. Caricature illustrating a certain interpretation of Roux and Metchnikoff's work on the syphilis of chimpanzees! The caption reads: "*THE BEST TESTIMONIAL: I cannot say that these young ladies have earned their diplomas, but they all come out of the* Institut Pasteur (where they were vaccinated)", as is written on the wall. (*L'Assiette au beurre*, no. 207, March 18, 1905.) (Author's document.)

It is likely that Diday's vaccination served no purpose; patients with chancroids were not syphilitic and, fortunately, the blood of the tertiary syphilitic patient he used as donor was not infected. This movement, not to call it a school, did not last long. Diday seems not to have had students. These efforts gave rise to various comments, particularly by Ricord, his old master, who on several occasions employed the term used by Diday himself, that is, "vaccination", in a polite manner that nevertheless clearly revealed his assessment of the value of this method: "*This vaccination, which has nothing in common with the other* (that of Auzias-Turenne), *is the dream of a well-meaning man; he is a scholar who wandered off, but who did no one any harm.*"[97]

Roux and Metchnikoff took a special interest in syphilis. They had the opportunity to contaminate monkeys and then rabbits, and to obtain infectious material from them. They achieved some protective effects. A laboratory assistant, who took care of the monkeys used in experiments, noticed that he had a small lesion on his lip. It seemed not to be syphilitic in nature. Yet three chimpanzees inoculated with samples from this lesion revealed its syphilitic character. But neither the assistant nor the monkeys developed secondary lesions. Roux and Metchnikoff concluded that the strain of Treponema employed was probably attenuated by its passage into monkeys. Later, they inoculated a Treponema strain passed in succession to five monkeys, to a consenting 79-year old man who had never had syphilis. The lesion he developed was a small local sore, with no general symptoms[98]. This test in a human being is surprising. Roux's behaviour in this instance is hard to reconcile with the long speeches on his hesitation (even refusal) to participate in the Pasteurian treatment of Joseph Meister... But years had passed since then! Today, it is unlikely that a vaccine against syphilis will be developed; work on satisfactory medical treatment has replaced the search for a vaccine.

Humans and Animals Are Inoculated (Variolated) with Almost Anything

Over the centuries, a great number of infectious diseases known to give long-term protection have been identified. Some have been inoculated. Perusal of the literature reveals traces of these experiments.

In Animals

In veterinary medicine, the inoculation of infectious diseases is said to be a very ancient custom in Africa and perhaps in Asia. Europeans adopted it willingly for sheeppox. During a great epizootic, 65,000 ovine animals were subjected to this immunisation method. In flocks that were not inoculated, about two thirds of the animals died; in inoculated flocks, only one third died[99]. In 1887, an English consul, Payton, described a somewhat similar method of inoculation: the insertion of a fragment of infected lung into a slit made on the ear of a goat. This practice was used in Morocco to avoid a contagious caprine pleuropneumonia called "*Bayoor*"[100]. Basset reported the use of

97. Ricord, 1856, p. 400.
98. Zinsser, 1918, p. 511.
99. Hutcheon, 1881, 1889; Borrel, 1903, p. 732.
100. Anonymous, 1887a, p. 227.

"variolation" to fight against swine pox in piglets, pustular stomatitis of small ruminants and avian pox[101].

In Tanzania, ruminants anthrax also became the object of a sort of vaccination (variolation?) consisting of injecting a concoction of tissue from animals killed by anthrax into the neck muscles of the animals to be protected[102]. Inoculation of catarrhal angina in horses did not give positive results. Finally, attempts made to prevent puppy distemper by inoculation were not very successful[103].

Inoculation of foot-and-mouth disease of hoofed animals, or "aphtisation", was used throughout the 19th century as a method of protection when the infection was already present in a stable. According to Ercolani, the first to use this method, in 1810, was Buvina of Turin, who also proved that it was possible to inoculate the disease using the saliva dribble of infected animals. The inoculation of the disease "*has the advantage of reducing the duration of the disease in a stable, and of moderating its intensity*"[104].

In Humans

On March 21, 1758, Dr. Home of the College of Edinburgh was the first (?) to inoculate measles in both arms, with no preparation, to twelve patients, protecting them from pulmonary accidents[105]. Many other authors agree that "artificial" measles is benign[106], but this method does not seem to have been used very much.

Valleix reports that preventive scarlet fever inoculation was proposed by Lehman and Mr. Miguel d'Amboise, in case of an epidemic, but the value of this method remains obscure[107].

In 1782-1783, Samoïlowitz sent several dissertations to the Academy of Dijon, proposing the inoculation of human plague as a method of prevention. The perpetual Secretary of the Academy, Dr. Maret, a man of great scientific and moral discernment, replied that the Academy appreciated his dissertations, but had reservations about the one dealing with human plague. In his long and determined answer, Samoïlowitz insisted on the fact that the plague is only transmitted by contact and does not recur in the same subject[108]. In fact, Dr. Samoïlowitz expresses his own hesitation about clinical testing: "*But who will be the first two to consent, one to be subjected to, the other to practice, the inoculation against the plague? When it* (the plague) *will have multiplied its murders, the government will be well-advised to designate a healthy criminal who, being condemned to death, will no doubt be happy to undergo this test in exchange for his life! As to the operator, I doubt that among physicians and surgeons there will not be one of these friends of humanity who will seize such a perfect opportunity to serve it, and to have his name immortalised. I dare to offer that I, myself, inoculate such a volunteer, if I am to treat plague sufferers again.*"[109] Samoïlowitz was made associate member of the Academy of Dijon, a distinction granted for the first time to a Russian. He was obviously overjoyed. The

101. Basset, 1936, p. 5.
102. Bizimana, 1994, p. 410.
103. Hurtrel d'Arboval, 1875, v. 2, p. 314; Rochard, 1888, p. 488.
104. Ercolani, 1858, p. 473.
105. Home, 1759, p. 253.
106. Buchan, 1802, t. 2, p. 320; Netter, 1903, t. VI, p. 777; Rosen de Rosenstein, 1778, p. 275; Stoll, 1809, p. 158; Tissot, 1768, p. 390; Valleix, 1860, t. 1, p. 182.
107. Netter, 1903, t. VI, p. 777; Valleix, 1860, t. 1, p. 211.
108. Samoïlowitz, 1782 & 1783.
109. Samoïlowitz, 1782, p. 12.

inoculation against the plague does not seem to have been pursued much further. Dr. Whyte died of the plague in Egypt, after having inoculated the disease into himself in an unfortunate "variolation" experiment. Blancou reports that in 1788 Eusebio Valli inoculated bovine plague into a man in order to protect him from human plague[110].

Inoculation of the yellow fever was proposed by Mr. de Humblot (also spelled Humboldt) in Cuba. The method, which used the venom of an ophidian, an indigenous snake, provoked symptoms presenting "*an analogy with those of yellow fever*"[111]. However, an official enquiry found a total lack of effectiveness, a fact that did not shake the conviction of partisans of the method[112]. Bérenger-Féraud testifies that inhabitants of Cuba and Mexico living in the interior sent their children to yellow fever zones on the coast to immunise them against this disease through a benign form[113].

In 1799, Valli from Livourne proposed a preventive treatment of rabies: a mixture of saliva from a dog with rabies, and of gastric juice from a frog. He claimed that inoculating this preparation had prevented rabies in dogs, and even cured two people bitten by dogs with rabies[114].

A benign skin disease, common in hot climates in the past, caused by a microscopic parasite called *Leishmania tropica*, described by Almroth Edward Wright, bore the name Oriental sore, Delhi boil or Biskara boil. Although it is benign and heals by itself, in most cases it leaves very ugly scars, especially on the face. Manson says that "*in general, a first attack is not followed by a recurrence. Having noted this fact, the Jews of Baghdad, in a certain period, practiced inoculation of the Oriental sore on their young children*"[115].

Most preventive inoculations were performed keeping in mind the welfare of the inoculated individuals. However, the truth is that some hazardous experiments were conducted on humans, and often on children. For example, Abilgaard and Wiborg inoculated smallpox to several animal species, unsuccessfully, and then to a monkey who presented the characteristic signs of the disease. The monkey experienced violent diarrhea and when he died: "*We inoculated small-pox matter from this monkey to three children: this inoculation produced no effect.*"[116]

Conclusion

The idea of immunisation was already familiar: "*Small-Pox inoculation prepared the way for vaccination; it is the introduction of the first that accustomed us to expose ourselves to a small danger to avoid a greater one, and taught us to calculate the probabilities of the outcomes of natural and inoculated Small-Pox, based on a more precise method, that was more suitable to our true interests. Therefore, the advent of inoculation will remain a memorable episode in the history of medicine and philosophy.*"[117] The association of variolation and vaccination prepared the way for the Pasteurian adventure.

110. Blancou, 2003, p. 161.
111. Manzini *in* Onghena, 1858, p. 194.
112. Guérin, 1863, p. 834; Sternberg, 1895, p. 313.
113. Leger, 1928, p. 970.
114. Blancou, 2003, p. 193.
115. Manson, 1908, p. 561.
116. Abildgaard, letter dated 1791 (1813).
117. Domenjon, 1801, p. 5.

Several fundamental elements of immunology and vaccinology were observed and reported as early as the eighteenth and nineteenth centuries: i) the use of a mitigated virus (Pessina, around 1800), that is, a virus with diminished virulence, created by man, for the purpose of variolating with smaller losses; ii) the particular susceptibility of the young to infections, for a certain period after birth: "*When inoculations in animals are practiced while they are still suckling, they usually produce complete effects; this does not happen when they are inoculated as adults or in old age*"[118]; iii) temporary immunity of young animals born of an immune mother, as Reinders discovered around 1770... However, the existence of immune defences of individuals against pathogenic agents was still unknown.

The role of the State in the protection of citizen from infectious diseases became defined slowly, over time. Working conditions in vaccine Services were often quite mediocre, despite their obvious usefulness. These Services represent, after all, one of the first attempts at individual preventive medicine, organised by the society.

The dream of a vaccine associated with every infectious disease was alive in many people's minds. Bourguignon pleaded for the discovery of a typhoid fever "vaccine", that he believed had to be looked for in cows... His argument ends with the statement: "*... The inoculation practiced to prevent sheeppox and contagious bovine pneumonia can serve to encourage us.*"[119] These are the two best-known classical examples in veterinary medicine, that were most discussed in the literature. In fact, these are examples of "variolation", not of "vaccination" on the model of Jenner or Pasteur. Variolation against various infectious diseases by inoculation of living pathogenic agents failed. This practice virtually disappeared with the arrival of the vaccines of the Pasteurian era. In veterinary medicine, some examples still exist, but they are marginal. A good vaccine is one which is effective and has no side effects.

History is disconcerting: just about the time when (give or take a few years) smallpox inoculation reached its fullest development, it was caused to compete with Jennerian vaccination, which disposed of it. This vaccination then went on to achieve such effectiveness and safety that the need for its use was eliminated! Both the "variolation" and the "vaccination" whose target was smallpox were discarded due to their success. This is the fate of effective methods... At the end of the nineteenth century, Louis Pasteur caused a great upheaval in vaccinology. He was not the only one, of course, but his work and especially his renown, and later that of his team, played a crucial role.

118. Sacco, 1813, p. 389.
119. Bourguignon, 1855, p. 544.

II
Pasteur and Vaccines

5
The Chicken Cholera Vaccine

"Science appears calm and triumphant when it is completed, but science in the making is only contradiction and torment, hope and disappointment."
Emile Roux.
Unveiling ceremony of Pasteur Monument in Dole, August 3, 1902.

When Pasteur embarked on the study of infectious diseases, he was already very familiar with micro-organisms and their culture, thanks to his experiments in spontaneous generation, and fermentation and from his search for the pathogens involved in silk-worm disease. Pasteur's view of micro-organism was very broad and not limited just to vaccine development. His interests ranged from anthrax in ruminants to puerperal fever, to furuncles in humans and a great deal in between. Given this breadth of experience and expertise it was therefore not surprising that Pasteur should have received a sample of chicken cholera bacteria from Pr. Henry Toussaint of the Toulouse Veterinary School, who had just discovered, or rather rediscovered the disease... and its causative agent.

Toussaint had heard of Pasteur's interest in his new bacteria from Henri Bouley, and spared no effort in feeding his research[1]. Several samples were sent to Pasteur's laboratory, but on receipt no infectious germ was detectable. As it turns out, this is because the bacteria had died in transit, before arriving at Pasteur's laboratory. Finally, on October 30, 1878, Pasteur received a viable sample. The sample was "*the heart of a young rooster who died after being inoculated with the anthrax of poultry*"[2], and it clearly revealed a new pathogen, namely chicken cholera, now called *Pasteurella multocida.*

The vaccine that resulted from Pasteur's subsequent work on chicken cholera has the distinction of being the first *de-novo* vaccine. Unlike the unaltered smallpox of variolation or the cowpox of Jenner's vaccination it was the result of further manipulation of the original pathogen. It therefore takes a place of great significance in the history of vaccines alongside cowpox. It is because of its significance in the historical development of vaccinology that the chicken cholera vaccine deserves close examination.

Pasteur's laboratory notebooks are very scrambled, written in very small handwriting that is hard to decipher. There are deletions, and additions that sometimes, but not always, bear dates, and which are sometimes, but not always, recognizable by a change in pen or ink. Each experiment usually takes up one page although it can be on several

1. NAF 18011, f.P. 4 & 13.
2. NAF 18011, f.P. 71.

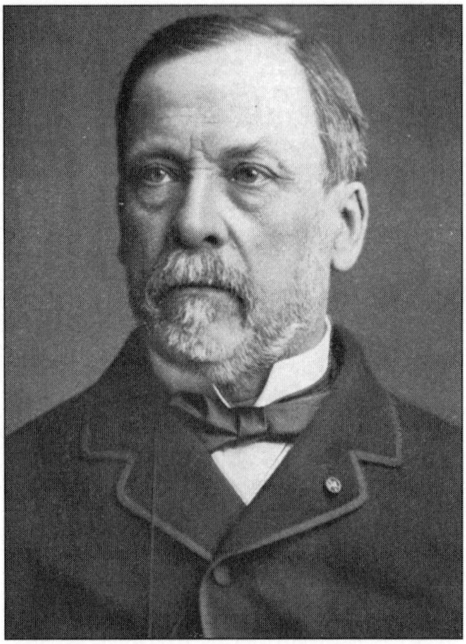

Figure 1. Louis Pasteur in 1884, at age 62, when he was working on vaccines. Photo Petersen og son, Copenhagen[3].

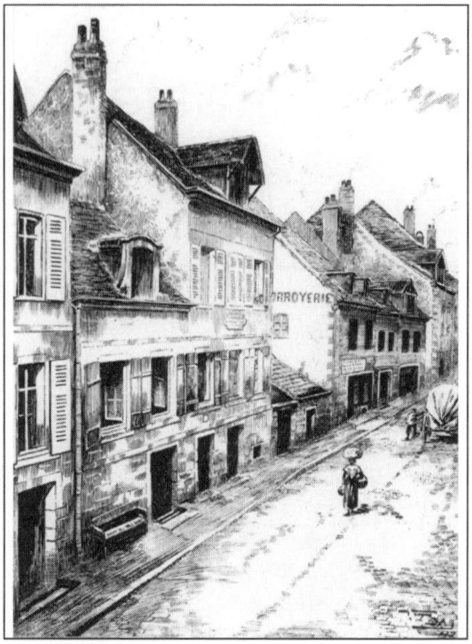

Figure 2. The house where Pasteur was born, with the modest commemorative plaque visible... Engraving published on the occasion of Pasteur's jubilee. *Le Patriote illustré*, November 8, 1893.

pages. Each new page is inserted into the same notebook or into the next, on the first available page. Each experiment is referred to by its page number, and is then described day by day in lengthy passages given in sequence.

As a result the interpretation of Pasteur's notes can be very difficult. For this reason, I have provided many verbatim quotations, keeping in mind the remark made by Noah Webster in 1799: "*I have discovered that many of the histories or rather abridgements and compilations which are almost the only authorities consulted by American readers in general are very incomplete; and no man who relies on them only, and neglects original writers, can acquire an accurate and comprehensive knowledge of history.*"[4]

It is worth starting with some of the codes used by Pasteur in his notebooks.

A new animal: one that has not yet been used in an experiment;

a pig: a guinea pig;

s.l.p.: subcutaneous;

ser.: syringe;

X^{bre}: the month of December.

In Pasteur's texts, always quoted herein in italics, the difficult-to-read words are given in parentheses and in Roman script, with a question mark, to stress their uncertainty. For example, (since?). Illegible words sometimes limited to a horizontal trait, are indicated

3. Thomsen, 1992.
4. Webster, 1799, p. 23.

(1 word). Page references marked "f.P." for "folio Pasteur" refer to page numbers inscribed by Pasteur, since he refers back to these numbers, and not to the printed notebook page numbers*. Where there is no special annotation, Pasteur refers back to pages of the same notebook or register; where there is, he indicates the page and the notebook. The number system of the French national library (*Bibliothèque nationale de France*), that contains thousands of documents, is obviously not the same as Pasteur's. Thus, Pasteur's 6th notebook is designated NAF 18011, to indicate "*Nouvelles acquisitions françaises*" (number) 18011; the 7th notebook: NAF 18012, and so on. Pasteur's writings on a single subject, most often bearing a date and sometimes even the hour, can be very dispersed in the notebooks. For example, in a paragraph shortly hereafter, I will present two quotes, one from the 6th notebook: March 3, 1879[5] and another from the 8th notebook: March 10, 1879[6]. Pasteur filled his notebooks very carefully, but in a precise order (disorder?), with numerous references. My own annotations in a quote are given in parentheses and in Roman script, to be clearly differentiated from Pasteur's writing. The Anglophone literature of the period also provides lengthy analyses of Pasteur's texts[7].

The Culture of the Chicken Cholera Germ: 1879

It is worth being clear upfront that chicken cholera (*Pasteurella multocida*) is totally unrelated to cholera (*Vibrio cholera*) in humans. Chicken cholera has limited economic interest as an infectious disease, compared to many other animal pathologens, however it provided Pasteur with a good model. It is a microorganism that transmitted a disease which was fatal in almost 100% of cases, in just a few hours, in a susceptible species such as a chicken. It was easy to buy lots of thirty to fifty chickens and roosters at the market. Because of the high case fatality rate there would be expected to be very few immune birds in the lots and because of the short incubation period there would be few apparently healthy birds incubating the bacteria. Finally and most importantly, there were only three infectious diseases, known at the time which were caused by pathogens that were visible under a light microscope: anthrax in ruminants and less often in humans, chicken cholera and acute experimental (laboratory) septicemia. Pasteur was no doubt very glad to have all three of them for his experiments.

The Extraordinary Discovery of the Chicken Cholera Vaccine: 1879-1880

When Pasteur received the "Toussaint germ" (this name did not persist for long in his notes, because his study of the literature revealed that this organism had already been described), he was only moderately interested. He continued his ongoing projects: septicemia, puerperal fever, and anthrax... In 1898, Duclaux reported: "*It was in the process of this research that he* (Pasteur) *noticed for the first time, in the septic vibrio, the virulence variations that have since acquired such importance.*"[8]

* To the knowledge of the present author, Pasteur, or his associates, or members of his family, did not remove pages from the laboratory notebooks covering the "vaccine" years. The notebooks are intact, with the original page numbers (printed) complete.

5. NAF 18011, f.P. 85.
6. NAF 18013, f.P. 1.
7. Williams, 1886, p. 549.
8. Duclaux, 1898, t. 1, p.51.

Pasteur's work on the septic vibrio was published in April 1878, as part of his famous lecture on the *Germ Theory*: "... *It is the ease with which the septic vibrio can multiply without showing the least movement, associated with a great reduction in virulence, although the latter is not absent... In our study of natural septicemia, we encountered a single vibrio, that our culture media can cause to change form, ease of propagation and virulence... We were able to bring the last cultures back to their initial virulence by changing the culture medium.*"[9] However, no vaccine was present at this stage, because strains varied with culture media; but Pasteur was already thinking of vaccination, as Roux points out: "*This question of immunity is essential throughout the history of infectious diseases; Pasteur continually returned to it in his experiments; he was always aware of it... As soon as we started to work in his laboratory, Pasteur often repeated to Chamberland* (entered the laboratory in 1875 or 1876) *and to me* (entered in 1878): *'We must immunise against the infectious diseases whose viruses we grow in culture.'*"[10] Starting with his earliest chicken cholera experiments, Pasteur often used the word "vaccination" in his laboratory notebooks; on March 3, 1879, he wrote: "*Have these meals vaccinated it?*"[11] Then, on March 10, 1879: "*Possible vaccination of the chickens...*"[12]. But he had no clear idea yet of the technique that might be used to vaccinate. However, he grew more and more enthusiastic about this microbe whose study would allow him to master the phenomenon of vaccination, in the sense given to the word by Pasteur.

As soon as he received the microbe sample, at the end of 1878, Chamberland inoculated two chickens. They were found dead the next morning[13]. This confirmed the virulence of the pathogen. The microbial strain was kept alive by successively inoculating chickens. At the same time he tried to culture it, without success in yeast culture medium (yeast water).

- **Finally, on January 15, 1879**, Pasteur wrote: "*We now have a culture medium for these little organisms.*"[14] It was, in fact, chicken broth. The resulting culture was inoculated into chickens that subsequently died. This was an important stage.
- **On January 20, 1879**, the team prepared two flasks of chicken broth, using diseased muscles (from the site of inoculation) and uninfected muscles from the opposite side of the same bird. The culture from the "diseased" flask did not develop; the team noted that this culture was considerably acid compared to the "healthy" flask[15]. **Pasteur's interest was drawn by the acidity of the culture medium, not a medium exposed to air, but a chicken broth whose composition itself was acid.**
- **February 15, 1879.** Pasteur applied to the chicken cholera bacilli the same approach he had taken with the anthrax bacteria to investigate: the mechanism of transmission of the microbe from one animal to another. In 1975, Wrotnowska wrote: "*In February 1879, Pasteur entitled an entry in his laboratory notebook: 'Study of the influence of food with Toussaint microbe on chickens.' On February 15, 1879, 2 chickens are placed in two cages and fed bread (12 to 20 small pieces) moistened with fluid from the microbial culture... Eugène (Viala, his assistant) gives it to them piece by piece, with a small clamp.*

9. Pasteur, O.C., t. VI, p.112.
10. Roux, 1896, p. 537.
11. NAF 18011, f.P. 85.
12. NAF 18013, f.P. 1.
13. NAF 18011, f.P. 71.
14. NAF 18011, f.P. 73 back.
15. NAF 18011, f.P. 74 back.

On the 20th, the chickens are still healthy, and another chicken is inoculated and remains well. Pasteur asks himself: 'This raises a question: either an initial inoculation protects, or the culture fluid has changed.' Pasteur continues the experiments and the inoculations; on March 3, 1879, he notes: 'We now have a chicken that ate contaminated bread and is well. Have these meals vaccinated it?' On the days that follow, the chicken is sick. 'On March 30, it is in very good health... Obviously then, an initial inoculation that does not kill but produces illness vaccinated the chickens.' These lines are very moving."[16] The last sentence is Denise Wrotnowska's comment. The text is quoted from Pasteur's 6th notebook[17]. The transcribed text is, of course, accurate, but its context should be clarified. In fact, a short time later, in one of the subsequent notebooks, an entry reads: "*March 10, 1879. Possible vaccination for chickens 1rst by inoculation that has not killed 2nd by contaminated meals that have not killed. We read at note p. 79, 6th notebook, that a chicken not killed by a first inoculation is not killed by a second inoculation; and at p. 85 that a chicken which ate meals of contaminated bread for 8 days, then two meals of microbe-infected muscle, subsequently inoculated, was very sick but did not die. The vaccination attempt by contaminated meals is repeated... Therefore, contaminated meals, even when* (2 words) *do not ordinarily vaccinate...*"[18]. **Thus, in March 1879, Pasteur is already aware of the phenomenon of resistance to cholera in chickens, but cannot define the conditions for obtaining it.**

The experiments continue: "*Microbe at 45°*"[19], "*Chicken microbe in a vacuum and in air*"[20], "*Non conservation of chicken microbe placed in dry plaster.*"[21] Then Pasteur interrupted his experiments for almost two months.

- **May 6, 1879.** "*Cultivation of chicken cholera microbe to continue the experiments, May 6, 1879. The incubator set at 30° contains two flasks of microbes in chicken broth, bearing the dates March 17 and March 31... it is sown in a new chicken broth flask.*"

- **May 7 [1879].** "*Development Cloudy flask in the March 31 flask - flask I No development in the March 17 flask, probably due to longer aging of the germ. This second flask developed on May 8. It was in fact the effect of the more advanced age of the germ.*"[22]

As early as May 1879, Pasteur showed that delayed bacterial growth in cultures is related to the age, a phenomenon of which he was perhaps already aware thanks to his previous fermentation experiments, so that the entry shows no surprise.

Also, "May 6, 1879 *Inoculation of the following resistant chickens... A Rooster inoculated three times B Chicken inoculated twice C Other chicken inoculated twice D Chicken inoculated twice E... F...*"[23]. "*See new inoculation of A, B, C on page 52, inoculation without result. It appears, then, that there was vaccination.*"[24]

- **May 7, 1879.** "*Vaccination attempt Apparent success in pig series* [i.e. guinea pigs] *of p. 6. May 7 Inoculation with 5 drops at a time microbes I page 29, to two pigs previously*

16. Wrotnowska, 1975, p. 274.
17. NAF 18011, f.P. 79 & 85.
18. NAF 18013, f.P. 1.
19. NAF 18011, f.P. 86.
20. NAF 18011, f.P. 87.
21. NAF 18011, f.P. 88.
22. NAF 18013, f.P. 29.
23. NAF 18013, f.P. 29.
24. NAF 18013, f.P. 29 & back.

inoculated twice with the microbe... They are most probably the pigs of February 4 p. 77 back of the 6th register... I believe there has been previous vaccination."[25]

- **May 17, [1879].** *"Study of resistant chickens and vaccination with chicken microbe..."*[26]
- **May 26, [1879].** *"Vaccination attempt..."*[27].

These experiments took place before Pasteur left on holiday. He arrived in Arbois between the 25th and the 28th of July 1879[28]; Roux had been left in charge of laboratory cultures. Pasteur was obviously not very preoccupied with the problem of a vaccine against chicken cholera. He returned to Paris around the 8th of October 1879[29], and the marriage of his daughter Marie-Louise to René Vallery-Radot was celebrated on November 4. Preparations for this event, which made him very happy, no doubt took up much of his time.

- When he returned to the laboratory, according to Duclaux's 1896 account, everything seemed to go wrong. "*The first chicken cholera experiments were conducted in 1879. They were interrupted by the summer holidays and taken up again afterwards; but they immediately encountered an unexpected problem. Almost all the cultures that had been left in the laboratory had become sterile. Because all of them were part of ongoing experiments, an attempt was made to revitalize them; to do this, germs taken from them were inoculated either into chicken broths or to chickens. Many had not produced cultures, had not altered the health of inoculated animals, and...*"[30]. Some inoculated cultures made the chickens more or less sick, but not sick enough to die. Why? Chickens arriving directly from "les Halles" were inoculated with "revitalized" cultures and demonstrated a reaction to the germs. Duclaux recounts: "*... We were about to throw everything out and start over, when Pasteur had the idea of inoculating a fresh new culture to these chickens that had proved to be so resistant, or so it seemed, to inoculations with cultures from the previous summer. To everyone's surprise, perhaps even Pasteur's, who had not expected such success, almost all these chickens were resistant...*"[31]. Pasteur is reported to have taken great interest in this chance event. Numerous testimonies similar to Duclaux's exist, probably based on his account[32].

Pasteur wrote to Roux several times from Arbois to give him instructions, and in October 1879 he pasted in his notebook a report from Roux about a series of experiments on anthrax bacteria, conducted before and during Pasteur's vacation. There is no mention of chicken cholera. In the weeks following Pasteur's return to the laboratory, between the end of the 1879 vacation period and December 5, there are no entries concerning chicken cholera. Pasteur was working on anthrax. The only exception is a page on December 6, 1879, where he mentions a thesis on puerperal fever written by Mr. Doléris, who was asking for advice[33].

Pasteur himself chose the 28th of October 1879 for the start of the work that was to lead to a vaccine against chicken cholera. On March 4, 1880 he wrote a summary of the beginning of his experiments, and later made several entries summarising previous

25. NAF 18013, f.P. 32.
26. NAF 18013, f.P. 52.
27. NAF 18013, f.P. 68.
28. Pasteur, Cor., t. 3, p. 98.
29. Pasteur, Cor., t. 3, p. 113.
30. Duclaux, 1896, p. 348.
31. Duclaux, 1896, p. 348.
32. Hannoun, 1999, p. 19; Metchnikoff, 1939, p. 6; Legroux, 1942, p. 42; Lagrange, 1954, p. 39, Cuny, 1966, p. 116 & many others.
33. NAF 18014, f.P. 18.

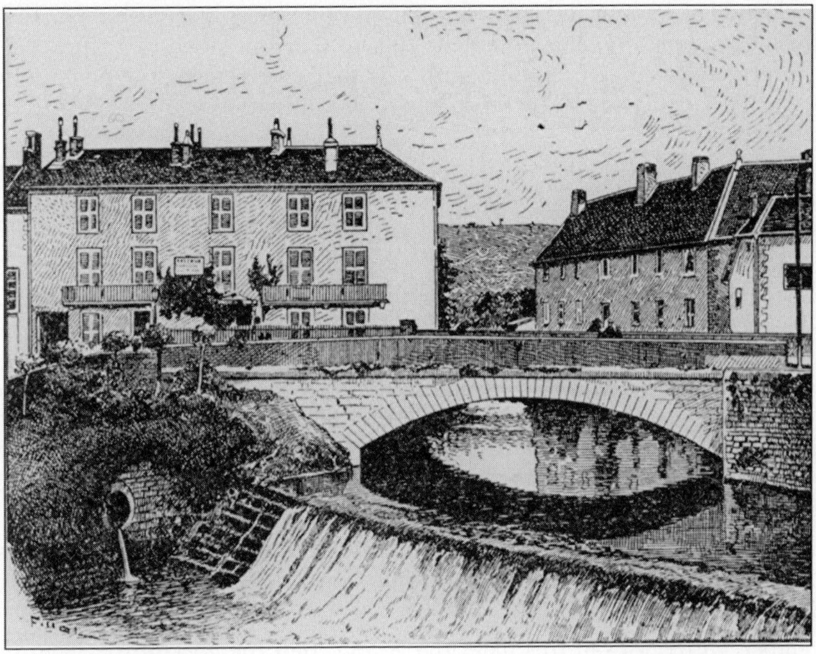

Figure 3. Pasteur's family home in Arbois, left, on the banks of the Cuisance. (Fraitot, circa 1900.)

work. The choice of experiments (*see below*) attempts to follow the sequence of Pasteur's ideas which led to the discovery of the first vaccine derived by man-made rather than natural manipulation. The sentences in bold (those in italics are taken from Pasteur's texts) summarize the main points and are intended to facilitate understanding. **A reader not familiar with this type of work is free to read only the passages in bold.**

• **Start of the work, October 28, 1879: "*Entry march 4, 1880 The opposite page records the early stages of the resumption of a study on chicken cholera. Start of the experiment with flask* X_1 *dated November 22, 1879 and originating from flask X of October 28, that came from a chicken which died the previous day.*** (These cultures of chicken cholera are not recorded, on these dates, in Pasteur's notebooks, although he was back in Paris.) *I had written to Roux from Arbois to recultivate four flasks of the microbe I had set aside when I left Paris, at the end of July. These four flasks were sown into flasks of broth kept in an incubator. These flasks produced cultures only on the second day, no doubt because they had become acidic. Believing that the microbe could no longer be cultivated, Roux inoculated the most recent as culture (of the month of July) to two chickens that were still alive 8 days later. Roux re-inoculated the two chickens with one of the recent cultures that had developed late. One of the chickens died on the 3rd day, the other one the 4th. The blood of one of them was used to inoculate a flask of broth, namely flask X of October 28.*"[34]

This text written in large letters was added subsequently, on the back of the October 28, 1879 page. It is intended as a personal reminder, and contains information on the following page, written without particular care by Pasteur[35].

34. NAF 18014, f.P. 20 back.
35. NAF 18014, f.P. 21.

In this addendum, Pasteur indicates the origins of cultures X (October 28, 1879) and X_1 (November 22, 1879). X is a virulent culture that has killed two chickens. X and X_1 are, in principle, virulent cultures with no other special features, and considered as such by Pasteur at the time. The procedure of re-cultivation was intended to preserve the bacterial strain.

• Roux tried to recover a virulent strain of chicken cholera microbe by inoculating two (author's note: probably new, but Pasteur does not indicate it) chickens that did not die. He re-inoculated the same chickens (Pasteur indicates that the interval between the two inoculations was at least eight days) with a culture similar to the first, but re-inoculated at least once, apparently, and the chickens died! Logically, after the first injection, Roux should have expected the death of both chickens if the culture was virulent; instead, no fatality occurred. The culture was probably more or less dead and was poorly immunogenic. The fact that the second injection, given at least eight days later, killed the two chickens after a clear delay shows that they were not, or were insufficiently, immunised, and that the second culture was virulent to some degree. Thus, Roux did not observe protection (still less of vaccination), because it was present. As for the delayed development of the chicken cholera microbe, Pasteur was already familiar with this phenomenon[36].

Pasteur was not particularly interested in the strain that came from the second inoculation ("*one of the recent cultures that showed delay*") and that had no other special features.

• December 5 [1879]. On this date, the X and then the X_1 culture, from flask X, that had remained in an acid medium from October 28 to December 5 (39 days), did not kill five resistant chickens from before vacation, nor five new chickens ("*including a beautiful rooster*")[37]. X_1 is harmless to the five new chickens, since Pasteur writes: "*on Xbre 11 none of the chickens became sick*"[38].

• On December 11, Pasteur re-inoculated the ten chickens already inoculated on December 5, with a three-day culture in neutral medium of the strain in flask X_1. "*Xbre 15 the chickens are in good health...*

Thus, the microbe cultivated in the neutral broth produced no more effect than the microbe cultivated in the broth that air had turned slightly acidic. ***The five chickens not inoculated before vacation ('new' chickens) appeared to be just as resistant as the five resistant chickens from before the holidays...*"[39].**

The ten chickens (five and five) are not affected by this new inoculation. Three days in neutral medium did not modify the virulence of X_1. Pasteur observes no clinical sign in these animals after their inoculations. He uses the word "resistance", because he still believes in the effective virulence of strain X_1 (inoculums of December 5 and 11). However, X_1 (in acid medium) and its derivative inoculated on December 11 (after three days in sterile medium) are not very virulent and have immunised the inoculated subjects, a fact that Pasteur was not yet aware of[40].

• December 12, 1879. "Effect of cold on chicken microbe. *Xbre 12... the microbe exposed to cold is the microbe used on Xbre11, p. 21, that had been re-inoculated Xbre 11*

36. NAF 18013, f.P. 29.
37. NAF 18014, f.P. 21.
38. NAF 18014, f.P. 21.
39. NAF 18014, f.P. 21.
40. NAF 18014, f.P. 21 & 21 back.

at 3 o'clock..." Chicken cholera and anthrax microbes were exposed for about an hour to temperatures between - 30 and - 38° C[41].

A culture re-cultivated from X_1 and exposed to cold killed a small chicken in 50 hours[42]. The reason for the recovered virulence of this strain by exposure to cold is not clear, in the absence of other technical details. Was this due to a mixing of strains? But this chance event gave Pasteur a culture with confirmed virulence, which was very fortunate at this stage in his experimentation*. It allowed him to assess without ambiguity the "resistance" of these inoculated chickens.

• December 15, 1879. "*However since on page 23 a small chicken was made sick with a microbe culture from a microbe exposed to cold at - 37°* (sic) *and to answer the question: is it possible that the cold made the microbe more virulent, the same 10 chickens were re-inoculated with 5 drops from the flask with microbe at - 38°.*

Xbre 16. The chickens appear to be in very good health (continued p. 24)[43].

***Xbre 30. The chickens are in good health*"[44]. Pasteur did not note any clinical sign of chicken cholera in the inoculated animals.**

"*There are two possibilities: the 10 chickens at p. 21 were all resistant and the small one on this page 23 was not, or exposing the culture to - 38° cold restored the virulence of the microbe.*"[45] Pasteur does not know the immune status of the chickens bought at the market, in terms of chicken cholera. Animals inoculated twice with re-cultivated culture X_1 fluids (one cultivated one whole month in acid medium, the other the same amount of time in acid medium plus three days in neutral medium), and tested with a virulent virus (that had killed a small chicken) did not die and are therefore "resistant". Why?

It is likely that Pasteur's first hypothesis reflects the idea of a natural resistance in certain animals[46]. In this experiment, the booster inoculation was performed six days after the first inoculation, and the test injection four days after the booster. These are short intervals. Pasteur had not yet considered the time factor in the success of immunisation[47]. He was to examine it a few weeks later: on January 13, 1880, he asked Roux how much time was needed for a smallpox vaccine to induce protection in the vaccinated subject. Roux answered that it takes about eight days; Pasteur checked this answer and noted in the margin: "*It is true Bousquet traité de la vaccine 1833 p. 117.*"[48] Strangely, this fact, well-known at the time, does not appear at the place in the Bousquet book indicated by Pasteur[49]!

• December 16, 1879, Pasteur wants to verify the virulence of the strain exposed to cold; he is not yet convinced: "*... new chickens were bought and we inoculated 4 with the same culture at - 38° which killed* (a small chicken) *at p. 23.*" This culture killed the four inoculated chickens[50]. The culture exposed to cold is indeed virulent.

---

* This origin of the virulent strain of chicken cholera used by Pasteur does not correspond to the one cited by Duclaux.

41. NAF 18014, f.P. 23.
42. NAF 18014, f.P. 23.
43. NAF 18014, f.P. 21 back.
44. NAF 18014, f.P. 21 back.
45. NAF 18014, f.P. 23.
46. NAF 18014, f.P. 80.
47. NAF 18014, f.P. 21 back.
48. NAF 18014, f.P. 64 back.
49. Bousquet, 1833, p. 117.
50. NAF 18014, f.P. 24.

• Key date. On December 18, 1879, Pasteur was intrigued by the results obtained with culture X_1 and imagined for the first time a vaccine: "*Study of the chicken microbe from flask X_1 Xbre 18 Content of flask X_1 It comes from a Nov. 22 culture made with germs from flask X - which comes from a chicken killed during vacation by one of the old microbe flasks. However cultures X and X_1 became acidic by contact with air, after having been neutral. It is the X_1 culture that was used at page 21 for the first inoculation of the 10 chickens. In fact the question is if at p. 21 this acidic culture had not presented diminished virulence that might have vaccinated* (underlined by Pasteur) *the 10 chickens at page 21 or at least the five (2°) at this page 21. Today Xbre 18 inoculation under the skin with this X_1 culture of two chickens in the series (series of 8) bought Xbre16 at p. 24 and which are certainly not resistant since at p. 24 two have already died and two others are very sick (note: they too have died). Shallow inoculation in thick muscle tissue.*

• *Xbre 19 The chickens are in very good health. No swelling; no whiteness at the inoculation site. It is strange. It appears then that the microbe from this culture X_1 in broth that became acidic by exposure to air is no longer active, although able to produce culture. Yet it is from this X_1 flask that germ was taken for culture in the neutral broth that was subsequently exposed to cold at - 38° at p. 29 and that proved to be active at p. 23 on the small chicken and at p. 24 on four new chickens.*

• *Xbre 20 The chickens are in very good health. X_1 is therefore probably no longer active to kill. Obviously they will not become sick.*

They were re-inoculated under the skin with 5 drops of crushed lardaceous muscle mixed with water from a chicken that died yesterday 19 at p. 24 (a lethal injection of chicken cholera microbes). *The aim was to find out if the first inoculation with X_1 vaccinated the two chickens, in which case it could be assumed that the five (rooster and 4 chickens of 2°) at p. 21 were also vaccinated by the first inoculation of Xbre 5 with X_1.*

N.B. *I want to specify however that if a first inoculation vaccinates, it might only do so after more than 48 hours; in the present case re-inoculation was performed after only 48 h.*"[51]

"*Xbre 21 One of the chickens shows signs of sickness. From time to time she closes her eyes. She is sad as is also the second. A little later we see them both eating.*

Xbre 22 A strange thing both chickens are doing much better...

Xbre 23 The two chickens seem to be healthy..."

This experiment was certainly crucial. But less than one week later, on January 1, 1880, one of the chickens became very thin, and could no longer stand up...[52]. For the first time, Pasteur was faced with the problem of the undesirable effects of certain inoculations against chicken cholera.

On December 20, Pasteur examined the problem of chronic infectious diseases[53] and the effect of inanition on anti-cholera immunity in chickens[54].

51. NAF 18014, f.P. 29.
52. NAF 18014, f.P. 29.
53. NAF 18014, f.P. 35.
54. NAF 18014, f.P. 37.

Between December 10 and 21, Pasteur pursued, in parallel with his work on chicken cholera, an experiment on "*earth and anthrax bacteridia*"[55].

• ***December 19, 1879. "Test of the virulence of flask X which at p. 21 was the source of X_1*** *(see p. 21 note December 5) Xbre 19, 1879 some fluid from this flask X (really X_1) was sown in neutral chicken broth. This was to give flask X_2 An error was made, we noticed that by mistake X was sown in acid broth. X_2 is therefore like X a culture in acid broth*".

In a note, Pasteur specifies that X is in fact X_1.

"*Xbre 22. X_2 is not developed. X_3 from X cultivated in neutral broth is not developed either (no see below on back).*"[56]

"*Xbre 24 Today a curious thing, there is weak but very clear devt in X_2. Thus, X was not dead (see X_2 continued page 40 then page 51).*"[57]

This example shows that there can be disorder in a laboratory, but that errors are (at least sometimes) identified. Pasteur was intrigued by the different rhythms of growth of these cultures, in relation with the acid or neutral character of the culture broths.

"Xbre 22 It appears at p. 24, note of Xbre 18, that blood from a dead chicken was sown in acidic broth (sic - the inoculum from this chicken was a culture taken from the one that was exposed to cold at - 38° C). ***This flask has the letter P inscribed on it*** (it was originally a virulent culture).

On Xbre 22 at 5 o'clock we inoculated flask P

1° in neutral chicken broth: it will be Pn

2° in acid chicken broth made acid by air (Pasteur specified "acide par air"): *it will be Pa*

At 11 in the evening Pn is already developed Pa shows nothing.

On Xbre 23 Pn and Pa are developed, Pn more than Pa, although the difference is small.

• ***Xbre 24 It can be concluded from this that a recent microbial culture*** **(1 word)** ***in acid broth can be obtained quickly in acid broth as well as in neutral broth. This is not so in the case of an old culture - Moreover the acid culture delays freshly inoculated culture (made acid by air)*** *(see Pn and Pa continued p. 49 on Xbre 31.*"[58]

Pasteur realized that, to obtain a culture with delayed development, the culture has to remain in acid broth for a long time.

Key date: "*January 4* [1880]. *X_2 was used to inoculate (see p. 51)...* [Author's note: "page 51, the origin of X_2: "*X_2 continued (acid broth) p. 33 back January 1, 1880 at 11 o'clock in the morning inoculation with flask X_2 at p. 33 back of page*"[59] *then see previous entry on December 19*]. ***I... II... III Culture from before vacation made acid by air, requiring for 5^{cc} 1^c.15 lime water*** (a method of measurement of the acidity of the medium)... ***Thus X_2*** (a culture derived from X) ***is still quite active but the microbe it contains is certainly different from an ordinary microbe by the slowness of its devt.*** (development) ***It is therefore legitimate to hope that microbe X_2 will exert an effect on the chickens to make them sick and that at the same time they will be receptive enough to the action of the medicating matter*** (Author's note: Pasteur wrote: "*matière*

55. NAF 18014, f.P. 25 & 26.
56. NAF 18014, f.P. 33.
57. NAF 18014, f.P. 33 back.
58. NAF 18014, f.P. 39.
59. NAF 18014, f.P. 51.

médicatrice") **not to die.** *In addition it can be seen clearly that culture made acid by air delays much more than the other crude* (Author's note: Pasteur wrote: "*naturelle*" then crossed out this word and replaced it with "*brute*") *acidity which does not really delay*" (Author's note: Pasteur probably refers to artificial acidity induced by ozone [Roux's idea][60] and/or, perhaps, by a few drops of an acid.)

"*Jan. 6 III of the broth made acid by air and inoculated with X_2 has developed during the night...*"[61].

The phrase: "*It is therefore legitimate...*" is explicitly related to Pasteur's new hypothesis: that a correlation exists between delays in development of certain cultures and the fact that they can induce benign diseases in the inoculated animals. As to the "*matière médicatrice*" (medicating matter), what is it exactly? A first reference to the future "*matière vaccinante*" (vaccinating matter) (see the chapter "Rabies")?

• **Key experiment: "*January 5* [1880]** *Bertrand has just brought 43 chickens.* ***We inoculate 48* (sic), *all with 3 drops.***

A. 12 with* (1 word) *blood of rooster that died yesterday p. 48 (Control series A, incorrect because of a technical error, was going to be done over and called A' on January 7 - 12 out of 12 chickens died January 11)[62].

B. 12 with culture from Pa flask *at page 39, which is a culture in broth made acid by air.*

C. 12 with culture from X_2 flask *on back of p. 33, also a culture in broth made acid by air, older than Pa.*

D. *12 are reserved.*

Jan. 8... in Pa series. Already 7 out of 12. In the X_2 series no chicken has died. They seem in good health except two."[63]

"*Jan. 13...* ***Today there are still eleven X_2 and 4 Pa (from Jan. 5).***"[64]

Pasteur confirmed his January 4 hypothesis: "*old culture in acidic medium / delayed microbe development / low virulence for the animal*". The next day he wrote:

• **Key date: "*January 14, 1880... When should the microbe be taken so that it will vaccinate? - X_2 vaccinated and perhaps Pa did a little (page 56)*** *- X_2 is a culture in broth made acid by air, developed after 4 days (Xbre 19-24 page 33 back)* [Author's note: that took 4 days to multiply, a very long time]; *and the germ came from X... this X_2 inoculated after 17 days of culture, that is, on Jan. 5 page 56, vaccinated or rather did not kill* (on January 13 there are 11 chickens left out of the 12 chickens inoculated on January 5, 1880). *Pa is very different from X_2. But it was a culture in broth made acid by air, that was only 14 days old (it dated back to Xbre 22 page 39)* (December 19 to January 5) *and above all its germ came from a culture only 4 days old* (December 18 to 22), *in acid medium. 14 days instead of 17 should not have much influence but* ***there is a big difference in the germs because one comes from a 4-day culture, the other from a two-month culture.***

Nevertheless, Pa which had 4 out of 12 chickens resistant to the disease seems to have provided some protection, since page 59 records 12 out of 12 deaths for the very

60. NAF 18014, f.P. 74.
61. NAF 18014, f.P. 54.
62. NAF 18014, f.P. 59.
63. NAF 18014, f.P. 56.
64. NAF 18014, f.P. 70 & back.

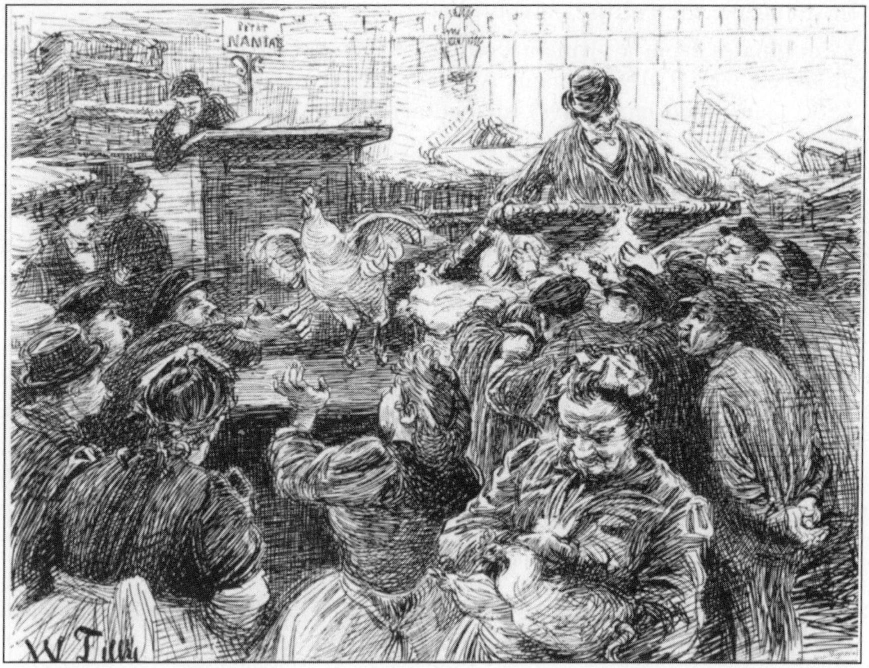

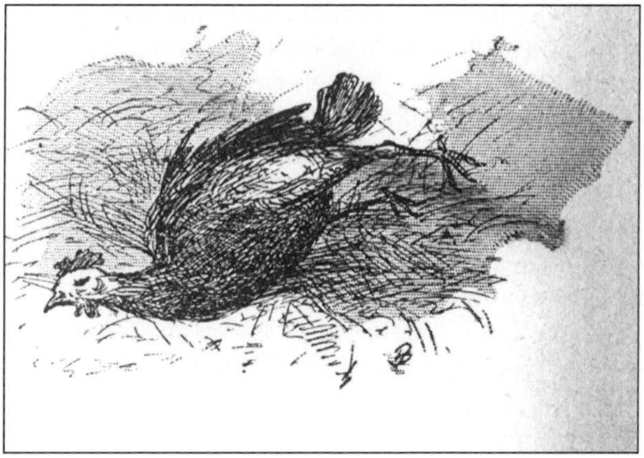

Figure 4. Chicken cholera. Top: sale of chickens at the market where Pasteur had his chickens bought, and some roosters (Strauss, 1892)[65]. Bottom: a chicken killed by cholera (de Préville, 1897)[66]. Images depicting chicken cholera are very rare. The subject was not of great interest, as Pasteur must have realized. He knew he had to apply his new method to a more talked-about disease. He succeeded better with anthrax, and marvellously well with rabies!

active microbe in fresh blood [series A'[67]]. ***This being so, because it is no doubt unnecessary, for having an*** X_2 ***that vaccinates, to take the germ from a two-month old acid culture and then inoculate after 17 days, I will use shorter intervals and study the delay in culture to see what happens..."***[68].

65. Strauss, 1892, p. 48.
66. de Préville, 1897, p. 94.
67. NAF 18014, f.P. 59.
68. NAF 18014, f.P. 71.

• In summary, the cultures involved are:

i) X_2 originates from a virulent culture of October 28, 1879 left in acid medium until December 19, 1879 (about two months in acid medium), then until January 5, 1880 (seventeen more days) in acid medium.

ii) Pa originates from the virulent culture of December 18, re-cultivated on December 22, 1879 (after four days) in acid medium, then until January 5, 1880 (fourteen days) in acid medium.

Pasteur realized that diminished virulence is the result of a long period spent in acid medium, and he planned to simplify the conditions in which these vaccinating strains could be obtained.

• January 14, 1880, *in footnote*: "***(1) For the moment, in a report to the Academy, it could be said: it*** (the vaccinating microbe) ***must be taken when there was noticeable delay in development compared to a very recent culture inoculated at the same time, in the same conditions, either in neutral culture or in acid culture.***"[69]

Pasteur had planned to reveal the important role of neutral or acid medium and the time the pathogen spent in culture, but not the method he used to obtain them, but on February 9, speaking before the Academies and the *Société Centrale Vétérinaire*, he revealed none of them.

Pasteur reconsiders his January 14 conclusions. He attempts to acquire certainty.

• Key date: "***Jan. 19*** [1880] ***Are the chickens of the series X_2 p. 56 eleven of which resisted while at p. 59, 12 out of 12 died*** (control series A') ***vaccinated?***

Yesterday Bertrand delivered 21 chickens and roosters. ***8 of the vaccinated chickens in series X_2 page 56, and 8 new chickens bought yesterday, were inoculated with 2 drops of fluid a 7th culture, the first of which came from infected chicken blood.*** *This 6th culture is from jan.16 and was inoculated on the 16th with the culture used p. 64 and which now proved to be very active on two new chickens...*" (Both died[70, 71]).

"***Jan. 20. For vaccination it is perhaps necessary that the disease be declared and visible the first time... (see above).***[72]

Jan. 21. This experiment appears favourable to the idea of a vaccination by an initial inoculation made 15 days previously: *the first was made Jan. on the 5, the second on the 19th but see below. The experiment of jan.5 on X_2 and its comparison* ***clearly shows that the microbe can be attenuated to the point of not killing anyone it makes sick, since eleven out of 12 resisted while the blood water*** (virulent bacteria) ***killed 12 out of 12.***"[73]

This experiment leads to two crucial conclusions: one, a little unfortunate, that a consistent feature of an efficacious vaccine is the induction of clinical signs. Pasteur himself would later re-examine this dogma, in the development of the rabies vaccine. In the present context of the chicken cholera vaccine, Pasteur used specific clinical signs (more or less benign) as indicators of future resistance in inoculated subjects; the second conclusion relates to the desirable lapse of time between the inoculation and the challenge test, that is, sufficient time to obtain immunity.

69. NAF 18014, f.P. 71.
70. NAF 18014, f.P. 64.
71. NAF 18014, f.P. 77.
72. NAF 18014, f.P. 77.
73. NAF 18014, f.P. 77.

• **January 20, 1880** *"... 4 flasks created today were seeded on the 20th at 2 o'clock with flask III of p. 54 which is an acid culture inoculated on January 4 with germ from X_2, that is, 16 days ago (see p. 101 for subsequent steps with one of these flasks)."*[74]

"January 22 [1880] ***Inoculation with blood of 19 chickens and roosters never before inoculated and of 8 chickens previously inoculated twice.***

Jan. 22. In the yard there are 5 chickens, 3 small roosters and 11 large roosters never before inoculated. 19 inoculations at noon...

All of them are inoculated with 2 divisions (of the syringe - always the same model) *of blood water (blood clots from crushed heart in a glass, and then with the same volume of water added) from a chicken that died the day before yesterday - blood full of microbe.*

In addition, we inoculate with 2 divisions (of the syringe) *of this* (2 words) *the 8 chickens remaining out of the nine at p. 64 and which were sick except three after two inoculations, and which have been labelled."* [Origin of the 8 chickens concerned, remaining from a lot of nine: *"January 1, 1880 Collecting together... of chickens which once inoculated were observed to be sick, sad, suffering and presenting swellings in the inoculation region..."*[75]; *"Jan. 9. Repeat inoculation of the nine chickens... (see p. 52) which have all been sick, with visible swelling after a first injection."*[76]]

"N.B. The aim is to verify by these inoculations if a very active microbial virus spares the chickens and roosters which have not been inoculated, if, in a word, there are naturally resistant chickens and roosters and finally, see if the 8 chickens already inoculated twice and sick both times, will show resistance to a very active microbe.

Jan. 23 - Out of 8 (5+3), five died at 9 this morning; two are dying, one seems healthy.

- Out of 11 roosters, three died, others are dying and the others sick.

- ***Out of the 8 vaccinated twice and which were sick, 8 alive seeming very well.*** **(in a footnote)** ***they eat except three which are sad. They have to be added to the 8 at p. 81. This gives 16 healthy against 8+11 = 19 dead (or?) dying after an initial inoculation."***[77]

And Pasteur rejoices:

• **Important key date: *"January 23* [1880]: *Proof of vaccination: sufficient intensity of disease is needed to prevent recurrence, that is, produce vaccination."*[78] Pasteur also tested the hypothesis that certain chickens could have natural resistance to chicken cholera, which does not seem to be the case.**

• **February 9, 1880. Exhilarated by these first results, that is, the immunisation of chickens against chicken cholera, Pasteur reports his results to the Academy of Sciences (Paris) (February 9, 1880) and then to the Academy of Medicine (Paris) (February 10, 1880). But he does not reveal his technique: *"Through certain changes in modes of culture development, we can reduce the virulence of the infectious microbe."*[79]**

• On February 12, 1880, Pasteur thanked the *Société Centrale Vétérinaire* (which became the French Veterinary Academy) for having made him a member, and he

74. NAF 18014, f.P. 74 back.
75. NAF 18014, f.P. 52.
76. NAF 18014, f.P. 64.
77. NAF 18014, f.P. 80.
78. NAF 18014, f.P. 80.
79. Pasteur, O.C., t. VI, p. 291.

included in his speech the report he had delivered to the two Academies to which he belonged[80]. **Did Pasteur have the necessary proof to announce his discovery, or not? It is a matter of opinion... But he had the genius to realize immediately what concrete benefits the generalisation of his "old cultures" results could bring to the investigations of all pathogens.**

- **Having published his crucial idea, Pasteur did not abandon it.**

"Feb. 14 [1880] *inoculations:*

Series II 8 (of batch) *N at p. 89...*

Series III 7 new chickens are also inoculated with the previous flask of attenuated microbe. Here the disease should be more pronounced than in the 8N of the previous series II... (series II and III are sown) *with a new attenuated microbe, taken from one of the flasks at p. 74 (back) of January 20, originating from III p. 54.* [a subculture originating from X_2 - *cf.* January 20, 1880].

Feb. 15. The 7 new ones are alive and well...

A very active virus was used, active enough to develop despite the first vaccinating inoculation* (sic)*. This shows the usefulness of vaccinating with two inoculations rather than one..."[81].

- **Pasteur is considering multiple injections to obtain good immunisation.**

"Feb. 20. Continued procedures for the 7 new chickens at page 101. I make a separate page here for the 7 new ones at p. 101, which are still healthy and are of real significance since they were inoculated once, without fatalities, 7 days ago, with the microbial vaccine that made them sick (except one) and thereby produced an initial vaccinating effect...

Feb. 21 These 7 chickens were re-inoculated with the neutral flask originating at p. 101 from the flask with attenuated virus that inoculated series II and III at this page 101..."[82].

February 28 [1880]: "*Microbe for vaccine virus research*. *Inoculation with 2 divisions (It is 5:30 in the afternoon)*

series I 10 chickens with the flask developed from muscle of chicken 2° killed yesterday, chickens in the series M'+N'+*etc...*

series II 10 chickens with flask* (1 word) *of February 25 p. 99, inoculated with acid* P4 *and which developed very late...

series III 10 chickens with flask of Feb. 7 p. 95 originating from flask A *of January 31* (all?) *containing very virulent virus...* ***To establish if this culture from very virulent flask A is attenuated by this stay in acid medium since Feb. 7; that is, for 3 weeks.***

series IV 10 chickens with the same flask of Feb. 21 p. 107 which inoculated 7 new chickens - It is a flask of attenuated virus, the vaccine virus... To obtain a new series of chickens vaccinated with the attenuated microbe, having received several inoculations of this weakened virus.

series V 10 chickens with the pus from an already present abscess in one of the pigs (guinea pigs) *p. 109 inoculated Feb. 21...*

80. Pasteur, O.C., t. VI, p. 287; Pasteur, 1880, pp. 125 & 204.
81. NAF 18014, f.P. 101.
82. NAF 18014, f.P. 107.

March 2 at 9 in the morning. Series I: All dead Series II: Two dead Series III: All dead Series IV: All alive one very sick will die Series V: All dead

Therefore cultures of inoculations I, III, V are very virulent. In other words… ***But IV proves that the vaccine virus remains attenuated and II seems to prove that the acid P4 flask reached the limit of its development on Feb.25, becoming a vaccine virus****; that the flask used for III was still a mixture of very virulent and attenuated virus, the latter being masked by the former. For the acid P4, only the latter remained."* [83]

• An essential point, series IV shows the stability of the vaccine virus in culture, at least in the conditions of the experiment. The hypothesis of a mix of viruses with different degrees of virulence is an attempt to explain the changes occurring in cultures, related to the characteristics of the mediums in which they develop. Pasteur will describe this hypothesis - which he discarded - in his October 26, 1880 presentation to the Academies, entitled "*On the attenuation of the chicken cholera virus*" [84]**.**

"March 4 [1880]. *Description of flasks p. 21 that I just found.*

P1 cultured from P of Xbre 20 [P is the acid flask in note at page 24, that produced all the P1 Pa Pn[85]].

Neutral P3… [P3 cultured from acid P2 from Xbre 22 to Xbre 31 is therefore eleven days fresher than P1 [86]].

Like acid P4, (cultured from acid P2 from Xbre 22 to Xbre 31 [87] *is dead, between the 25th and 28th* (February 1880) *as noted at p. 99 (back)* [88]. *But P3 was originally neutral and is probably still active and perhaps even P1…*

March 5, flask cultured from P1 stayed clear.

Flask cultured from P3 developed…

March 6 flask cultured from P3 developed well. Cloudiness.

Flask from P1 is still only slightly developed, no cloudiness… This seems very strange. Is the microbe present? External appearance indicates it, but the delay and speed of development are unusual. I believe the microbe must be very weakened.

March 7. It is strange, the acid P1 flask does not develop at all, no progress since yesterday. On examination, double points are observed. Thus the microbe is dead and there was an impurity. Fortunately P3 has developed well. It was started Xbre 31. P1 is from Xbre 20. Only an eleven-day difference

In any case, there is now a dead microbe in neutral broth after 2.5 months…

N.B. We will test the virulence of the flask cultured from P3.

March 8 [1880]. *10 new chickens are inoculated, each with 2 divisions of flask from P3 of March 4.*

March 10. All 10 chickens seem healthy. If this continues the result will be very important; because what is present here is the origin of P3 at the limit of its possible development; this is proven by P1. In fact, having reached its limit (of development) *it has lost its virulence.*

---

83. NAF 18014, f.P. 113.
84. Pasteur, O.C., t. VI, p. 323.
85. NAF 18014, f.P. 21 back.
86. NAF 18014, f.P. 21 back.
87. NAF 18014, f.P. 21 back.
88. NAF 18014, f.P. 99 back.

March 10 There is confirmation. ***Here is a new weakened microbe that seems much more weakened than the previous one cultured from the X. I will call it vaccine P and the previous one vaccine X."***[89]

Pasteur now has two vaccines, P and X, of different virulence, whose origins he knows and whose virulence he believes to be stable.

A note written on March 4 summarizes Pasteur's ideas: "*N.B. March 4, 1880: it is safe to conclude that flask X contained a weakened microbe because out of the 10 chickens five had not yet been inoculated.* [In fact, culture X, of October 28, 1879, was rather virulent and had become "avirulent" on January 5, 1879, after two months in acid medium.]

At p. 23 this microbe is exposed to cold at - 38° An ulterior culture kills (a) little chicken.

At p. 24 this culture kills four out of four chickens. It can therefore be concluded that the virus has been made more virulent by the cold to which it was exposed.

At p. 24 (and in the note) the blood of one of these 4 dead chickens produces a culture which, at p. 35, when inoculated to two chickens, killed one and made the other very, very sick.

Thus, the microbe is really virulent.

At p. 39, this flask, cultured from the blood of one of the 4 dead chickens, is called flask P and is used to start Pn and acid Pa of Xbre 22.

At p. 49, with this Pn flask Pn1 is started and Pa1 is started with Pa.

At p. 56, the culture from Pa of p. 39 caused 8 deaths out of 12 in the B series. This is further proof that a microbe is present here that recovered its virulence by exposure to cold initially or, in any case, through one of the 4 dead chickens at p. 24.

Finally at p. 113 it can be noted that this microbe from acid P4 (series II) has been brought back, probably by the long stay of this acid P4, lasting from Xbre 31 to February 28 **[60 days],** ***to an attenuated state once again...***"[90].

Note in the margin: "*Flask P was started Xbre 19 as recorded by the note p. 24 and at p. 39. This flask is at the origin of P1 in neutral broth* (P1 started Xbre 20, 1879), *then acid P2 (cultivated in acid medium between December 22 and 31, 1879) which gave neutral* P3 (P3 was started Xbre 31, 1879) *and acid P4* (culture also inoculated on December 31, 1879) *but all these P flasks come from X, whose virulence was restored by exposure to cold and by passage through chickens; this virulence was then weakened again in acid P4 during the period between Xbre 31 and February 28...*"[91].

- **Around March 4, 1880, Pasteur had defined the fundamental elements of his "artificial" vaccine. He was careful not to reveal his method, probably for fear of being copied. At this stage, he certainly did not want this to happen. But the concept of a vaccine that Pasteur presented on February 9, 1880 was to be applied to the anthrax of ruminants by Henry Toussaint as soon as May 1880 and disclosed on July 12, 1880, to the great surprise (and confusion?) of Pasteur and his assistants...**
- **On October 26, 1880 Pasteur revealed his method of preparation of his vaccine against chicken cholera[92a], and on February 28, the details of his technique - a year after his first preparation[92b].**

---

89. NAF 18014, f.P. 115.
90. NAF 18014, f.P. 21 back.
91. NAF 18014, f.P. 21 back.
92a. Pasteur, O.C., t. VI, p. 323.
92b. Pasteur, O.C., t. VI, p. 332.

• Pasteur is careful, conscientious and meticulous in his work. He proceeds by stages, one hypothesis at a time, experiment after experiment... Among his collaborators, only Roux is cited in his notes pertaining to this research period, *a priori* without playing a major role. There is nothing original about his participation in the experiments of the summer of 1879. There is no reference to a crucial experiment; Pasteur himself never alluded to one. Reality is more banal, but also more amazing. Pasteur's genius created, in the space of a few weeks, a new discipline, vaccinology, which has benefited a great portion of humanity and of the animal world. A century and a quarter later, vaccinology is still flourishing.

For the first time, on April 26, 1880, Pasteur used the word "to vaccinate" officially: "*In order to explain more clearly and more succinctly the results I reported, I would like to use the word "vaccinate" to refer to the act of inoculating a chicken with the attenuated virus.*"[93] On August 8, 1881, speaking at the international medical Congress in London, Pasteur ended his presentation on vaccines against Chicken Cholera and Splenic Fever by saying: "*I gave the term vaccination an enlarged meaning that science, I hope, will consecrate as an homage to the merit and immense services rendered by one of the greatest men of England, your Jenner. What Joy for me to glorify this immortal name on the very soil of the noble and hospitable city of London!*"[94] Pasteur was no doubt aware of the work of Diday and Auzias-Turenne who had used the term "to vaccinate" to describe their immunisation procedure against syphilis. Pasteur was paying homage to his forerunner, Jenner, and also borrowing from the syphilis researchers without naming them. It must also be remembered that the scientific and humanitarian glory of these men had considerably faded with time.

Pasteur continued to study chicken cholera. In November 1880, he tried "*to restore virulence to a culture* (of chicken cholera bacteria) *no longer virulent for the chickens*", and he used "*a coral-beaked bird (?), a silver-beaked Tanager, a green parrot, a goldfinch, a canary, two guinea pigs 2 months old, 2 old guinea pigs, 2 beautiful rabbits*"[95]. He also used white mice and quails.

In December 1880, Pasteur re-oriented his research in another direction: he started a long series of inoculations of the chicken cholera bacteria in sparrows: at least 41 successive inoculations, but he was to lose the strain[96]. This method of virulence attenuation of a pathogenic virus specific to a species by passing it to another animal species was based on the classical idea of attenuation of the smallpox virus by passage through cows, an idea never formally confirmed. We now know that the two viruses, smallpox and cowpox, are related, but different.

Obviously, Pasteur was not satisfied with his vaccine against chicken cholera. Its side effects often produced discomfort and could even be disabling. Its preparation was going to be difficult. Finally, the cost was prohibitive. In 1880, Victor Galtier, professor at the Lyon Veterinary School, analysed the value of this mode of protection - he did not call it vaccine - as follows: "*But thanks to a method of culture he did not reveal, Monsieur Pasteur has succeeded in attenuating the deathly power of the cholera microbe, so as to be able to inoculate it without causing death, and to induce immunity in the inoculated animals... The immunity conferred to chickens by this method is quite real... Some inoculated chickens, after having been very sick, recover relative health, then lose weight and die weeks*

93. Pasteur, O.C., t. VI, p. 304.
94. Pasteur, O.C., t. VI, p. 388.
95. NAF 18016, f.P. 1.
96. NAF 18016, f.P. 9 & 18.

or months later, presenting the cholera parasite, whose virulence is in no way attenuated, and which had long been lodging, no doubt, in tissues not readily lending themselves to culture. Moreover, sometimes the chickens given immunity develop an abscess somewhere in the body, and this abscess contains the cholera microbe."[97] Clearly, this is not a very enthusiastic assessment. Pasteur must not have been very happy to read this text, which nevertheless probably reflects reality quite closely. This could explain the strained relations between the two men, as well as Pasteur's attitude toward Galtier's work.

Later, in 1892, Galtier reiterated his opinion. It was no more favourable, but it was based on a greater quantity of results: "*However, the vaccination* (against chicken cholera) *can sometimes be associated with more or less serious accidents. Death can result sometimes quickly, sometimes slowly... and immunity can actually be conferred sometimes, although certainly not to the majority of the animals vaccinated; it is also certain that local lesions at the inoculation site cause the animals great suffering, and that immunity develops too slowly to make it possible, by means of vaccination, to check a cholera epizootic that can ravage a chicken coop in a few days; that the inoculated animals can spread the disease, transmitting it to healthy, non-vaccinated animals through their excrement, epidermal pellicles and feathers fallen from the inoculated region. And let us not forget that the price of vaccinations is too high...*"[98]. An even more severe assessment... Some of the problems related to this vaccination, such as an abscess at the inoculation site or a chronic form of the disease, are well-known[99] and have been pointed out by Pasteur himself, who minimised them[100]. In 1897, Galtier again expressed numerous reservations about the use of Pasteur's chicken cholera vaccine, but he ended his text with the admission: "*Some veterinarians have obtained good results when using preventive vaccinations.*"[101] This shows a softening of his previous judgement.

More disturbing still, Nocard, a collaborator of Pasteur's, expressed a similar opinion: "*Despite its unquestionable efficiency, this vaccine has not been widely used in practice.*"[102] In 1914, things have still not progressed. Courmont and Panisset stated: "*This vaccination procedure has not become wide-spread despite its effectiveness.*"[103] Years later, Lesbouyries, renowned specialist of avian pathologies, delivered the final blow to this ground-breaking vaccine: "*This path opened by Pasteur's genius and which proved to be so fruitful, soon ended in an impasse for the chicken cholera vaccination. Difficulties arose with the predictability of attenuation and with maintaining virulence at an established and constant degree.*"[104] Finally, conferred immunity did not last very long, varying between a month and a year at the most[105]. The chicken cholera vaccine was greeted with no particular enthusiasm, other than among a small number of specialists. It was more a laboratory model than a usable vaccine, and Pasteur no doubt considered it as such, although his laboratory was producing it and offering it for sale.

The fact remains that the chicken cholera vaccine was the first artificial vaccine. In medicine, this is a major achievement. Through this experiment and the conclusions he drew from it, Pasteur opened the way to a scientific discipline that has been among

97. Galtier, 1880, p. 303.
98. Galtier, 1892, t. 2, p. 745.
99. NAF 18014, f.P. 35.
100. Pasteur, O.C., t. VI, p. 312.
101. Galtier, 1897, p. 1261.
102. Nocard, 1896, p. 17.
103. Courmont, 1914, p. 705.
104. Lesbouyries, 1941, p. 340.
105. Pasteur, O.C, t. VII, p. 55.

the most fruitful for humanity. In 1880, just when Pasteur revealed the vaccination against chicken cholera, the editorial [probably written by Charles Richet (Nobel prize, 1913) or at least with his consent] of the *Revue scientifique* reported on Pasteur's work in its February issue: "*However - and this is the fundamental discovery of the great academician - the chickens poisoned in this manner by the weakened infectious virus, will no longer be able, after their recovery, to contract cholera again... In short, we can say that the weakened cholera virus behaves in relation to the virulent virus like cowpox in relation to smallpox.*"[106] The editorial was right. The hope was to artificially create a "cowpox vaccine" for every infectious disease. The transition from idea to reality was to be long and difficult and, a century later, still imperfect and incomplete.

But Pasteur's explanation of the mechanism of the immunity afforded by his chicken cholera vaccine was inaccurate. "*As to the cause of an absence of recurrence, we cannot overlook the idea that for the microbe, agent of the disease, the body of the animal becomes a culture medium and that, for the sake of its own vital needs, it alters or destroys, which amounts to the same thing, certain elements, either by creating them for its own benefit or by burning them using oxygen taken from the blood.*"[107] On August 6, 1880, Pasteur wrote to Dumas: "*Good or bad, this explanation is satisfactory at the moment because it accounts for the first achievements. As long as it will be perceived in this light, it will be wise to look for experimental confirmation of the deductions it invites.*"[108] Pasteur was content with this explanation for a time, before he found others.

There is almost no trace left of the actual chicken cholera vaccine, because it was never efficient and was soon replaced by the slaughter of contaminated animals, to avoid the spread of the disease. The concept of a vaccine prospered throughout the world and brought Pasteur immense and well-earned glory.

Pasteur's Discovery and Related Controversies

Pasteur's initiation of the discipline of vaccinology gave rise to endless discussions and even serious disagreements among his contemporaries. The idea of vaccinating with a microbial strain with attenuated virulence was not easily accepted. As soon as it appeared in print, Pasteur was subjected to criticism, particularly from German scientists. Koch and his assistants became his permanent, declared adversaries. "*In 1881, Löffler asserted that if a culture loses its virulence, it is because it is impure, because a foreign organism accidentally entered it from the outside and took the place of the pathogenic agent.*"[109] In the same year, Buchner also declared that the anthrax bacillus, through successive cultures in different mediums, comes to resemble the hay bacillus, *Bacillus subtilis*[110]. "*Here we have the attenuated anthrax bacillus transformed into the hay bacillus. Then Buchner starts with the real hay bacillus and through successive cultures, by educating the microbe... in the end he observes all the morphological attributes of the anthrax bacilla and at the same time their essential quality, virulence. This is transformational theory at its purest.*"[111] In 1887, Flügge wrote, referring to Pasteur's work on the chicken cholera vaccine:

106. Editorial, 1880, p. 789.
107. Pasteur, O.C., t. VI, p. 305.
108. Pasteur, O.C., t. VI, p. 315.
109. Quoted by Bouchard, 1889, p. 52.
110. Gradle, 1883, p. 100; Bouchard, 1889, p. 52.
111. Bouchard, 1889, p. 53.

"*Pasteur's results have not been confirmed by Kitt, among others. Cultures on potatoes and on gelatine, six months old and constantly exposed to outer air, showed the same virulence as recent, pure cultures. It is possible that in Pasteur's cultures, always developed in liquid medium, there could have been pollulation of foreign bacilla that caused the reduction of virulence.*"[112] The last sentence is representative of the intention of Pasteur's Germanic competitors: to demonstrate poor technique.

Does the invention of a vaccine, a concrete product, start with the idea of its conception or with its first, awkward application, or only with its more or less industrial-scale development? Traditionally, an idea and its application can be patented if they are not obvious.

The description must be explicit enough to allow a qualified person to reproduce the invention. Pasteur's procedure of presenting his chicken cholera vaccine to the Academy of Sciences on February 9, 1880 was daring and risky. He had the idea and some proven elements for its application, but no vaccines strictly speaking. However, he had a real intellectual head start in the field, compared to his contemporaries.

Was Pasteur Secretive and a Fraud, or a Selfless Genius?

When he first presented his chicken cholera vaccine, why did Pasteur choose not to reveal its mode of preparation? It is hard to say, but this was a common practice at the time. His August 5, 1880 letter to Lister, in which he clearly admits his insufficient mastery of the preparation of chicken cholera vaccine[113], gives an adequate reason for not revealing his method. In 1880, only a few months later, Toussaint attempted to hide the method of preparation of his anthrax vaccine, and only revealed it under pressure from the Academy of Medicine and because of the moral pressure (probably) exerted by Bouley. Toussaint also had an unproven method. In 1885, Ferran would not reveal to official foreign Commissions the mode of production of his anti-cholera vaccine, but he had admittedly described it previously. In 1889, Grancher (senior physician ("*Professeur*") at Pediatric diseases clinic, Faculty of Medicine) submitted a sealed envelope - with secret content - to the Academy of Medicine; it described "*a method for the cure of tuberculosis, based on an inoculation system*"[114]. The treatment and the vaccination method in question were only revealed after nine months of secrecy[115]. In 1890, Koch kept secret the method of fabrication of tuberculin for over six months: from August 4, 1890 to January 14, 1891[116]. Thus, Pasteur's behaviour is similar to that of other researchers of his era.

There are no known documents to date depriving Pasteur of the glory of having discovered the concept of a vaccine by artificial and stable (?) modification of the virulence of a pathogenic agent, a fact which in no way detracts from the competence and merit of his assistants Chamberland and Roux. Did Pasteur count his chickens before they were hatched? At the time of his first presentation, the preparation of the vaccine was not entirely well controlled, but some of his experiments were valid. In the past few years, Pasteur's role in the discovery of the chicken cholera vaccine has been

112. Flügge, 1887, p. 218.
113. Pasteur, Cor., t. 3, p. 155.
114. Anonyme, 1890a, p. 7.
115. Grancher, 1890, p. 333.
116. Arloing, 1891, p. 365.

seriously challenged[117]. The historical foundations of these dilatory comments are very far removed from the original contents, given on the preceding pages, of Pasteur's laboratory notebooks, which can be consulted at the *Bibliothèque nationale de France* (French National Library).

What was Pasteur's contribution to the field of protection against infectious diseases? At the time, two procedures were known: those classified as "variolation" against smallpox, sheeppox and contagious bovine pleuropneumonia; and Jennerian vaccination. The latter always raised the question of the relatedness of the cowpox virus to the smallpox virus. A number of other clinical assays had been conducted, with no practical results. Pasteur's chicken cholera vaccine offered the advantages of an artificial, man-made "cowpox vaccine". It raised the hope that every infectious disease whose pathogen is known can have its own "cowpox vaccine".

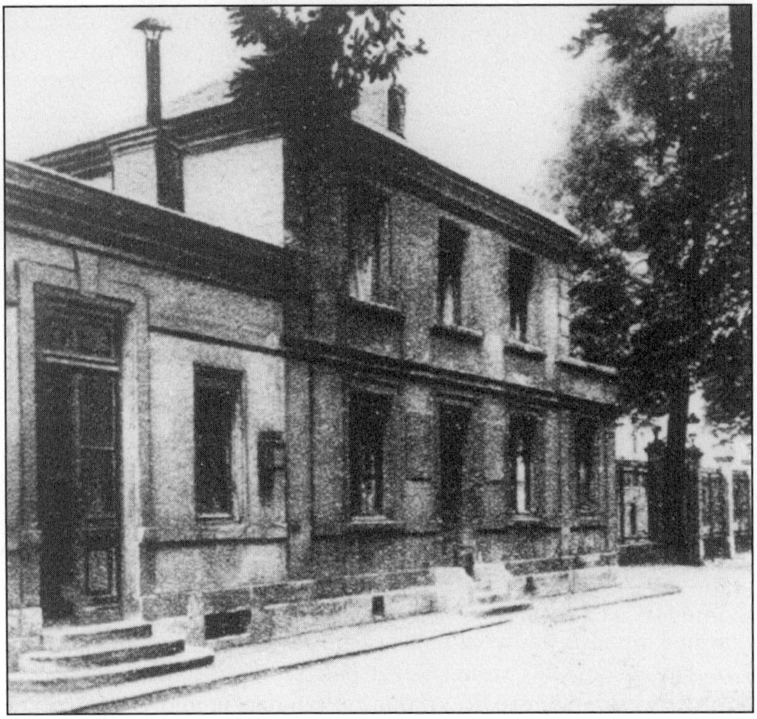

Figure 5. Catetaker's quarters: Pasteur's first laboratory at the *Ecole Normale Supérieure*.

The idea of a vaccine was gaining ground at the time. The first artificial vaccine was created in Pasteur's laboratory, at the *Ecole Normale Supérieure*, on Ulm Street in Paris. Pasteur found a specific vaccine against a disease, chicken cholera, by cultivating its agent in particular conditions. He was hoping with all his heart to be able to extend the field of application of his first vaccine, using his initial method - the one by oxygen - to which he remained strongly attached. But to be remembered as "the saviour of chickens" was not the glory that Pasteur sought. Something else was needed to impress

117. Cadeddu, 1985; Decourt, 1989; Geison, 1995; Robin, 2002; etc. My commentary on their opinions will be the subject of an upcoming work.

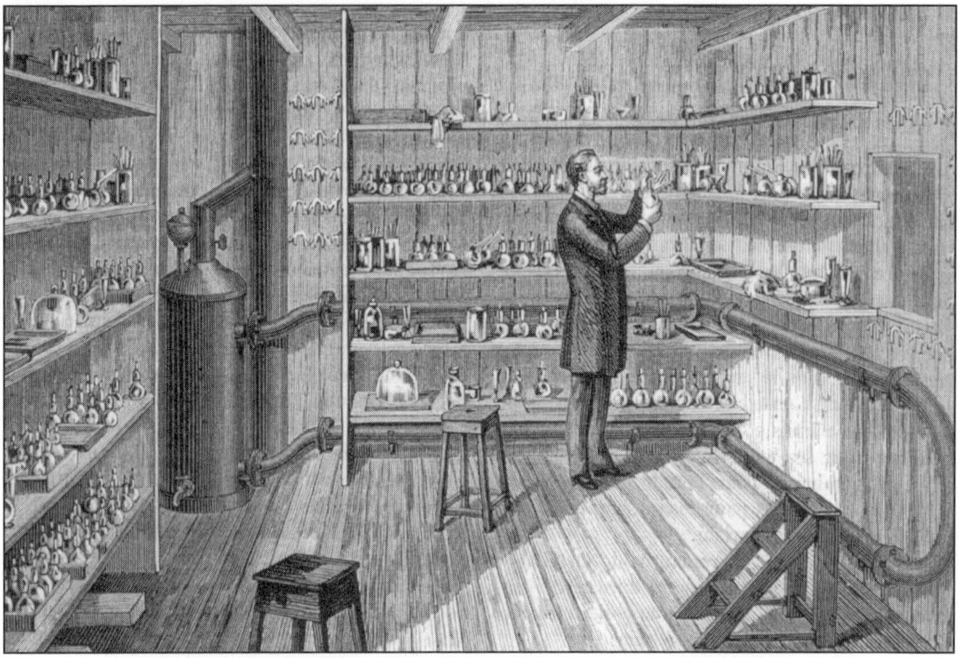

Figure 6. Pasteur's laboratory at the *Ecole Normale Supérieure*. Incubator for microbial culture.

the world. He had to go on to something better. The adventures involving the anthrax vaccine were arduous for the team, because Pasteur took risks in order to achieve what he wanted. He eventually triumphed, but not without effort, and not without finding himself in conflict with the unfortunate Toussaint, who ended up taking the heaviest losses.

If we want to define Pasteur's role in the proliferation of so-called Pastorian vaccines starting in 1880, it is fair to say that he was the first to present the idea of a vaccine prepared from a virulent virus specific to a disease, whose virulence was attenuated or eliminated by man. His idea was built on results acquired thanks to an uncertain vaccine of limited interest; this would no longer be the case for the three other vaccines developed by Pasteur and his team. Nevertheless, his initial idea began a veritable revolution in the world. The studies of Burdon Sanderson and Greenfield on anthrax at the Brown Institution in London are highly interesting, but did not open to the so-called Pastorian Vaccine. They will be analysed in another book.

6
Cattle Anthrax and Splenic Fever in Sheep: 1880-1881...

Pasteur hoped to find a way of modifying the virulence of any pathogenic agent, so as to produce a vaccine for any infectious disease, as he had done with chicken cholera. He chose to concentrate on anthrax; in fact, since his work on this disease had already received financial support, he was obliged to carry it out. In common language, this disease was known as cattle anthrax and splenic fever of sheep. Epidemics, catastrophic for animal breeders, raged in most areas of the world. The disease led to septicaemia, which caused convulsions, hematuria (presence of blood in the urine), fever... and death. Very rapidly, the disease decimated herds of bovines and sheep, as well as many other animal species, even elephants among them[1]. "*The 'charbon' is called anthrax by the Greeks, and 'carbo' or 'carbunculus' by the Latins... And in fact the 'charbon' burns like hot coals, & has the colour of extinguished embers; for it is a burning tumor, & has a black crust.*"[2] "*... In common use in England is splenic fever... The names applied to the disease when it occurs in horned cattle seem to be commonly, black quarter, mal noir, glossanthrax...* (In humans) *the disease, in England, has received the trivial names of woolsorters disease, and malignant pustule.*"[3] Human anthrax, caused by *Bacillus anthracis*, was common in areas where men worked with cattle or the crude products of cattle breeding. Pasteur, son of a leather tanner, must have been familiar with this zoonosis. Most often, human anthrax started with a pimple that developed at the site of a skin infection. The infection was usually contracted by contact with substances containing anthrax spores. Left untreated, the disease spread throughout the body and, in most cases, led to the death of the patient. Bacterial anthrax is caused by Davaine's bacillus or *Bacillus anthracis*, called "bactéridie" by Pasteur himself after the name proposed by Davaine. "Bactéridie" was translated as "Bacteridium" [Davaine] in the Billings Medical Dictionary[4], and will appear as "bacteridium" in the present text.

There is also a disease of cattle called symptomatic anthrax, which will be discussed separately at the end of this chapter. Pasteur and Toussaint's studies concern only the bacterium *Bacillus anthracis*, the agent of bacterial anthrax.

The treatment of human anthrax was well known: the affected area was to be "*eliminated by repulsive or resolutive remedies... That if despite the above the malignancy still persists, Galen orders immediate or potential cauterisation...*"[5]. Later, the approach was even more direct: "*Physicians of the Beauce who have occasion to treat malignant anthrax daily* (true anthrax, not simply a furuncle), *usually prefer a sublimate, and some of them potash. With a lancet, they make a cross-shaped incision in the pustule until they reach healthy tissue, use scissors to detach the four flaps of mortified skin, stop the flow of blood and*

1. Kengragsat, 1926, p. 13.
2. D'Aquapendente, 1649, p. 140.
3. Williams, 1886, p. 549; Black's veterinary dictionary, 1967, p. 41.
4. Billings National Medical Dictionary, 1890, vol. 1, p. 141.
5. D'Aquapendente, 1649, p. 140.

immediately pour in the cavity they have obtained one to two grams of powdered sublimate. This causes the patient to experience a very sharp burning sensation..."[6]. We can easily imagine...

The anthrax bacterium, *Bacillus anthracis*, still has special status today. This germ that is inhaled into the lungs with the air we breathe is one of the most dreaded weapons of bacteriological warfare. Certain countries have produced bombs filled with the spores of this germ, intended to be dispersed without being killed when the bombs explode. But this germ has played other roles in the past. "*Because it was discovered at the dawn of bacteriology, because of the ease with which it lends itself to experimentation, and because of the considerable economic interests linked to knowledge of anthrax, for a long time Bacillus anthracis was the favourite microbe to use in laboratory studies.*"[7]

Veterinary vaccines against anthrax, and above all proper elimination of the bodies of animals that died of anthrax, have made it possible to eradicate the disease almost entirely in developed countries. However, the disease still occurs in certain regions of France, in animals. Human cases are rare. In France, an 11-year old girl died of anthrax on February 5, 1996. The origin of the infection was never clearly established[8].

The History of Ruminant Anthrax

The transmission of anthrax from animal to animal was discovered a very long time ago. In 1863, Davaine wrote: "*In 1850, I examined with Monsieur Rayer several cases of this disease* (splenic fever), *both in his Paris laboratory and during an excursion to Chartres, where I accompanied this venerable master... In the course of a first observation, the blood examined under a microscope eight to ten hours following death presented a very large number of bacteria; in healthy living sheep, or sheep killed for consumption, such Infusoria are never found...*"[9]. But this observation did not lead the two authors to associate the phenomenon with anthrax etiology. Pollender stated that he had seen these corpuscles before Rayer, in 1849, but only described them in 1855, after Rayer did. This explains the fact that some German-speaking authors attribute the discovery to Pollender[10]. Subsequently, Delafond d'Alfort was to show that these corpuscles are living organisms that can be cultivated *in vitro* and multiply in this setting. However, their role was still seen as simply accessory rather than causal.

Linking the origin of infectious diseases with these stick-like organisms was a completely original idea that would not be readily accepted. From today's perspective, we can see that the elaboration of current infectious germ theory was a very lengthy, collective effort. In 1546, Fracastor formulated the hypothesis of infinitely small beings, Van Leeuwenhoek described them, and in 1845 Semmelweis assigned them a role in pathology, without identifying them. The crucial idea arrived in 1863. Davaine was still puzzled by the enigmatic corpuscles that he had observed

6. Rengade, 1879, p. 173.
7. Kengragsat, 1926, p. 16.
8. Vaissaire, 2001, personal communication.
9. Davaine, 1863, p. 220.
10. Kolle, 1918, t. 1, p. 210.

with Rayer; they were still in the back of his mind. When he read Pasteur's writings on fermentation, he asked himself if, by any chance, the tiny filiform organisms in animals killed by splenic fever could not be the cause of the disease, rather than an artefact. In 1863, he wrote: "*I had not yet had occasion, and other tasks did not allow me* (Davaine was a practicing physician with a private clientele), *to look for it* (the cause of deterioration of the blood and, as a result, the death of the animal) *actively, when Monsieur Pasteur, in February 1861, published his remarkable work on butyric ferment, a ferment consisting of small cylindrical sticks, having all the characteristics of vibrions and bacteria. The filiform corpuscles I saw in the blood of sheep with splenic fever having a shape very similar to that of these vibrions, I was led to investigate if analogous corpuscles... These reflections intensified my desire to examine a new the blood of animals with splenic fever, but two summers passed without any possibility that I might obtain a sheep with this affection... These corpuscles obviously developed during the infected animal's life, and they were no doubt related to the disease that caused its death.*"[11] But only two weeks after Davaine's communication, a letter written by Signol, read before the Academy of Sciences, complicated the problem: bacteria are present in numerous diseases, so that they are probably artefacts...[12]. This argument was used over and over to oppose Davaine, together with the notion of a hypothetical virus existing alongside the pathogenic bacteria. Guipon, the author of an excellent study on anthrax written in 1867 (four years after Davaine's communication), remained very skeptical about the idea of an infectious germ. "*Regarding Monsieur Davaine's theory of bacteria or bactéridies, which asserts that these Infusoria constitute a constant and quite specific property of anthrax diseases, since not only are they found in large numbers in animals naturally affected with the disease, but can also be detected in the blood of animals to which the disease was inoculated, and this within a very short time, we wish to express a more reserved opinion, first because even if these organisms are specific to anthrax, nothing proves that they are not its result rather than its cause; and second because similar corpuscles have been found in the most diverse fluids...*"[13]. As long as it was maintained that bacteria represented an effect of the disease and not its cause, they were not assigned a role in infectious pathology.

It was at this time that Weigert discovered the staining of bacteria with aniline and Schroeter dyes, and the possibility of differentiating bacteria an solid media. Koch put these valuable discoveries to good use[14]. He also demonstrated that certain bacteria have the ability to sporulate. He definitively confirmed their role in anthrax, a role already more or less established by Davaine and Pasteur.

Pasteur Investigates Ruminant Anthrax

Pasteur began his studies of anthrax in 1877. How could animals be protected from anthrax? When bacteria are placed in unfavourable conditions, they sporulate to protect themselves from the external medium. They can survive for ten minutes at a temperature of 99-100° C[15]. Anthrax spore virulence does not change over time.

11. Davaine, 1863, p. 220.
12. Signol, 1863, p. 348.
13. Guipon, 1867, p. 135.
14. Frankland, 1898, p. 145.
15. de Varigny, 1884, p. 277.

Pasteur examined the problem of protection against anthrax, first by hygiene [the accursed fields ("*champs maudits*")] and the role of earthworms that push up the spores of carelessly buried cadavers], then by the development of a vaccine that was to become his major endeavour. In 1878, Pasteur and Toussaint were asked separately by the same authorities to study anthrax in order to reduce its ravages. This imposed competition did nothing to improve their long-term relations.

Henry Toussaint: an Intruder in the Field of Vaccines

In 1880, when the summer holidays arrived, Pasteur left Paris for Arbois, as he did every year. Suddenly, he was amazed to learn the incredible news that Toussaint had succeeded in immunising sheep and dogs (that is, producing a protective effect) against anthrax, using a vaccine he had created. Pasteur was advised of this by a letter from Bouley, which arrived in Arbois on August 9, and which contained newspaper clippings and Reports of the Academy of Sciences. Toussaint's presentation before the Academy of Sciences, referred to by Bouley, took place on July 12, 1880.The subject of the presentation was preventive inoculation of dogs and sheep: "*My experiments involved eleven of these animals* (of the Lauraguais breed, very susceptible to anthrax). *Five were inoculated against anthrax one time only, but at different times and died in two or three days... The six remaining animals were inoculated preventively. After a single vaccination, two were inoculated with anthrax, and one of them died with the usual symptoms. I vaccinated the remaining five again and, over the past month, I gave each one a subcutaneous inoculation of anthrax-infected blood from a dog, a rabbit, a ewe; and an inoculation of spores, without producing any local or general symptoms.*"[16] Toussaint specifies that he had started this work on the protection of animals against anthrax in April or at the beginning of May 1880[17], and that the idea was inspired by Pasteur's work on the vaccination against chicken cholera, published on February 9, 1880. The first reliable data on ruminant immunisation against anthrax were provided by a study commissioned by the Minister of Agriculture, and conducted by Pasteur and his team. The objective of the study was to test a new anthrax treatment invented by a Jura veterinarian, Mr. Louvrier. An experiment took place in the summer of 1879. Some cows, treated or not, recovered spontaneously from the inoculation of anthrax bacteria, and proved not to be receptive to a subsequent test dose, as some sheep cured of anthrax in the Beauce in 1878 had already shown. Pasteur commented: "*We know of a virulent parasitic disease* (chicken cholera) *that tends not to recur. We now have a second example, consisting of anthrax disease.*"[18] Pasteur and his associates imparted this key notion to Toussaint in 1878, near Châtres, during their respective missions to study anthrax[19]. This could have put Toussaint on the track of an anthrax vaccine, since he knew that post-infectious immunity could exist in this disease.

On July 12, 1880, Bouley presented Toussaint's results to the *Académie des sciences* (Paris). The method of preparation of the vaccine was kept secret; Toussaint entrusted a sealed envelope containing this information to the Secretarial Office of the Academy

16. Toussaint, 1880a, p. 135.
17. Toussaint, 1880a, p. 135; Toussaint, 1880c, p. 574; Toussaint, 1883, pp. 207 & 297.
18. Chamberland, 1883a, p. 97.
19. Pasteur, O.C., t. VI, p. 254.

of Sciences. This procedure had long been employed in France (and might still be), to protect the priority of discoveries. But a few months earlier, Pasteur himself had not done this with his vaccine against chicken cholera! He had not said anything at all. On July 27, 1880, Bouley presented Toussaint's communication to the Academy of Medicine[20], where it provoked a violent reaction among opponents of the germ theory, because Toussaint's method was not revealed. Faced with this outcry, Toussaint quickly revealed the secret of his preparation.

On August 2, 1880, the perpetual Secretary of the Academy of Sciences read, before the assembly, the sealed letter Toussaint had entrusted to him on July 12, 1880, entitled "*Procédé pour la vaccination du mouton et du jeune chien*" (*Procedure for the vaccination of sheep and young dogs against anthrax*)[21]. This letter was read by Bouley at the August 3, 1880 meeting of the Academy of Medicine; Bouley added some comments[22]. Toussaint explained that his procedure makes use of anthrax-contaminated blood, difficult to handle, because the technique of anthrax bacteria culture is unknown to him. He described his failure with filtration of anthrax-contaminated blood, then his recourse to defibrinated blood heated to 55° C for ten minutes. During the March 1, 1881 session of the Academy of Medicine, Colin presented a communication entitled "*Sur un prétendu moyen de conférer l'immunité contre le charbon*" (*On a supposed means of conferring immunity to anthrax*)[23], in which he tried to ridicule Toussaint. Colin's text was malevolent and unfair. Not only did this gesture lack elegance, but his arguments were scientifically incorrect. Toussaint replied to them through Bouley[24].

At the meeting of the *Association française pour l'avancement des sciences* (French Association for the Advancement of Sciences), held that year in Reims, Toussaint provided detailed explanations. On August 9, 1880, he described his study of the pathogenesis of anthrax infection in the bodies of inoculated animals: "*I observed, moreover, that in several species the lymph node can stop the bacteridia, act as a sort of filter; this occurs in pigs and most often in adult dogs. When this takes place, the lymph node is inflamed, and enlarges to ten times its normal size; then, in a few days, five or six, these phenomena disappear and the bacteridia present die; the inflamed lymph node returns to nearly its previous size, but retains considerable firmness and greater consistency, which confer it a certain impermeability to parasites. Making lymph nodes impermeable was the objective of my first studies. I used filtered anthrax-contaminated blood... To test the above hypothesis, I had to inoculate each lymph-node region. Eight to ten inoculations were practiced at points on the external surface of the regions corresponding to these lymph nodes. The first inoculations of fresh anthrax-contaminated blood were made on the fifteenth day after the filtered blood injection... The absence of local or general phenomena indicated complete immunity.*"[25] Toussaint's studies had already demonstrated, concerning lymph nodes "*which receive lymph from the inoculation site, that these lymph nodes are swollen, bruised, surrounded by more or less pronounced oedema; and that they contain such a considerable accumulation of bacteria that the structure of the lymph node seems modified*"[26].

20. Tousaint *in* Bouley, 1880a, p. 753.
21. Toussaint, 1880d, p. 301.
22. Bouley, 1880c, p. 791; Toussaint, 1880c, p. 574.
23. Colin, 1881, p. 279.
24. Bouley, 1881a, p. 300.
25. Toussaint, 1881a, p. 1021.
26. Toussaint, 1879, p. 1143.

Toussaint was attempting to obtain killed bacteria, so as to use their phlogistic action (producing inflammation) on lymph nodes. As he himself said[27], he used the procedures described by Davaine in 1873: heating to 55° C for ten minutes, or the effect of diluted carbolic acid[28]. Paper filtering, apparently Toussaint's own idea, did not allow him to be certain of eliminating all bacteria. Heating was the method providing the best results. Toussaint concluded: "*These experiments show that, when we inject in the subcutaneous conjunctive tissue of a young dog, a sheep or even a rabbit, a small quantity of anthrax-contaminated blood, diluted and filtered through twelve filters, or subjected to 55° heat or to carbolic acid, we produce a state thanks to which bacteridia inoculated subsequently no longer produce any local or general phenomenon.*"[29] Toussaint started with a false hypothesis and arrived at an accurate result. Bouley was delighted with Toussaint's results. He obtained permission from the Minister of Agriculture to use twenty sheep taken from the Alfort Veterinary School flock to test the effectiveness of Toussaint's vaccine[30].

Toussaint arrived from Toulouse with two vials of his vaccine. On July 28, 1880, he "*collected from a dying sheep a sufficient quantity of blood, that was prepared, as I just said, with dosages of one to one-and-a-half per one hundred parts of carbolic acid. After 9 days of preparation (August 6) during which I tried it on rabbits, I used it on ewes. Six ewes were inoculated, three with one percent carbolic acid solution, and the other three with the solution containing one and a half grams of carbolic acid, for one hundred grams of blood (N° 1 of the Alfort series)... on the same day, I left for Paris...*"[31]. Once in Paris, Toussaint continued his account: "*I had brought from Toulouse two vials containing 100 grams of anthrax-contaminated blood, treated with 1.5 gr of carbolic acid since July 28. The two vials only differed from each-other in that solution 1 had been filtered through paper, while solution n° 2 had only been passed through a cloth towel.*"[32] Toussaint's vaccine procedure is often associated with 10-minute heating at 55° C, although this was not the case for his best-known test, that of Vincennes/Alfort (known as Alfort, where the major part of the experiment was conducted), although Roux, who spoke with Toussaint many times during that period, states that the Toussaint vaccine was heated for 10 minutes to 55° C, and then mixed with carbolic acid[33]. This was Toussaint's second method involving carbolic acid and very basic filtering that did not eliminate bacterial organisms. Twenty sheep were inoculated with solution 1, at the Vincennes farm, on August 8, 1880[34]. On August 9, these animals were taken to Alfort where Piot, later known as Piot Bey, and Cadiot, from Professor Trasbot's Service, kept them under observation. Four sheep died rapidly, during the "*first four days*"[35], on the 3rd and 4th day[36], or the 4th and 5th day[37] after inoculation... Some of the sixteen remaining sheep were adversely affected by the vaccine, but survived. And yet the flock was not in the best of health, having just recovered from a

27. Toussaint, 1881a, p. 1021.
28. Davaine, 1873a & b, pp. 726 & 821.
29. Toussaint, 1881a, p. 1021.
30. Bouley, 1880b, p. 942; Bouley, 1880c, p. 791.
31. Toussaint, 1883, p. 256.
32. Toussaint, 1883, p. 256.
33. Roux *in* Nicol, 1974, p. 336.
34. Toussaint, 1883, p. 256.
35. Bouley, 1880d, p. 457.
36. Toussaint, 1881a, p. 1021.
37. Toussaint, 1883, p. 256.

foot-and-mouth disease epizootic, according to Toussaint[38]. Bouley says that the animals were "*beautiful specimens*", which seems contradictory, but Bouley was diplomatic: he did not want to offend the minister who had authority over the Alfort flock, property of the State[39]. On August 22, six new sheep were inoculated with Toussaint vaccine from the second vial, and reacted very well. The twenty-two surviving sheep (sixteen after the August 8 inoculation and six after August 22) had no ill effects after test injections of virulent anthrax bacteria[40]. On October 13, two new ewes were inoculated with the same "solution"; one died on October 19, the other developed an abscess of anthrax bacteria, but survived[41]. It must be noted that the "Toussaint" sheep received a single vaccinal injection, and therefore cannot be directly compared to the sheep vaccinated using the two-injection Pasteur method employed at Pouilly-le-Fort. Toussaint's vaccine is alive (at least partially), since the animals that died after the first vaccination had living bacteridia in their blood. This vaccine was later considered by its inventor to be in the same category as the chicken cholera vaccine[42], a live attenuated vaccine, that is, containing a pathogenic agent with attenuated virulence. The fact is that it is difficult to arrive at a firm opinion based on the very incomplete data available to us. However, the overall result was twenty-two immunised sheep out of twenty-six inoculated with a single injection, or twenty-three out of twenty-eight if we include the last two of the month of October, which all reacted well to a test inoculation.

Pasteur made his presentation on the chicken cholera vaccine before the Academy of Sciences on February 9, 1880; Toussaint made his on July 12, 1880. Toussaint had lost no time: only about five months had passed since February! He even specifies, in his note read to the Academy of Medicine on July 27, that he had practiced immunisations "*nearly three months ago*"[43], that is, at the beginning of May[44]. The idea of vaccination comes from Pasteur's work on chicken cholera, as Toussaint himself states[45], but not the method. Pasteur had not yet revealed his preparation technique at that time. He had only revealed his results.

At the September 27, 1880 meeting of the Academy of Sciences (Paris), Pasteur and his assistants revealed that cattle and sheep can become refractory to anthrax, a finding emerging from their work on Louvrier's treatment of anthrax in the Jura. They were lagging behind Toussaint, and were no doubt frustrated by this. It was the start of fierce competition between Toussaint and the Pasteurians. Toussaint was already known at the time, but Pasteur's reputation was even more solidly established. Toussaint had two reputable allies: Chauveau and Bouley, both of whom also had great respect for Pasteur and his studies. Pasteur had dozens of allies... The rivalry soon became heated. Pasteur was clearly passionately involved, as was Toussaint, who was encroaching on someone else's territory. All eyes were on him. And secrecy reigned. The competition for first place in this race created growing tension and firmly held positions in the two camps.

38. Toussaint, 1883, p. 256.
39. Bouley, 1880b, p. 942.
40. Toussaint, 1883, p. 256; Bouley, 1880b, p. 942.
41. Toussaint, 1881a, p. 1021.
42. Toussaint, 1881a, p. 1021.
43. Toussaint, 1880b, p. 753.
44. Toussaint, 1880c, p. 574.
45. Toussaint, 1883, p. 207.

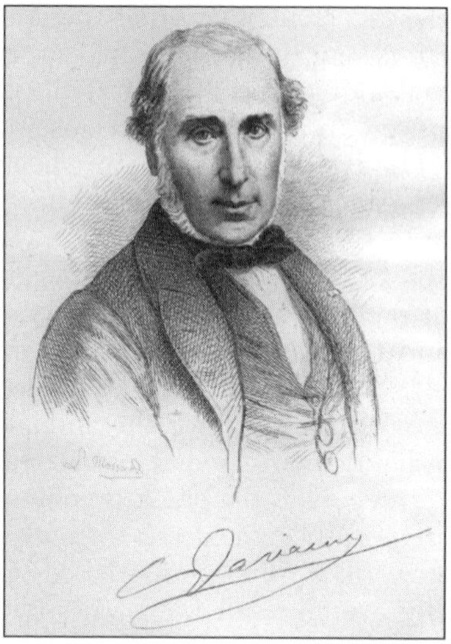

Casimir-Joseph Davaine (1812-1882). Portrait published by Dr. A. Davaine in 1889 with *L'Œuvre de C.-J. Davaine* at the J.-B. Baillière et Fils Librairie in Paris.

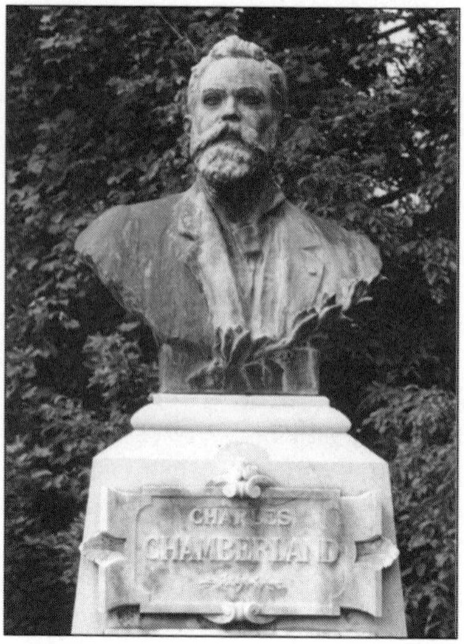

Charles Chamberland (1851-1908). Funeral monument of the bacteriologist, erected in Chilly-le-Vignoble (Jura). (Photo kindly provided by Mr. Gilles Béjot.)

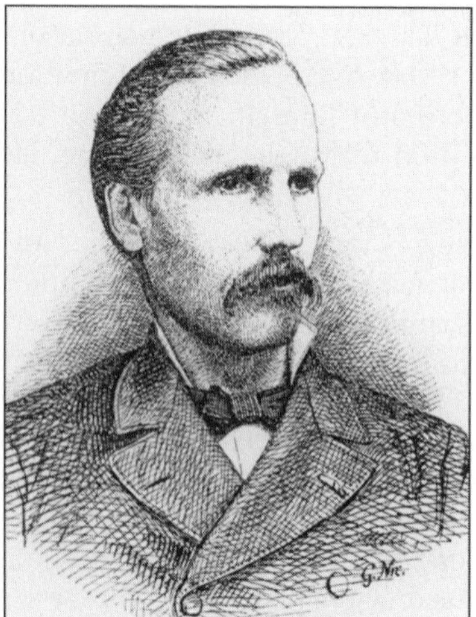

J.-J.-H. Toussaint (1847-1890). According to his contemporaries, not a very good resemblance. Still, the man deserves admiration. He was a brilliant researcher who struggled with various difficulties. Although he ventured too far in his writings, he was a remarkable pioneer in the field of infectious disease prevention. (Neumann, 1896, p. 383.)

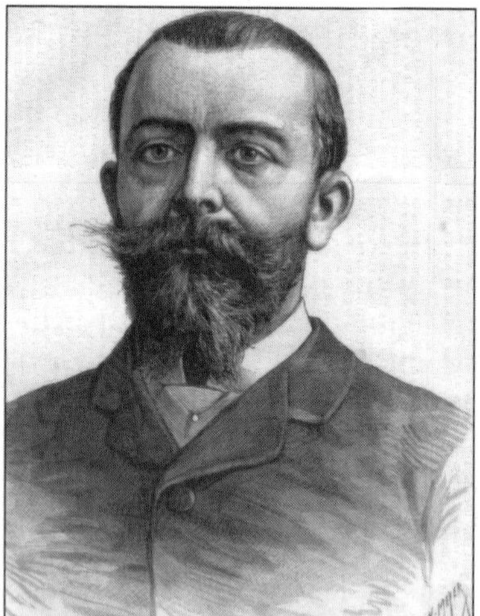

Louis Thuillier (1857-1883). Having gone to Egypt to study cholera, as a member of a French scientific mission, this collaborator of Pasteur died of the Epidemic in Alexandria at the age of twenty-six. Drawing by Henri Meyer, Photograph by Pierre Petit. (*Le journal illustré*, n° 7, October 1883.)

Figure 1. A few protagonists in the discovery of the anthrax vaccine.

What is of capital importance is that Toussaint made two interesting observations which clearly supported his work. On the one hand, the test injection with the greatest load of bacteridia, given "*without provoking any local or general phenomenon*" in the vaccinated animals[46]. On the other hand, the fact that "*the vaccinal effect is only complete after twelve to fourteen days*"[47], which showed the development of an immune response. Chauveau had already noted that the protection conferred by a first anthrax bacteridium inoculation only appeared after a few days[48]. This lapse of time was already known to exist in the case of smallpox vaccinations. This was one of the earliest measurable observations in immunology. Finally, animals could have true protection. Toussaint vaccinated. At first, he maintained that his vaccine was dead, with all the consequences this had for Pasteur's theory of exhaustion, which Toussaint was attacking. Not only was he invading Pasteur's domain, but he went so far as to question Pasteurian immunity theory.

"*At first, these experiments led me to conclude that a substance secreted by a parasite, a product of excretion, had a vaccinal effect on the disease caused by this parasite. It was the first time that such a fact was observed in physiology.*"[49] This statement can be interpreted as an acceptation of Chauveau's immunity theory (*see Glossary*), or as the notion of a chemical vaccine. It indicates Toussaint's uncertainty about the physiological mechanism explaining the effect of his vaccination procedure.

Pasteur Mounts a Counter-Attack, without Amunition

On August 10, 1880, Pasteur wrote to Bouley: "*I dreamed of it asleep or awake all night long.*"[50] He was evidently displeased that a young professor from a provincial Veterinary School should rise to his level. He had been working for years on ruminant anthrax, and this little scamp was surpassing him. Clearly, Pasteur and his team had trouble accepting competition from Toussaint. Pasteur's immediate reaction was to have Toussaint's experiments reproduced. He addressed his pressing request to Roux in Paris and to Chamberland, who was in his Chilly-le-Vignoble summer residence (not far from Lons-le-Saunier, in the Jura).

Pasteur made the trip from Arbois to Chamberland's residence to undertake with his assistant the reproduction of Toussaint's experiment[51]! They concluded, rather rapidly, that Toussaint's results were scarcely or not at all reproducible[52].

In the meantime, Pasteur was still searching for a vaccine.

• **November 21, 1880:** "*Anthrax Test of bacteridium attenuation by air... Blood sample is taken from this sheep... this blood is used to seed 8 flasks of chicken broth and 2 flasks of yeast solution. It is 10 o'clock in the morning. Tonight the flasks will be taken out of the incubator and placed in the basement next to a thermometer. I hope that these bacteridia that have not had time to produce spores will be exposed to air in this state without ever forming spores and be attenuated by the action of oxygen. Unfortunately on the 24th the basement*

46. Toussaint, 1880c, p. 574.
47. Bouley *in* Toussaint, 1880c, p. 574.
48. Bouley, 1880b, p. 942.
49. Toussaint, 1881a, p. 1021.
50. Pasteur, Cor., t. 3, p. 158.
51. Pasteur, Cor., t. 3, p. 160.
52. NAF 18092, item 128.

thermometer rose to 13°. November 25. Still 13° and 14° in the basement. This temperature must produce spores. This test will be repeated when the cold sets in."[53]

• **January 5, 1881:** "*Anthrax. Culture of the bacteridium in cold temperature at 16° and at 41°. Comparison of virulences... in flasks at 17°... nowhere did I see spores... Flasks at 35° and 41°5 are very similar... with very clear spores in both cases... Culture at 43° at 45° at 47° at 50°... will have to be developed.*"[54]

• **January 14, 1881:** "*Anthrax. Culture of bacteridium at high temperature. See previous p. 35. January 14 evening*" Anthrax *bacteridia* are sown in chicken broth, veal broth and yeast solution... "*and are placed in d'Arsonval incubator set at exactly 43°.*" At the bottom of the page, Pasteur noted that the thermometer reading was inexact, that the temperature was really 42.6° C. At the bottom of the back of a page covered with small writing in pale ink... a note: "***Very important Here is something very important on February 19, the flask at 43° of January 14 developed culture from the 15th to the 16th, but on the 17th, it no longer did. The test was repeated on the 18th still no culture. Finally the last culture of the 15th is not very abundant, cloudy but only slightly (see p. 70) thus no germs at all before death occurs...***". This is probably the first indication of the temperature to be used in the laboratory work.

Pasteur also studied the virulence of these cultures: "***January 30. The guinea pig inoculated on the 24th with the culture developed at 43° presents no symptoms. Therefore after 10 days, the 43° culture has no effect, is very weakened... February 19. Seeing that 4-day old guinea pigs do not die and thus present no reaction, a small white mouse, born in the laboratory 15 days ago, was inoculated. It was inoculated with the last culture developed on February 15... On February 20, the little white mouse is found dead...***"[55].

• **January 26, 1881:** "***Anthrax for attenuation, see previous page 42. Bact. at high temp. Jan. 28... Culture at 43° and at 35° to compare... virulence later... Very important*** *February 9 the guinea pig inoculated with the culture in the tube incubated at 43° from Feb. 3 to 4... is found dead - The other one inoculated from the flask* (i.e. in contact with air) ***is very well and appears healthy. This guinea pig is still very well on Feb. 15... Thus air has an effect at 43° to attenuate the bacteridium since, without exposure to air, a tube, a culture without possible*** (contact?), ***retains its virulence and the corresponding culture in the flask loses it on February 11 and 12 In Fact the culture in the tube incubated (at 43°) killed a sheep on the 3rd day. Virulence is maintained This is very important.***"[56]

• **January 26, 1881:** Pasteur's inquisitive mind turns to another subject: "*Rabies. Search for the organism of true rabies, in the medulla oblongata*[57]*. January 26, 1881. M. Bourrel sent two dogs killed by rabies...*"[58]. This is the start of rabies experiments after a failed attempt in 1880.

• **January 28, 1881:** "*P. 42 indicates that bacteridium flasks cultured at 43° become attenuated very rapidly. On the 26th a culture was developed with a flask cultured at 43° since January 14. It developed very well. This culture from the 26th was re-seeded in chicken*

53. NAF 18016, f.P. 4.
54. NAF 18016, f.P. 35.
55. NAF 18016, f.P. 42 & 42 back.
56. NAF 18016, f.P. 53.
57. "Bulbe" is translated in "*medulla oblongata*" (Billings Medical Dictionary, 1890, vol. 2, p. 124).
58. NAF 18016, f.P. 67.

broth - The culture made on the 20th from the same flask at 43° was also re-seeded. ***The intent is to find out if the weakening observed p. 42 persists in the new cultures and if spores will form in the new successive cultures..."***[59]. Pasteur indicates no such result on this page.

• **February 4, 1881:** "*Still continuing from page 53 Culture of bacteridium at 43° Study for spores... At page 59 there is the study of fls. at 43° from January 28. Every two days, one of these fls. at 43° is used to seed a chicken broth flask that is heated to 35°. Thus we have flasks of culture at 35° originating from the flask at 43° on dates February 4, 7, 9, 11, 13, 15... 21 then March They are* (studied?) *for spore formation and for their virulence. On March 2 Flask of Feb.18 originating from that of February 7 Very important vaccine probable by action* (1 word) *at 42°-43°... A new sheep is inoculated... March 18 The sheep registers 40°.6. It is very well. Obviously, it will be vaccinated... March 23 The sheep is inoculated again, that is after 13 days, with the February 4 culture that has recently killed two sheep and that nevertheless does not kill all guinea pigs every time... March 31, 1881... It* (the sheep) *has now returned to its normal temp... On April 13. The above sheep of April 1rst that received the February 7 culture on March 10 and the Feb. 4 culture on March 29 is re-inoculated with very virulent 4-year old bacteridium It showed no signs on the following days. Thus, at least sometimes, the bacteridium of the 7th followed by that of the 4th vaccinates. See pages 102 and 103.*"[60]

• **February 25, 1881:** "*Return to virulence Continued from last line of p. 42 back.*" After inoculating mice and guinea pigs with *bacteridium*, Pasteur writes: "*On this flask I wrote: probable vaccine, by return to virulence*". Pasteur indicates among his cultures several "*probable vaccines*". "*Therefore using the original culture at page 42 back and p. 70 with the label... the series with return must be repeated in a mouse or in guinea pigs. A pause will be made for vaccine after the first guinea pig, so that after the 2nd virulence is left for the sheep.*" Pasteur was in fact very quickly losing (all?) the virulence of his bacteridia by developing them in culture at 43°, and he was now searching for a vaccine by return of virulence after passages to mice or guinea pigs of different ages. In a note: "***It is clear that there are two modes of returning to virulence for very attenuated bacteridia****;*

1° by using guinea pigs but only when they are 1-day old and gradually larger guinea pigs

2° by using mice and after several generations in mice, passage to guinea pigs."[61] Pasteur often used this technique, referred to in Chamberland's February 18, 1881 note (*see below*), and which gives an idea of the relative stability of his vaccine...

• **February 28, 1881**, Pasteur makes another presentation aiming to ensure his glory and his success. Very sure of himself, he writes: "*... We will demonstrate all the difference between the two methods, the uncertainty of one* (Toussaint's published method), *the reliability of the other...*", his own, of course, which he has to specify in the same text: a week or more at 42°-43° C[62]. In fact, his method is still at the experimental stage, and although the experiments are promising, the method would only be ready to use a few (weeks?) later. In this instance, Pasteur acted (at least) incorrectly because, two months later, on April 28, 1881, when he signed the Pouilly-le-Fort experiment protocol, he was thinking of Chamberland's "bichromate" method (very probably developed in collaboration with Pasteur and Roux), and not of the "oxygen" method he

59. NAF 18016, f.P. 54.
60. NAF 18015, f.P. 78 & 78 back.
61. NAF 18016, f.P. 77 & 77 back.
62. Pasteur, O.C., t. VI, p. 332.

was praising. This is not strictly speaking a lie, since he wrote in the future tense ("*we will demonstrate*"), but his action is questionable.

• **March 12, 1881:** "*As was said p. 78 every two days the flask is cultured at 43° since January 28. At p. 78 it was noted that the February 9 culture is no longer virulent for older guinea pigs... However p. 71 (note) indicates that the February 19 culture (10 days later) was very much weakened and did not kill a 1-day old guinea pig... On March 5, the flask at 43° continues to develop. On March 7 the flask at 43° is still developing. On March 9, 3 div.* (divisions) *of this culture are used to inoculate a young mouse but* (1 word) *young... On March 12 it* (mouse) *is still well. If it does not die the attenuation achieved is such that a return is not conceivable... March 13. The mouse is very well... March 14. The mouse is very well It has been 5 days...* ***This is the first weakened bacteridium that does not kill mice.***"[63] The word "*mice*" is perhaps a slight exaggeration, since only one mouse was inoculated, but the result is real: there has been attenuation of the anthrax bacteridium using the oxygen method. Pasteur did not yet know this result when he made his February 28 presentation.

• **March 18, 1881:** "*New comparative trials of vaccination between 3 cultures originating from the flask incubated at 42-43° since January 18 It is a series from page 78.*"[64]

Each culture is inoculated to two sheep, two rabbits and two guinea pigs. The February 4 culture killed the sheep, the rabbits and one out of two guinea pigs, the one from February 7 killed the sheep, but not the rabbits or the guinea pigs; the one from February 9 killed the two sheep, one guinea pig out of two, and spared the rabbits. At the bottom of this page, Pasteur wrote: "*I take the culture developed on March 18 with spores (originating in a February 4 culture after heating to 90°) spores which served above to inoculate a sheep, and with this culture from these spores I prepare a tube of chicken broth, in a tube with two points in order to maintain this state...* (to preserve the strain from contact with air)."[65]

Pasteur knows how to apply a procedure of virulence attenuation "*from heat*", but the procedure is very rapid and does not make it possible to obtain a vaccine with known virulence. Moreover, his method of assessment based on a small number of subjects belonging to three or four animal species, of various ages, is not discriminating enough. He uses cultures of bacteridia without spores, but also cultures from the cultivated spores of attenuated bacteridia heated to 90° C.

• **March 21, 1881**, Pasteur makes a presentation before the Academy of Sciences, aimed at tearing Toussaint's work to shreds: "*At the end of no more than three weeks, our predictions had already come true. We were convinced that as far as Mr. Toussaint's results were concerned, some lacked precision, others were incorrectly interpreted...*"[66]. Pasteur's communication was, to say the least, aggressive toward Toussaint. Perhaps Toussaint didn't understand what he was doing, but neither did Pasteur. It was Bouley's intervention in Toussaint's favour that influenced Pasteur and made him show indulgence (?) toward this daring opponent who admittedly surpassed him. Bouley is a kind man, and this is evident in the mediatory role he plays between Toussaint and Pasteur[67]. All things considered, it is difficult to detect great benevolence in Pasteur's behaviour. He is elegantly ferocious.

63. NAF 18016, f.P. 91.
64. NAF 18015, f.P. 98.
65. NAF 18015, f.P. 98.
66. Pasteur, O.C., t. VI, p. 339.
67. Nicol, 1974.

• March 30, 1881 "*Continuation of pages 78 and back and see also p. 98 March 30 inoculation of 4 new sheep with February 7 culture (the same as that (filaments) used on March 18 p. 98...* A B C D (are four sheep) *April 13, inoculation of two of these sheep A and B with culture from the* 7th (2 words) *two preventive inoculations will protect them, later, from the culture of the* 4th*... rise in temperature... They are back to normal.*

Inoculation of the other two, C, and D March 30 above Chamberland's culture B. This culture has killed 2 out of 4 sheep and was used on March 18 to test Chamberland's sheep. For both there was a rise in temperature 40°.2 the next day and 41°.1 the day after that... they must already have been vaccinated.

***Thus, this experiment tends to prove that the bacteridium from the* 7th *which does not vaccinate against the bacteridium of the* 4th*, still too virulent (see p. 98 April 1) vaccinates against a bacteridium that killed 2 out of 4 sheep (Chamberland's. The bacteridium of the* 4th *killed more than 2 out of 4 sheep; I do not remember how many just now). Therefore, it was not the vaccine of the* 7th *that had no protective virtue but the culture of the* 4th *that was too virulent for a* 2nd *experiment.*"**

Experiments conducted on April 13 with the 4-year old bacteridium: the two Chamberland sheep C and D survive, A dies on May 1, B survives. Pasteur concludes that: "*The bacteridium from the* 7th *only vaccinates one time out of two. Therefore it is not a reliable vaccine.*"

New vaccination experiments conducted between April 3 and May 6: "*4 new sheep were inoculated with February 9 culture (spores) that was used on March 18 at p. 98. This test was performed because page 98 indicates that today there are deaths with the use of the February 4 bacteridium. This time, we began with the culture from the* 9th*, continued with that of the* 7th*, as a second vaccination, and went on to that of Feb. 4. It is likely that this time, the inoculation with that of Feb.4 will no longer kill... These experiments show that the culture from the* 9th *followed by the culture from the* 7th *does not vaccinate against a virulent bacterium like that of the* 4th*.*"[68a] This laboratory notebook is devoted to anthrax only and goes on to discuss the project agreed upon with the Agriculture Society of Melun.

At this stage of his search for an anthrax vaccine, Pasteur had anthrax bacteridium strains that were only slightly or not at all virulent; he was seeking to obtain vaccinal strains either by reducing their virulence or, essentially, by recovering their virulence through passages to animals. He admits that he has no vaccine that is perfect, but he vaccinates in some cases.

The conflict is clearly one-sided: Pasteur and his team are highly competent, and they have money and renown on their side. When Toussaint made his presentation in August 1880, Pasteur's group had everything... except a real vaccine against anthrax. And yet Bouley wrote to Pasteur on August 27, 1880: "*But the Toussaint phenomenon retains all its importance and I would not be surprised to see an inoculable solution prepared that, extemporaneously used, will act as a vaccine and convey immunity in infected regions.*"[68b] Bouley is still willing not to call vaccine Toussaint's "*inoculable solution*" that "*acts as a vaccine*", so as not to offend Pasteur, but he hopes to be able to immunise animals

68a. NAF 18016, f.P. 102 & 103.

68b. Nicol, 1974, p. 339.

susceptible to the anthrax bacterium. He is not concerned with the conflict, he is only thinking of possible benefits for farm animals, and of the reputation of his profession. Over and over, Bouley states and restates his observations following Pasteur's presentations: "*I am happy to have heard M. Pasteur testify, with the authority carried by his opinion, to the truth of M. Toussaint's discovery.*"[69] Chauveau, professor at the Lyon veterinary school where Toussaint was his student, also lent him his support. After repeating Toussaint's experiments, he published results that agreed with those of the latter. In a communication submitted to the Academy of Sciences, he wrote: "M. *Toussaint's initial research, confirmed and explained by* M. *Pasteur, showed that heating anthrax-infected blood is likely to significantly attenuate the virulence of the bacilli this blood contains.*"[70]

• **About May-June 1882** (Pasteur's note is not dated), Pasteur shows great reserve about Toussaint's work, in his personal notebooks: "*Note on work presented by* M. *Toussaint. Summary of a Toussaint dissertation addressed on May 25, 1882 to the* Institut *for the Vaillant prize.*" Pasteur comments on Toussaint's lack of sincerity at the Reims conference, then: "... *he is not any more honest* (when) *he says that he became aware of his error because of the bacteridia in the blood of 4 sheep that died at Alfort. These deaths due to preventive inoculation were something he had seen many times in Toulouse and he found explanations for them* (spores?)... M. *Toussaint is unwell, 'ta...pis'* (sic, probably stands for the French expression '*tant pis*', meaning 'too bad'.) - *Very painstaking and in this respect praiseworthy, but lacking scientific rigour. I have known it since our St. Germain experiments* (at Mr. Maunoury's farm) *near Chartres, in 1878... Be that as it may, what he puts forth in the 2nd part of his May 25, 1882 communication to the Academy must be verified and he must be given the Vaillant Prize if he is right. Note Chamberland and Roux are more displeased than myself with the little scientific refinement shown by* M. *Toussaint.*"[71] Pasteur does not seem inclined to make allowances for Toussaint's state of health. But is he even aware of it? The fact is that he himself has serious health problems. However, it was not altogether fair to write: "*These deaths due to preventive inoculation were something he had seen many times in Toulouse and he found explanations for them* (one word: spores?)..."[72], because Toussaint had already indicated that he had inoculated six sheep, one of which died of anthrax[73]. Then, describing the Alfort carbolic vaccine: "*After 9 days of preparation (August 6) during which I tried it on rabbits, I used it on ewes. Six of these animals were inoculated, three with one percent carbolic solution, and the other three with the solution containing one and a half grams of carbolic acid per one hundred grams of blood (N° 1 of the Alfort series)... I was leaving for Paris the same day, but I was kept informed, and I knew that they were all in good health ten days after the vaccination.*"[74] *A priori*, Toussaint only had one sheep that died in his laboratory, unless he tested other formulations of his vaccines on other ewes... without reporting his results. An article by Wrotnowska contains many interesting details on Toussaint-Pasteur relations[75].

Later, in 1883, Bouley, rapporteur of the Commission awarding the Vaillant Prize of the Academy of Sciences, made the following evaluation, with his colleagues Pasteur,

69. Bouley, 1881e, p. 668.
70. Chauveau, 1883a, p. 553 & 1883b, p. 612.
71. NAF 18017, f.P. 7.
72. NAF 18017, f.P. 7.
73. Toussaint, 1880c, p. 574.
74. Toussaint, 1883, p. 256.
75. Wrotnowska, 1975.

Bert, Vulpian, Gosselin: "*The process used by M. Pasteur and his assistants was not yet known, M. Toussaint was developing a process of his own... by the application of heat... This process of attenuation, put to the test in practice, proved to be effective...*"[76]. Such a conclusion must have been difficult to accept for Pasteur, but he did not want to upset Bouley whose almost unconditional support was most valuable to him. And in any case, competition from Toussaint was no longer a threat.

Toussaint's Work as Seen by his Contemporaries

For a few years after Pasteur discovered his first vaccine (against chicken cholera), most authors attributed the discovery of the vaccine against anthrax to Toussaint. Bouley and Chauveau took Toussaint's defence at every opportunity. And what about the others? Even those close to Pasteur admitted Toussaint's merit. Duclaux, one of the master's followers, very close to Pasteur, declared: "*As far as anthrax is concerned, it was M. Toussaint who first obtained a virulent fluid, unquestionably possessing the character of a vaccine, that is, transmitting a benign protective anthrax.*"[77]

Chamberland, Pasteur's collaborator, wrote: "*Heat, before killing microbes, also seems to change their virulence, as M. Toussaint was first to show for the anthrax bacteria.*"[78] In 1893, Dr. Grancher, a follower and later a friend of Pasteur's, went so far as to say: "*M. Toussaint had already observed that heat attenuates the anthrax bacteridium and transforms it into a vaccine.*"[79] Obviously, many of his contemporaries saw Toussaint as the inventor of the first vaccine against anthrax[80]. It was Chauveau who had the last word in this situation; in 1882 he wrote: "*... The inventor of the first anthrax vaccine, momentarily incapacitated by illness, was unable to give his discovery all the developments it can have. Toussaint's former teacher felt it was his duty, while his student recovered, to show the public through new experiments the full importance of M. Toussaint's discovery... It* (Toussaint's vaccination method) *is considered, in any case, to be much less reliable. I intend to show this opinion to be mistaken. If it is used in accordance with certain rules that I will lay out, heating, very briefly, blood infected with bacteria, transforms this fluid into a vaccine as reliable as M. Pasteur's vaccine.*"[81] The large-scale application of this procedure was to be carried out by Piot in the Middle East, to fight cattle plague.

The Wind Shifts: Toussaint Loses Favour

Unfortunately, the fact that the paternity of the anthrax vaccine had first been attributed to Toussaint was soon forgotten or worse, denied by Pasteur's team and its admirers. First by Pasteur himself, who delivered the first blow, writing to Bouley on August 20, 1880: "*In all of this there is no vaccine strictly speaking, nothing mysterious, nor extraordinary.*"[82] Pasteur himself was soon to modify the meaning of the word "vaccine" based on his results and the interpretation he gave them. Moreover, Pasteur's laboratory work

76. Bouley, 1883, p. 914.
77. Duclaux, 1882, p. 144.
78. Chamberland, 1882, p. 459.
79. Grancher, 1893, p. 678.
80. Arloing, 1891, p. 305; Courmont, 1914, p. 343; de Varigny, 1884, p. 276; Magne, 1883, p. 803; Richet, 1923, p. 97; Roger, 1915, p. 69; Trouessart, 1886, p. 134; Trouessart, 1891, p. 120.
81. Chauveau, 1882, p. 337.
82. Pasteur, Cor., t. 3, p. 165.

was still not flawless. On August 27, Bouley informed Pasteur that an anthrax bacteridium culture supplied by Roux had been unable to contaminate the sheep used in Toussaint's experiment at Alfort... "*Unfortunately, the product supplied to M. Toussaint by M. Roux last Sunday, has proven totally ineffective. We had inoculated two sheep from the batch of 16 sheep, and a rabbit as control; the inoculation had no effect on the rabbit: we therefore concluded that M. Roux's virus was without virtue* (virulence)... *Toussaint should be sending me from Toulouse a virus certain to be reliable.*"[83a] An occasion for Bouley to retaliate for the fact that Roux is ruthless in his criticism of Toussaint. However, Roux offers justification a few days later[83b].

From the start of the confrontation, members of the Pasteur family and later some of his associates, adopted an attitude that cannot be said to do them honour. René Vallery-Radot, his son-in-law, showed little generosity toward Toussaint: "*Toussaint's claims were hasty. Pasteur did not fail to notice this... Pasteur wrote a rather cutting note setting things straight. His need for rigour in experiments sometimes made him too critical... He* (Bouley) *remarked that Pasteur had had "the discretion of abstaining from any detailed criticism in order to give M. Toussaint a chance to make his own rectifications.*"[84] This text was published in 1900. René Vallery-Radot added nothing to attenuate his comments, that he knew to be mistaken in the light of Chauveau's work. In 1951, Pasteur Vallery-Radot, his grandson, wrote in a note added on the occasion of the publication of a letter written by his grandfather: "*During the March 21, 1881 session of the Academy of Sciences, Pasteur presented his experiments testing Toussaint's so-called vaccine.*"[85] This comment shows even less objectivity, since its author had greater perspective. Pasteur's brilliance left no doubt; there was no need to attack Toussaint... in 1951, especially with false data and in possession of his grandfather's notebooks...

Numerous scientific books, some of them written by Pasteur's collaborators on his work on the anthrax vaccine, ignore Toussaint's work altogether, or discredit it. In 1892, Nocard wrote: "*Toussaint's procedure seems simple, practical and universally applicable, but unfortunately this is not the case: if eight or ten sheep are inoculated with Toussaint's vaccine, some of them are killed by the vaccination and among those that survive, some will not withstand the virulent inoculation*"[86], and this despite Chauveau's studies demonstrating the contrary. Pursuing this perspective became a tradition. Lépine, in 1975, takes up the biased view of Pasteur, disregarding Loir's 1938 account of these events[87]. The next step is outright omission. Straus and Dubary, in their long article on anthrax in Berthelot's *La Grande Encyclopédie*; Duclaux in *L'Histoire d'un esprit*; Roux (1896) in *L'Œuvre médicale de Pasteur*[88]; Metchnikoff in 1901, in *L'Immunité dans les maladies infectieuses*[89]; in 1909, Charpentier in *Les Microbes*[90]; and Hannoun in *La Vaccination*[91], do not mention Toussaint.

Outside of France, there were those who protested, Koch among them, of course, and many others. And a recent opinion, strongly expressed in *The Observer*, in 1993 by

83a. Nicol, 1974, pp. 341 & 343.
83b. Nicol, 1974, p. 339.
84. Vallery-Radot, 1900, p. 437.
85. Pasteur, Cor., t. 3, p. 167.
86. Nocard, 1892, p. 72.
87. Lépine, 1975, p. 8.
88. Roux, 1896, p. 538.
89. Metchnikoff, 1901, p. 490.
90. Charpentier, 1909, p. 219.
91. Hannoun, 1999, p. 20.

McKie is worth quoting: "*Louis Pasteur: Genius, pioneer and Cheat. Historian* (Gerald L. Geison) *claims France's greatest scientist was fraud. Dr Geison has discovered that Pasteur - famed for showing that micro-organisms cause disease - not only falsified data, but stole ideas from other researchers, and even rigged public demonstrations of his discoveries. This revisionist view has gone down like a lead bacillus with the French. 'The authorities in Paris were not at all thrilled when they realised what I was doing' said Geison. 'It took me a long time to get myself re-established with them.'... So he simply appropriated the work of a M. Toussain* (sic), *a veterinarian who had found a way to attenuate - i e cripple - viruses using potassium dichromate... These viruses could then be used as a vaccine... Pasteur was not very pleasant*", says Geison. "*He was eager to push rivals aside for the sake of acquiring fame and, to a lesser extent, fortune. So he lied, took shortcuts and stole others' ideas.*"[92] There is nothing to add. It is true that the Toussaint vaccine was far from fully developed. But the first Pasteurians were often biased. Toussaint is indeed the indisputable inventor of the second artificial vaccine discovered, imperfect of course, but valuable nevertheless. However, Pasteur's vaccine is not derived from Toussaint's. However, Toussaint is the inventor of the first published method of producing an artificial, man-made vaccine.

Why the Change of Attitude among Pasteurians?

At least two points of friction divided the two camps. Toussaint's announcement on August 2, 1880[93] that acute septicaemia and chicken cholera were the same disease amused Pasteur, who did not believe this to be true for an instant, and said so immediately, with reason. Toussaint's discovery of the sheeppox microbe had become somewhat contested over time[94]. The second point of disagreement was most certainly Toussaint's vaccine against anthrax. Toussaint published his findings rapidly, retracted himself, became lost in his explanations... His original method was valid. But, at this time, in the eyes of Pasteur's followers a living strain with unstable virulence was not a vaccine, any more than a culture of dead bacteria would be... On August 22, 1880, Roux wrote to Pasteur: "M. *Toussaint and* M. *Bouley would no doubt love to drop in to the laboratory one day to catch a glimpse of the method that produces the famous cultures which trip them up.*"[95] On the same date in August, Pasteur wrote to Bouley: "*How is it that* M. *Toussaint did not try to culture his so-called vaccinal blood...*" Pasteur is right to ask the question, but he forgets that at that time Toussaint had not mastered the technique of anthrax bacillus culture... known to the Pasteur group, but not revealed. And Pasteur's letter continues: "*... and why call vaccine something that was not proven to reproduce indefinitely while keeping its protective properties.*"[96] On this last point, Pasteur is faithful to his first idea of a "vaccine", based on the smallpox vaccine. He was to admit the existence of inactivated or chemical vaccine when Roux and Chamberland demonstrated its existence to him several years later (after the Americans Salmon and Smith), and from then on he used the term "vaccine" in a larger sense. At this time, Pasteur considered that Toussaint had only failed once: in his attempt to immunise chickens with a filtrate from chicken cholera bacterial culture. Pasteur was sincere in his opinion, but he was wrong.

92. McKie, 1993, p. 4.
93. Toussaint, 1880d, p. 301.
94. Toussaint, 1881b, p. 362.
95. Nicol, 1974, p. 336.
96. Pasteur, Cor., t. 3, p. 167.

In short, the Pasteurians seemed irritated with Toussaint's behaviour, which threatened to discredit the orientation of their research on vaccines. On September 3, 1880, Pasteur wrote to Bouley: "*The development of germ theory still has so many battles to wage that its advocates should be careful not to lend arms to the enemy.*"[97] In fact, they were probably worried about this competition.

Toussaint's Meanderings

Toussaint described and/or used several different vaccines: 55° C for 10 minutes (Toulouse), a low percentage of carbolic acid (Toulouse and Alfort), 55° C for 10 minutes with 0.5% carbolic acid (Cambridge), culture medium without bacterial agent (Cambridge). Toussaint arrived in Paris with his two vials of carbolic acid vaccines on the 6th or 7th of August 1880. His vaccine was transported in unfavourable conditions. After analysis, Roux found it to be contaminated by all kinds of bacteria...[98], but Roux was very critical of Toussaint. The Alfort experiment (Vincennes farm and then Alfort Veterinary School) started on August 8, 1880, with the inoculation of twenty sheep. Toussaint left Paris without knowing that four sheep were going to die following this inoculation. He attended the Cambridge meeting of the British Medical Association, held between August 10 and 13, as well as the Reims meeting held from August 12 to August 19. Toussaint conducted one experiment after another, went from one conference to another: he presented a communication in Cambridge on the 12th, and in Reims on August 19, 1880. The report summarising the Cambridge session where he spoke indicates that he remained cautious: "*With regard to the method of vaccination, he* (Toussaint) *thought it better not to make it known until he had ascertained that it was not likely to cause death to the animals vaccinated.*"[99] In his introduction to the section where Toussaint makes his communication, Lister is much less restrained. Obviously, Toussaint met Lister before the session and revealed his results to him. Lister described Toussaint's methods of anthrax immunisation: production of bacteria by culture in an animal, puncture for blood, dilution and paper filtration or destruction of bacterial virulence. Lister also spoke of a procedure consisting of heating to 55° C to kill the bacilli, then adding carbolic acid to prevent putrefaction of the vaccine. Lister then predicted: "*I need hardly remark on the surpassing importance of researches such as these* (Robert Koch, Louis Pasteur et Henry Toussaint). *No one can say but that, if the British Medical Association should meet at Cambridge again ten years hence, some one may be able to record the discovery of the appropriate vaccine for measles, scarlet fever, and other acute specific diseases in the human subject.*"[100] In these reports, neither Toussaint nor Lister specified that the vaccine could be chemical rather than live, but the idea was implicit. Clearly, this point did not disturb those attending the meeting, who were less aware of this problem than the Reims meeting participants.

On August 12 in Cambridge, Toussaint only knew the few results obtained in Toulouse before his last experiment on August 6. He might have been informed by telegram, before he went to Reims, of the fact that the Toulouse sheep survived for at least ten days[101]. In Reims, he delivered his presentation on August 19. If he received the good

97. Nicol, 1974, p. 349.
98. Roux *in* Nicol, 1974, p. 336.
99. Toussaint, 1880e, p. 385.
100. Lister, 1880, p. 363.
101. Toussaint, 1883, p. 256.

news (from Toulouse), he must have felt justified in his views on inactivated vaccine; however, the four deaths in the Alfort experiment (inoculation on August 8 - deaths on the 11th and 12th, or 12 and 13th of August), of which he probably learned at the same time, should have made him more cautious. "*It was proof that the inoculated liquid was not devoid of bacteridia.*"[102] At Reims, Toussaint certainly presented his theory of vaccine without living bacteria, but did he reveal the death of the four Alfort sheep and propose the other explanation: that of a Pastorian vaccine with attenuated virulence?

According to Roux, who is not easy on him, when Toussaint returned from Reims he became very confused and embroiled in his explanations[103]. Was his health starting to deteriorate? *A priori*, this was not the case, because in September 1880 he went to Luchon to study a malignant anthrax pustule that had developed on a hospital patient in that city[104]. Moreover, Lister visited him in Toulouse, probably in September as well: "*Soon after the Cambridge meeting he* (Lister) *visited Professor Toussaint at the Ecole Vétérinaire in Toulouse. He wished to perform additional experiments on the resistance of blood to putrefaction, and required the Jugular vein of living donkey in which to do so. He said that he went because the antivivisectionist legislation forbade him to do research in England, but there may have been another reason why it was convenient to work in Toulouse. He had received a 6,000 franc prize* (about 19,000 euros) *from the French Academy of Sciences, a one-time bequest by a M. Boudet, to be given in 1880 to the man who had contributed most effectively to medicine in the field of Pasteur's work. Lister may have determined to spend the money in France because in September, when the experiments at Toulouse were completed, he and Mrs. Lister took their holiday in the Pyrenees.*"[105] He returned to work again in October. Lister received the Boudet prize with the following mention: "*The Academy discerns the Boudet prize to Mr. Lister for the very beneficial changes he introduced in the treatment of wounds.*"[106] On July 28, 1881, Bouley submitted, on behalf of Toussaint, "*1° the manuscript of a dissertation on anthrax immunity; 2° the manuscript of a dissertation on anthrax, chicken cholera and acute experimental septicemia (with seven plates), and 3° an ès sciences doctoral thesis entitled: Experimental Research on Anthrax Disease.*"[107] There is every reason to believe that Toussaint is really the author of this thesis. Bouley remarked, on August 1, 1882, that Toussaint had fallen ill some time ago and had had to interrupt his teaching[108]. Henri Toussaint's serious and very unfortunate health problems occurred in the latter part of 1881 or in the beginning of 1882, but according to Neumann, they progressed relatively slowly, and he was only placed on availability in 1887[109].

The Pasteurians were very critical of Toussaint's relative lack of experimental and even scientific rigour. He changed his mind about his vaccine's mode of action: dead vaccine or attenuated live vaccine. Worse still, in 1880 or 1881, Toussaint wrote (for the *Montyon - Académie des Sciences and Barbier - Académie de Médecine* 1881 prizes): "*... In the August 19 session of the field of Medicine section of the "Association française pour*

102. Bouley, 1880d, p. 457.
103. Nicol, 1974, p. 338.
104. Bouley, 1880b, p. 942; Toussaint, 1883, p. 297.
105. Fisher, 1977, p. 265.
106. Gosselin, 1881b, p. 546.
107. Bouley, 1881c, p. 847.
108. Bouley, 1882b, p. 861.
109. Neumann, 1896, p. 383.

l'avancement des sciences" (French Association for the Advancement of Sciences) *held in Reims, after being informed on the 18th by M.Bouley of some important facts to which I will return later, I expressed formal reservation about an immunity procedure I had indicated earlier, and I agreed that vaccination, as M. Pasteur had demonstrated for chicken cholera, was due to an attenuated virus and not to fluid secreted by parasites."*[110] Toussaint seemed to be in good health. Further in this belated description of his work, he continued: "*This result implied extremely important consequences for vaccination theory, and when M. Bouley informed me of it on August 18, when I returned from a voyage to England, I unhesitatingly changed my perspective on the interpretation of the immunity results observed so far... Given the Alfort results, on August 19, 1880, at the last session of the 'Association pour l'avancement des sciences', in the field of medicine, I formulated formal reserve before several members of the Academy.*"[111] The text is a little difficult to interpret; Toussaint writes: "*I admit that the vaccination... was caused by an attenuated virus...*" Then: "*I did not hesitate to change my mind about the interpretation...*" and to express "*formal reserve*". At the Reims meeting, Toussaint was (perhaps) able to propose, orally, the two interpretations of his results, but he had still not applied what he wrote: "*I unhesitatingly changed my perspective on the interpretation of the immunity results observed so far...*"[112].

When exactly did Toussaint change his mind? Certainly after the Alfort experiment in which four sheep died of anthrax septicaemia. There is no record of Toussaint's itinerary from Cambridge to Reims (Cambridge meeting of the British Medical Association between August 10 and 13, then the Reims conference from August 12 to 19). Did he stop in Paris? Had he been advised of the faith of his four unfortunate sheep? It is almost certain that he had[113], and precisely on August 18[114]. But if he did not stop in Paris until he was on his way back from Reims, where he spoke on August 19, he would not have learned of the death of his four sheep until the 20th. This, however, is unlikely, because Bouley gave formal credence to Toussaint's statement that he expressed reservations about the interpretation of his immunisation experiments in his Reims presentation on August 19[115]. Thus, Toussaint had been advised of these deaths while he was in Paris between the Cambridge and Reims meetings. Nevertheless, on August 18 he was still not convinced... He was holding on to his original idea.

Roux believes that Toussaint changed his mind not on August 18, but on Saturday, August 21, 1880, as shown in a letter mailed to Pasteur in Arbois the next day, from Paris. Since he referred to the Reims meeting, the Saturday in question can only be the 21rst: "*On Saturday morning M. Toussaint admitted that he could not understand the death of the Alfort animals... But I saw him the same evening and he was speaking very differently, he was saying that he did not know what to think and that he had just expressed reservations to the Reims Scientific Association* (August 12 to 19) *about his original opinion.*"[116] Toussaint and Bouley met with Roux on the morning of the 21rst. Roux must have been quite clear: no protection without virulence attenuation of living bacteria... based on Pasteur's theory. Toussaint left Ulm Street with Bouley, who had witnessed the conversation. After thinking it over, he decided to change his mind,

110. Toussaint, 1883, p. 207.
111. Toussaint, 1883, p. 256.
112. Toussaint, 1883, p. 256.
113. Bouley, 1880d, p. 457.
114. Toussaint, 1883, p. 256.
115. Bouley, 1880b, p. 942; Bouley, 1881e, p. 668.
116. Roux *in* Nicol, 1974, p. 337.

but seems to have added a lie or made an error, presenting this change of opinion as having occurred before his Reims communication... He was to repeatedly reproduce in writing this false or erroneous version of the facts... Was Bouley an accomplice in this falsification or mistake?... It does not seem so. There is no serious reason to doubt his good faith. But it is surprising to note that he is wrong about the dates of the Alfort experiment, which he says started on August 26[117], when in fact it started on August 8. This approximately twenty-day error made by Bouley in September 1880 about an event that took place in August is puzzling. Was he trying to confuse the facts and the dates, or was he making an innocent mistake? In the same text, he stated that the concentration of carbolic acid in one of Toussaint's two vaccines "*does not seem right*"[118]. In fact, Bouley continued to create confusion: he specified that Toussaint learned that sheep had died of anthrax after their first vaccination (supposedly on August 26). This result could have led Toussaint to change his opinion of his vaccine, and to present his new point of view... at the Reims meeting on August 19. Toussaint's reservations about his initial view were perhaps formulated in Reims (August 19, 1880), but it is more likely, as Roux says, that this did not occur before the 21rst of August. Unless the 26th cited by Bouley is a printing error...

Toussaint's statements concerning his presentation at the Reims conference on August 19, 1880 are mistaken. During his speech on that date, Toussaint "*repeated his allegations concerning vaccinal matter. I learned it from colleagues who were present at the session. But nothing like this appears in conference summaries. M. Bouchut and M. Landowski's comments on this subject, presented in the report, deal with soluble vaccinating matter. But there is no reference to vaccinating matter in the printed text of M. Toussaint's communication... This is because between the time when M. Toussaint presented his communication and the time when the written text was submitted to print, a change had taken place in his perspective.*"[119] Bouchut's comment, written after Toussaint's presentation, is explicit: "M. *Bouchut requests some details about this new method of performing vaccinations with fluids containing no figurations of bacteria. These new experiments constitute a revelation of sorts in the history of inoculations, since until now it was admitted that they could only be performed with fluids containing such components.*"[120] Clearly, Toussaint described his vaccine formula without bacterial agents. The summary of this session, published in *Le Progrès médical* on August 28, 1880, confirms that Toussaint's position was unchanged when he made his oral presentation in Reims, in light of the responses made by M. Bouchut and M. Landowski[121]. However, the same summary goes on to say: "M. *Toussaint gave an important communication on anthrax vaccinations. He presented specifically the results of numerous vaccinations performed over the past fifteen days in Toulouse and in Vincennes with anthrax virus, without bacterial components. Only a few of the animals succumbed so far, probably because the serum used was not absolutely free of bacteria. Animals vaccinated in this manner become refractory to subsequent inoculations.*"[122] Toussaint was aware of the problem posed by the death of "vaccinated" sheep, but he persisted in his opinion on immunity induction through a bacteria-free vaccine, in the surviving sheep. It is possible that in Reims he expressed conflicting opinions. He was to change his mind

117. Bouley, 1880b, p. 942.
118. Bouley, 1880b, p. 942.
119. Bouchard, 1889, p. 120.
120. Bouchut, 1880, p. 1025.
121. Blondeau, 1880, p. 712.
122. Blondeau, 1880, p. 712.

later. In a letter addressed to Pasteur on August 27, 1880, Bouley remarks: "*He* (Toussaint) *is deeply troubled about his special vaccine, although he holds on to some slight hope that he was not wrong. This hope is founded on the immunity shown by lambs born of mothers inoculated with anthrax during the last term of gestation. Because the placenta, according to Davaine, is a filter that does not allow the passage of any blood components, neither blood cells nor bacteria, if a lamb born of an inoculated mother remains unaffected by anthrax inoculations that do not even produce local irritation, it means that it has received immunity from the mother through something that her blood let pass through the placenta, that is, through a fluid without blood components. This is the argument to which Toussaint is still clinging.*"[123]

Toussaint's written communication is somewhat different from his oral presentation. Yet his text, dated August 19, 1880, is supposed to reproduce the speech he made the same day. But some of the events described are dated August 22, and even go as far as October 19, 1880! He does not conceal this, and the text produces a curious impression. According to the rules indicated in writing at the beginning of meeting reports, the texts had to be sent to the secretary by December 1 following the Meeting, without alterations. Moreover, at the Cambridge meeting, Lister congratulated Toussaint publically for his discovery of a new method of immunisation against ruminant anthrax, using infected blood with the anthrax bacteria removed[124].

Toussaint indicated a number of times that his change of perspective occurred on July 19, 1880. He first indicated this in the dissertation written for the Montyon prize of the Academy of Sciences and the Barbier prize of the Academy of Medicine, in 1881; the article was written thirteen of or fourteen months after April or May 1880[125], some time between May and July 1881, well after the events in question and the submission of his Reims meeting manuscript. Of course, Pasteur noticed the discrepancy. In his March 21, 1881 note to the Academy of Sciences, he remarked: "*I read in the March 8, 1881 Bulletin of the Academy of Medicine, page 302, that* M. *Toussaint has rectified his initial Notes to the Reims meeting on August 19, 1880. There must be an error in the date: the rectification must have occurred in the last days of August 1880.*"[126] Pasteur seized this opportunity and showed no indulgence... but he was right. Toussaint changed his opinion officially most probably on August 21, and Pasteur knew it from Roux's letter. Toussaint exposed himself to criticism through his conduct, but his fault would be of no consequence for the development of vaccines.

On August 21, faced with Roux's firm stand and Bouley's presence, Toussaint found himself in an untenable position. He quickly retreated from his previous position and accepted to join the Pasteurians, admitting that his preparation was live, in the report from the Reims meeting: "*We can therefore conclude that the immunity observed was not, as I had announced, due to the effect of the liquid on the animal, but due to an attenuated state of the parasite, which slows its action and allows the economy to tolerate it for a time and to vanquish it.*"[127] Years later, it would be demonstrated that immunisation against anthrax in domestic animals could be obtained using killed bacilli and adjuvants[128].

---

123. Bouley *in* Nicol, 1974, p. 339.
124. Fisher, 1977, p. 264.
125. Toussaint, 1883, p. 297.
126. Pasteur, O.C., t. VI, p. 342.
127. Toussaint, 1881a, p. 1021.
128. Boivin, 1947, p. 343.

Pasteur and his group lent no importance to Toussaint's experiments and lost no advantage. As to Bouley, in a letter addressed to Pasteur at the time he wrote: "*The Alfort experiment indicates that the vaccine tried in Toulouse, and which proved to be inoffensive, had acquired greater intensity in the twelve-day period before it was used at Alfort, because the bacteridium, momentarily made inert by the carbolic acid, had had time to waken and pullulate despite this acid.*"[129] Bouley had found a plausible explanation but was it accurate? The Toulouse experiment began on the 6th and the Alfort experiment on the 8th of August. Where is Bouley's "twelve-day period"? It must be remembered that Toussaint's vaccine was not heated, and that the bacteria were only subjected to the action of the carbolic acid.

Toussaint Has Good Intentions but Is Overwhelmed

Toussaint was a professor at the Veterinary School in Toulouse; he was talented and full of promise, internationally recognised and fervently supported by Chauveau and Bouley, two very influential figures in his field. As early as March 31, 1875, on Chauveau's advice, Toussaint began studies on anthrax. In 1878, he was entrusted with a mission by the Minister of Agriculture and Commerce, to study anthrax in Beauce. The same Minister entrusted Pasteur with an almost identical mission. This placed them in a competitive situation, although at the time their relations appeared to remain cordial. In the meantime, Toussaint embarked on the study of tuberculosis[130], swine fever, chicken cholera[131] and finally sheeppox[132]. All this was too much for one man, who seemed to have few collaborators or technical assistance. Toussaint's entourage was not always reasonable when it encouraged him to undertake so many projects at once.

However, Toussaint did not claim to be the discoverer of artificial vaccines. In the summary he sent to the Academies for the Montyon and Barbier prizes, he was absolutely clear: "*In any event, these anthrax experiments that followed upon M. Pasteur's experiments on chicken cholera, demonstrated that the most powerful viruses can be attenuated and that, in the case of proven parasitic affections, immunity follows disease that has not killed.*"[133] When was this article written? At the end of it Toussaint wrote: "*There is no better way to end this dissertation than by recalling what my dear and honoured master M. Chauveau did for me in regard to the subject I just discussed; knowing that my health did not allow me to continue the experiments involving heating of the virus, he took up this work, and the notes published at the Academy of Sciences* (in 1882) *and reproduced in this journal show that this procedure can have practical applications.*"[134] Toussaint did not forget to defend his work and to thank those who helped him. This text was probably written after the onset of Toussaint's serious illness. The idea that Pasteur might appropriate portions of his work did not seem to have occurred to Toussaint. In his *Biographies vétérinaires*, Neumann writes: "*Pasteur had just shown, without disclosing his procedure, that it was possible to vaccinate chickens against cholera... Toussaint was working on bestowing artificial immunity to French ovines by inoculating them with attenuated cultures;*

129. Parodi, 1941, p. 21.
130. Toussaint, 1881e, p. 281; Toussaint, 1881f, p. 322; Toussaint, 1881g, p. 350; Toussaint, 1881h, p. 741.
131. Toussaint, 1881d, p. 219.
132. Toussaint, 1881b, p. 362.
133. Toussaint, 1883, p. 207.
134. Toussaint, 1883, p. 297.

he was the first to make this important discovery."[135] This author's opinion carries weight; he was a professor at the Toulouse Veterinary School, and his ideas and judgements directly reflected those of his contemporaries. On April 2, 1883, the Vaillant prize was awarded to Toussaint by the Academy of Sciences, acknowledging that his attenuation procedure could be applied without identifying, and above all without cultivating, the pathogenic agent. The rapporteur suggested cattle plague, cattle pleuropneumonia and sheeppox as illustrative possibilities[136].

Cattle plague was a good example because, in fact, Toussaint's vaccinal preparation method was to have at least one application. In 1881, Piot, a member of the Alfort faculty, was named head veterinarian of the domains of the Egyptian State, in Cairo. In 1880, Piot and Cadiot had been assigned to survey the sheep inoculated in Alfort with Toussaint's anthrax vaccine[137]. In 1883, Piot, who was familiar with germ theory, met the Pasteurian group entrusted with studying cholera in Egypt. The day before Thuillier died of cholera, Roux was recounting in a letter to Pasteur that Thuillier and Nocard had attended, along with Piot, the autopsy of an animal that had died of cattle plague[138]. Piot was well aware of Toussaint and Pasteur's work on vaccinations. He apparently organised successful vaccinations against cattle plague, also called "contagious typhus of horned cattle", in Egypt and then in Great Lebanon. Piot's method for producing his vaccine consisted of heating virulent blood (source of the virus), as Toussaint and later Chauveau recommended[139]. Piot's results seem interesting. He was criticized locally (jealousy?), but he was thanked warmly by local authorities, who bestowed the title of Bey on him, showing their appreciation of his vaccination campaigns.

Pasteur Races against Time: the Search for an Anthrax Vaccine

At the start of 1881, Pasteur found a chink in the armor of anthrax bacteria: they cannot produce spores (their classic defence in difficult conditions) when they are cultivated at the maximum temperature of about 42° C, at which they can still survive. Duclaux (1896) explains: "*Thus, what was needed was to prevent the appearance of spores, while keeping the baccilus alive. This could be achieved by various means, of which the first to prove successful was the action of antiseptics. But Pasteur was not satisfied. He wanted a repeat of the chicken cholera...*"[140].

Rossignol, editor in chief of *La Presse vétérinaire*, was unknowingly going to be helpful to the Pasteurians in the testing of the method on a large scale, so as to make it known... and indirectly crush Toussaint. Rossignol's initiative was primarily meant to help the lion eat the tamer, rather than the contrary, because he had been, from the start, rather unfavourable to Pasteur, to whom he refered as a "microbiatrist". In 1881, he had written in his Journal, under the title "*Reflections*": "A *new species has just been added to the collection of microbes; if you agree, dear reader, we will shut the lid... Microbes*

135. Neumann, 1896, p. 385.
136. Bouley, 1883, p. 914.
137. Toussaint, 1883, p. 256.
138. Lagrange, 1954, p. 61; Vallery-Radot, 1900, p. 540.
139. Brocq-Rousseu, 1935, p. 213; Piot, 1883, p. 487.
140. Duclaux, 1896, p. 358.

are to be had everywhere, to our heart's content. Today, microbiatry is in fashion, it reigns over our lives; it is an indisputable doctrine, to be accepted without argument, especially since its great priest, Pasteur, has spoken the sacramental word: I decree. The microbe alone is and must be the description of any disease; it is agreed that from now on germ theory must predominate over pure clinical observation; only the microbe is eternally true, and Pasteur is its prophet. If God grants life to the illustrious M.Pasteur, we are sure to know in the next twenty years which microbe causes each particular disease... the veterinarian of the future will no longer need today's cumbersome pharmacy... we will indeed no longer have veterinarians, but inoculators... For you see, inoculation is the thing. Amen. H. Rossignol."[141] The agreement between the *Société d'Agriculture de Melun* (Melun Agriculture Society), represented by Baron de la Rochette and Pasteur, was signed on April 28, 1881. A public experiment would be conducted at Pouilly-le-Fort, near Melun, on a farm belonging to the very same Mr. Rossignol. A flock of sixty sheep would be divided into three groups, twenty-five would be vaccinated with attenuated cultures, and twenty-five would receive no preventive treatment at all. Both groups would be tested with virulent bacteria. The remaining ten would serve as controls. In addition, the experiment included two goats and ten bovines that contributed little to the results; "*La Presse vétérinaire*" announced this experiment with some ceremony: "*In a few days, experiments on anthrax will be attempted in Briard; we will keep our readers informed of their progress... If he* (Pasteur) *succeeds, he will bring a great benefit to his country and his adversaries, like the slaves of Antiquity, will have to bind their foreheads with laurel and prepare to follow, bent and in chains, the chariot of the immortal victor. But first he must succeed, triumph demands a ransom. Let M. Pasteur remember that the Tarpeian rock is close to the Capitoline* (sic)."[142]

Pasteur did not reveal his vaccinal preparation method[143] nor the use of a bacteria inactivation technique using an antiseptic. Loir's book written in 1938 specifies that the vaccine used was the one prepared by Chamberland and Roux, using potassium bichromate: "*While he* (Pasteur) *was aiming for the attenuation of the anthrax vaccine by oxygen in the air, Chamberland and Roux were trying the action of different antiseptics on this microbe.*"[144] The comparative action of various antiseptics on microorganism development had already been studied in Pasteur's laboratory. Chamberland had recorded the following observations: "*February 18, 1881... The confirmed results obtained by cultivating bacteria in chicken broth containing potassium bichromate are as follows:*

10 broth + 2 bichrom. at 1/100 does not develop bacteridium,

10 broth + 1 bichrom. at 1/100 develops bacteridium but poorly,

10 broth + 1/2 bichr. at 1/100 develops quite well, but produces spores.

All experiments were conducted in flasks containing 10 parts chicken broth and 1 bichrom. at 1/100.

Weakening of bacteria. After four days the flask killed the pigs but only one out of two sheep, the other was very sick. At twelve to fourteen days the flask killed the pigs but not the sheep and vaccinated the latter. At about twenty-five days it sometimes killed the pigs and sometimes not - did not kill the sheep and vaccinated them After forty days killed neither pigs nor sheep

141. Rossignol, 1881a, p. 50.
142. Redaction, 1881, p. 174.
143. Kuntz, 1881, p. 170.
144. Loir, 1938, p. 18.

and did not vaccinated the latter. Subsequent cultures were inoffensive. No germs were present…

Return through white mice The 40-day cultures inoculated to white mice killed them and often, as with the small pigs, no bacteridia were present in the blood. After 4 or 5 inoculations to mice the bacteridium still had no effect on large pigs and vaccinated sheep… (signed) *Ch.*"[145] This was the signature Chamberland used in the Pasteur laboratory. On February 25th, Pasteur made a note of these two modes of return to virulence in his bacteridium[146]. Who had the idea: Chamberland, Roux or Pasteur? It is hard to say. But increased virulence by passage to animals had already been achieved. Similarly, bacteria culture development with chemical substances had already been used (May 1879) at the Pasteur laboratory before this work[147] and perhaps much earlier, during the experiments on fermentation. The summary recorded by Chamberland (with Roux? Who did not sign, but this might not mean anything), doubtless addressed to Pasteur, clearly indicates experimental results, and particularly those of experiments on sheep. It is hard to believe that Pasteur did not participate in the elaboration of the protocol of this long experiment that lasted about two months, and that he would not have been aware, day by day, of experiments on mice, (guinea) pigs and especially sheep that had to be bought! According to his laboratory notes, Pasteur was using only a limited number of sheep at that time.

Pasteur returned from the Academy where he had signed the Pouilly-le-Fort experimental protocol and, according to Loir's description: "*When he was back in the laboratory where he made the announcement, his assistants asked, presenting arguments, which vaccine he would use. He answered: 'The one with potassium bichromate.' Indeed, this was the vaccine used. In any case, the protocol did not reveal his method of obtaining attenuation.*"[148] It must be remembered that Adrien Loir arrived at the Pasteur laboratory at the end of October 1882, as he himself indicates[149]. Loir did not witness this scene, which took place in 1881. Roux recounts in his memories: "*The Société d'agriculture de Melun* (Melun Agriculture Society) *proposed that Pasteur conduct a public test of the new method. The procedures of the experiment were established on April 28, 1881. Chamberland and I were on vacation. Pasteur wrote us to come back at once, and when we all met in the laboratory he read us the description agreed upon.*"[150] No vaccine preparation protocol is included. In Pasteur's 10th notebook, there is reference to a project proposal, accepted on April 28 by the Baron de la Rochette, president of the *Société d'agriculture de Melun*. The 3rd point specifies: "*25 of these sheep will be given two vaccinal inoculations at 12 or 15-day intervals with attenuated anthrax virus.*" Nothing more[151].

Pasteur's 10th notebook also contains the following: "*Continued from pages 106 and 107 Vaccination of sheep and cows near Melun, at the farm of Mr. Rossignol, a veterinarian, commune of Pouilly-le-Fort. May 5. The bacteridium used as first vaccine; this May 5th, in the presence of M. Tisserand, Bouley, Foucher de Cariel, Baron de la Rochette, Rossignol, Poirier of the General Board, de Roussigny, Signon, the last two from the Chamber of Agriculture of Seine and Oise as well as other persons, veterinarians and farmers etc. etc. was a bacteridium*

145. NAF 18092, item 129.
146. NAF 18016, f.P. 77.
147. NAF 18013, f.P. 2, 8, 51, 55.
148. Loir, 1938, p. 18.
149. Loir, 1938, p. 10.
150. Roux, 1896, p. 539.
151. NAF 18016, f.P. 106 & 107.

attenuated by Chamberland with bichromate and which no longer kills at all, was reinforced by three successive passages in three mice. This bacteridium is stored in a tube with two points seeded by me on May 10 and placed in the incubator for conservation. I also store in a tube with two points the bacteridium that will be used on May 17, 13 days after the vaccination it is a bacteridium originating directly from the bichromate after only a few days. Once, it killed one out of two sheep and on several occasions, when used on sheep after the bacteridium, above from the three mice - it vaccinated very well for the 4-year old bacteridium, very virulent inoculated for the 3rd time (virulence test). (In a note Pasteur wrote: "*Once, it killed one out of two sheep*" [he is probably referring back to one of the experiments in Chamberland's February 18, 1881 note, the one describing bacteridia stored for 4 days in a bichromate culture] "*and on several occasions used on sheep after the above-mentioned destruction of germs in three mice, it vaccinated very well for 4-year highly virulent germ, given as the 3rd inoculation*"). I (the author) found no trace of these experiments in Pasteur's notebooks, but there is no reason to think that they did not take place. They were possibly conducted by Chamberland. *May 17. On Tuesday May 17 departure for Melun at 11: 55. The culture of the bacteridium above developed between the day before yesterday and today, that killed 2 out of 4 sheep (Bacteridium B) will be inoculated. It presents as rather slender long threads. Each day starting on the 18th their temperature will be taken (See general temperature table) May 28 Inoculation with 4-year old bacteria (recent culture) is given to one of the 25 sheep vaccinated and to one of the 25 unvaccinated sheep May 29. The vaccinated one showed almost no change in temperature. It only increased by 0°.1. It increased by 2°.3 in the unvaccinated one. It died in the night between the 29th and the 30th (oedema). A vaccinated 7-8 month - old lamb and an unvaccinated one are reinoculated. May 30 the Temperature of the vaccinated one rose by 0°.2. The rise in the unvaccinated one was 0°.3 (oedema). It died during the night of the 30th or 31rst. May 31 General meeting for autopsy of the two dead sheep and general inoculation of the 23 vaccinated and the 23 unvaccinated sheep with 4-year old bacteria.*"[152] One goat and six bovines were also inoculated.

These four-year old bacteria are discussed in Pasteur's 10th notebook: "*4-year old anthrax. Rapid culture developed in a few hours between 12-18h. January 10, 1881. This tube is in the incubator with the labels I am copying exactly...*" Spores from portion A of the tube are cultured: "*Here is an almost 4-year old bacteridium that is easy to cultivate. January 11... At 5 o'clock a new sheep is inoculated with 3 divisions* (of a syringe) *of this culture... January 13 the sheep was found dead this morning... Therefore spores from bacteridium 4 years old less 2.5 months are very virulent. January 15 what is extraordinary, is the abundant development in the flask of this 4-year old bacteridium, and very pure.*"[153] Pasteur used it several times between the month of January and the Pouilly-le-Fort experiment as a very virulent anthrax bacteria. He called it "*the 4-year old* bacteridium".

Pasteur had the temperament of a gambler. He was willing to take risks. He was a fighter, full of daring, trusting his good fortune. The use of this vaccine called "*from bichromate*" (*sic*) was still referred to in 1882 by Thuillier in correspondence to Pasteur; Thuillier used this designation to differentiate this vaccine from the so-called "*from heat*" vaccine, whose name indicates its origin. However, the Pasteurian vaccinal protocol was not yet well defined.

Thuillier wrote to Pasteur: "*The contradiction between your Vincennes results and my Packisch results makes me think that double vaccination is only preferable to one-time*

152. NAF 18016, f.P. 113.
153. NAF 18016, f.P. 36.

vaccination when 2 vaccines are of the same origin: either 2 heated vaccines without passage to Guinea pigs or mice, 2 bichromate vaccines also without passage, a 1rst of mice with a 2nd, having finally had a passage to a few mice, or a 2nd, of Guinea pigs with a 1rst having had a passage in a young Guinea pig. It seems that development in different living or dead cultures differentiates bacteridia more and more, and that they then cause more and more distinct diseases and do not originate from each-other."[154] These procedures were not at all well defined and Thuillier's comment makes no contribution. Chamberland and Roux published two articles on the attenuation of anthrax bacterium virulence, and on the effects of antiseptic substances in the *Comptes Rendus des séances de l'Académie des sciences* in 1883[155].

Bouley, who spoke on Pasteur's behalf before the Academy of Medicine starting in 1880-1881, stated repeatedly: "M. *Pasteur then asked himself if the microbe, that when cultured in heated medium no longer produced spores, might not produce them again if they were placed in cold medium again... So that, through methodical cultures, it became possible to constitute, so to speak, different races of anthrax bacteria, that is, to obtain this result... that virulence attenuation be transmitted through heredity...*"[156]. Obviously, this is a very important point for the production of Pasteur's vaccine, giving it undisputed superiority over Toussaint's, if indeed this valuable quality was present.

Toussaint's publication presents three procedures (vaccines being killed or attenuated while alive, according to the successive versions of their author): filtering, exposure to heat or action of diluted carbolic acid[157]. In July 1881, before he became ill (see his bibliography), Toussaint himself said of Pasteur's anthrax vaccine: "*His method* (the little that was known about it, *i.e.* the culture of germ with attenuated virulence) *is with absolute certainly the last word on the question.*" Chamberland and Roux's subsequent publications[158] refer to the action of carbolic acid, potassium bichromate and sulphuric acid (with unclear results for the latter) for obtaining stable virulence attenuation. Texts published at the time do not make a clear distinction between the method of sporulation suppression and that of virulence attenuation. On the one hand, Pasteur's team used antiseptics in an attempt to stop sporulation for a time, during culture development (aging); on the other hand, Toussaint used antiseptics to kill bacteria (which he achieved only in part) and gave no indication of culture development, since he had no technique for it.

Pasteur's decision to postpone revealing his procedure is understandable. There is every indication that he truly believed in aging by exposure to air as a method of attenuation. This was going to be, *a priori*, the procedure used later to prepare the commercial vaccine. But can it be said that the Pasteurians copied Toussaint, as McKie claimed and Geison, at the very least, suggested[159]? Loir, who was not an actual witness, gives no indication to confirm this. Did Toussaint's communication set Pasteur's team on the path of antiseptic use? It seems doubtful, since the Pasteurian team had already used this type of substance in previous years. The Pouilly-le-Fort vaccine was not the same as Toussaint's, who did not use potassium bichromate. Superficial perusal of the facts could give the impression that copying was involved, but a careful reading

154. Thuillier, 1882 (1968), p. 132.
155. Chamberland, 1883b & c, pp. 1088 & 1410.
156. Bouley, 1881b, p. 803.
157. Toussaint, 1881a, p. 1021; Toussaint, 1881c, p. 163.
158. Chamberland, 1883b & c.
159. McKie, 1993, p. 4.

certainly dispels this impression. Pasteur and his associated did not copy Toussaint's anthrax vaccine, nor did Toussaint copy Pasteur's team, unless it be the concept of a vaccine, which had been published and overtly referred to by Toussaint.

The Pouilly-le-Fort Experiment (1881): Fortune Smiles upon the Daring

On May 5, 1881, a number of professionals, local officials, physicians, pharmacists and, above all, veterinarians, gathered at the Pouilly-le-Fort farm. Roux, Chamberland and Thuillier inoculated the first vaccine, the one containing highly attenuated anthrax bacteria. Pasteur, who never lost an opportunity to publicize his work, gave a little improvised speech to a half-skeptical, half-convinced audience[160]. The second vaccination was administered without any problem. It was Biot, veterinarian from Pont-sur-Yonne (a neutral participant) who inoculated the two groups to be tested, on May 31. Four times the mortal dose of anthrax bacteria was to be administered to each animal, in the vaccinated group and the control group. When Colin crossed paths with Biot, he intimated to the latter to shake the experimental bacterial culture well before inoculating the sheep, in order to avoid all bias in the experiment[161]. The next day, fever was observed in some of the vaccinated animals. Fortunately for Pasteur and his colleagues, on June 2 there was reason to rejoice: all the vaccinated sheep were in good health and all the unvaccinated sheep were dead! The goat and the bovines that had been vaccinated were in good health, while the unvaccinated goat was dead and the unvaccinated bovines were very sick. It seems that Pasteur had a great fright, because the first news he heard about the experiment was alarming. Apparently, vaccinated sheep had been killed by the vaccine. Thankfully, this was a false report! Pasteur, who had been despairing, upon learning of his success recovered his assurance and arrived at the site proclaiming: "*You see, men of little faith.*"[162] The Pouilly-le-Fort experiment had wide-ranging repercussions. Many well-known figures from the medical, agricultural and veterinary fields, as well as a *Times* correspondent had followed it with great interest and diffused it world-wide. Of course, the unfortunate Toussaint was far from all the noise and bustle.

Pasteur's reports announcing this victory were sent in rapid succession to the Academy of Sciences, to the Academy of Medicine and to the French national Agriculture Society. The account of the event was taken up over and over in all kinds of medical and agricultural newspapers or weekly publications. The interest of the experiment surpassed by far the agricultural and veterinary fields, arousing hopes of infectious disease prevention in humans. But Pasteur's own accounts do not give many details concerning his methods: first inoculation "*culture of attenuated anthrax virus*", a second inoculation "*attenuated anthrax virus again, but more virulent than the previous one*" and "*on May 31 the very virulent inoculation was performed, that was to determine the effectiveness of the May 5 and May 17 preventive inoculations*"[163]. A wave of criticism arose at the Academy of Medicine when a gestating ewe carrying a dead foetus died a few days after the inoculation of the smallpox vaccine. This criticism was headed by Depaul,

160. Chamberland, 1883a, p. 126.
161. NAF 18092, items 164-165.
162. Nicolle, 1932, p. 65.
163. Pasteur, O.C., t. VI, p. 346.

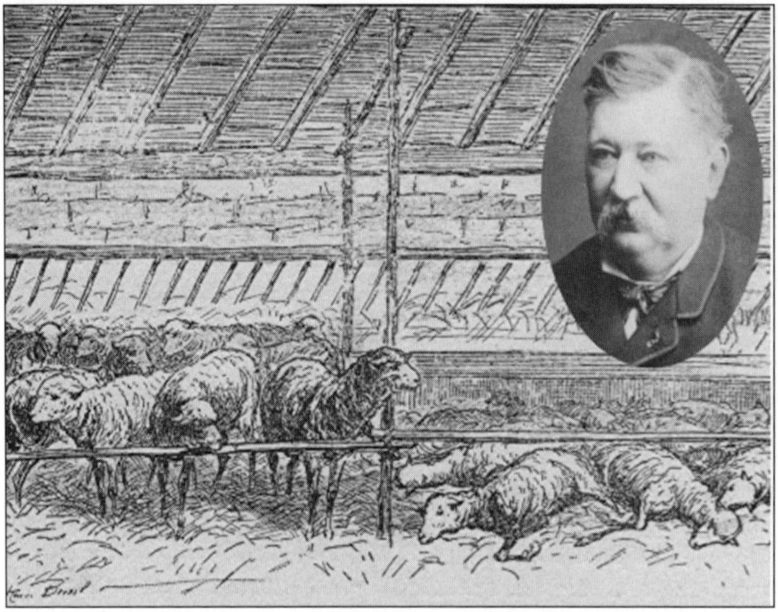

Figure 2. The Pouilly-le-Fort farm is famous, but the building itself is quite ordinary. Illustrators focused on more eloquent images: after the test inoculation, on one side can be seen the vaccinated sheep in good health, on the other, the unvaccinated sheep killed by anthrax (Desplantes, about 1900). Top right, in medallion, portrait of Hippolyte Rossignol, instigator of the experiment. (Photograph courtesy of Jean Rigoulet of the "*Association centrale d'entraide vétérinaire*", where Rossignol had served as president for a time).

the great master of smallpox vaccination, and by Colin, enemy of all scientific advances, supported by colleagues of lesser stature. This rear-guard skirmish revealed a certain small-mindedness; but Pasteur's good fortune persisted.

The anthrax vaccine was not any more unanimously acclaimed in other parts of the world. In 1883, Gradle in Chicago takes up Koch's arguments and explains to his students that vaccines are not always "attenuated" correctly and, above all, that animals infected naturally "*the natural infection with anthrax through the intestinal canal...*" are not adequately protected. "*The 'natural' mode of infection is therefore the most dangerous to the animal and cannot be absolutely prevented by protective vaccination.*"[164] The argument is valid, but the objections presented are not based on enough perspective to be objective. Salmon et Smith wrote in 1892: "*Protective inoculation was first introduced by Louis Pasteur about ten years ago, and has been quite extensively practiced in France and to some extent in other European countries. The fluid used for inoculation consists of bouillon in which modified anthrax bacilli have multiplied and are present in large numbers. The bacilli have been modified by heat so that they have lost to a certain degree their original virulence. Two vaccines have been prepared. The first or weakest for the first inoculation, and the second or stronger for a second inoculation some twelve days later.*

These vaccines have been used for cattle and sheep. Their power to prevent an attack of anthrax subsequently has been the subject of controversy ever since their use began. The

164. Gradle, 1883, p. 84.

French claim that the vaccines are successful in protecting cattle and sheep and that the losses from anthrax in France have been much reduced by their persistent application. According to other observers there are several difficulties inherent in the practical application of anthrax vaccination. Among these may be mentioned the variable degree of attenuation of different tubes of vaccine and the varying susceptibility of the animals to be inoculated. It would be impossible at present to decide from published statistics as to the relative value of these anthrax inoculations in preventive losses. While some authorities regard the vaccination of sheep of little use because of the losses directly due to the vaccination, they admit that vaccination of cattle is accompanied by fewer losses, and that it seems to be protective and of use in localities where the disease regularly appears every year, and is, so to speak, bound to the soil.

It is very important to call attention to the possibility of distributing anthrax by this method of protective inoculation, since the bacilli themselves are present in the culture liquid. It is true that they have been modified and weakened by the process adopted by Pasteur, but it is not impossible that such modified virus may regain its original virulence after it has been scattered broadcast by the inoculation of large herds. No vaccination should therefore be permitted in localities free from anthrax."[165] Of course, this is not very favourable to Pasteurian endeavors, but Smith, the co-author of this text, was of German origin and educated in Germany!

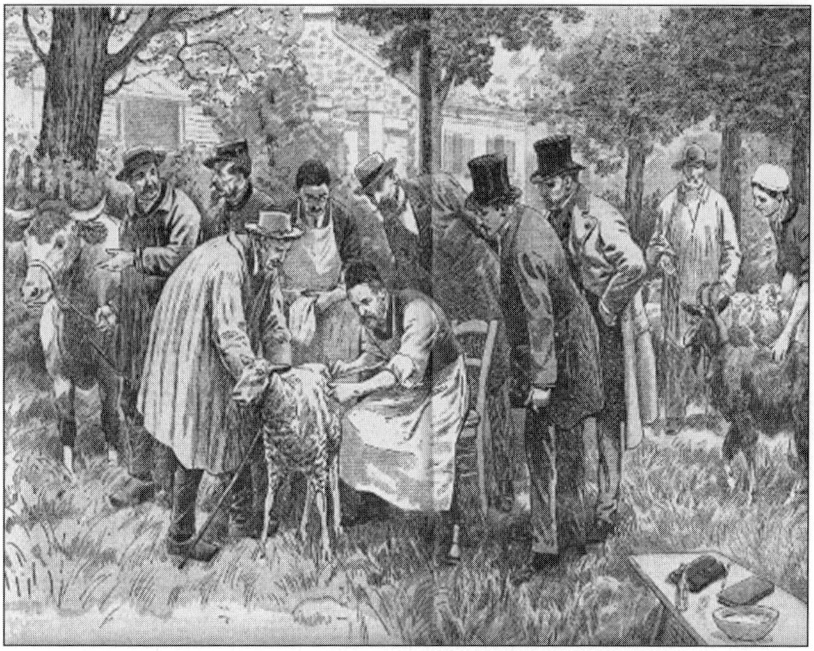

Figure 3. At the request of the Melun Agriculture Society, Pasteur conducted a successful experiment, at Pouilly-le-Fort, trying out his anthrax virus on a flock of sheep, cows and goats. Drawing by Damblans. Illustration published on the occasion of the hundredth anniversary of Pasteur's birth. (*Le Pèlerin, nº 2333,* November 5, 1922.)

165. Salmon, 1892, p. 422.

Immediate Application of Anthrax Prevention

Pasteur continued to conduct experiments to improve his anthrax vaccine for a long time. In June 1881, he went to the Alfort School with two vaccinated sheep, to present his method. He was greeted warmly by the students and by a group of professors (but not by Colin and his followers). The 300 sheep on the farm next to the School were to be vaccinated, 225 with a weak vaccine, followed by a stronger one, as had been done at Pouilly-le-Fort. The remaining 75 sheep were to receive an intermediary vaccine[166]. The use of a single injection to vaccinate, as Toussaint had done, would have been a significant improvement, but this procedure seems to have had limited application. Vaccinations were carried out in the Brie and Beauce regions. Pasteur was heading a young and loyal team, which carried out his orders and diffused his teaching and his vaccinations. Requests poured in. Dates were set. Two by two, Chamberland, Thuillier, Roux, Nocard and Eugène Rozoy would take the train early in the morning to arrive at a station from which a rented car would take them to a farm. Once there, they needed help to assemble the animals, sheep, bovines and horses that had to be inoculated twice, fifteen days apart. A lot of work! But the message was spreading. Numerous demonstrations were requested and were carried out everywhere on farm animals: at Fresne (Loiret), Barjouville near Chartres, Artenay (Loiret), Toulouse, Nevers, Mer (Loir-et-Cher), Montpellier, Bordeaux, Angoulême, Clermont-Ferrand, Budapest and Kapuvar (Hungary), Packish (Austria-Hungary), Torino, Elvaux-Herve (Belgium), Bern, England and Spain[167]. Most of these demonstrations were successful, but some had mixed results. Those who made the requests were not always in good faith, experimental conditions were sometimes modified without good reason, and animal species were changed arbitrarily. Deaths occurred after the first or second vaccination. Thuillier was sent to Hungary and then to Germany to conduct public experiments not free of unfortunate incidents. On May 8, 1882, he wrote to Chamberland who was preparing the vaccines in Paris: "*Hidden in the depths of your laboratory, you have no worries, whereas I, when a poor animal seems to lower its head a little, see all eyes going from the head of the animal to mine and back again. I can assure you that this situation is not amusing. And it is all the worse when I must lead the mourning for vaccinated animals that have died by my hand, and must make a speech at the grave about their receptivity (Roux's touchy point). Naturally, most people don't notice anything.*"[168] Of course, one could not confide such things to the master, but only to one's colleagues. On June 1, 1882, about three hundred thousand animals had already been vaccinated; 25,000 of them were bulls and cows[169]. Pasteurians almost always prepared two vaccines to be inoculated one after the other. Experience in vaccine preparation was still very limited; the vaccines were not always perfect. Either the first vaccine proved to be too virulent and killed some of the animals, or they were not virulent enough and did not induce sufficient immunity to prepare the animals for the second inoculation. Finally, some animal species were more sensitive than others to the virulence of Pasteurian vaccines. Vaccinal strains required constant attention, because they were not completely stable. Shortly after the Pouilly-le-Fort experiment, Pasteur noted: "*Test of vaccines used during the months of February and*

166. Bouley, 1881d, p. 854.
167. Anonyme, 1883b, p. 724.
168. Thuillier, 1882 (1968), p. 160.
169. Chamberland, 1883a, p. 293.

March 1882. March 30. The old vaccines from the months between May and September 1881 having been recognized to be weakened when the work was continued in November December January, the first was passed to 2 mice and the 2nd to 2 (guinea) *pigs...*"[170]. This kind of empirical reasoning is a little difficult to explain, even using modern molecular biology concepts...

The vaccines were made in an annex of the laboratory, on Vauquelin Street. Chamberland and his laboratory assistant Rebour were in charge of production. Boutroux was the commercial agent of the laboratory. He took care of shipping[171]. This did not fail to create confusion. In 1882, Pasteur wrote to Duclaux: "*The failure you bring to my attention is incomprehensible. A similar situation occurred near Meaux after the Thursday 22nd vaccination: 28 deaths out of 150* (almost the same mortality rate as in Toussaint's Alfort experiment!); ... *Chamberland who prepares the tubes does not understand an error occurring on his part. But it must have happened. He must have sent the second vaccine instead of the first...*"[172]; and also: "*The reports about the virulence of the first* (vaccine) *and of the second* (vaccine) *are not what I expected. The first is too strong and the second not strong enough. Someone should really attend to nothing but this. It is the task with which I entrusted Chamberland, but the sacred fire sometimes goes out.*"[173] To take Chamberland for a Vestal guardian of the fire required a stretch of the imagination. Chamberland, with his long, full beard and his pipe... held an advanced degree diploma in physics, landed in medicine by chance and lacked any clear vocation. In truth, his passion concerned sterilization ovens, incubators, filters and materials, and not particularly bacterial virulence. Poor Chamberland, relegated to preparing vaccine for cows and fowl, until the time would come for pigs! And the saga continued; in 1885, Pasteur wrote to Roux: "*I find that the anthrax vaccines have given rise to many complaints and accidents in the last while, particularly deaths in the flocks that were vaccinated last June* (sic)."[174] Anyone who has prepared biological products knows that it would have been very surprising for Pasteur and his associates not to encounter difficulties in their work, especially given the equipment available at the time. In fact, it was officially recognized that Pasteurian vaccination could create new loci of disease. Article 8 of a French Ministerial decree issued on July 28, 1888 specified that: "*Farm owners who wish to make use of preventive vaccination* (Pasteurian vaccine) *must first advise the mayor of the commune of their intention. A certificate from the performing veterinarian, indicating the date when the inoculation was completed, shall be submitted to the mayor immediately following the operation. The mayor shall inform both the perfect and the public health veterinarian of the circonscription; the latter shall, within a period of fifteen days, not counting the date of the last operation, have the animals inoculated under his supervision. For the duration of this supervision period, it is forbidden to have the inoculated animals leave for any destination.*"[175] To make matters worse, Chamberland and Boutroux did not always get along: "*I am very displeased to learn of the unpleasantness between M. Chamberland and M. Boutroux.*"[176] This too must have affected the quality of the work.

170. NAF 18016, f.P. 185.
171. Loir, 1938, p. 16.
172. Pasteur, Cor., t. 3, p. 297.
173. Pasteur, Cor., t. 3, p. 316.
174. Pasteur, Cor., t. 4, p. 31.
175. Conte, 1895, p. 320.
176. Pasteur, Cor., t. 3, p. 369.

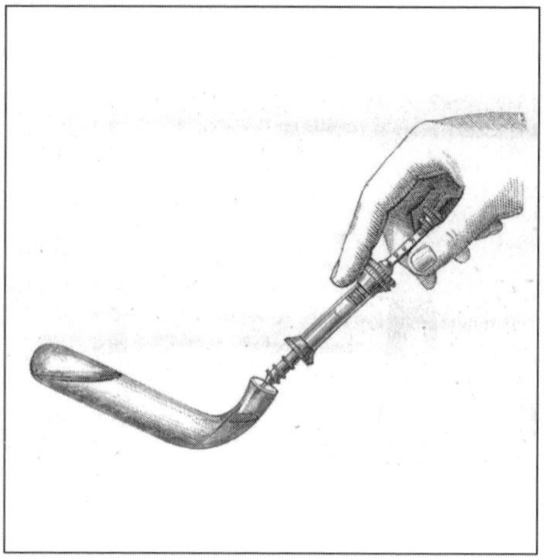

Figure 4. "*Practice of the anthrax vaccination: ... once the tube is opened, the liquid is aspired slowly by lifting the piston. In general, after the first aspiration a rather large air bubble is left under the piston...*" Chamberland's explanations were meticulous because the art of injection was not yet routine practice for veterinarians. (Chamberland, 1883)[177a].

But overall, results were favourable. Between 1882 and 1886, 116,248 animals were vaccinated, and 404 of them died. When compared to the 5% average mortality rate from the natural disease, this 0.34% ratio is a positive result.

All this led Pasteur to conceive another idea: "*The best thing would be to vaccinate with a guarantee. If we retained 10 centimes on the price of each vaccination, we would collect sufficient funds to reimburse all the losses.*"[177b] This was an excellent idea and was, in fact, implemented, at least in some areas. In 1882, Duclaux achieved a victory in his beloved Cantal (his birth place!), with help from some official grants: "*Now, a farm owner in the Cantal can have his herd vaccinated without cost, and if an animal dies he is reimbursed. My region has something to be proud of.*"[178] Insurance companies offered special favourable rates for animals vaccinated against anthrax[179]. Centres producing anthrax vaccine based on Pasteur's procedure were already in existence in Torino, Vienna, Madrid and Buenos Aires[180].

Pasteur was working to achieve personal recognition, as well as recognition for his country, *a priori* without concern for personal financial gain, although he was always mindful of providing for his family. He thought of marketing his vaccines on a large scale, but gave up the idea after consulting Dumas[181]. His greatest concern was the wide application of his method. Therefore, in June 1890, Loir opened an Institute on a small island, in a cove near Sydney, to prepare anthrax vaccine; by the middle of 1892, 400,000 vaccinations had already been performed[182]. Loir mentions no financial returns for Pasteur or for his Service in France. Details are easily available on Internet.

Pasteur's achievements were quickly diffused throughout the world. As early as 1887, India created bacteriology laboratories that, among other activities, prepared anthrax vaccine. Burke makes no distinction between vaccines associated with Toussaint, Pasteur, Chauveau, Chamberlain (*sic*) and Roux, Gibier, Kitt, Perroncito and others...

177a. Chamberland, 1883a, p. 297.
177b. Pasteur *in* Chamberland, 1883a, p. 284.
178. Quoted by Duclaux (Mary), 1906, p. 165.
179. Keser, 1889, p. 182.
180. Anonymous, 1887b, p. 227.
181. Loir, 1938, p. 150.
182. Loir, 1938, p. 115.

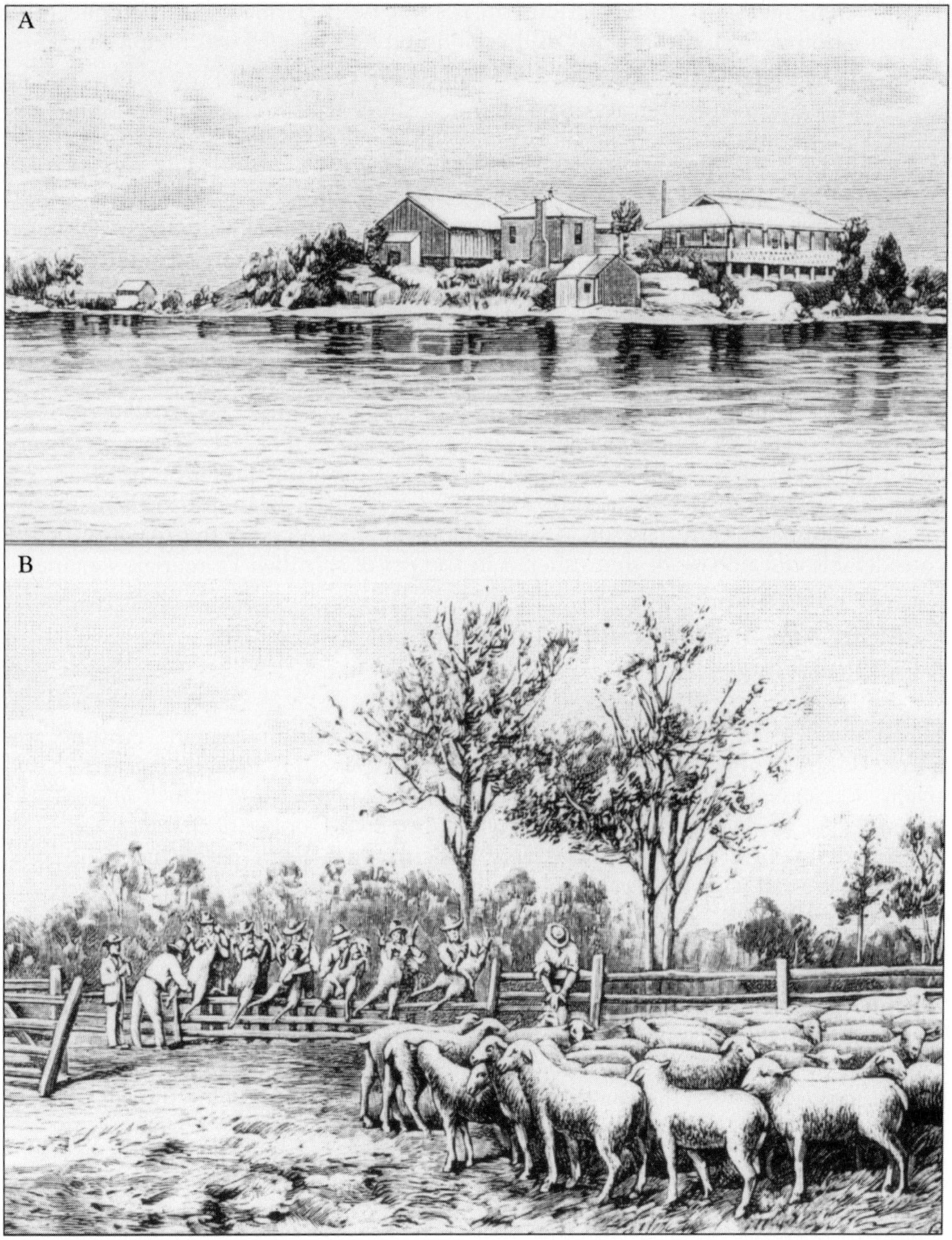

Figure 5. A. The *Institut Pasteur* in Australia. Rodd Island in a cove near Sydney. B. Anthrax vaccination as it was practiced in Australia. In September 1888, Loir, sent to Australia by Pasteur to kill rabbits there, conducted an anthrax vaccination experiment similar to the Pouilly-le-Fort experiment, on thirty-nine sheep and six cows. His demonstration was completely successful. When he was back in France, Australians asked him to return to their country to prepare anthrax vaccine. Settled on a small island in a cove near Sydney, Loir produced vaccine for several years before stopping for personal reasons. (*La Nature*, n° 997, July 9, 1892.)

The different methods of preparation had not yet been clarified, but the concept of immunisation against anthrax was well established[183]. The idea was taking shape.

An article by W.D. Tigertt designated William Smith Greenfield of the Brown Animal Sanatory Institution as the inventor of the anthrax vaccine, before Toussaint and before Pasteur, of course[184]. This idea was taken up and developed by Peter C.B. Turnbull, who attributed the discovery to Chauveau and Toussaint (spelled several times 'Touissant' and never 'Toussaint')[185a]. Toussaint's priority over Pasteur and his team in the development of the anthrax vaccine is undeniable[185b]. However, Chauveau's is not, since he himself always made it clear that it was his student, Toussaint, who made the discovery[186]. W.S. Greenfield's work is undoubtedly interesting. He might or might not be credited with the first anthrax vaccine; historically, this is of little importance. On August 17, 1880, Lister, who described Greenfield and Toussaint's work respectively, did not takesides in the matter of granting priority to one or the other. But he insisted on Buchner's hypothesis that *Bacillus anthracis* and the Hay-bacillus could be the same organism modified depending on external circonstances[187]. Although Greenfield is to be credited* with the very good idea of attenuating virulence in pathogenic agents in order that they be used to immunise, and although he used this technique on a few animals before Pasteur, it is the latter alone who gave the impetus for the considerable research work that ushered in the era of so-called Pasteurian vaccines.

Pasteur's Search for Human Subjects to Vaccinate: a Difficult Task

It had always been Pasteur's dream to perform vaccination on humans. Anthrax was a dread disease, affecting primarily "*... shepherds, whittawers tanners, butchers, blacksmiths, veterinarians, that is, humans who had constant contact with animals infected with anthrax: those who prepared their skins, sectioned their bodies, or looked after their health*"[188]. Treatment of infected humans was very difficult. In a letter dated June 26, 1881, Pasteur, obsessed with the desire to vaccinate humans, wrote to René Vallery-Radot and his daughter: "*... In the meantime I am vaccinating monkeys* (against anthrax) *and this is going very well. I am always hoping that some veterinarians will ask to be vaccinated. There is no danger, absolutely none, I am sure of it.*"[189] One veterinarian vaccinated himself against anthrax with Pasteur's vaccine: "*This veterinarian from the Yonne department inoculated himself with the two vaccines, with no ill effect other than a slight fever. His* family *had to use all its persuasive power to prevent him from inoculating himself with the very virulent virus.*"[190] This man was probably the first human being inoculated with

---

* Greenfield's data are very dispersed and require lengthy and precise analysis that is beyond the scope of the present work. For example, they are not in the "Garrison". The controversial discussions (Lutaud, Decour, Théodoridès, Cadeddu, Geison, etc.) conducted on the subject of Pasteur's work will be the theme of a separate book.

183. Burke, 1887, p. 22.
184. Tigertt, 1980, p. 415.
185a. Turnbull, 2010, p. 57.
185b. Bazin, 2008, ch. 6.
186. Bazin, 2008, p. 159.
187. Lister, 1880, p. 363.
188. Bayle, 1870, t. 1, p. 332.
189. Pasteur, Cor., t. 3, p. 216.
190. Vallery-Radot, 1884, p. 315

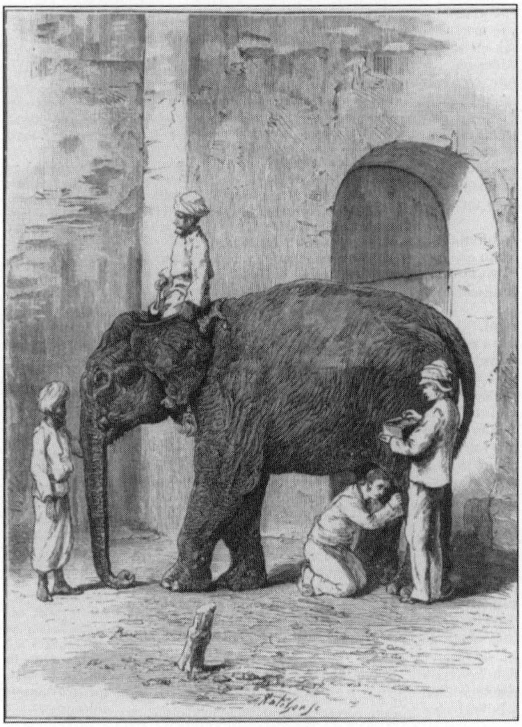

Figure 6. ***"Inoculation of elephants: Hindu veterinarians applying Pasteur's method."*** **(*Journal des voyages*, n° 778, June 5, 1892.) Because anthrax was raging in India, Indian students who had finished their studies at the Cirencester College of Agriculture came to learn the Pasteur method and were soon "*dispensing the vaccine and inoculating elephants as well as bulls and other animals*". Pasteur's bacteridian anthrax vaccine was quickly used in distant lands.**

Pasteurian vaccine. According to Kruif, his name was Biot[191], but the author gives no details and his book embroiders on historical facts. The person in question must remain "the unknown vaccinated"... one who unfortunately lost his chance to go down in history. The anthrax vaccine was to follow a very successful path. The number of animals inoculated, in the millions, proved it to be unquestionably effective[192]. The Pasteurian anthrax vaccines were replaced to advantage by Sterne's 34f_2 Strain[193]. Today, human vaccination against anthrax is of concern again, due to fears associated with bioterrorism.

A Forgotten Competitor: Symptomatic Anthrax Vaccine, 1882

It must not be forgotten that at about the same period when anthrax (splenic fever) vaccine was being developed by Toussaint and Pasteur, a competing vaccine, at least in terms of notoriety, was placed on the market...

The symptomatic anthrax vaccine was only distinguished from anthrax (splenic fever) vaccine at a later date, in 1880, by Arloing, Cornevin and Thomas[194]. This was a disease of bovines, only rarely transmitted to other species and never to man. The disease is characterised by the sudden appearance of a tumor or of general symptoms:

191. de Kruif, 2006, p. 209.
192. Paget, 1914, p. 66.
193. The Merk Veterinary Manual, 1986, p. 359.
194. Arloing, 1880b, p. 1302.

fever, generalised stiffness, absence of rumination and digestion, shaking, chills, dejection, lack of appetite... sometimes followed by limping due to a tumor. Local infection develops due to an anaerobic bacterium: *Bacterium chauvoei* or *chauvaei* (today *Clostridium chauvoei*). This infection generally ends in death.

Intravenous injection of virulent matter (in practice, tumoral serosity) was the first form of immunisation against the disease, discovered in 1880 by Arloing, Cornevin and Thomas[195]. It was, in fact, variolisation, that is, the use of a virulent pathogenic agent, or one that was still wild. The risks associated with this method of administration, given the material available at the time, explain the fact that the method never became commonly used. Arloing and his colleagues attempted to attenuate germ virulence. By heating fresh serum for more or less long periods to between 65° C and 70° C, they obtained vaccinating solutions. Unfortunately, the procedure was uncertain, and virulence varied greatly due to slight changes in heating conditions. Residual virulence was often too great. The experimenters noticed that when the serum was dry, it became more malleable: temperatures between 60° C and 100° C, and a few hours of heating, allowed easy and reproducible control of experimental parameters[196]. The vaccine took the form of a powder to dilute before use. It was tried in the field on 250 bovines; the experiment was financed by "an animal insurance company"[197]. It was used for the first time in Vesoul (France), in 1882... then shortly afterwards in Switzerland, Austria, Germany and Holland... According to Arloing, this vaccine reduced losses by 2.15% in vaccinated animals, knowing that losses in unvaccinated animals reached between 10 and 17 percent, in areas where the disease was present[198]. This vaccine was truly successful. In 1891, Arloing, Cornevin and Thomas shipped quantities of it sufficient for over 50,000 bovines, 30,000 of them in foreign countries. In January 1893, Strebel counted 158,579 preventive inoculations, with 107 deaths caused by the procedure[199]. Metchnikoff referred to 400,000 bovines already immunised by the "Lyonnese method" in 1901[200]. In France, legislation identical to that applying to bacterium anthrax vaccine was issued for the symptomatic anthrax[201].

But after some time, around 1900, legislation governing all veterinary vaccines of the period seems to have fallen into disuse: bacterium anthrax, symptomatic anthrax and erysipelas. Rivalry in methods of vaccination, concomitant and coming from research in Lyon (and Toulouse), concerning essentially veterinary practice, partially explains the climate of competition that caused Pasteur to publish results rapidly... without specifying the methods he used to obtain them.

195. Arloing, 1880a, p. 561.
196. Arloing, 1891, p. 309; Nocard, 1896, p. 211.
197. Bouley, 1881a, p. 300.
198. Arloing, 1891, p. 352.
199. Nocard, 1896, p. 216.
200. Metchnikoff, 1901, p. 493.
201. Conte, 1906, p. 315.

7
The Swine Erysipelas Vaccine: 1883

The pig, alas, does not enjoy a very glorious image, except in cartoons or when it takes the form of cured meat. Most Pasteur syncophants quickly relegated it to oblivion, turning over this page they considered lacking in prestige. However, this building stone in the Pasteurian edifice is far from negligible.

Swine erysipelas affected mainly the South-Eastern region of France. Pasteur spared no effort to carry out his studies of this disease successfully. On March 15, 1882, Louis Thuillier, sent by Pasteur to the region where the disease was present, identified the bacillus, which was independently discovered by Detmers in Chicago[1]. However, Ramon believed that the bacillus discovered by Thuillier was not that of swine erysipelas, but rather that of a swine *Pasteurella* infection. Löffer was to be the one to identify the erysipelas bacillus later[2]. The erysipelas bacillus is very small, much smaller than the anthrax bacterium. Pasteur and Thuillier described it, seen under a microscope, as being colourless and shaped like a figure eight. They were mistaken. When Straus brought back a bacteria staining technique from Germany in 1884, Roux used it to observe swine erysipelas bacilli cultivated in the Pasteur laboratory, and noted that the cultivated bacillus was shaped like a stick and not like a figure eight. Thuillier and Pasteur cultivated the right bacillus, as was confirmed by Loir; but its initial description had been mistaken[3], as Flügge points out[4]. Pasteur and Thuillier proceeded to attempt to modify swine erysipelas virulence by successive passages to susceptible animals, specifically pigeons. They succeeded in increasing bacillus virulence in pigeons as well as in pigs. No vaccine was in sight yet, but they had a stable and highly virulent bacterial strain. By passing it to rabbits, animals that were not very receptive to this bacillus, they developed an attenuated strain for pigs, which they described in November 1883: "*When erysipelas is inoculated from one rabbit to another, the microbe adapts to rabbits. All the animals die and death occurs in a very few days… When pigs are inoculated with the blood of the last rabbits, as opposed to blood from the first rabbits in the series, virulence is observed to diminish gradually, between the first rabbit and those that follow. Soon rabbit blood inoculated to pigs no longer causes death, but makes the animals sick. Once they have recovered, they are inoculated against deathly erysipelas.*"[5] A vaccine against swine erysipelas had been found. It was the first example of a vaccine obtained by reducing germ virulence through successive passages to another animal species, that was, of course, not very receptive.

This idea is similar to Jenner's explanation of the modification of the horsepox virus for humans, by the passage of this virus from the horse to the cow, then from the cow

1. Herter, 1904, p. 58.
2. Ramon, 1957, p. 489.
3. Loir, 1938, p. 36.
4. Flügge, 1890, p. 309.
5. Pasteur, O.C., t. VI, p. 533.

to humans[6]. Pasteur himself was very familiar with this phenomenon that he had already seen in two different microbes[7].

The erysipelas vaccine was to know various faiths. Chamberland started to market it in 1886, as a product of the Pasteur laboratory. Between 1886 and 1894, 111,437 animals were inoculated, with losses of 1.45 percent[8], a low figure for a vaccine of this type. The French government took measures to encourage the use of the erysipelas vaccination, but results were disappointing. Was Chamberland responsible for this? "*On this Xbre 22, 1884, I asked Chd to look after the erysipelas vaccinations and I gave him this note: The Charente Vet. Society has been discouraged once again by erysipelas vaccinations due to a failure it experienced in October... Oct.85 Chambd has done nothing about erysipelas - too busy with his filter.*"[9] Elsewhere, vaccinations against erysipelas were being performed at a steady pace. Poor Pasteur! "*In Hungary, during 1890 alone, almost 250,000 pigs were vaccinated, while in France the overall vaccination figures never rose above 20,000.*"[10] Sternberg considers the swine erysipelas vaccine valuable in endemic areas, but he advises stamping out whenever possible[11].

Many living vaccines were to be modelled on this technique developed for swine erysipelas, in its original form consisting of passage to animals, followed by modification by successive passage in cell cultures. Molecular biology was going to demonstrate that this technique makes it possible to select mutants that have lost all or part of their pathogenic power for the targeted species.

6. Jenner, 1798 (1805), p. 52.
7. Pasteur, O.C., t. VI, p. 391.
8. Chamberland, 1894, p. 571.
9. NAF 18018, f.P. 140.
10. Conte, 1895, p. 347.
11. Sternberg, 1895, p. 186.

8
Rabies or Hydrophobia Vaccine

"Of all the diseases to which animals are subject
& which they communicate to humans,
the one which inspires the greatest dread, repulsion and alarm is rabies."
Enaux and Chaussier, 1785[1].

Since 1876-1877, Pasteur had been studying numerous animal and human diseases, but the progress he had made with rabies was so significant that he dedicated most of his remaining energy to this disease. Why rabies? It was probably a mere matter of chance, for Pasteur was simultaneously conducting studies on several microbes and several diseases: fowl cholera, anthrax, swine erysipelas, saliva microbe, human typhoid fever[2], equine typhoid; the agents of smallpox and of the vaccine[3], diphteria[4], human typhoid fever[5], furuncles, osteomyelitis, puerperal fever[6], yellow fever[7], sheeppox[8], chancroid[9], finger panaris (from Pasteur's own finger)[10], human tuberculosis[11], chicken diphteria[12], contagious bovine pleuropneumonia[13a] and probably others...

But rabies had a number of major advantages for Pasteur:

- it was transmitted to animals and humans;

- it was relatively frequent in dogs, making it possible to conduct experiments on the natural disease. Dogs bought at the dog pound (and later rabbits at the Paris market "les Halles") were not expensive;

- finally, this disease inspired great dread, was present everywhere in the world, and no treatment for it existed; once the infection was present, the outcome was always fatal, leaving a window for experimentation on compassionate grounds.

Rabies was a first-choice disease for its publicity value, unlike chicken cholera! Between 1850 and 1880, most scientific or popular publications contained one or more articles on rabies each year. Pasteur probably did not choose rabies deliberately. Puerperal fever or yellow fever would have served the purpose just as well.

---

1. Enaux and Chaussier 1785, p. 9.
2. NAF 18016, f.P. 1.
3. NAF 18015, f.P. 49, 57; NAF 18016, f.P. 10; Pasteur, O.C., t. VI, p. 391.
4. NAF 18015, f.P. 81.
5. NAF 18017, f.P. 112 & 127.
6. NAF 18013, f.P. 8; Chamberland, 1882, p. 450; Lucas-Championnière, 1880, p. 243; Pasteur, O.C., t. VI, p. 147.
7. NAF 18016, f.P. 119, 136 & 166.
8. NAF 18016, f.P. 140.
9. NAF 18016, f.P. 142.
10. NAF 18016, f.P. 144.
11. NAF 18016, f.P. 158.
12. NAF 18016, f.P. 167.

13a. NAF 18015, f.P. 59; NAF 18016, f.P. 179.

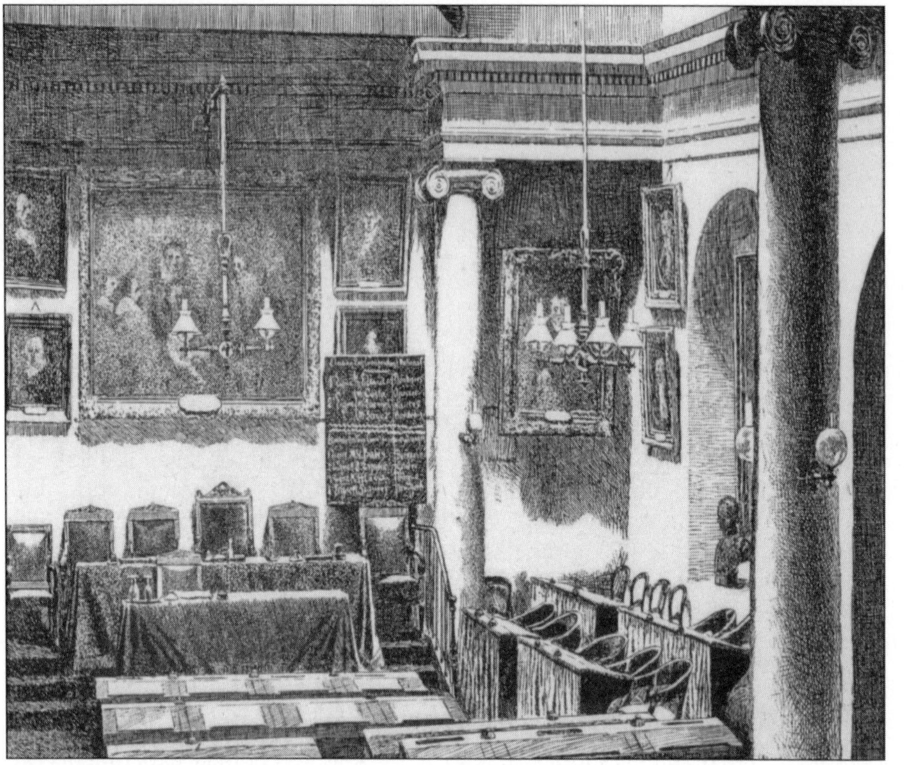

Figure 1. "*Conference room of the Academy of Medicine*." (Strauss, 1892, page 346.) The meetings of the Academy of Medicine took place in the former chapel of the Hospital of Charity, at the time Pasteur frequented the Academy. The room is very small... lit by gas lamps. To the right of the Academy podium can be seen the blackboard where Pasteur drew the microbes he suspected of causing puerperal fever, during the March 11, 1879, meeting: "*Well then, with the Academy members' indulgence, I will draw before their eyes the dangerous microbe to which I now tend to attribute the existence of this fever*." (Pasteur)[13b]. Pasteur was ahead of his time in his conception of infectious diseases, as expressed in his "germ theory"; his work on ruminant anthrax and chicken cholera is ample confirmation of this. He studied many other infectious human and/or animal diseases. He had to deal with medical opposition that became stronger in reaction to his treatments of rabies in humans. Fortunately, he had supporters as well as opponents.

Although rabies was less frequent in our part of the world than other infectious diseases, it was not exceptional in Western Europe. Rabid wolves were particularly feared, with reason, because they were extremely aggressive in their attacks on men and on animals of all kinds. Mortality among persons bitten by these animals was very high. Accounts describing the disease were always terrifying. In 1753, near Dijon, a she-wolf with rabies killed a child and wounded seventeen people by biting them. The wounds of those bitten were cauterised with a hot iron, and they received mercury orally as well as mercury rubs. Despite this treatment, eight of them died[14a]. Around 1855, Dr. Michel from Salle described the case of forty-seven people bitten by the same rabid wolf; forty-five died of rabies, and only two, who were cauterised with butter of antimony,

13b. Pasteur, O.C., t. VI, p. 133.
14a. Hoin, 1761, p. 99.

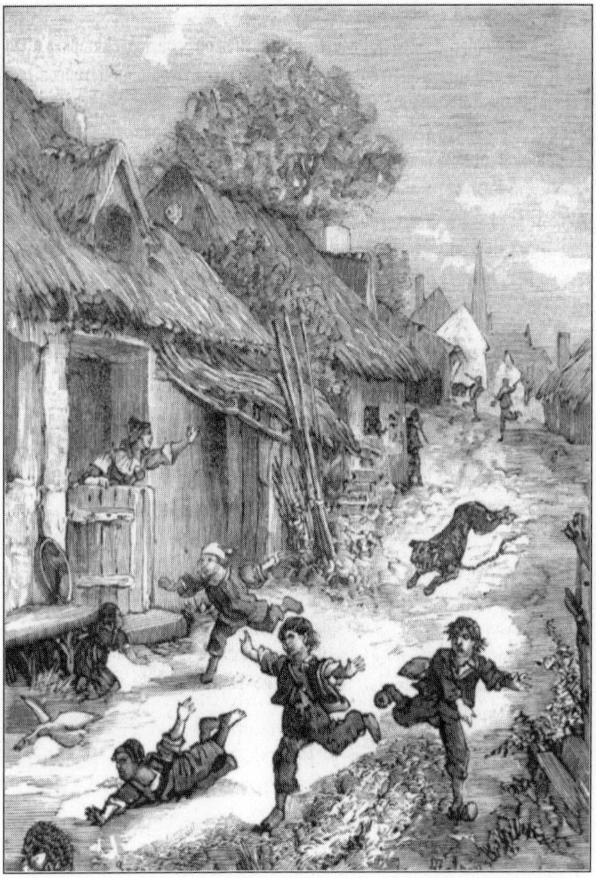

Figure 2. "*If there was ever a dread disease, a disease that never spares its victims, it is certainly rabies.*" (Clerc)[14b].

survived[15]. The number of cases was limited, but it was sufficient to maintain a climate of collective terror. In Western Europe, rabies caused by wolves became rare when this animal virtually disappeared, after being persistently pursued and hunted, with everyone's blessing.

The most common form of rabies was that found in dogs, and perhaps in domestic animals like cats, and in farm animals. The disease occurred often enough to keep the fear alive and to provide (infectious) material to a few scientists interested in this disease. Enaux and Chaussier's definition of rabies, formulated in 1785, clearly reflects their perplexity as to the cause of the disease, but not its transmission: "*Rabies is a kind of nervous fever that attacks the vital principle, & produces in all the humors, & particularly in the saliva, such depravation that the bite of an affected animal communicates the disease to another.*"[16]

14b. Clerc, about 1900, p. 737.

15. Duboué, 1879, p. 120.

16. Enaux, 1785, p. 11.

Spontaneous or Transmitted Origin of Rabies

Up until the middle and almost to the end of the nineteenth century, whether rabies was spontaneous or transmitted, both in men and animals, was a subject still open to debate[17]! "*Whether this disease* (rabies) *arises spontaneously in the body, or results from a specific contagion, rabid animals are capable of communicating the infection, through the medium of their teeth and saliva, to others, and also to the human species. In this form it still retains the appellation of canine madness; but, in appropriate medical language, it is termed Hydrophobia, literally signifying 'dread of water'.*"[18] At about the same time, in 1808, de la Vergne wrote: "*Rabies, also known as hydrophobia, originates either in internal causes, being called spontaneous in that case, or is produced by external causes, in its transmitted form. The animals most susceptible to spontaneous rabies are dogs, wolves, foxes and, in general, all carnivorous quadrupeds. The disease is extremely rare in other animals; however, its existence cannot be denied, even in man...*"[19]. In 1812, Thacher was not taking a clear stand: "*Does an actual and idiopathic hydrophobia ever arise in the human body; independent of the action of contagion, for its production? This position has been contested, and in the opinion of some of its opponents, completely refuted.*"[20] But he contested spontaneity based on the model of smallpox and measles. At the end of the 19th century, there were still advocates of the spontaneous origin of rabies, at least in animals, but their numbers were dwindling[21].

And yet, a century earlier, careful observers had already brought this old concept into question. "Mr. *Meynall, a celebrated sportsman in England... has paid particular attention to this disease among his dogs, and is confident that madness never originates from hot weather, putrid provisions or any other cause than a bite; he never knew the distemper to commence without being able to trace it to that source, and it was never introduced into the kennel, but by a bite of a mad dog. He has for many years preserved his dogs from the disease, by subjecting every new hound to a quarantine before he was introduced to the pack.*"[22] This practice remained in effect and proved efficient in Great Britain for a long period of time.

As knowledge developed, hydrophobia was gradually differentiated from rabies. It was accepted as a spontaneous condition, not always fatal, while rabies was slowly recognized as having a viral origin, in the modern sense, at least in humans.

Clinical Signs of Rabies

What does an animal suffering from rabies look like? There are two main forms of clinical rabies in dogs, the animal species most affected by this disease: "*The disease shows itself in one of two forms: 1. furious or delirious madness; by far the commonest. 2. Dumb madness. In the furious form note:*

17. Weyland, 1844, p. 86
18. Thacher, 1812, p. 15.
19. de la Vergne, 1808, p. 26.
20. Thacher, 1812, p. 53.
21. Americanized Encyclopedia Britannica, 1892, vol. VI, p. 3313.
22. Thacher, 1812, p. 42.

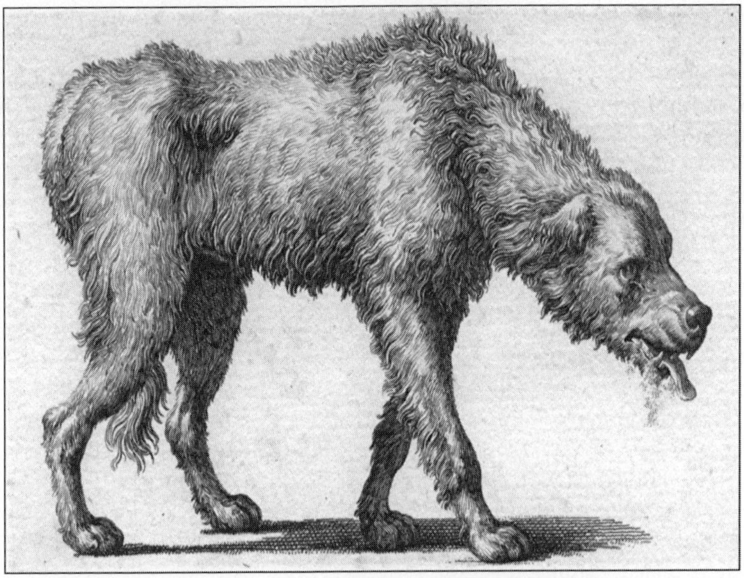

Figure 3. Rabid dog (*Magasin universel*, August 1835). The article accompanying this illustration is entitled: "*About Rabies... This disease is likely to develop spontaneously in dogs, wolves, cats and foxes that can then transmit it to other quadrupeds or to man.*" The article accurately describes rabies in dogs and in wolves, and particularly the treatment to be given to people or animals bitten by a rabid animal. As was often the case, the article has a moralizing tone: "*If our hopes are not too unrealistic, we could, by means of a notice to the population, repeated often and in a most persuasive manner, establish a helpful balance between the care the wounded person can give himself immediately following the incident, and the medical care he can receive subsequently; this collaboration would prove, by its successes, that medicine is the true human science, as much as the exercice of any virtue.*" This illustration accompanied a "*Notice about rabies*" written in Dijon in 1785 by Chaussier and Enaux in response to a request from the States of Bourgogne; the notice was distributed throughout the province to inform the population.

a) A change in the usual ways and habits of the animal. He becomes dull and voiceless, crouches down in the dark and quiet corners. He tries to sleep, but is often perturbed in his sleep as if by painful dreams and delusions; he rises and walks about, then lies down again. He is in a continuous state of restlessness and agitation. In some cases he is not agitated, but sleepy and careless of whatever is going on near him. If perturbed, he growls and shows no inclination to stir. In either case he still obeys the voice of his master and has no tendency to bite yet. The agitation increases. In his kennel he piles up the straw, lays his chest on it, then rises in anger and scatters the litter about. In apartments, he tears and tosses the cushions, carpets, &c. Occasionally there is a manifestation of intense and unwonted sulkiness to some other animal, or to the people of the household; or he is seen constantly to lick cold objects. He is haunted by visions and hallucinations, he barks, snaps and growls at imaginary beings. But still he knows and obeys the voice of his master and has no tendency to bite him. Nevertheless, his saliva is already virulent, and his caresses dangerous. The saliva is virulent eight days, and possibly longer, before the disease is plainly evident. Often, too, in this early stage, dogs will bite a stick thrust at them. So also will they often bite people when worried but slightly.

b) The mad dog has no horror of or repulsion for water. On the contrary, at all periods of the malady, he drinks eagerly or tries to drink. When he fails to swallow the water it is only owing to spasmodic contraction of the throat. The appetite may be at first and for a short time increased. But very soon it diminishes and is quite lost and replaced by marked disgust for all kinds of ordinary food and a thorough perversion of the sense of taste. He tears everything that he meets, carpets, trees, grass, and swallows fragments of anything, including his own excreta, urine, earth, bits of straw, chips of wood, anything. As a consequence of this there is not unfrequently present a certain quantity of blood in the vomited matter, vomiting being a common phenomenon at this stage. The saliva of the mad dog is not usually over-abundant, and may even be quite normal in quantity.

c) The bark of the mad dog is quite characteristic, and is never forgotten when it has been heard once. Bouley says of it: 'Instead of bursting out with its usual sonority and of being made up of a succession of notes equal in duration and in intensity, it is hoarse, veiled, lower in tone, and after a first full-mouthed bark there follows immediately a succession of five, six, or eight howls coming far back from the throat and during which the jaws are never completely closed, as they are ordinarily after each bark.' It is not unlike the voice of dogs chasing a hare; it is something intermediate between a bark and a howl, made up of the two, with something more added, strange and sinister.

d) The sight of another dog at once and invariably puts the mad dog in a fit of passion. This is therefore, an easy and valuable test method... The mad dog is analgesic, i.e., his general sensibility is blunted to a considerable degree. He now seems to feel only the very intensest pains. He no longer expresses pain by the usual nasal sound or sharp cry which is so familiar. He can be beaten, pricked, and even slightly burnt, without stirring and without uttering any sound at all... The sexual instincts also are greatly excited and increased...

e) Confirmed rabies. In a few cases the animal remains tame and unaggressive to the end, but as a rule he is in a state of delirious rage about which there can be no mistake as to its significance...

Dumb madness. Inoculations of this form of madness often reproduce the disease in its furious form, and vice-versa, showing that the two are only different manifestations of one and the same malady. The stages a, b, c, are very much the same as in the furious type, perhaps less marked. Then, d, e, the voice is quite lost, and even in the first stages it is more exclusively a howl, with no admixture of a bark. The mouth is constantly gaping, owing to the paralysis of the lower jaw; the eyes open, without expression, constantly fixed in the same direction. The predominant symptoms are muscular weakness and cerebral depression. The animal is constantly lying down or sleepy, has neither the will nor the power to bite. His saliva is quite as virulent as in the other form. In the immense majority of cases hydrophobia in a dog ends fatally..."[23].

In general, three criteria have always been taken into consideration: "*saliva drooling from the mouth, lack of interest in food* (lethargy), *& horror at the sight of water*"[24], but these signs cannot constitute a definite diagnosis. Loir, Pasteur's nephew, points out the disturbing nature of the barking of rabid dogs, in the courtyard of the

23. Suzor, 1887, p. 9.
24. Colombier, 1785, p. 196.

former Rollin College, where Pasteur kept the many dogs used in experiments. "*One characteristic sign is the particular nature of the howling, that resembles the cry of a rooster, a bark produced by the sudden closing of the jaws, coming from the back of the throat and becoming a jerky howl in three notes, sharper than ordinary barking.*"[25] These howls were so distinctive that Pasteur would order that dogs at this stage of the disease, no longer useful to his experiments, be put to death. In fact, the only practically absolute criterion was the death of the animal, most often in less than eight days, so that Pasteur and his colleagues had to be willing, and above all be able, to wait.

In humans, symptoms were very similar. James gives a description of human rabies that is far from pleasant: "*The symptoms of this distemper* (rabies) *vary so much in different persons, that it is not possible to describe it with that accuracy which the importance of the subject should seem to demand. And it is somewhat more difficult, because the disorder is providentially so rare, that no physician has seen a number of cases sufficient for so ample an information as is requisite for drawing an exact picture of the disease...*

... those who are just about to fall into an hydrophobia, are seized with a certain anxiety, without any evident reason, are prone to anger, have their bodies rendered uneasy, and subjected to preternatural and unusual motions. Their sleep is either restless and disturbed, or they are affected with perpetual watching. Their aliments become corrupted, their stomachs oppressed and they are inclined to stretch out their legs and arms. They are afflicted with a continual oscillation, and a violent nausea, or inclination to vomit. They make unaccountable complaints, with respect to the weather, as thick and rainy, when at the same time the state of the air is pure, serene, and clear. They are rendered uneasy, fretful, and discontented, by showers and falls of rain, and have small appetite to drink. When the disorder comes on they are afflicted with a violent and insatiable thirst, but, at the same time, are struck with an unaccountable terror and dread, not only at the sight, but also the sound or name of water. Then they become afraid of fomentations of oil used for their relief and their pulse is thick, small and irregular. Some are seized with a slight fever, convulsive throws of the stomach, a torpor and numbness of the joints, a preternatural elevation of the Praecordia to the superior parts, and a costive state of the belly. Then they discharge their urine frequently, and by little at a time, and are seized with a trembling and convulsions. Their voice becomes hollow, and resembling the barking of a dog. The posture of their bodies is like that of a dog when lying asleep on the ground. Their respiration is difficult, and their whole body is rendered highly restless, and uneasy, upon the entrance of any person into the room, for fear he should bring water with him. Their eyes and countenance become red, their bodies slender, and the superior part of it pale, and covered with sweat. The tongue hangs out of the mouth and, in men, the Penis is seized with a frequent tension, accompanied with an involuntary emission of the seminal fluid.

The last stage of the disorder is attended with an hiccup, and a vomiting of bile, which is generally of a blackish colour..."[26].

Thierry adds: "*Once one has seen a man die of rabies, the picture never leaves his mind and he never wants to see such a thing again.*"[27]

25. Littré, 1908, p. 1407.
26. James, 1760, p. 52.
27. Thierry, 1897, p. 692.

Is There a Rabies Virus?

The existence of a rabies virus was the subject of passionate debate for many years. In 1808, in a letter published in the *Journal de Paris*, Dr. Bosquillon, Regent of the former Faculty of Medicine of Paris, expressed strong opposition to this idea[28]. But others held an opposing view. According to Saint-Martin's account, "*on June 19, 1813, Messieurs Magendie and Breschet inoculated saliva from a rabid man to two dogs; the man, called Surlu, died the same day at Hôtel-Dieu: one of the dogs became rabid on July 27 and they had him bite other dogs, who also became rabid; in this way, they spread the disease the entire summer.*"[29]

It was not until the 19th century that the origin of rabies was attributed to the action of an infectious agent. Paul Bert and Nocard demonstrated that this infectious agent did not pass through plaster filters, and was, therefore, a solid matter[30]. Later, Rivolta and Peuch noted that the rabies virus does not pass through a Chamberland filter[31]. In fact, the virus in question was only visible under an electronic microscope. However, many microbes were designated as being the agents of rabies, creating confusion in the research conducted in this field. Several researchers believed they had found the rabies virus: Ferran[32], as well as Dr. Noguchi of the Rockefeller Institute, who came to Paris to present his discovery[33].

Pasteur also believed he was able to see the rabies virus, which takes the form of slender particles. "*Show M. Pasteur or one of his colleagues two brains, one healthy, the other rabid; they will tell you, upon simple inspection of the medulla oblongata under the microscope, which one belongs to the rabid animal.*"[34] Loir confirms this statement, saying that only Pasteur had this special ability to observe accurately. He was rarely wrong[35].

A priori, there was only one virus. Pasteur was certain of it. It had been known for a long time that rabies was transmitted by the bite of rabid animals. It was also known that "*there is less risk when the person is bitten on clothed areas. Bites to the hand & other uncovered areas have always been followed by death*"[36]. Therefore, there was direct transmission.

Rabies Diagnosis

How was this terrible disease diagnosed? Many different tests existed. For example: "*A nobleman who does every thing with adroitness, that generally results from a good understanding, was one day last summer informed, that a strange mad dog in his park had bit some of his dogs, and that his keepers were endeavouring to shoot him. This he forbid, and directed that they should catch him in a net. This was put in execution; the*

28. de la Vergne, 1808, p. 1.
29. de Saint-Martin, 1823, p. 149.
30. Nocard, 1896, p. 733.
31. Peuch, 1890, p. 499.
32. NAF 18094, item 187.
33. Anonyme, 1913, p. 3; Garisson, 1966, p. 588.
34. Cartaz, 1886, p. 211.
35. Loir, 1938, p. 56.
36. Darlue, 1756, p. 274.

dog was confined, so as to render it impossible for him to do any mischief, till he died extremely raving. Mean time, he ordered a cur dog to be procured at the neighbouring village, who was confined three days without food, having only water allowed him. Then a piece of roasted veal was rubbed on the mouth of the dead dog, and offer'd to the half-famished cur. This he would not touch, but avoided it with signs of the utmost consternation. Another bit of the same veal, which had not been near the mad dog, was immediately after offered him, and he ate it very greedily."[37] Enaux and Chaussier (1785) proposed the use of the method of a certain Mr. Grüner: "*An incision, he says, must be made on a healthy dog, rubbed with saliva from the dead animal... If after several days & even a week, there is no symptom of the disease, it can be concluded with certainty that the suspected animal was not rabid.*" Unfortunately, these worthy authors advise an observation period that is much too short to be useful. However, they add: "*This experiment is no doubt very decisive; but the result cannot be obtained before several days* (in fact, too short a time), *& time is valuable... If the test is for a man, he is tormented by uncertainty: therefore, in all suspicious cases, it is best to start treatment early...*"[38].

In practice, it was difficult to obtain a definite diagnosis. First, the animal that had inflicted the bite had to be found, dead or alive. Most often, the animal was declared rabid based on observation of his behaviour, and sometimes following surprising tests. In 1890, Peuch wrote: "*Testing the dog consists of placing the suspected dog in the presence of another dog, to see if a rabies-triggered attack occurs. If the suspected animal shows no aggresivity, it can be assumed that he is not rabid.*"[39] Of course, *a posteriori*, if a bite transmitted the disease to other animals or to humans, the diagnosis left little doubt. Finally, in France animals had to be killed routinely as soon as they were declared rabid, or simply suspected of having rabies. Suspected animals were those that had been bitten or rolled over, that is, known to have been in direct contact with a rabid dog. It was said of dogs that they had been "rolled over" because when a rabid dog met another dog, the healthy dog was most often knocked down and bitten in the scuffle that ensued[40]. However, the distinction between a rabid dog and one suspected of being rabid was highly subjective, and killing suspected dogs eliminated all possibility of observing the evolution of their symptoms.

Autopsies yielding valuable results were performed relatively early. The first description of the autopsy of a dog suspected of having rabies is probably that given by the Englishman Richard Mead in 1709[41]. One relatively reliable indication, although still not specific, was finding inedible substances in the animal's stomach, such as stones, pieces of wood, etc. "*According to statistical figures provided by Bruckmuller, professor at the Vienna Veterinary Institute in Austria, out of 375 rabid dogs, that he autopsied over a period of 20 years, he only came upon foreign objects 199 times, that is, in about 54 cases out of 100.*"[42] This is why this criterion could only serve as an indication.

37. James, 1760, p. 263.
38. Enaux, 1785, p. 21.
39. Peuch *in* Bouley, 1890, t. 18, p. 490.
40. Conte, 1895, p. 283.
41. Blancou, 1994, p. 362.
42. Bonjean, 1878, p. 85.

On the basis of experiments conducted by Pasteur and Roux, cerebral matter from the suspected animal was inoculated to a control animal, most often a rabbit, intra-cerebrally (Roux and Pasteur), or intravenously as Galtier recommended, or into the anterior chamber of the eye anesthetized with cocaine (Gibier), the procedure recommended by Peuch[43]. But these techniques were not described in veterinary manuals until the 1890s, and even then not in all manuals.

Possibly the first attempt at making a diagnosis using intracranial inoculation to rabbits appears to have been recorded by Pasteur on March 22, 1884: the cadaver of a dog who bit the face of a person was brought to the laboratory located at the *Ecole Normale Supérieure*. His stomach contained four strands of straw, fragments of skin and a 5 to 6-centimeter length of rope. "*Trepanation is performed on 2 rabbits with his medulla oblongata... On April 29, the 2 rabbits are in good health... They leave like new.*"[44] This should be understood to mean: "*Trepanation is performed on 2 rabbits and a sample of the medulla oblongata from the dog suspected of being rabid, diluted in physiological solution, is inoculated into the rabbits' dura mater... April 29, the 2 rabbits are in good health... They leave like new.*" This last statement is not very clear. Were the rabbits killed, resold, given to whom? "*Like new*" intimates that these animals were considered as new... On December 31, 1884, the Pasteurians received a bear's head. The inoculated rabbits died of rabies after an eighteen-day incubation period. Pasteur concluded: "*It is possible that the bear attenuated the virulence* (of the virus) *of the dog that bit it [yes, there seems to be no doubt of this based on what follows].*"[45] Pasteur was still thinking of the phenomenon of virulence attenuation by passage of the virus to a host... to be discovered for the rabies virus. The bear was indeed rabid, but passages of the virus to bears would have been hard to accomplish. Pasteur noted: "*Eugène wrote me on December 15, 1886: I have trepanned and inoculated* (these two words are abbreviated) *a rabbit with the optic nerve of an Italian child killed by rabies... This rabbit showed signs of rabies on October 15, the 99th day after trepanation.*"[46] Intracranial inoculation to arrive at a diagnosis was sometimes a slow process.

Clinical evolution of rabies in the dog that inflicted a bite allowed a sure diagnosis, but the animal inflicting the bite had to be captured alive. The dogs invariably died in 5 to 12 days after the onset of clinical signs[47a]. The introduction of Pasteurian intracranial inoculations made diagnosis by means of a fresh cadaver possible. However, neither of these two methods of diagnosis eliminated the need for treating as early as possible, with cauterisation and/or Pasteurian inoculation. On the other hand, a correct negative diagnosis for rabies was extremely useful for reassuring the person or persons bitten by an animal suspected of having rabies.

43. Anonyme, 1889, p. 64; Peuch *in* Bouley, 1890, t. 18, p. 493.
44. NAF 18018, f.P. 72.
45. NAF 18018, f.P. 138.
46. NAF 18020, f.P. 23.
47a. Americanized Encyclopedia Britannica, 1892, vol. VI, p. 3313.

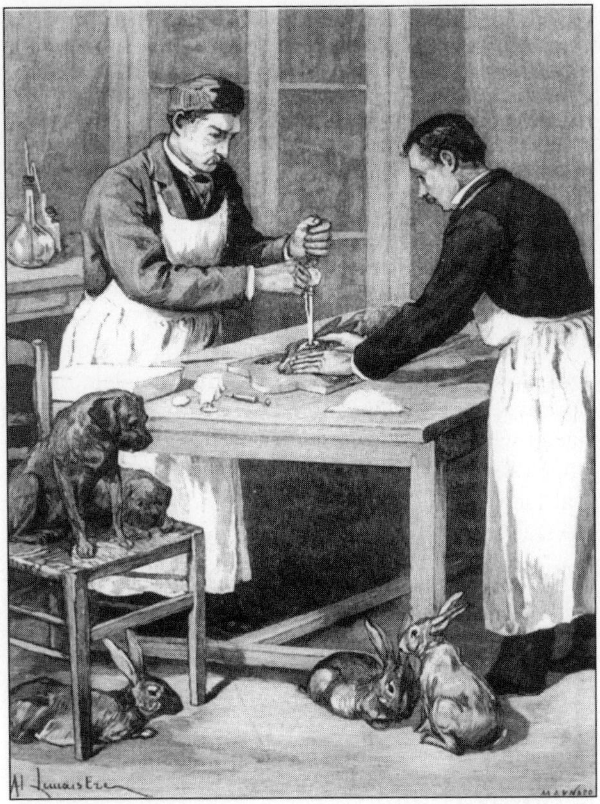

Figure 4. Trepanation of a rabbit. The rabbit is put to sleep with chloroform, "*the surgeon cuts off a square of fur on the top of the head, then makes an approximately three-centimetre incision in the skin... removes a circle of bone the size of a twenty-centime piece... and then takes a Pravaz syringe filled with rabies virus and inoculates the virus directly into the rabbit's brain...* (before) *re-sewing the skin...*" (Lemaistre, 1896)[47b]. The artist who made the drawing no doubt portrayed the other animals sitting around the operating table as a deliberate sign of reciprocal good-will reigning in the laboratory. A slight exaggeration, to say the least!

Preventive and Curative Rabies Treatments

"The man who still has much to learn thinks he knows everything; the one who does know is not afraid that doubt will cast dishonour upon him."
Chabert, 1809[48].

Numerous and varied therapeutic attempts were carried out on people and, sometimes, on animals. Unfortunately these experiments were always conducted on a limited number of subjects, many of whom (two thirds?) were not contaminated, even if they had been bitten by a rabid animal. It is impossible to fully resume all the attempted treatments in a few pages: medicinal plants, mercury, baths, pilgrimages to holy places, particularly Saint Hubert in the Belgian Ardennes[49], etc.

Interestingly, secret remedies were bought from their inventors by governing authorities in many countries. "*It appears that Mr. Crous was in possession of a secret composition, which he avowed to be a never failing remedy in canine madness. The legislature of New-York, in the spirit of philanthropy and benevolence, resolved to purchase the secret for the benefice*

47b. Lemaistre, 1896, p. 218.
48. Chabert, 1809, p. 277.
49. Bazin, 2007, p. 104.

of the community... 'State of New-York, Comptroller's office' Pursuant to the direction, of an act, entitled, 'an act for granting a compensation to John M. Crous, for discovering and publishing a cure for the canine madness, passed the second day of February, 1806... Cure for the bite of a mad dog... 1rst. Take one ounce of the jaw-bone of a dog, burned and pulverized, or pounded to a fine dust. 2nd. Take the false tongue of a newly foaled colt; let that be also dried and pulverized; and 3rd. Take a scruple of the verdigrise which is raised on the surface of old copper by lying in moist earth: the coppers of George I or II are the purest and best. Mix these ingredients together, and if the patient be adult, or full grown, take the common tea-spoon a day... but if after the symptoms appear, a physician must immediately be applied to, to administer the following viz. Three drachms (180 grains) of verdigrise, of the kind before mentioned, mixed with half an ounce of calomel, to be taken at one dose." Mr. Crous received 1,000 dollars for his trouble, paid by the citizens of New-York State[50]. The literature abounds with examples of these false remedies, for sale or not, published more or less with the approval of local authorities. This clearly shows that the populations and the officials faced with rabies were desperate; rabies was a mysterious, terrible affliction, with no hope of recovery unless it be cauterisation, which was sometimes prevented by anatomical factors. For instance, how could cauterisation be carried out next to a large blood vessel?

Inventive minds found solutions but only for those cases where there was something to be done: "*All these considerations lead us to conclude that we must rely heavily on excision of the bitten part, whenever possible; on washing and dilation of wounds... on scarification-producing suction... cauterisation..., hot iron... caustic substances borrowed from the field of chemistry...*"[51]. As medical technology progressed, electrocautery came into use during the period immediately preceding Pasteurian treatment, rendering this treatment obsolete.

If Contracted, Rabies Was Always Fatal

Once rabies was contracted, it was almost always fatal. Cases of recovery were extremely rare. Death sometimes occurred amidst horrible suffering that could not be relieved at the time, except by suffocating the patient between two mattresses or by bloodletting to the utmost extent (euthanasia, rather than fear of biting behaviour since rabid individuals were very rarely aggressive). These practices lasted into the early years of the 19th century; the last case reported in the press occurred in 1816[52]. In most countries, this type of euthanasia was legally prohibited around 1800, but according to Rommelaere, one case occurred around 1870 near Brussels[53].

Public Health Measures for Rabies Prevention

Rabies prevention in the public domain has always consisted in attempts to restrict dogs from roaming freely; muzzling, capture, poisoning or euthanasia of stray dogs, compulsory castration of male dogs (a measure that was never applied), filing down of teeth: incisors and canines. In 1892, French legislation demanded that dogs wear muzzles, and that stray dogs be captured and put to death. Rigorous observance of the

50. Thacher, 1812, p. 208.
51. de la Vergne, 1808, p. 32.
52. Bonjean, 1878, p. 9.
53. Rommelaere, 1889, p. 251.

measures established against stray dogs in Paris resulted in Roux's observation that the number of Parisians treated for rabies had fallen from ten new cases a day to a single case. About 25,000 stray dogs were killed. These measures were stopped after a short time due to protests[54], and anti-rabies treatments were again dispensed to a greater number of people. Finally, wolves were exterminated with the approval and the financial support of the State, as well as the consent of the population. In France, the number of people bitten by wolves decreased very rapidly.

Rabies in Europe at the Start of Pasteur's Studies

Human rabies mortality statistics are difficult to analyse. Between 1850 and 1860, rabies caused about twenty deaths per year in Prussia, four in Bavaria, three in Belgium, ten in England, one in Scotland, four in Sweden. In France, between, 1850 and 1872, there were 30 deaths per year. All authors agree that the figures underestimate the situation, but nobody knows by how much[55].

The frequency of rabies transmission from a rabid animal to man or to another animal is also poorly understood. Figures abound; indeed, they are available in sufficient quantity... to reveal total confusion. They reveal considerable disagreement between different authors. Renault, Director of the Alfort Veterinary School, estimates that at most one third of the individuals bitten by rabid dogs and left untreated contract rabies[56]. Bouley cites a 90% mortality rate for bites to the face by rabid animals (based on 32 cases studied) and 63% for bites to the hands (based on 73 cases studied); 28% for bites to the upper limbs (except hands) out of 28 cases studied, and 29% for bites to the lower limbs (based on 24 cases studied)[57]. Pasteur himself provides the following figures: 20% of dogs bitten by rabid dogs become rabid themselves, and 10% or 15 to 20% of bitten individuals contract rabies[58]. Some exceptions are also cited in the literature: "*John Hunter mentions one remarkable instance in which of twenty-one persons bitten by a rabid dog only one subsequently died from hydrophobia.*"[59]

However, among people bitten by wolves and left untreated, the mortality rate was two thirds, according to Renault (254 people bitten) and to du Mesnil (800 people bitten)[60].

Rabies Experiments Before Pasteur's Era

Attempts to transmit rabies from one animal to another started long ago. In 1804, G. Zinke succeeded in transmitting rabies by applying saliva from a dog killed by rabies on incisions made on another dog[61]. In 1813, Magendie and Breschet transmitted human rabies to a dog[62].

54. Conte, 1895, p. 283.
55. Brouardel *in* Dechambre, 1874, 3rd series, t. 2, p. 192.
56. Renault, 1853, p. 384.
57. Bouley, 1870, p. 62.
58. Pasteur, O.C., t. VII, p. 363; Pasteur, 1890, p. 166.
59. Americanized Encyclopedia Britannica, 1892, vol. VI, p. 3313.
60. Suzor, 1887, p. 26.
61. Kolle, 1918, t. 2, p. 376.
62. Hurtrel d'Arboval, 1877, t. 3, p. 322.

When Pasteur started his work on rabies, others were engaged in this work as well: Galtier, Duboué, Gibier, Raynaud, Fol and probably many others in France and elsewhere... The competition existing between them cannot be overlooked.

Vaccine is the Goal; Preventive Vaccine is the Dream

"*Rabies is the disease that makes the fewest human victims. But Pasteur chose it because the rabic virus was always considered the most mysterious of viruses and also because rabies is considered the most terrifying and dreadful disease.*"
Dr. Roux, 1922[63].

Very likely, Pasteur had been interested in rabies for a long time, given that it had no effective treatment other than cauterisation, which was only possible if the number of bites allowed it, if they were not too deep, not located near a vital organ, etc. Perhaps childhood memories - cauterisation of people bitten by a rabid animal, performed in the blacksmith's forge in Arbois - motivated his interest in this cruel affliction.

In December 1880, he was informed that a child had died of rabies on Dr. Lannelongue's ward at the Trousseau Hospital. Samples of saliva revealed an unknown microbe, to which Pasteur refers in many places in his laboratory notes. This incident showed Pasteur the limitations of the use of saliva as a source of rabies virus. He then went on to explore nervous tissue[64], knowing that it is bacteriologically sterile (characterised by absence of bacterial germs), as he had learned when he studied so-called spontaneous generation. He noted: "*Rabies. Search for the organism of true rabies, in the medulla oblongata. January 26, 1881. M. Bourrel sent two dogs killed by rabies...*"[65]. It was a gift to Pasteur from Bourrel, Parisian veterinarian, specialized in the treatment of animals suspected of having rabies.

Thanks to the remarkable experiments conducted by Galtier, professor at the Lyon Veterinary School, Pasteur knew that it was possible to make sheep refractory to rabies by injecting them intravenously with saliva from rabid dogs. "*I was the first to reveal, in various communications, starting on January 25, 1881, the effects of intravenous injections of rabies virus on herbivorous animals... It was thanks to this important discovery that the idea of vaccinating against rabies was conceived.*"[66] The procedure was not really a vaccination, but a sort of variolation (see Glossary). The virus used had normal virulence and it was (only?) the intravenous method of introduction that produced immunisation in herbivores, without infecting them with rabies. Injecting virulent matter intravenously to induce immunity in animals was not an entirely original idea, especially at the Lyon Veterinary School, where it was practised routinely. "*When Mr. Galtier obtained immunity against rabies for the first time (February 1881), there was nothing in his method that contradicted our theoretical notions; it was the application to rabies of a general method perfected at the Lyon school.*"[67a] Galtier's work was innovative as it applied to rabies, and Pasteur's attitude was questionable when, at the December 11, 1882 meeting of the Academy of

63. Roux, 1922, p. 723.
64. Cartaz, 1886, p. 211.
65. NAF 18016, f.P. 67.
66. Galtier, 1892, t. 2., p. 115.
67a. Bouchard, 1889, p. 167.

Sciences, he announced: "*Although it does not kill, intravenous inoculation of rabic saliva or blood to dogs does not prevent subsequent rabies infection, nor death following a renewed inoculation of pure rabic matter, by means of trepanation or intravenous injection.*"[67b]*

Earle, Raynaud... and perhaps others[68] had already succeeded in inoculating rabies to rabbits by using rabic human saliva. But in 1881 Galtier was the one who was by far the most knowledgeable about rabies in rabbits. He had identified the rabbit as the best species in which to study this disease. In effect, rabbits often contracted rabies after a shorter incubation period, and most often presented paralytic symptoms. Rabbits were inexpensive and docile. The Pasteurians conceived the idea of cultivating in rabbits the pathogenic agent they had not been able to isolate. This had been the method used to produce certain infectious agents not yet isolated, like that of cowpox in heifers or sheeppox in sheep, when they were both unknown agents.

Studies on rabies carried out by Pasteur and his team covered a period starting in 1881 and lasting until at least 1886; it is difficult to identify them without making an attempt at classification. They fill most pages of about ten 150-page registers... It would be impossible to summarize all the experiments. At most, the major experiments can be described briefly to show the abundance and variety of ideas the Pasteurians put into practice during this period. The dates of the experiments are given, so they can be situated chronologically. The laboratory notes do not allow the reader to determine the role of each of Pasteur's associates, and particularly that of Roux. Their names are sometimes mentioned in the notes, but rarely and most often in connection with a specific task carried out by one of them. In addition to Pasteur's personal notebooks, there are sometimes more or less detailed reports concerning tasks performed by Roux (not necessarily initialled by him), by Chamberland, Thuillier, etc., these last bearing signatures.

Tackling Rabies: Where to Start?

• **At the start of 1881**, Pasteur and his team began their methodical study of the rabies virus, looking for the best way to transmit the disease in a reproducible manner and with a reasonable inoculation time. Galtier had spoken of an incubation period of five to twenty days in rabbits[69], but later he modified his own data by citing a period between five and forty days, and even two to nine months or more...[70]. This uncertainty must have made it difficult to interpret experimental results. In addition, Galtier wrote: "*In my own studies, I inoculated numerous times, and in various ways, the product of lingual nerves, of medulla oblongata, of the protuberance, of the brain and of the spinal cord, without inducing rabies.*"[71] Imagination and an innovative spirit led

* In a note, Pasteur wrote: "*These results contradict those announced by Mr. Galtier before this Academy on August 1rst 1881, based on experiments on sheep.*"[67c] In fact, Pasteur's results do not contradict Galtier's, they merely limit their scope. Much later, Galtier responded in writing: "*In a word he* (Pasteur) *by speaking of 'dogs' while I was speaking of 'sheep and goats' made it look as if my conclusions were wrong; but this was not so, and their truthfulness is fully recognized today...*"[67d]. In 1888, Nocard and Roux conducted experiments that validated Galtier's work, and published their results[67e].

67b. Pasteur, O.C., t. VI, p. 575.

67c. Pasteur, O.C., t. VI, p. 575.

67d. Galtier, 1892, t. 2, p. 136.

67e. Nocard, 1888, p. 341.

68. Brouardel *in* Dechambre, 1874, 3rd series, t. 2, p. 197; Doléris, 1881, p. 451.

69. Galtier, 1880, p. 780.

70. Galtier, 1892, t. 2, p. 125.

71. Galtier, 1880, p. 776.

Pasteur and Roux to think that inoculating contagious matter, particularly *medulla oblongata* and spinal cord matter into the surface of the nervous system, could be more effective than injections into any subcutaneous tissue[72]. According to Bordet, this was Roux's idea[73], and he was the one who put it into practice. Trepanation is an ancient surgical technique: "*This doctor* (Hippocratis) *who advises the use of the crowned trepan, does not claim to have invented it... The very ingenious invention of the crown trepan... dates back... to before the fifth century* B.C."[74] Once the instrument, a trepan, was obtained, the method was quickly perfected. "*The hair covering the crown of the head is cut off with scissors, - a procedure resembling the preparation of condemned men - then the skin is incised with a scalpel over a length of a few centimetres. The cranium is now exposed; placing a trepan crown over the centre of this incision, a round portion of bone the size of a lentil is removed using a few turns of the crown; this exposes the covering of the brain called dura mater. This membrane is delicately pricked with the needle of a small Pravaz syringe, and a few drops of its content are introduced into the surface of the brain...*"[75]. This method proved to be reliable and very important for Pasteurian studies. Pasteur's notebooks mention rare cases where rabbits died after one or two days, indicating bacterial infection. For instance, at the end of October 1884, one rabbit died after two days. Roux took a bacterial sample and Pasteur noted: "*Roux stains them and* (1 word) *the culture which develops quickly and easily and which he will photograph later.*"[76]

• **March 27, 1881.** Pasteur's notes speak of a (first, probably) dog subjected to trepanation on March 27, 1881 and inoculated with crushed *medulla oblongata* matter mixed with chicken broth, from a dog that died of rabies on the 25th; the dog died of rabies on April 11, after a fourteen-day incubation period[77]. Culture of the rabies virus in the rabbit's nervous system represented considerable progress. Animals died of rabies in 100% of the experiments, after an incubation period of about two weeks. It was possible to cultivate rabic virus uncontaminated by bacteria, and to preserve it using successive passages from rabbit to rabbit.

• **December 2, 1881.** Roux used trepanation to inoculate three rabbits with a portion of *medulla oblongata* from a man who died of rabies at Hôtel-Dieu, and on December 3rd he inoculated three dogs from the pound[78]. All these animals died of rabies; the first rabbit died after thirteen days, and the first dog after sixteen days. In an added note undated, Pasteur concluded: "*Easy transmission of rabies to rabbits and dogs.*" This appears to have been the first use of trepanation to transmit human rabies to animals.

As usual, Pasteur tried to obtain the most virulent strain of the germ under study, and then to reduce this virulence until he reached the degree he needed. The Pasteurians started to carry out successive passages to rabbits in order to obtain a source of "fixed rabies virus". The present text only reproduces a limited number of entries giving dates and page references. The rest of the passages are easy to find in Pasteur's notebooks.

---

72. Nocard, 1892, p. 235.
73. Bordet, 1934, p. 73.
74. Littré, 1841, p. 150.
75. James, 1886, p. 33.
76. NAF 18018, f.P. 97 back.
77. NAF 18016, f.P. 99.
78. NAF 18016, f.P. 143.

• **December 13, 1882.** "*Rabies Series of rabbits with cerebellum of the cow that died December 12 p. 58 back Successive series of rabbits December 13 with the medulla oblongata of the rabbit with cerebellum that died on the 11th in the evening or during the night, inoculation by trepanation of 2 rabbits and a female dog (new) in the right shin, 1/2 syringe. Rabbits are intended for a rabbit to rabbit series to intensify rabies in rabbits and weaken it in dogs. The dog will serve to evaluate virulence for dogs at the start of inoculation with the first rabbit. Present virulence will be compared to subsequent virulence.*"

On December 28, 1882, the two rabbits were paralysed in all four limbs. 1rst passage. Incubation period for rabbits: 15 days[79]...

On May 7, 1884, 43rd passage. Incubation period: 9 days[80]...

On May 10, 1884, "*on May 10 the 43rd passage to rabbits was repeated.*" Incubation period: 9 days[81]. Pasteur did not attribute a number to this series. It is a second series, a "bis"...

On March 20, 1884, 50th passage. Incubation period: 6 days[82].

On July 29, 1884, 50th "bis" passage. Incubation period: 8 days[83]...

On March 20, 1885, 72nd passage. Incubation period: 6 days. "*The passages at page (85-42) are not continued. Only those at p. 88. See this page in notebook 12.*"[84] Therefore, only the "bis" series was preserved...

On December 26, 1885, 100th "bis" passage. Incubation period: 7 days[85]...

On July 16, 1887, the 155th passage was carried out, incubation period of the 154th passage: 6 days[86]...

The passages were performed continuously. The method was reliable. But it is clear that several times there were simultaneous passages of a series, perhaps as a safety measure. Incubation periods slowly decreased. This strain of rabies virus became the "fixed virus" adapted to rabbits, by contrast to the "stray-dog virus" of common rabies. Although this is not specified in writing, it is likely that the virus used to treat little Joseph Meister came from the cerebellum of a cow killed by rabies.

In a presentation given at a conference, Bouley explained Pasteur's method: "*The first question to answer was whether the rabies virus can have various intensities, as the anthrax virus and the chicken cholera virus do; for in order to induce a refractory state against any infectious disease, a method must be found to modify by stages, as it were, the energy of the virus causing the disease, and thus to establish immunity by gradual steps: letting the virus at its lowest intensity prepare the body to withstand the action of a more intense virus. But by what indication... could various intensities of the rabies virus be recognized?... Mr. Pasteur found this indication in the duration of the incubation period after inoculation performed during trepanation and using the highest dose of virulent matter, so as to avoid duration variability associated with low doses.*"[87a]

79. NAF 18017, f.P. 81.
80. NAF 18018, f.P. 85.
81. NAF 18018, f.P. 88.
82. NAF 18018, f.P. 85.
83. NAF 18018, f.P. 88.
84. NAF 18019, f.P. 42.
85. NAF 18019, f.P. 68 back.
86. NAF 18020, f.P. 17.
87a. Bouley, 1884, p. 364.

Throughout his experiments involving the passage of the rabies virus to different animal species, Pasteur tested viral virulence on other species: most often one dog, two rabbits and two guinea pigs, more rarely chickens or even animals of other species. Pasteur never really clarified the question of a prolonged rabies incubation period produced either by inoculation of a small quantity of virus or by a virus strain with attenuated virulence. At that time, there was no method allowing the quantification of viral doses, unless the experimenter had recourse to dilutions and comparison to a more or less well defined standard, impossible to keep except by passage on animals. But this method was highly approximate, since accurate results could not be obtained without knowing the initial quantity of virus. As Bouley reported, Pasteur used a maximum dose, but was this always the case? In fact, Pasteur used a "simple" experimental structure: a large quantity of infected "matter", but really an unknown quantity, and if there was viral virulence "attenuation" the incubation period would have been prolonged in the inoculated rabbit and would have remained so on the occasion of a second transfer; if "small quantities" were used and the inoculated rabbit died of rabies, the virus would be present in normal quantities and would have retained the same degree of virulence, and therefore normal incubation time, that is, not prolonged when the virus was passed to another rabbit.

In the course of these series of passages of the virus, viral strains are lost when the inoculated animals do not die of rabies. Pasteur and his associates conducted all sorts of experiments. Very quickly, they went beyond the limits of the established scientific data available at the time. They were exploring vast, unknown territories. For at least two years, they stumbled in the dark, going from one disaster to another.

"*Rabies Rabies Vaccination. Series of passages from dog to dog - (the 1rst dog with street rabies.) etc...* **May 13, 1882**, *p. 3, 11th notebook, trepanation of a dog inoculating street rabies from mad dog. This dog shows symptoms* after 21 days - On June 9 p. 11 trepanation of a second dog with the medulla oblongata of the previous one. This dog shows symptoms* after 11 days...*" A third dog shows symptoms* after 15 days... a fourth after 10 days... a fifth after 12 days... a sixth after 8 days...

"**Sept. 1rst** [1882] *Two rabbits are inoculated by trepanation with the medulla oblongata of the previous dog* (the sixth). *Both rabbits become rabid, one after 15, the other after 16 days Conclusions. Passage of rabies virus, virus originating from stray dogs, increased virulence when passed from dog to dog... (no); but this virulence that promptly reaches the maximum for the dog - (in six passages - no) transferred to rabbits turns out to be as weak (and perhaps even weaker) than in a direct passage from the street dog to the rabbits.*"[87b] The two "no"s have been added by Pasteur after his initial notation. A note specifies: "*Written* **May 11, 1884**. *In fact, although successive trepanations from dog to dog, with medulla oblongata from stray dogs seemed to transmit rabies faster to the latter dogs than to the first, the virus does not appear to become more virulent. In fact, reverting to rabbits again the incubation period is about 13 to 15 days. This must be so if the street virus has reached a maximum through successive passages from dog to dog.*"[88] The street virus seems best suited to "maximum" virulence in this species.

* Pasteur spent hours observing his laboratory animals. When he writes "*prendre*", he is refering to the onset of clinical signs, not to contamination or infection, which are terms used in relation to inoculation.

87b. NAF 18018, f.P. 75. This page is reproduced in Hannoun, 1975.

88. NAF 18018, f.P. 75 back.

• **December 9, 1882.** After one year of work, Pasteur is still very cautious: "*Rabies: tests for vaccination or rather for no relapse, today Dec. 9, 1882...*"[89].

July 30, 1883, Roux presents his thesis to The Faculty of Medicine of Paris, before embarking on the unfortunate expedition to Egypt where Thuillier was to die. Roux felt he would need the title of doctor of medicine overseas. He observed: "*There are now four dogs in Monsieur Pasteur's laboratory to whom we have not been able to transmit rabies, even by inoculating them several times in the arachnoid cavity...*"[90]. The inoculation protocols are not described. Were they known? This was, after all, a decisive stage. Of course, as Roux indicates, this work was carried out collectively in the laboratory.

May 14, 1884. Pasteur is searching for an attenuation method, in rabbits, by removing and inoculating tissues such as lacrimal glands: "*NB It seems very likely that virus from the lacrimal gland can be attenuated relative to the inoculated virus.*"[91]

August 19, 1884: new hope: "*NB If as everything seems to indicate the pancreas gland attenuates and if this is true for the other glands, it might be possible to attenuate the canine virus, by passage in the glands, do the same in monkeys... it remains to be seen...*"[92]. Pasteur was probably referring to a small quantity of virus...

January 23, 1885, Pasteur inoculated six new dogs under the skin with half a syringe of *medulla oblongata* from passage 66 to rabbits. Five of them died of rabies, one survived and was resistant to a dose of virus injected under the skin[93]. The virus from the 66th passage to rabbits (well adapted to this species, incubation period of about seven days) was still very virulent for dogs. In this series, virulence attenuation was absent or very slight.

The experiment did not produce any conclusions. The Pasteurians tried many rabic virulence attenuation techniques, clearly somewhat randomly and not very successfully. Passage of the rabic virus to monkeys held great promise for them.

Passage of Rabic Virus from Monkey to Monkey

Pasteur's notebooks describe many inoculations of street rabies virus to monkeys. Rather than the death of inoculated animals, the team's criterion is still the duration of the incubation period, that is, the lapse of time between inoculation and appearance of the first symptoms. The notebooks indicate that Pasteur himself observed these animals very closely. But his perspective was rather subjective. In summary, Pasteur's work involving monkey's comprises:

- December 6, 1883 to May 29, 1884: a series of seven passages, with virus from a deceased man;
- June 20, 1884 to January 31, 1885: a series of thirteen passages, with virus from the 46th passage to rabbits;
- November 12, 1884 to December 31, 1885: a series of eighteen passages, with virus from a dog killed by street rabies;
- June 8, 1885 to September 4, 1885: a series of seven passages, with virus from a man killed by rabies.

89. NAF 18017, f.P. 78.
90. Roux, 1883, p. 42.
91. NAF 18018, f.P. 94.
92. NAF 18018, f.P. 122.
93. NAF 18019, f.P. 4.

Four trials were stopped after the first passage (March 10, April 29, June 13, August 29, 1884). The first series, conducted on December 6, 1883, was the most promising, since it achieved a prolongation of the incubation period in monkeys. This experiment clearly raised Pasteur's hopes, but in vain.

• **December 6, 1883**, the first monkey is inoculated with the *medulla oblongata* of a dog killed by rabies, inoculated on November 6 with "*nerve bundle from the armpit of bitten arm*" of a 7-year old child who died of rabies on November 5, 1883[94]. The monkey died on December 20. Inoculation period: 11 days; rabbits, 19 and 16 days; guinea pigs, 11 days[95].

On December 1883, virus from this monkey was inoculated to a second monkey, who died on January 7, 1884. Incubation period: 11 days; rabbits: 13 days and 2 days (microbial infection); guinea pigs: 11 days[96].

January 7, 1884. The same virus was inoculated to a third monkey, who died on February 5. Incubation period: 23 days; rabbit: 16 days[97].

On February 5, 1884, the virus used in this series of passages was re-inoculated to a fourth monkey, who died on March 3. Pasteur described his dying as follows: "*The monkey is still alive. He is closer to death than yesterday, barely breathing. He died in the middle of the day.*" Incubation period: monkey, 20 days; rabbits, 26 and 31 days; guinea pigs, 25 and 29 days[98].

March 4, 1884. Virus from this monkey was inoculated, using trepanation, to a fifth monkey, who died on March 26. Incubation period: monkey, 17 days; rabbits, 28 days[99].

March 28, 1884. The virus is passed to a sixth monkey: "*(Very nasty, according to the keeper in the animal park, who brings him.* [This site is a Paris park where exotic animals and plants were kept for acclimatation.]), *2 new rabbits, 2 new guinea pigs, 2 new dogs... April 29 The monkey died on the spot. Of the two March 28 rabbits, one died, the other is dying. The second dog subjected to trepanation on March 28 is still in good health, after 32 days. This is a long period after trepanation. If he does not become rabid, he will no doubt be vaccinated. This will be as important as it is curious...*"[100].

"April 29 [1884] *the medulla oblongata of the 6th monkey is used to trepan a small monkey, the 7th...*". On May 29, the monkey was still in good health[101]. There have been seven successive passages to monkeys. The strain seems to have been lost after the last passage. Pasteur does not seem to have recovered it from the rabbits or guinea pigs inoculated at the same time as the last monkey. He conducted three more long series of passages of the rabies virus to monkeys, with inconclusive results: that is, with a rabies incubation period that remained almost unchanged. The results of his first series were not reproduced.

During his first series of passages to monkeys, on May 19, 1884, Pasteur stated, before the Academy of Sciences: "*In passages from dog to monkey and subsequently from monkey to monkey, rabies virus virulence weakens after each passage. When virulence has been*

94. NAF 18017, f.P. 159 & 161.
95. NAF 18018, f.P. 44.
96. NAF 18018, f.P. 33.
97. NAF 18018, f.P. 33 back.
98. NAF 18018, f.P. 44.
99. NAF 18018, f.P. 59 back.
100. NAF 18018, f.P. 74.
101. NAF 18018, f.P. 74 back.

reduced by these passages from monkey to monkey, if the virus is transferred to dogs, rabbits, guinea pigs, it remains attenuated."[102] Pasteur relied for a long time on these passages of rabies virus to monkeys to defend his work to the outside world. His results were not very brilliant, but they were the only ones he had... Moreover, adapting stray-dog rabies virus to monkeys reduced (?) its virulence in dogs. But would it have produced the same effect in humans, a species genetically close to the monkey? The question is worth considering.

• **May 28, 1884**: date of the creation of the "Commission de la rage" (Rabies Commission) in response to a request addressed by Pasteur to the Minister. Pasteur has completed his first series of "monkey" passages...

How many dogs were immunised, before or after inoculation of rabies by the bite of a rabid animal or in the course of an experiment? On August 10, 1884, at the International Conference of Medical Sciences in Copenhagen, Pasteur described his results, before the Rabies Commission. Among the twenty-three dogs vaccinated and then tested, there was not a single case of rabies. Among the nineteen dogs in the control group, there were fourteen cases of rabies. Pasteur's exceptional results earned him great esteem. The dogs in question had been vaccinated using a virus with attenuated virulence achieved by successive passages to monkeys[103], a method neither very reliable nor reproducible.

Where to House Experimental Dogs?

Other problems connected with the experiments arose... The Pasteurians used many animals in their experiments: monkeys, chickens, rabbits, guinea pigs and, above all, dogs. Some dogs were housed in the basement of Pasteur's laboratory, others at the Alfort School or in the shelters of two Parisian veterinarians, Frégis, director of the Montmartre kennel, and Bourrel, at number 7 Fontaine-au-Roi Street; their names appear frequently in Pasteur's laboratory notebooks. Pasteur was also given part of the premises of Rollin College, a school recently closed. On these sites there were sheep with anthrax, horses with meiloidosis, chickens with cholera and rabid dogs[104a] - a sinister menagerie that, according to Loir, disturbed the neighbours with its cries and caused repeated complaints from the other occupants of the buildings.

Pasteur wanted to keep the experimental dogs for a certain period of time, especially the "Rabies Commission" dogs. It was proposed that he set up a kennel in the woods of Meudon, which angered the residents of the area, who denounced by every conceivable means the dangers associated with Mr. Pasteur's dogs. The *Figaro* of May 26, 1884 published a long satirical poem on the subject, written by Gaston Jollivet. The stanza below illustrates the tone of the poem.

> "*Quoi! C'est en plein bois de Boulogne;*
> *Que les gens du gouvernement;*
> *O Pasteur, t'ont dit sans vergogne:*
> *Choisissez votre emplacement.*"

(*What? It's right in the Boulogne Wood That those who govern our nation, oh Pasteur, told you: "Feel free to choose your location."*)

102. Pasteur, O.C., t. VI, p. 586.
103. Pasteur, O.C., t. VI, p. 590.
104a. Lemaistre, 1896, p. 204.

This project was quickly abandoned... In the end, a location was found in Villeneuve-l'Etang in another Paris suburb, where the same protests arose. But this time they were quickly subdued, since they came from the residents of a retirement home, the "Grateful Home" or Brézin Residence, after the name of its founder (the original structure of the present-day Garches Hospital). The experiments continued. The site was in fact what remained of the Villeneuve castle, fallen to ruin, where Napoleon III and Eugenie started their wedded life together. The servant's quarters were in better condition and the first floor was used to house the experimental dogs. Pasteur had a few rooms modestly furnished on the floor above, so that he could rest there in the summer.

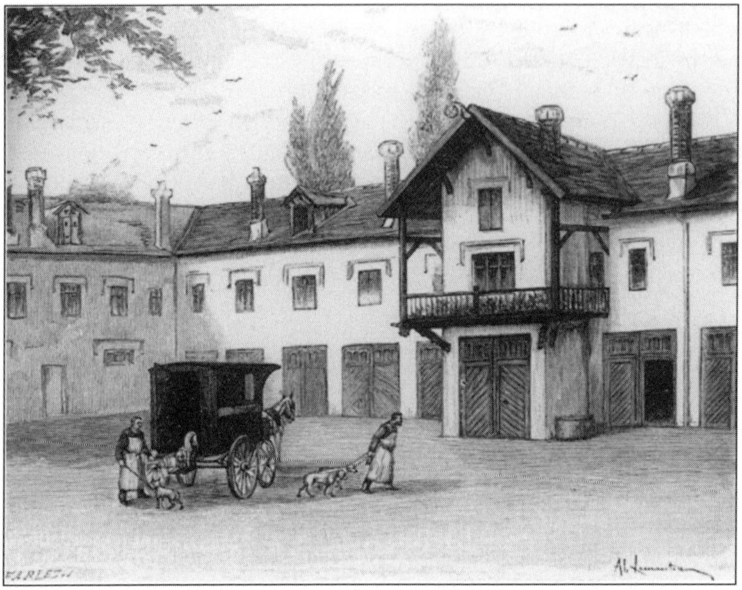

Figure 5. The *Institut Pasteur* in Villeneuve-L'Etang (A. Lemaistre, 1896)[104b]. The illustration shows the arrival of the dogs bought at the pound *"for a sum of between 2 francs and 2 fr. 50 on average"*, and taken to the kennel located in the new annex of the *Institut Pasteur*.

Was Rabies the Only Focus?

Pasteur's work is often described as perfectly orderly. In reality, Pasteur was interested in all sorts of problems, and his projects were not always carried through. For instance, a long list "*written on August 30, 1884*" enumerates thirty-five subjects he planned to investigate, most of them focusing on the new method of immunisation against rabies. But the list also includes many ideas concerning swine erysipelas, canine distemper, a combined anthrax/erysipelas vaccine, cattle pleuropneumonia, foot-and-mouth disease... and other, more surprising questions:

"*24th test of Ct. Fotocki's plant...*"

"*34th - If what* M. Romanes (Revue scientifique *Oct. 18, 1884*) *says about the effects of taming on the instincts, especially for dogs, I feel certain that rendering dogs refractory to rabies over several generations will result in breeds of dogs refractory to rabies. My current experiments on dogs and guinea pigs should clarify this.*" [Romanes's article deals with

104b. Lemaistre, 1896, p. 241.

learned traits in domestic animals. The breeds used as examples are hunting dogs and shepherds[105].]

"*35th Propose to M. Grancher collaboration in the study of rabies remedies.*" [Pasteur is mindful of finding a subject of study for Grancher, who entered his laboratory a few days earlier.]

There are also material concerns: "*Set up barns for cows, calves... in Villeneuve l'Etang.*" Then, below: "*Monkey rooms have to be set up first in Villeneuve l'Etang.*"[106]

• **October 8, 1884.** Pasteur's mind never rests, not even when he is on vacation. He imagines all sorts of experiments, and takes notes to remember his ideas:

"*Experiments to conduct in 1884-1885 - written in Arbois on Oct. 8, 1884.*

- Study of pleuropneumonia to find vaccines. Culture microbes and their virulence. Pass natural virus found in stables from calf to calf. Is there attenuation. Transmission tests in animals that are smaller and less expensive than cows and calves...

- Study of rabies and its attenuation, see other experiments to try p. 119 (back)...

- Multiple passages of virus, mostly from rabbits, to calves. From calves pass to rabbits and from calf to calf, and again to rabbits after each death of rabid calf. [at p. 119 back, there are 35 suggestions for experiments including Inoculations subc. - use street virus to 12 dogs - id. id. id. Rabbit virus maximum to 12 dogs - to evaluate comparative mortality... Set up barns for cows, calves... in Villeneuve l'Etang.]

- Go back to swine erysipelas...

- True vaccine Pass smallpox virus to calf and form calf to calf until proof of attenuation. Pass to monkey and from monkey to monkey.

- Foot-and-mouth disease. Does it recur? If so look for remedy and not vaccine - operate on very young calves to cause death and look for microbe.

- Abortion disease in cows - trials of frequent injections in the vagina and frequent lavage with 3% boric acid fluid - use of this fluid for lavage of reproductive organs of bulls during the days preceding mounting (half of the animals in each barn - leaving the other half in their natural state)."[107]

Obviously rabies was not Pasteur's only interest, and neither were vaccines, ten months before the first vaccination attempt on Joseph Meister!

Pasteur Wants to Make the Leap from Animals to Humans, but he Knows the Risk

Very quickly, Pasteur announces that he is convinced if the effectiveness of his anti-rabies treatment, based on the results he obtained in passages to monkeys, knowing this involved some risk for the patients (it is certain that he was thinking of treating humans) and, above all, for his reputation; or perhaps wanting only to give himself some publicity... On the one hand he keeps repeating that passage from animals to humans is a feat equivalent to crossing the Rubicon, requiring caution and reflection. To illustrate, on May 15, 1884, he declares: "*But it is not easy to experiment on human beings. For a long time, I was considering condemned criminals: it became difficult to sustain*

105. Romanes, 1884, p. 499.
106. NAF 18018, f.P. 119 & 120.
107. NAF 18018, f.P. 141 & 142.

this line of thought."[108] On the other hand, still in May 1884, Pasteur declares his faith in the value of his (first) method, which consisted of repeated passages of the virus to monkeys. He was reaching the end of his first series of seven passages, started on December 6, 1883, not knowing that it would end in May 1884.

In effect, the May 18, 1884 *Figaro* wrote: "*An indiscretion that is, at the same time, good news. As we all know, the day before yesterday in the evening (May 15 or 16) the Hôtel Continental hosted the monthly banquet of the Paris branch of the Association of alumni of the Ecole centrale. This banquet was presided over by Mr. Pasteur; in this regard, several newspapers reported that, at dessert, the illustrious scientist announced to his audience, whose discretion he requested for a few more days, a new discovery that would bring great benefits to humanity. We believe that this discovery is the remedy for rabies that Mr. Pasteur has been seeking for a long time and that he declares to have found.*"[109]

A few days after his announcement at the Hôtel Continental, on May 19, 1884, in a communication submitted to the Academy of Sciences, Pasteur declared: "*Using inoculations with blood from rabid animals, in specific conditions, I was able to simplify greatly the vaccination procedure and to induce in dogs the most pronounced refractory state.*"[110] It is hard to know what these inoculations of blood could have been. Was Pasteur deliberately creating confusion to mislead potential competitors? Further in his text, he expressed appropriate caution concerning passage to humans. He added: "*The first experiments were very favourable to this view, but demonstrations have to be infinitely multiplied on various animal species, before human therapeutics might dare to attempt this prevention in men.*"[111] But that same day, Monday, May 19, 1884, the *Figaro* published a long interview with Pasteur in his laboratory, in which he stated: "*From now on, any person bitten by a rabid dog can simply come to the Ecole Normale laboratory and ask for M. Pasteur's treatment, which will make him refractory to rabies, and therefore unharmed...*"[112]. He provided details about his method of rabies prevention: "*First, I took virus from the brain of a dog killed by rabies; I inoculated it to a first monkey, who died: I inoculated his virus, already attenuated, to a second monkey, and the virus of the second to a third; after what I would call this third passage, I obtained a virus with an almost complete degree of safety* (sic); *I inoculated this virus to a first rabbit: it gained some strength; to a second, in whom it became even stronger; to a third, to a fourth, until it reached its maximum strength. In this way, I obtained viruses with very different strengths, - exactly as I had obtained more or less harmful anthrax microbes by developing them in chemical cultures. Only here, I developed the rabies virus, - and the as yet unknown rabies microbe, whose existence seems certain, - in animal mediums, each animal showing a different aptitude to contract and to withstand the disease... Knowing this, here is how I treat, or rather prevent, rabies: I make the animal - or the person - refractory. For example, I give a dog three inoculations of virus from my rabbits starting with the lowest virulence, then using an intermediary virulence and finally, after a few days, the highest virulence. Afterwards, if I inoculate rabies from any dog to the dog I have just subjected to the above treatment, he will not become ill: he will be refractory... But the discovery does not end there: I inoculate two dogs with rabies virus; I leave one untreated; after a few days, seven or eight, sometimes more, sometimes less, the dog becomes rabid, either with furious rabies or with dumb rabies; I take the*

108. Pasteur, O.C., t. VII, p. 363.
109. Anonyme, 1884c, p. 1.
110. Pasteur, O.C., t. VI, p. 586.
111. Pasteur, O.C., t. VI, p. 587.
112. XXX, 1884, p. 1.

other dog and give him successive inoculations of my virus at different degrees of virulence, from the lowest to the highest, before the initial incubation period is over, that is, within about a week; the second dog recovers, or rather, does not fall ill... I will be able to prevent the incubation of the rabies virus in any person who, after being bitten by a rabid dog, is willing to accept my three little incubations."[113]

"*Three little inoculations*", Pasteur says; but he does not know if the virus passed to monkeys is stable. How can this low-virulence virus be preserved? The fact that this virus can recover its virulence by successive passage to rabbits, as Pasteur himself asserts, precludes the possibility of using this method to preserve it. At the time, passage to animals was the only know method of virus conservation...

The *Figaro* news item was reprinted in the newspaper *La Science pour tous* on May 24, 1884. This paper, however, left the responsibility for the content to the *Figaro*, remarking that Pasteur's official texts are very different from Pasteur's declarations to the *Figaro*: "*But it does not seem possible that the Figaro announced a cure for human rabies, or rather the neutralisation of the rabies virus thanks to M. Pasteur's method, without the latter's autorisation.*"[114] Clearly, this possibility intrigues (shocks?) the journalist. However, in the account (specified as a stenograph) of the same speech (made at the May 15, 1884 banquet) and published in the paper *Génie civil* on June 28, 1884, Pasteur is reported to have said: "*This being so, could we not render the dog refractory to rabies before he contracts the fatal disease from a bite!... If so, why not do the same in humans, that is, try to render human beings refractory to rabies after being bitten!*"[115]

Soon after, the May 29, 1884 issue of the *New York Magazine Life* quotes Pasteur's declarations: "*Mr. Louis Pasteur, the celebrated savant, claims to have discovered an antidote for hydrophobia by inoculating the patient with the virus of a rabid animal. His experience is thus described by himself: 'My method is as follows: I took the virus direct from the brain of a dog that died from acute hydrophobia. With this virus, I inoculated a monkey. The monkey died...'*"[116].

Pasteur was always reserved in his official writings. For instance, in the same presentation, no mention is made of the call for candidates to be treated against rabies. The end of the official text of his discourse, published in *Génie civil*, shows great reserve: "*Since I am not a physician, I appeal to a physician to be kind enough to help me, so that I do not practice illegal medicine; I repeat that I will not conduct these experiments until I have carried out the same tests many times on animals, on dogs, monkeys and especially on bovines, who seem to contract rabies much more easily than humans or dogs after a bite.*"[117]

In the same way, when he spoke before the Academy of Medicine, with Chamberland and Roux, on May 19, 1884, he only described experiments on dogs. In his correspondence, several letters discuss his great apprehension at the prospect of inoculating a human being with his attenuated rabies virus. On August 10, 1884, at the International Conference of Medical Sciences in Copenhagen, he exclaimed: "*But the experiments authorized on animals are criminal when they are carried out on men.*"[118] In its August 23, 1884 issue, *La Nature* reports that M. Pasteur has began the experiments aimed at establishing if an anti-rabies vaccination can counteract the effect of a dog bite. This

113. XXX, 1884, p. 1.
114. Editeur, 1884, p. 161.
115. Pasteur, O.C., t. VII, p. 370.
116. Anonymous, 1884, p. 296.
117. Pasteur, O.C., t. VII, p. 371.
118. Pasteur, O.C., t. VI, p. 591.

work was being observed by the Commission. For the moment, Pasteur was experimenting on dogs: dog owners brought dogs to board with him and be vaccinated. Results did not always live up to expectations. On July 24, 1884: "*Vaccinations of bitten dogs. Rabies. July 24* M. *Béranger, gamekeeper for* M. *Janin* (?) *in Combes la Ville (Seine et Marne) brought to the laboratory a Griffon hunting dog (value 300 francs) he believes was bitten by a rabid dog... The Béranger dog was returned to his owner well vaccinated on January 10, 1885 [;] 6 inoculations the last on November 28 p. 115 back.*"[119] Pasteur writes in a subsequent note: "... *He died of rabies at his owner's residence.*"[120] This raises questions about the treatment proposed by Pasteur in May 1884 for "*those who are bitten*"; but it is true that this dog was treated late, over a month following the bite. Incidentally, both Pasteur and M. Béranger were committing an infraction by disregarding the ministerial ordinance of August 20, 1882[121], stipulating that any cat or dog suspected of having rabies must be put to death.

Next, Pasteur tried to find "guinea pigs" outside of France, as his famous letter of September 22, 1884 to the Emperor of Brazil, Pedro II, testifies: "... *I think that my hand will shake when I will have to go on to man. It is here that the initiative of a high and powerful head of State could intervene very usefully for the greatest benefit of humankind. If I was king or Emperor or even President of a Republic, this is how I would exercise the right to grant pardon to those sentenced to death. On the eve of the execution, I would propose to the solicitor of the condemned man a choice between imminent death and an experiment consisting of inoculations to prevent rabies. If he agreed to these experiments, the life of the condemned man would be spared.*"[122] Pasteur did not propose test injections, only preventive inoculations. But in the case of Joseph Meister, his treatment protocol made no absolute distinction between them, as Pasteur himself admits. The Emperor very politely refused this proposition, pointing out that in his kingdom, Brazil, capital punishment had been abolished. Evidently, Pasteur did not speak in the same terms in all circumstances. As a member of the Academies, he was extremely cautious, but at the same time he tried to recruit candidates for inoculation in order to validate his experiments. It is hard to know what to think of his assertions, since he also refused to experiment on volunteers who came to him, when they were not likely to contract rabies following bites by suspicious animals. "*Already, on several occasions, persons asking to receive preventive inoculations came to me... But as I said earlier... I will give in to the temptation to try this prophylaxis, but only when I will be certain of being able to prevent the disease in dogs.*"[123] Pasteur wrote to Mrs Astié de Valsayre "*who, for the love of science, offered to subject herself like a mere poodle to the experiments of the savant* Mr. *Pasteur: 'It would be very dangerous, Madame, to try the experiment to which you have the courage to expose yourself.' Mrs Astié de Valsayre insisted.*"[124] Pasteur was unwilling to undertake this type of endeavour. The danger to which he accepted to expose his first inoculated subjects had to be compensated, either by avoidance of a death sentence or by the elimination of the risk of rabies after a suspicious bite. Pasteur's position was not rigid or definite. In a letter to his son Jean-Baptiste, dated March 31, 1885, he wrote: "*In fact, I continue my research,*

119. NAF 18018, f.P. 116.
120. NAF 18019, f.P. 0.
121. Conte, 1895, p. 286.
122. Pasteur, Cor., t. 3, p. 438.
123. Pasteur, O.C., t. VII, p. 370.
124. Anonyme, 1884b, p. 374.

trying to advance, to discover new principles and to fortify myself by habit and conviction in order to dare to try preventive inoculations on human beings who have been bitten."[125] These writings are ambiguous; they cannot at all be said to be proof that Pasteur has the confidence to prevent rabies in a person during the incubation period of the disease. But one thing is certain: he is eager to advance.

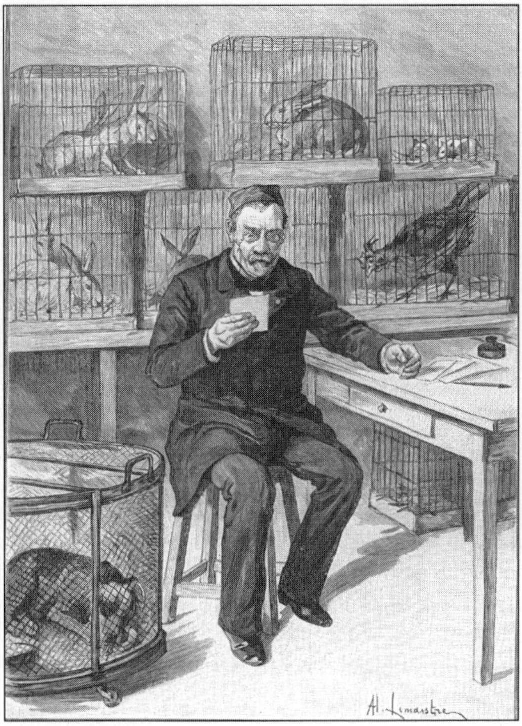

Figure 6. Pasteur in his laboratory. Publicity poster for the book "*L'Institut de France et nos grands établissements scientifiques*", by Alexis Lemaistre, published in 1896. Illustrated volume containing 82 engravings based on the author's drawings. Pasteur is reading, his left hand resting on the table, surrounded by chickens, guinea pigs, rabbits and a dog...

The Ministerial Rabies Commission

At this stage, the Pasteurians had developed a method of immunisation that was successful in a certain percentage of inoculated dogs, even after exposure to the virus of street rabies. Pasteur submitted a request to the Ministry of Public Instruction for the creation of a Control Commission. The Commission was composed of Mr. Béclard, dean of the School of Medicine; Mr. Paul Bert, professor at the Faculty of Sciences; Mr. Bouley, professor at the Museum of Natural History; Mr. Tisserand, Director at the Ministry of Agriculture and State Advisor; Mr. Villemin, professor at the School of Medicine and Military Pharmacy; and Mr. Vulpian, professor at the School of Medicine. This Rabies Commission, very favourable to Pasteur's work, was created on May 28, 1884; it chose Bouley as President and Villemin as secretary. The Commission's mission was to verify Pasteur's results and "*implement rabies prophylaxis in bitten dogs, by inducing, during the incubation period, an immunity that can prevent the virus of the bite from causing rabies*"[126]. The Commission went to Pasteur's laboratory without delay to

125. Pasteur, Cor., t. 4, p. 14.
126. Bouley *in* Pasteur, O.C., t. VI, pp. 753-758.

start its work, and supervised experiments comprising twelve sessions, within one month. On August 6, 1884, it sent a long letter signed by Bouley to the Minister of Public Instruction and Fine Arts, in which it declared: "... *We are happy, Mister Minister, to testify before you today that* Mr. *Pasteur has made no assertions that are not absolutely true. Yes, he has been able to use science to solve the problem of rendering dogs refractory to rabies by a preventive inoculation with the attenuated virus of this disease... But more experiments must be conducted, particularly for the purpose of establishing the duration of the immunity conferred to dogs by the preventive inoculation and above all to solve this other problem, so important for the prevention of human rabies: the question of whether after a bite the preventive action of the inoculation with attenuated virus can effectively counteract that of the virus inoculated by the bite...*"[127]. The report included with the letter provided details about the Commission's observations: "*Up until this time, the Commission has observed experiments of various types, involving 42 dogs, 23 of which were described by Mr. Pasteur as refractory to rabies and 19 acting as controls who did not receive any preventive or vaccinal inoculation... After being bitten by rabid dogs, 3 out of 6 cases of rabies occurred among the nineteen control dogs. Six cases of rabies out of eight after intravenous inoculations. Finally 5 cases of rabies out of 5 after inoculation by trepanation. By contrast, among the 23 vaccinated dogs there was not a single case of rabies...*"[128]. This was followed by a cautionary comment about one of the refractory dogs who died "*after diarrhoea with black excretions*", and from whose brain samples were extracted and inoculated to three guinea pigs and a rabbit, who were then closely watched. This report was published in the August 8, 1884 issue of the *Journal officiel.*

• **August 31, 1884.** Pasteur keeps exact count: "*In summary, on this August 31* [1884], *22 refractory housed by Frégis 12 refractory at Bourrel's total 34 refractory, and over 20 are in preparation at Vauquelin. This makes about 60 refractory dogs that I possess, of which only 22 aside from the 23rd who died on July 13 (not of rabies) have been tested by the Commission...*"[129]. The dogs have indeed been immunised, but the method used is still random. On February 2, 1885, Pasteur counts once more the refractory dogs housed by Frégis and Bourrel, and in Villeneuve-l'Etang[130].

"*Rabies 11th session of the Commission - April 17, 1885 Our presence (no one came.)* (sic)... *May 23, 1885 12th session of the Commission Presence of Mr. Béclard, Mr. Villemin.*"[131]

The sessions of the Rabies Commission take place regularly. The refractory dogs remain refractory. "*In 1887, Mr. Villemin recounted that it* (the Commission) *had continued its work in 1885; in March it had failed to transmit rabies to six dogs who had been found refractory the year before, while three dogs in the control group became rabid; that it had administered the Pasteur treatment* (virus adapted to monkeys) *to two dogs bitten one day before, to three other dogs bitten five days before and one bitten two days before, and that it had saved all of them, except one among the three that had been treated starting on the third day.*"[132] The Commission studied the duration of the immunity conferred to the dogs, and started the study of rabies treatment following a bite. These six dogs seem to be the only ones treated after being bitten, at the time of the treatment administered to Joseph Meister. Five dogs

127. Anonyme, 1884d, p. 258.
128. Pasteur, O.C., t. VI, p. 757.
129. NAF 18018, f.P. 118 back.
130. NAF 18019, f.P. 13.
131. NAF 18019, f.P. 57.
132. Galtier, 1892, t. 2, p. 149.

survived - a ratio equal to the normal ratio of animals saved when vaccinated, after exposure, with present-day vaccines. However, Pasteur's treatment, consisting of vaccination plus test(s), was very different from modern vaccination.

The Pasteurians Study Rabid-Animal Nervous Tissue Virulence Preservation

The Pasteurians possessed samples taken from dogs, rabbits and guinea pigs killed by rabies. They let them age in sterile containers, tubes with two points and double-headed flasks, in carbonic acid, or ordinary or dried air, at room temperature in the laboratory (in the scale room), or in the incubator (between 37° C and 40° C). Metchnikoff, a close associate of Pasteur's (but not an eye witness to his work on rabies) explains the dried-out condition of these tissues "*In the laboratory, they had set aside a whole stock of jars containing rabbit spinal cord in which they had tried in vain to cultivate the rabies virus, and these spinal cords had dried out over time; Pasteur asked his assistant Eug. Viala to determine their degree of virulence, hoping to find a preventive substance, an 'antirabies vaccine'.*"[133] Among his ideas for experiments, Pasteur listed, on June 28, 1882 and again in October of the same year, thirty-six suggestions including "*XIV: It is possible that rabic matter loses its virulence very quickly when exposed to air and that this explains why there is no culture in a flask, nor under vacuum because a vacuum is always imperfect and above all because culture must be slow, even at 38°...*"[134].

It is at this time that Pasteur conceived the possibility of a culture *in vitro* of rabies virus from spinal cord. In fact, on February 25, 1884, he wrote: "*We have made many attempts at developing the rabies virus, either in cephalospinal fluid, or in other substances, and even in spinal cord extracted, in a pure state, from sacrificed healthy animals. To date, we have not succeeded.*"[135] And again on August 10, 1884: "*It seems however, Gentlemen, that this Communication is lacking an important element: I do not speak of the rabies microbe. We do not have it. The process needed to isolate it is still imperfect and the difficulties of its culture outside the bodies of animals have not been dispelled, even by the use of fresh nervous matter as a culture medium.*"[136]

• **Key date: January 27, 1883.** Pasteur places spinal cord from a rabid dog in sterile glass tubes, hermetically sealed. They are stored at a temperature between 30° C and 35° C, or between 39° C and 40° C. The virulence of this spinal cord inoculated to rabbits is lost in twenty days. But Pasteur realizes that the samples of spinal cord were not tested to ascertain that they were rabic before the experiment... The work will have to start over, he notes[137]. He has started his series of passages of rabies virus to rabbits; the third passage is in progress[138].

• **November 27, 1883.** On loose-leaf pages, Roux clarifies his ideas. He takes notes based on Pasteur's notebooks: "*Series of tubes stored - Summary of November 27, 1883 results... in sealed tubes, at 33° the rabic matter preserved its virulence for 18 days... In these experiments, despite compounding, the virulent matter seems irregularly distributed in the tubes... The tubes are kept either in an incubator at 33°, or in the scale room - results*

133. Metchnikoff, 1939, p. 62.
134. NAF 18017, f.P. 49 & 50.
135. Pasteur, O.C., tome VI, p. 579.
136. Pasteur, O.C., tome VI, p. 590.
137. NAF 18017, f.P. 100.
138. NAF 18017, f.P. 81.

hard to reproduce... Rabies virus in salivary glands." Roux also notes that very small quantities of virus do not transmit rabies but do not confer protection either. He also remarks that the virulence of rabbit *medulla oblongata* stored at - 35° C to - 45° C for ten hours, or at between - 40° C and - 50° C for eight and a half hours is not attenuated[139].

Between the end of 1883 and the beginning of 1885, Pasteur conducted numerous experiments which included the passage of rabies virus to monkeys.

• **Key date: January 13, 1885.** On page 3 of his register 13[140] and then again on page 10[141], Pasteur draws a double-headed flask like the one depicted by Edelfeld in his famous painting where Pasteur is seen contemplating spinal cord in the process of drying out. Pieces of potash are represented in both cases, and potash is mentioned in the caption of the second drawing. Pasteur describes how he placed 10-centimeter cylinders of spinal cord from a dog killed by rabies in this new dried-air conservation system (usually called, in his notes, dry flask as opposed to humid flasks or tubes without potash). Rabbits subjected to trepanation and contaminated with this dog spinal cord dried for sixteen days died of rabies in eight days. After the experiment, Pasteur noted: "*NB On this May 5, 1885, in the course of the procedures above, I was very surprised to read that very virulent spinal cord was stored for sixteen days in a dry flask, preserving its full virulence. But this clearly observed and indisputable fact must be admitted* (*note* [in different ink] *This must be due to the low January temperature*)." These notes written by Pasteur differ from Loir's account, that links the first use of double-headed flasks with the time when Pasteur started his experiments with rabbit spinal cord, and the anti-rabies immunisation of dogs with the protocol that would be applied to Joseph Meister. The page has been reproduced[142].

• **February 4, 1885.** On January 26, 1885, a rabbit was inoculated with *medulla oblongata* from a female monkey killed by rabies; the rabbit was found dead on February 4. "*A cylinder of its cord is conserved to be dried in 2-headed flask.*"[143]

• **February 7, 1885.** "*The second guinea pig is dead. Its spinal cord is conserved as well as some spinal cord. This is 16-17 day guinea pig spinal cord.*" This guinea pig had been inoculated with rabic virus from a bear, previously passed to a rabbit. The storage mode is not mentioned[144].

• **March 4, 1885.** "*Rabic spinal cord samples stored see previous p. 10 March 4 1° Two new rabbits are subjected to trepanation and inoculated with rabbit spinal cord sample conserved since February 4 at page 2. This has already been recorded in the margin at p. 2. After 28 days of dry-flask storage. 2° Two new rabbits are given by trepanation a spinal cord sample conserved since February 7 at p. 138 of 12th notebook - guinea pig spinal cord (16-17 day guinea pig) After 25 days in dry flask...*". One of the rabbits died shortly of diarrhea, the other three died after long incubation periods[145a]. On April 25 Pasteur revised these results in a *Nota Bene* (*see below*). Thus, at the start of 1885, Pasteur was using several double-headed flasks, at least one of which contained rabbit *spinal cord* on February 4, 1885. Loir's recollections differ.

139. NAF 18094, items 268 to 354.
140. NAF 18019, f.P. 3.
141. NAF 18019, f.P. 10.
142. Hannoun, 1995, p. 156.
143. NAF 18019, f.P. 2.
144. NAF 18018, f.P. 138.
145a. NAF 18019, f.P. 27.

• **April 9, 1885.** Pasteur studies the virulence of spinal cord from rabbits killed by rabies. He has the spinal cord of a rabbit used in the 73rd passage cut into three segments called "superior", "middle" and "extremity", and has them placed in dry flasks.

On April 25, the two rabbits inoculated by trepanation (spinal cord conserved from the 9th to the 14th, for five days) on April 14 are in good health, and on the 26th: "*The two rabbits trepanned on the 14th show some signs* (of rabies). *Therefore the spinal cord used on the 14th was still active. It is the 12th day for a 73rd - passage spinal cord at 7 days. This could be due to attenuation or small quantity. We will see.*"[145b] In a note in the margin: "*Very important if there is truly attenuation.*"[145c] On the back of the page: "*Note of April 30. One of the rabbits of April 14 with spinal cord* (one word) *from April 9 died at 2 o'clock. Its spinal cord was given by trepanation to 2 new rabbits, to see if the 12 days of inoculation in this rabbit of April 14 are due to virus attenuation achieved by five days of dried-air attenuation in dry conditions, or due to small quantity. If the cause is attenuation the result has great importance. Because it would be a mode of artificial attenuation produced by air, by air alone, due to virulence preservation in CO2... the 2 rabbits trepanned on April 30 with April 14th rabbit spinal cord, from rabbit who died on the 30th, are in good health. This is the 8th day. The spinal cord used in their trepanation on the 30th apparently did not have 7-day virulence. We will see if this lasts, in which case, the 12-day incubation period in the April 14 rabbits cannot be attributed to small quantity but to true attenuation by air acting on dessicated spinal cord. No this period is not prolonged... In the rabbits at 12 days at p. 52 by stored spinal cord there was no true attenuation. It must have been a matter of small quantity.*"[146] Pasteur is a man of stature. He has a seat at the "*Académie française*". His laboratory notes record his reflections solely for himself and his assistants. The text above has clearly been written at different times. Pasteur was reaching his objective. Five days of drying out were not sufficient. But the question of attenuation *versus* small quantity remained pending.

• **April 14, 1885.** On April 13, Nocard brought Pasteur dogs bitten by a rabid dog: "*1rst inoculation, April 14. These 4 dogs are inoculated subc. with 1 syr. dog spinal cord (street rabies) from dog found dead this morning p. 20 marrow from this dog stored. 2nd inoculation April 15, subc. Inoculation with one syr. spinal cord stored yesterday from dog p. 20, to these 4 dogs...*"[147]. These dogs received eight nervous tissue inoculations from dogs killed by street rabies. Three dogs died of rabies. One was still alive on June 4. He was soon put to death with an injection of strychnine. There is a constant shortage of space in the kennels for experimental dogs. As Geison rightly points out[148], the (apparently?) immunised dogs do not take up much room in Pasteur's notebooks. After the classic incubation period, most of them are subjected to euthanasia. This method of making room in the kennels for animals needed for new experiments can be seen as overly expeditive. But the number of cages is limited. Many of them are occupied by dogs in the Rabies Commission experiments, and are therefore untouchable. Pasteur uses the remaining cages, which have to be freed at the end of each experiment for the next experiment to be conducted.

145b. NAF 18019, f.P. 52.
145c. NAF 18019, f.P. 52.
146. NAF 18019, f.P. 52, back.
147. NAF 18019, f.P. 55.
148. Geison, 1995, p. 243.

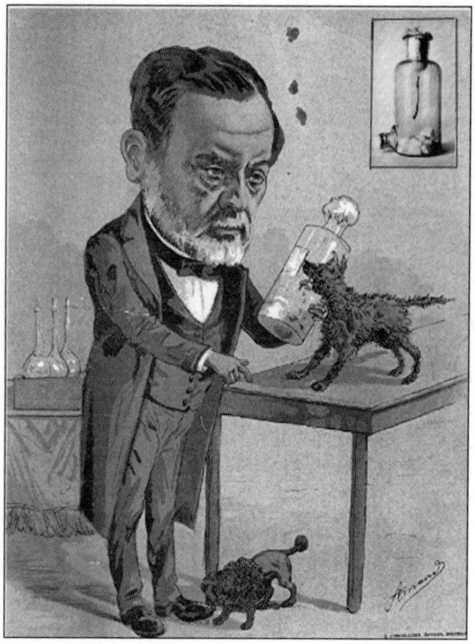

Figure 7. "*Pasteur*", caricature by Amani, E. Lyon-Claesen, editor, Brussels. Pasteur, serious as usual, holds a flask in his left hand, more or less identical to those used to dry out rabbit spinal cord (*see insert at right of Figure*); he seems to be pointing out with a finger, as an example to a wild-looking, threatening dog, a poodle shaven to resemble a lion, very proper, who is tamely licking his shoe. Illustration representing Pasteur and his work on rabies. (Author's document.)

• **April 14, 1885.** And what about the dogs immunised after being bitten? Have they acquired protection or not? On April 14[149] Pasteur accepted from Mr. Rouilly "*a privately owned dog*" that had been bitten by a rabid stray dog. This dog was given more or less the same treatment as the April 13 dog. He was returned to his owner with the assurance that he was immunised and out of danger, but he died in Bourrel's shelter on July 25, 1885.

• **April 20, 1885.** Pasteur still does not have a reliable method of immunisation against rabies. He tries "*to reinforce the refractory state of these rabbits*" by inoculating them for eight days with one injection a day of inactive spinal cord emulsion: "*April 20. Since several rabbits who received stored spinal cord by trepanation showed no signs, I asked myself if the inferior portion of these cord samples might have vaccinated them. I placed the 2 rabbits trepanned on April 1 p. 46... in the same cage... and this is what I did first, to try to reinforce a refractory state in these rabbits if it is not already present as it was in the rabbit on the back of p. 10 April 21. Each day starting on April 21, the next inactive segments from the ends of cord samples stored in dry flasks are cut off. They are all placed in the same heat-resistant glass container and are dissolved in broth, and each of the above rabbits is inoculated with one subc. syr. of this liquid, hoping to inoculate the soluble and perhaps vaccinating portion of these spinal cords, which would reinforce their refractory state if present or would induce it if they do not yet have it - This will be verified by subsequent inoculation at trepanation of all the rabbits with street rabies virus.*" Pasteur concluded (later): "*No vaccination wsover took place.*"[150]

Key date: April 25, 1885. Pasteur imagines a new procedure for the attenuation of rabic virus: March 4 experiment continued: "*NB The rabbits are now at 23 days incubation with dry guinea pig spinal cord at 16/17 days. This seems to be proof of virus attenuation by dessication, as previously at p. 41 in the margin. However we did not verify now*

149. NAF 18019, f.P. 56.
150. NAF 18019, f.P. 58 & back.

or at that time whether it was not a question of small quantity. But it is unlikely that it was a matter of small quantity ***and these results are perhaps indicating a procedure for rabic virus attenuation, without passages to monkeys or any other animals. Very important to do (written April 25, 1885).***"[151] Pasteur is alerted to the possibility of a new procedure for rabic virus attenuation...

• **May 4, 1885.** Another day, another experiment. "*Trial vaccination of 6 new dogs see previous p. 41, 44, etc. May 4, 1885 with medulla oblongata from dog who died this morning p55 (dog with owner killed by stray-dog rabies): 1rst inoc May 4 subc. inoculation one syr. to 6 new dogs from the Pound and storage in dry flasks of section of superior cord for the following days. 2nd inoc. May 5 inoculation part of stored section of this cord - one syr. subc. to the 6 dogs...*" between May 7 and 13 the dogs received the same treatment. "*The experiment is stopped after 10 inoculations.*" May 22: One of the May 4 dogs is paralysed, the other five are in good health. "*June 4 - the five remaining dogs are well. It is the 31rst day since May 4 and the 22nd day since May 31. Obviously these five dogs are refractory. Because the cages are needed, these dogs are sacrificed with strychnine.*"[152] This immunisation protocol is an "inversed Meister" protocol, since the animal is contaminated first, then vaccinated with more and more attenuated virus. Geison explains that in this experiment and in other similar protocols Pasteur began inoculating in the most infected tissues and went on to the least infected, which is the opposite of the method used in his previous experiments on chicken cholera, anthrax or swine erysipelas vaccines. Geison attributes this change to Pasteur's new conception of immunity[153]. He could be right, but it is also possible that there was simply a shortage of *medulla oblongata* from animals killed by rabies. The same *spinal cord* is used throughout the experiment because it is the only one the laboratory has. Thus, these tissues stored in dry flasks are one day, two-day, three-day old, etc. Pasteur always remembered to test the virulence of his rabies virus used in passages to rabbits. Perhaps he was already thinking that it would be useful to always have supplies of virus from different passages, to serve as vaccine with more or less attenuated virus. It is hard to know... Often, Pasteur specified the objectives of his experiments. But not in the case of these experiments; he was probably proceeding by trial and error.

The same day, May 5, 1885, a man suffering of rabies, by the name of Girard, arrived at Necker Hospital. He was placed on Dr. Rigal's ward. Pasteur was called; he went to Necker with Roux and Loir. On December 11, 1882, Pasteur wrote, concerning rabies in dogs: "*We have seen cases of spontaneous recovery from rabies only after the first rabies symptoms appeared, never after the appearance of acute symptoms.*"[154] He made his treatment recommendation with the approval of the medical staff. "*An inoculation is given under* (?) *ribs on the right under the skin a full Pravaz syringe* (1 centicube) *of diluted spinal cord from the morning p. 52 of April 14 p. 52.*"[155] Everything was prepared for a second, identical inoculation to be given the same evening... but the Social services ('*Assistance publique*', the Paris hospitals administration) were alerted and prevented the procedure... These nervous tissues inoculated came from a rabbit in the 73rd passage, paralysed by rabies in eight days, and whose spinal cord was stored in dried air for five days. New rabbits, inoculated with the same spinal cord, were paralysed in twelve days.

151. NAF 18019, f.P. 27.
152. NAF 18019, f.P. 63.
153. Geison, 1995, p. 245.
154. Pasteur, O.C., t. VI, p. 575.
155. NAF 18019, f.P. 62.

Pasteur concluded that there had either been attenuation or a "*matter of small quantities of virus...*" A few days later Girard felt better and soon left the hospital. Rigal believes that he had not been infected with rabies. Dujardin-Beaumetz still thinks he did have rabies (according to the hospital file), but he is close to the Pasteur team... On May 25, 1885 Pasteur wrote: "*We must wait to see if Girard will continue to be well. If he develops rabies, it could be due to the bite or to the inoculation. We would ascertain this by studying virulence after his death. I believe, on the contrary, that the inoculation could have cured him of the rabies he had already developed. This is the opinion of Dr. Duj. B. as well as Dr. Rigal, with whom I have, however, not spoken these past few days, since he returned to his original idea that Girard arrived at Necker sick with rabies.*"[156] Pasteur is saying that his treatment (one injection) could have cured a patient with rabies. He is clearly very optimistic... since none of his experiments on animals authorizes him to hope for such a result. The outcome remains unknown because the trace of the patient is lost. It is not likely that he died of rabies, since this information would (most probably) have been made public. The terrible death of most rabies sufferers did not go unnoticed. But nothing is certain.

A New Immunisation Method: Spinal Cord from Rabbit Stored in Dry Flask

• **Critical key date: May 16, 1885. Pasteur begins** (a new experiment, not entered in his laboratory notes until May 28) ***daily or almost daily storage, in "dry flask", of spinal cord from rabbits killed by rabies...*** for a future experiment[157]. He does not explain the reason for this new protocol. It is probably the application of his April 25 idea and the continuation of his storage in dry flask experiment of January 13, 1885. This new technique was to bring success. But rabbits killed by rabies were needed almost every day. The task was sizeable and imposed heavy constraints. The dedication of Pasteur's team was a key factor in achieving success...

• **Critical key date: May 28, 1885.** Major disruption: the first "Meister-type" protocol is carried out on ten dogs, vaccinated with more and more virulent spinal cord. The writing is big, very easy to read. Pasteur is meticulous. He clearly believes he has solved the problem. He is surprisingly sure of himself: "*Different method of vaccination. Since May 16 (1885), we have been able to collect each day, from rabbits subjected to numerous passages and therefore maximum virulence: on 7th day, superior cord segments that were stored in dry flasks with potash fragments. Once this was done, after 10 dogs from the Pound were assembled at the Frégis kennel, each one was inoculated subs. with one Pravaz syr. 1rst inoculation May 28 with May 18 cord that is, after 11 days of storage... 13th inoculation June 9 with June 8 spinal cord one-day old. The experiment was stopped after these 13 inoculations...*"[158].

"***... June 18,*** *2nd rabbit trepanned May 28 after 17 days, is dead. Using its medulla oblongata 2 new rabbits are trepanned. It will be very useful to know if there will be an incubation period of 7 days or longer, in which case, there would be attenuation by air... Here the proof is certain, absolute, the 17-day incubation period of the inoculator* (sic) *rabbit of May 28 who died June 18 was due to small quantity. Therefore air does not attenuate during dry-flask storage. It gradually destroys virulence, but the virulence still present is full virulence. Why*

156. NAF 18019, f.P. 62.
157. NAF 18019, f.P. 73.
158. NAF 18019, f.P. 73.

then is the method of refractory state production at pages 72, 74 successful... There must be vaccinal matter that is still active in the stored spinal cord samples and even in the one with the smallest quantity of virulent matter still present and even in the inactive one."[159]

The spinal cord samples had been stored 12, 11, 10, 9, 8, 7, 6, 5, 4, 3, 2, and 1 days. "*June 4... the 10 dogs are taken to Vauquelin* (former Rollin College), *for fear that they catch rabies and have an accident, from the Frégis kennel, where the keeper and his wife are terrified of rabid dogs.*"[160] Pasteur thinks of everything, even the smallest details. But transporting ten dogs from Montmartre to the Latin Quarter, after only six day of the experiment, seems like a task that could have been avoided. Perhaps there was a shortage of cages at Rollin.

• **June 3, 1885.** The first experiment was not yet completed; Pasteur began a second without waiting for the results of the first. "2nd *trial of the method at page 73 June 3 at Bourrel's shelter 10 new dogs from the Pound were assembled, I sent Eugène... 1rst inoculation... 14-day spinal cord*" then *spinal cord* stored 13,12,11,10,9,8,7,6,5,4,3,2,1,0 days, from rabbits of the 77th, 78th and 79th passages. Eugène conducted the experiment alone. He had the master's total trust. On June 23rd the dogs were in good health[161].

• **June 5, 1885.** "*One of the rabbits trepanned May 28* (1rst series) *with spinal cord from the 16th (12 days of storage) shows some signs, it is the 11th day of incubation. NB Perhaps the spinal cord used was not sufficiently dessicated. Instead of the May 16th spinal cord, perhaps on May 28 we should have started with spinal cord from May 14 for instance. But nothing is lost because none of the 10 dogs is infected! Moreover, it is likely that the May 28 spinal cord was attenuated or contained a very small quantity of virus since on the one hand the rabbit infected on the 28 is the only one and its companion is healthy and the contamination (at eleven days) instead of 7 incubation days which was the spinal cord virulence at the start of storage.*"[162] Pasteur has found a method of vaccination, but he is not yet sure of it. He is still hesitant about the number of dessication days for the marrow samples used in his treatment.

• **June 12, 1885.** Pasteur expresses his convictions clearly. On June 12, 1885, in a letter to Mr. Quintard, mayor of Levier, a village in the French Jura, he writes: "*... I have not yet tried to induce the state refractory to rabies in human subjects, as I do easily in dogs, even after they have been bitten; I shall soon dare to do it in men but the present stage of my research does not yet allow me to treat human beings... Death is inevitable as soon as the first symptoms appear, usually after six weeks, two months. Therefore there is no reason to hesitate, although I know that at this time it is already too late to intervene.*"[163] Pasteur is very confident about his results, after contamination in six dogs. He is basing his conclusions solely on his "virus passage to monkeys" experiments conducted before contamination. Pasteur writes in the future tense and speaks of compassionate treatment. And yet he inoculated Girard with virulent spinal cord more than a month earlier! But he believed Girard to have the clinical signs of rabies.

A former intern on Dr. Dupuy's ward at the Saint-Denis Hospital, Dr. Mourret, recounted (in 1895, on the occasion of Pasteur's death) the admission of an 11-year

159. NAF 18019, f.P. 73 & back.
160. NAF 18019, f.P. 73.
161. NAF 18019, f.P. 74.
162. NAF 18019, f.P. 73.
163. Pasteur, Cor., t. 4, p. 21.

old girl, Julie-Antoinette Poughon, on June 22, 1885. She presented the characteristic symptoms of rabies, after being bitten by a rabid dog. Since Pasteur's work on rabies had been widely publicised, Pasteur was informed of the case by Dr. Grancher. He arrived very quickly, with Dr. Leroy des Barres and several city physicians. "*The physicians present did not hesitate to confirm the symptomatic rabies diagnosis and, since there had never been any true cases of cure after the onset of rabies, Pasteur attempted treatment as a humanitarian gesture.*"[164] The child died the next morning, in Pasteur's presence, after having received two injections of the first preparation, a seven-day old spinal cord. Pasteur was very moved, but when he was no longer in the presence of the girl's body and of her mother, he made pleasantries - probably a means of emotional relief. "*He* (Pasteur) *described his work on rabies, the results obtained with dogs and the immunity conferred to them by vaccines (1884 experiment) - But the dogs were immunised before, while human beings had to be immunised after the bite, with the probability of a cure inversely proportional to the time elapsed since the bite... The case quoted above was a desperate attempt, since it was too late to counteract the damage. Pasteur had already inoculated another subject: a man who had begged to be inoculated, but who had not been infected with rabies and who got well. It was Pasteur himself who recounted this incident.*"[165] Pasteur did not reveal these attempts officially, but he did not hide them - at least not the first, of which he spoke freely. He did not consider them failures, but unsuccessful attempts.

• **June 25, 1885.** Third experiment between June 25 and July 9 with 13,12,11,9,8,7,6,5,4,3,2,1,0-day spinal cord. Once again, it is Eugène who inoculates. On July 11, the dogs are in good health[166]. Pasteur feels that success is imminent. He is sure of himself, and he is right... He skips stages.

• **June 27, 1885.** Pasteur continues his major experiments. He has assembled "*10 new dogs at Rollin*", and he sends Eugène to inject them with 13,12,11,10,9,8,7,6,5,4,3,2,1,0-days spinal cord[167].

• **July 2, 1885.** The ten dogs of the first May 28 series are in good health. "*Today, trepanation of 2 of these 10 dogs and of 2 control dogs with spinal cord from the June 10 rabbit p. 76 who died July 2 (rabbit at 19 days) killed by rabic human spinal cord. Today we have no street rabies virus. July 16, one of the July 2 control dogs is infected, very rabid and biting, it is the 14th day... July 23 The second control is infected... But one of the 10 dogs, trepanned July 2... is also infected, very aggressive and biting... July 26, the 2nd of the ten, who appeared agitated, is well and eats well... August 8, he is in good health...*"[168]. This makes one refractory dog out of two when using the "Meister" method, but inoculation by trepanation is not natural and is very invasive.

A fifth experiment is planned in the register, and crossed out[169]. Pasteur probably considered it unnecessary. He went on from dogs to human beings. No use bothering with monkeys and bovines... as it was previously thought[170] to ensure the safety of the method, before going on to man![171]

164. Mourret, 1895, *in* Madeline, 1996, p. 160.
165. Mourret, 1895, *in* Madeline, 1996, p. 160.
166. NAF 18019, f.P. 75.
167. NAF 18019, f.P. 80.
168. NAF 18019, f.P. 73 back & 74.
169. NAF 18019, f.P. 81.
170. Pasteur, O.C., t. VII, p. 371.
171. Pasteur, O.C., t. VI, p. 587.

• **September 22, 1885.** "*Because we have to make room and because the experiment of this page 74 is completed* (1rst series), *I asked Eugene to go to Bourrel's kennel and sacrifice all the dogs p. 74, keeping only two.*"[172]

• **August 2, 1886**, the dog wearing collar 104, vaccinated by the "Meister" method between June 3 and June 18, 1885 (second series) was tested by inoculation of *medulla oblongata* tissue from rabid dog (street rabies) by trepanation. He died August 21, indicating that he lost his immunity in thirteen months[173].

Success: the Roses with their Thorns

But, unexpected competition came from the South...

• **July 4, 1885.** Since the Toussaint vaccine had been abandoned in France or diluted in many protocols published by many scientists, and given that the vaccine against symptomatic anthrax had little notoriety, Pasteur was the uncontested master in the field, when an unexpected competitor made his appearance. On July 4, 1885, the cover of the *Monde illustré* proclaimed: "*Spain. Anti-cholera vaccination, using Dr. Ferran's method, in the Murcie region (Drawing by Mr. Atalaya)*". When this issue of the weekly magazine came out, Ferran had already vaccinated 4,700 people against cholera, while Pasteur had vaccinated chickens, sheep, cows and pigs, but no human beings (except perhaps the "unknown vaccinated man" against anthrax). Pasteur knew about Ferran's vaccinations, since he had given the Brouardel Mission a letter dated June 26, 1885 to give to Ferran (*see below*). Pasteur was a winner... he did not like to see others enter the competition. On July 6, the arrival of little Joseph Meister, bitten by a dog in Alsace, a province lost by France after the Franco-Prussian war of 1870-1871, was heaven-sent, although the decision to treat him remained difficult.

Joseph Meister was treated, Pasteur left on summer holidays and Ferran's accomplishments were more and more widely publicised. He was on the cover of *L'Illustration* (highly illustrated French-language weekly of the period, with wide circulation for that time: 21,425 copies per week in 1885, distributed in many countries) of July 25, 1885, then on the cover of the August 2, 1885 *Journal Illustré*, whose caption read: "*Dr. Ferran, the Spanish vaccinator.*" The August 1, 1885 *L'Univers illustré* published a long, illustrated article on Ferran's vaccinations. On August 8, 1885, *La France illustrée* published the article "*Cholera in Spain: Dr. Ferran's vaccination*", with an attractive double-page illustration showing Ferran vaccinating. This was truly impressive: all the major French-language weekly magazines, all of them illustrated, were informing their readers of Dr. Ferran's exploits. The commentary was not always favourable, but the publicity created fervent interest in vaccinations. There were no doubt other articles in the daily papers. Pasteur was confronted with a real competitor. Cholera was the infectious disease on everyone's mind at that time. The last epidemic (1884) had broken out in Marseille and Toulon, and the story was carried on first page in the press. In Paris, in December 1884 and January 1885, the cholera caused between 600 and 800 deaths; the disease ravaged Spain, where there were 120,000 fatalities. Grancher had advised Pasteur that he was expected to produce a cholera vaccine, but the Pasteurians did not have such a vaccine at the time... The story of Ferran's "artificial vaccine", the first to be used in large human populations, will be recounted in a subsequent chapter (*see chapter on Cholera*).

172. NAF 18019, f.P. 74.
173. NAF 18020, f.P. 7.

The First Complete Rabies Treatment: Joseph Meister, July 6, 1885

On July 6, 1885, Joseph Meister, a 9-year old boy, arrived to Pasteur's laboratory... René Vallery-Radot, Pasteur's son-in-law, recounts the events (and almost all authors reproduce his account): "*On a Monday morning, July 6, Pasteur received the visit of a little Alsacian boy, 9 years old, bitten two days earlier by a dog with rabies. The boy's mother was with him. She explained that her son was walking alone on a little side road to the Meissengott school, near Schlessadt, when a dog jumped on him. Lying on the ground, unable to defend himself, the child's only reaction was to cover his face with his hands. A mason, who had witnessed the scene from a distance, came running, carrying an iron bar. He hit the mad dog repeatedly and forced him to let go. He lifted the child, who was covered with blood and saliva. The dog went back to his master, Théodore Vone, grocer in Meissengott, and bit his arm. Théodore Vone took hold of his gun and killed the dog. When the animal was autopsied, straw, hay and fragments of wood were found in his stomach. When little Joseph Meister's parents learned all this they were extremely worried and went, the same evening, to Schlessadt, to consult Dr. Weber. After cauterising the wounds with carbolic acid, the doctor advised Mrs. Meister to leave early next morning for Paris. There she was to recount what happened to someone who was not a physician, but could judge, better than a physician, what was the best thing to do in such a serious case. As for Théodore Vone, worried both about the child and about himself, he insisted on making the trip. Pasteur reassured him. His clothes had shielded him from the dog's saliva, and the sleeve of his shirt had not even been pierced. He could take the first train back to Alsace. He did not wait to be told twice.*"[174]

André Dubail, Alsacian historian, wrote a beautiful account (1985) based on a long and detailed study conducted in Joseph Meister's family. His account differs from that of René Vallery-Radot in several ways. Joseph Meister was the eldest son of the baker of the Alsacian village of Steige, which had been under German rule since the end of the Franco-German War of 1870. He had been bitten two days earlier, on July 4 around 7 in the morning, by a dog that jumped on him while he was walking to the Meissengott brewery, near Schlestadt, to buy yeast, which his father needed for baking his cakes. A locksmith who was passing by saved the child from the "mad" dog. Little Joseph Meister knew this hunting dog. The animal returned home and immediately attacked his master, Théodore Vone, grocer in Meissengott. The child's wounds were washed abundantly with water by the Vones, who patched his clothing and sent someone to buy the yeast he needed. The child was also given one mark to buy candy. All this had taken place rather quickly, and the child had to walk back to his house, two kilometres away. "*My wounds hurt terribly and I had to sit down on the grassy bank on the side of the road almost every 10 meters...*"[175], said the poor little boy. Théodore Vone, worried about his own "bite", had locked the dog in his barn; when he learned that the dog had bitten other dogs, as well as cows and pigs, he was very disturbed. He started off with the guilty dog to go and see the Schlestadt veterinarian. It seems that on the way the suspicious behaviour of the muzzled dog attracted the attention of an agent of the Gendarmerie, who shot the dog on the spot. After all, the second paragraph of Article 10 of the July 21, 1881 law prescribed: "*Dogs and cats suspected of rabies must be killed immediately.*"[176] In this particular case, the interpretation of the law

174. Vallery-Radot, 1900, p. 600.
175. Meister *in* Dubail, 1985, p. 109.
176. Percheron, 1885, p. 132.

was no doubt correct. But the region was under German rule. What laws were enforced? How did Mr. Vone explain his dog's behaviour to the agent? Once the dog was dead, Vone carried the body the rest of the way, very worried about this turn of events. The veterinarian autopsied the dog and found straw, hay and fragments of wood in his stomach; at the time, this was considered a characteristic sign of rabies. The dog had been rabid, at least in the opinion of the medical expert.

In fact, an autopsy has never been sufficient to make a definite diagnosis of rabies. According to Pasteur, an inquest conducted by the local German authorities, at a time when they could not be suspected of showing indulgence to the French and to Pasteur, concluded that the dog had indeed been rabid, probably based on autopsy results and the circumstances surrounding the event. Perhaps bitten dogs had become, in turn, rabid. But there were only oral accounts. No written traces supporting the inquest results exist. However, an official inquest almost certainly took place, since Pasteur speaks of it in a letter dated November 27, 1885, addressed to little Joseph[177], and mentions it in a presentation to the Academy of Sciences[178]. It is unlikely that Pasteur invented such a story in support of his cause. Of course, this argument arrived too late to justify, on its own, Joseph Meister's treatment. It only served as an indication among others.

On the evening after the boy was bitten, his parents (who had no doubt learned the details of the death of the dog that had attacked their son) requested the assistance of the physician of Schlestadt, the nearest city, who cleaned the child's wounds with carbolic acid. This treatment was given late, in any case, twelve hours after the bite. But in the meantime, Théodore Vone, while waiting for the stagecoach to return home, recounted what happened to some people he encountered and who told him about Pasteur and his work on rabies. Back in Meissengott, perhaps feeling some remorse, he apparently went to the Meister's house to enquire about the boy's health. Faced with the threat of dying of rabies, that concerned not only Joseph, but to a lesser extent himself, Théodore Vone and the Meisters immediately decided to go to Paris to see Pasteur. The Meisters had, in fact, met and married in Paris. Thus, the city was not unknown to them. But at that time travelling from Meissengott to Paris was not easy: about 465 kilometres to cross, including the border between Alsace (German territory at that time) and France. This border was routinely crossed by residents in the area, and customs officers did not impose strict rules. The boy and his mother, as well as the grocer Vone, had to pack their bags quickly; the boy's father would stay home with the other children. They left at dawn the next morning, by charabanc, and arrived in Saint-Dié two hours later. From there, they took the train to Nancy, and then to Paris. In the capital, they apparently had trouble finding Mr. Pasteur, who was not seen favourably in every quarter. Many medical practitioners must have considered that referring a patient to Pasteur was to encourage to some extent the illegal practice of medicine. After all, Pasteur's laboratory was located at the *Ecole Normale Supérieure*, not in a medical setting. His reputation relative to infectious diseases concerned animal pathologies. In any case, on the morning of July 6 the Alsacian patients reached their destination[179].

The two versions of these events are not really contradictory, but why would René Vallery-Radot stray so far from the truth? André Dubail explains that Steige, little

177. Ducout, 1995, p. 315.
178. Pasteur, O.C., t. VI, p. 612.
179. Dubail, 1985.

Joseph Meister's village, was French-speaking; in Meissengott, on the other hand, German (Alsacian dialect) was spoken. Was the boy going to a school whose language he did not know, since he came from Paris? How could Pasteur know the details concerning Vone's shirt sleeve? From Vone? "M. *Vone had heavy bruising on his arms, but M. Pasteur assured him that the dog's teeth had not gone through the shirt. As there was nothing to fear…*"[180]. Pasteur must have examined Vone's arm rather than his shirt. The detail of the "side road" is strange as well, because the shortest distance between Steige and Meissengott is the main road, as anyone who has been there knows.

When Pasteur saw little Joseph Meister with fourteen bites on his legs and thighs, and the pitiful state he was in (he could hardly walk), he must have been very pained. In addition, the boy was an Alsacian, one of those whom the Francfort Treaty had wrested away from France; this must also have counted for Pasteur. He reassured Mr. Vone and sent him home, since his dog's teeth had only caused contusions. As to the boy and his mother, he had them settle in at the former Rollin College, near his laboratory, which provided them with an inexpensive shelter and allowed Pasteur to keep an eye on the wounded child before the Public Assistance or the Faculty could interfere. Loir recounts that he went with Pasteur to buy two iron beds and bedding. All this was taken to the annex on Vauquelin Street, which had many uses, including that of infirmary.

In the afternoon, Pasteur attended the weekly meeting of the Academy of Sciences, where he was sure to see Vulpian, a great Professor of medicine, expert on nervous diseases and member of the Commission entrusted with writing a report on Pasteur's experiments on rabies and on the treatment he applied to dogs. Vulpian would be able to advise him. In effect, Vulpian saw the wounded boy around eight that evening and, learning of the circumstances of the accident, the lapse of time since the bites were inflicted and the relatively late cauterisation with carbolic acid, he advised Pasteur to try his treatment. How did Vulpian know that cauterisation had been performed with carbolic acid? "Pure" carbolic acid is a very powerful caustic substance, not recommended for use in such cases. On the other hand, carbolic water has little effect if it is too diluted[181]. It is hard to assess the value of the treatment administered to the boy. His mother, who had been present when Dr. Weber treated the child, knew what had been done, but was not necessarily aware of this detail. In any case, the cauterisation was probably not carried out rigorously, given the great number of wounds and their location, and the child's age. At the time, Dr. Cartaz qualified this treatment as being "illusory"[182]; he might have possessed more detailed information. Correctly performed cauterisation left scabs that fell off between the 5th and 7th day[183]; but no one mentioned such scabs in reference to Joseph Meister. Most likely, cauterisation of little Joseph's fourteen wounds had been light and would not have saved him from rabies if he was contaminated. His one chance of survival was Pasteur's treatment by multiple injections of more and more virulent rabbit spinal cord, only tried on dogs with no previous contamination, and too recent to really be evaluated.

The 1936 *Almanach du Pélerin* provided some details whose veracity cannot be verified. First, Joseph Meister is said to be a shepherd, and the grocer who owns the dog is said

180. Pasteur, O.C., t. VI, p. 603.
181. Nocard, 1892, p. 250.
182. Cartaz, 1886, p. 213.
183. de la Vergne, 1808, p. 40.

to be called Théodore Volney! It's possible, but none of the evidence supports this. However, the article does say that Joseph knew the dog well, and that he received no help from the residents of Meissengott. Joseph's mother specifies that when they arrived in Paris, they first went to see her father, a policeman in the capital [Grancher speaks of an uncle[184]. Is it the same person?]. As to how Mrs. Meister obtained the address of Pasteur's laboratory, she and her father went from one pharmacy to another, until someone told them at last to enquire at the Cochin Hospital, not far from Ulm Street. There, they were given Mr. Pasteur's address. When they arrived to Ulm Street, Pasteur first had a meal served to his guests in the kitchen (*sic*), which is quite possible, since Pasteur was living in the main building of the *Ecole Normale Supérieure*, only a few meters from his laboratory. Joseph's mother begged Pasteur: "*Save him, implored the mother. Try! Insisted Vulpian.*"[185] This version generally agrees with Dubail's, but differs from that of René Vallery-Radot.

Pasteur's notes, at page 83 of the Register[186], specify that Vone "*had a shirt that was not pierced*", that the dog "*at autopsy had hay, straw and wood fragments in his stomach*", and then that "*I settled in the mother and the child at Vauquelin. She did not want to go to the hospital.*" Pasteur does not have spinal cord samples ready each day, but every second day. He solves the problem by inoculating little Joseph at 9 in the morning or at 6 in the evening. He crossed out in his laboratory notebooks all the figures indicating the drying out duration of the spinal cord samples, and replaced them with the figures seen today. He probably wanted to present a more rational impression of his treatment by using a more regular series of numbers from 15 to 1. He did not modify the dates or times of inoculations, or those indicating when the samples were taken; nevertheless, it is easy to see that he adjusted a little the figures related to duration in the first few days. What is surprising is that he changed all the dates, since *a priori* their exactness causes no ambiguity!

"*We stop after these 13 inoculations. On the evening of the 12th, the child had a convulsion, the day after the 6-day spinal cord, the day of 5-day* [6 and 5 have been retouched by Pasteur]. *Redness around the injection site started to appear on July 10 and on the following days. The first virulent spinal cord is that of the 11th, a 6-day spinal cord.*"[187]

Who Discovered the Rabies Vaccine: Pasteur or Roux?

It is important to go back to Loir's account: "*Attempts to develop rabies microbe remained unsuccessful, but we knew that the virus was located in nervous matter (spinal cord and brain). Pasteur's objective was to attenuate the hydrophobia virus: but in the meantime we were attempting to see how long this virus would survive in nervous matter. Each one of us was free to conduct the experiments he saw fit. Pasteur had had me place cord fragments in tubes through which I then passed a carbonic acid current...*". In short, Loir recounts what Pasteur had noticed by chance: "*When I turned around, I saw Pasteur standing before a 150-centimeter cube flask with double head, one at the bottom and one at the top, intended to establish a current of air inside the flask. Suspended in the flask by a thread, could be seen a fragment of rabbit cord. We were all conducting experiments on the conservation of the rabies virus.*" Pasteur requested that more similar flasks be bought, but bigger, with 2-liter capacity.

184. NAF 18103, item 404.
185. P.A., 1936, p. 69.
186. Reproduced *in* Balibar, 1995.
187. NAF 18019, f.P. 83.

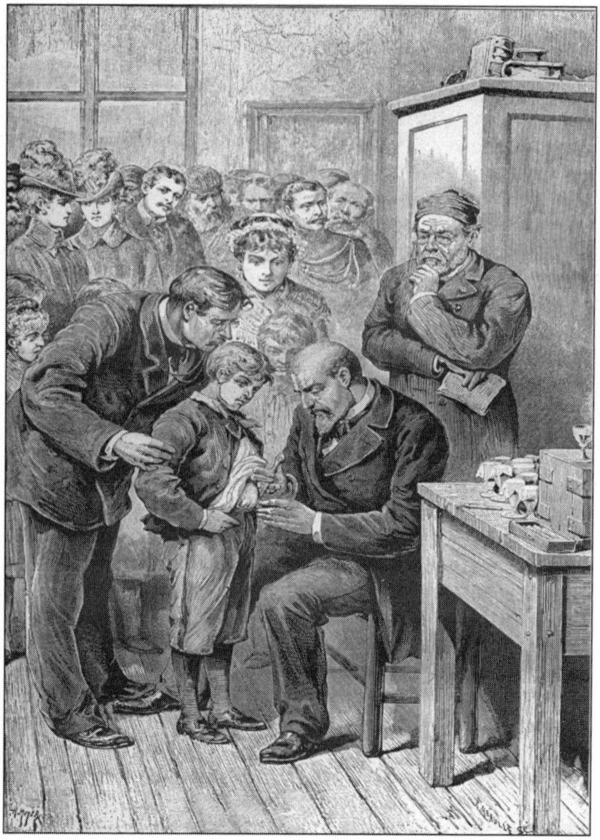

Figure 8. Inoculation of rabies vaccine to young Meister. From left to right: Mr. Viala, Joseph Meister, Dr. Grancher and Mr. Pasteur. *"The treatment was supposed to consist simply of an injection under the skin at the bottom of the ribs, with a virus that Mr. Pasteur considered able to preserve the Meister boy from rabies."* (Bournard, 1896)[188].

Table I. Summary of the inoculations received by Joseph Meister

Day in the month of July 1885	Hour	Spinal cord from	Drying out duration
6	8:20 evening	June 21	15 days
7	9 morning	June 23	14 days
7	6 evening	June 25	12 days
8	9 morning	June 27	11 days
8	6 evening	June 29	9 days
9	11 morning	July 1	8 days
10	11 morning	July 3	7 days
11	11 morning	July 5	6 days
12	11 morning	July 7	5 days
13	11 morning	July 9	4 days
14	11 morning	July 11	3 days
15	11 morning	July 13	2 days
16	11 morning	July 15	1 day

188. Bournard, 1896, p. 79.

"The next day, when Pasteur arrived, I saw him look through his experiment notebook. After studying it at length, he asked me to go to the basement to get one of the rabbits used for passages, a specific one that had just died.

I dissected this rabbit in his presence, and he made me cut the spinal cord in three parts. Each segment was placed in a flask, suspended by a white thread with a slipknot. Then the three flasks were deposited in the holy sanctuary of room-temperature culture." When Roux saw Pasteur's flasks, he burst into a fit of anger and left the laboratory, slamming the door behind him.

"A dramatic event had just taken place, as I understood later. I never heard Roux say anything at all to Pasteur about these flasks, and I don't know if they ever talked about them in private; I don't think so.

But from then on Roux never worked on rabies again. He stopped his investigations and stopped coming to the laboratory.

At that time, he used to go to Val-de-Grâce, to his friend Vaillard's laboratory, where they were studying the septic vibrion and the tetanos agent."[189]

This passage in Adrien Loir's text is very difficult to take at face value because it is hard to make Loir's description fit chronologically with the facts given in Pasteur's register. Roux went to see Girard, the first human being inoculated (treated) by Pasteur, on May 5, 1885 (or May 2[190]). Pasteur noted: "Mr. *Roux trepanned on May* 6 (1885) *a rabbit with crushed spinal cord from a tube and dried by* CO^2 *current..."*[191]. At the *Ecole Normale Supérieure*, the first attempts at storing dog spinal cord infected with rabies virus (not rabbit spinal cord) in glass tubes were probably carried out on January 27, 1883[192]. The first drawing and the text by Pasteur referring to the new storage procedure say *"in dry flask"*, and go back to January 13, 1885; once again, the spinal cord used is dog[193]. According to Loir, the conflict between Roux and Pasteur was sparked by the first use of dry flasks by Pasteur to dry out spinal cord from a rabbit killed by rabies. Supposedly, he never worked on rabies again before November 26, 1886, when he came back and assisted Pasteur after the death of the Rouyer child. But Roux was working with Pasteur in early May 1885, well after storage in dry flask of dog spinal cord on January 13, of rabbit spinal cord on February 4, of guinea pig on February 7, and even of the three segments of rabbit cord on April 9, 1885. Who and what can be believed: Pasteur's daily notebooks or Loir's account written in 1938 without notes, as he himself admits?

In a public address given in Brussels, Jules Bordet, a Pasteurian who spent six years at the *Institut Pasteur* in Paris between April 1894 and 1900, said: "*In this context, let us point out that Roux always remained in retreat and constantly attributed to the sole genius of his master the entire honour of the projects in which he participated."*[194] Bordet, who had direct contact with Metchnikoff and Roux, is a very credible witness, since his deep attachment to both Pasteur and Roux makes him impartial. It is particularly interesting to know that he considered Roux in retreat vis-à-vis Pasteur, and that he always kept this in mind. The simplest analysis of Loir's original text clearly shows perceptible or

189. Loir, 1938, p. 66.
190. NAF 18019, f.P. 62.
191. NAF 18019, f.P. 71.
192. NAF 18017, f.P. 100.
193. NAF 18019, f.P. 3.
194. Bordet, 1934, p. 73.

obvious differences between Roux's and Pasteur's texts: volume of the flasks, potash, temperature... Finally, Loir specifically says that Roux was studying duration of virus preservation, while Pasteur was working on virulence attenuation. Loir describes Roux's angry reaction to Pasteur's procedure, but he gives no precise reason for it, and it is likely that he does not know the reason.

An abrupt conflict, with door slamming, between Roux and Pasteur, is only reported by Loir, who relates it to certain elements (double-headed flasks, rabbit cord...) that do not correspond to any point in the laboratory notebooks. Mary Cressac only speaks of Roux's refusal to sign the first publication, on October 26, 1885, of Pasteur's description of the treatments he administered to Meister and Jupille. It seems that Roux considered that the lapse of time after treatment was not long enough to confirm its value. Pasteur himself had written, on February 25, 1884: "*In my previous Lecture on rabies, I explained that we had encountered in dogs cases of disappearance of the first rabies symptoms, with the recurrence of the disease quite some time later. We recognized the existence of this phenomenon in rabbits. Here is an example: A rabbit is stricken with rabic paralysis thirteen days after trepanation; over the following days, he recovers completely; the paralysis returns forty-three days later and the rabbit dies of rabies on the forty-sixth day. But these occurrences are very rare in rabbits and in dogs, although we have seen them often in chickens...*"[195]. Roux's refusal to co-author a text published too quickly is also recorded by Pasteur Vallery-Radot[196], given that street rabies could have a long incubation period lasting between six and twelve months, contrary to the rabies injected to dogs in the laboratory. Roux was certainly aware of the liberties Pasteur took with his notes (laboratory notes). It is possible that he did not want to be part of this. According to Mary Cressac, Roux returned to work in the laboratory in December 1885, after the tragic death of the little Pelletier girl[197]. Although it might have been serious, the misunderstanding between Roux and Pasteur certainly did not last long. It is true that Roux's name does not appear officially on Pasteur's publications on rabies between October 17, 1885 and November 2, 1886. But on August 4, 1885 Pasteur sent Roux news about various matters, and about Joseph Meister in particular[198]; he also sent instructions, on August 24 and then on September 2, 1885[199], about the ceremonies surrounding the repatriation of Thuillier's body, dead from cholera in Egypt. Pasteur received a letter from Roux and spoke of it in a letter to his friend Versel, on October 9, 1885[200]. On August 17, 1886, he wrote to his son: "*We have entrusted the rabies Unit to Dr. Roux, Dr. Chantemesse and Dr. Charrin.*"[201] Roux's refusal to sign the first publication (October 17, 1885) concerning Pasteur's treatment of Meister and Jupille could have offended Pasteur, but the duration of the conflict is difficult to determine. It might have lasted from the middle of October to the middle of December 1885[202], or until August 1886, at most, because Pasteur recorded an exchange of ideas with Roux at that time[203]. The correspondence between Pasteur and Roux does not portray the disagreement between them as taking the proportions that Loir suggests and, most

195. Pasteur, O.C., tome VI, p. 579.
196. Pasteur Vallery-Radot, 1968, p. 45.
197. Cressac, 1950, p. 81.
198. Pasteur, Cor., t. 4, p. 31.
199. Pasteur, Cor., t. 4, pp. 35 & 36.
200. Pasteur, Cor., t. 4, p. 41.
201. Pasteur, Cor., t. 4, p. 82.
202. Cressac, 1950, p. 81.
203. NAF 18020, f.P. 9.

importantly, the dates given by Loir do not agree with the facts at all. There is little doubt that this part of Loir's recollections is inexact and cannot be taken at face value.

In his October 26, 1885 communication, Pasteur stated: "*Rabies prevention, as I described it in my own name and that of my associates in previous notes* (those of May 1884), *certainly constituted a real advance in the study of this disease, but an advance that was more scientific than practical. Its application involved the risk of accidents. Out of 20 dogs treated, I can only claim to have rendered 15 or 16 refractory to rabies.*"[204] As Pasteur himself admits, the procedure was imperfect and very different from his previous descriptions. Pasteur then describes his new method of dessication of rabbit spinal cord, in dry air and at room temperature, and his method of immunisation by injecting dogs with more and more virulent crushed spinal cord, against rabies. "*By using this method* (the dry flask method, described in detail), *I had succeeded in rendering fifty dogs of all ages and races refractory to rabies, without a single failure, when unexpectedly, last Monday, July 6, three persons from Alsace arrived at my laboratory.*"[205] According to the 13th register[206], ten dogs were given the "Meister" vaccine protocol between May 28 and June 9, and ten others between June 3 and 18, with observation periods of 27 and 18 days respectively, at the time when Joseph Meister received his first treatment on July 6. This period was probably sufficient to ensure that the dogs were properly immunised against rabies thanks to the last inoculations (subcutaneous), but it still left a considerable degree of uncertainty.

These experiments are particularly well described and easy to read, which is not the case for most of the pages of the notebooks. Immunisation of twenty additional dogs was only completed on July 9, 1885. But we are still quite short of the fifty dogs Pasteur himself claims to have immunised by this "Meister" method: "*By using this method...*"[207]. Pasteur's notes also refute this. Had there been dogs not recorded, or treated by other people? Perhaps by Roux and/or Chamberland? It is not very likely, but remains conceivable... At the end of the experiment, a total of twenty dogs had been treated. Two dogs from the first batch had received a test inoculation with street rabies virus (normal, wild), intra-cranially, four days after the July 2 treatment, on July 6[208]. One of the dogs developed rabies on July 28. However, the last injection of the treatment was, in a manner of speaking, a test inoculation, but with an uncertain incubation period. The dogs were inoculated subcutaneously; subsequently, Joseph Meister and the people who followed were inoculated in abdominal, subcutaneous tissue, a site distant from nervous centres and relatively poorly innervated. "*The child* (Meister) *is injected in the hips, a little above the abdomen, in the hypocondria.*"[209] As to dogs vaccinated after being bitten, at the time these animals were treated with virus attenuated by passage to monkeys. Once Pasteur discovered a much better method of vaccination, he admitted that these first results were far from conclusive[210]. A parallel can be made between Pasteur's twenty dogs and Jenner's sole vaccinated patient, who caused Home to say that he would have wished that there be twenty or thirty![211]

204. Pasteur, O.C., t. VI, p. 603.
205. Pasteur, O.C., t. VI, p. 603.
206. NAF 18019.
207. Pasteur, O.C., t. VI, p. 603.
208. NAF 18019, f.P. 73 back & 74.
209. NAF 18019, f.P. 83.
210. Pasteur, O.C., t. VI, p. 603.
211. Home quoted by Baxby, 1999, p. 109.

In the communication Pasteur submitted to the Academy of Sciences on October 26, and to the Academy of Medicine on October 27, 1885, he wrote: "*Given that the child's death seemed inevitable, I decided, not without serious qualms, as you can imagine, to try on Joseph Meister the method that always succeeded when I used it on dogs. It is true that my fifty dogs had not been bitten prior to my determining their refractory state to rabies, but I knew that this circumstance should not be of concern because I had already induced a state refractory to rabies in a large number of dogs after they were bitten. The members of the Rabies Commission have witnessed, earlier this year, this new and important advance.*"[212] Pasteur was combining the results obtained by using these two methods of immunisation: dogs immunised with virus attenuated by passage to monkeys, and dogs immunised with virus dried out in "dry flasks". Most commentators took Pasteur at his word. Grancher, who had not been a close collaborator of Pasteur's in the months preceding the Meister case, testified as follows: "*During the first half of 1885, he (Pasteur) conducted a series of experiments that were more and more successful, and finally arrived at the one which served as the basis for human vaccination, I mean the experiment on 50 dogs, carried out using the following method. Day by day, 50 dogs were inoculated successively with more and more virulent spinal cord, starting with 15-day spinal cord and ending with fresh spinal cord, the spinal cord from the day of autopsy. The 50 dogs prepared in this manner proved to be refractory to subcutaneous or even intracranial injection of the most virulent virus; by contrast, among the 50 control dogs, the proportion of dogs that developed rabies represented the usual percentage associated with various modes of inoculation.*"[213] Many authors of the period believed Pasteur unreservedly and repeated his declarations: Cartaz, Peuch, Pierret, Trouessart, Vulpian[214] (*see below*), and probably others.

In his laboratory notebook, Pasteur wrote: "*First human subject treated*", and then "*Induction of refractory state in a child very badly bitten by a rabid dog. On July 6, 1885, I received...*"[215]. This heading is audacious... In his communication to the Academy, Pasteur also wrote: "*The child's death seemed inevitable...*". Pasteur did not offer any proof for this statement, and seemed to want to convince himself. Was the child contaminated? It was not certain. But his wounds were serious, and some had been inflicted on bare skin; moreover, Vone, and therefore Pasteur, knew the results of the dog's autopsy. In addition, it had been known for a long time that wounds to the head and the hands were the most likely to transmit rabies[216]. The circumstances were clearly more indicative of a rabid dog, rather than simply an angry animal. And finally, the most crucial factor was that symptomatic rabies was always fatal. Even considering the lowest statistics, a ten-percent risk of dying of rabies was still a considerable ratio! Once the disease became symptomatic, it would have been, very probably, too late to administer the Pasteurian treatment. Therefore, treatment was started immediately. Vulpian refused to inoculate, arguing that he was not a practicing physician, which was not strictly speaking true. Loir, Pasteur's nephew, was sent to bring Grancher, who took the (legal) risk of inoculating, in his role as physician[217], a treatment that, *a priori*, was not legally authorised; but it is not certain that this requirement existed (*see below*).

---

212. Pasteur, O.C., t. VI, p. 606.
213. Grancher, 1886, p. 33.
214. Cartaz, 1886, p. 213; Meunier, 1885, p. 351; Peuch *in* Bouley, 1890, t. 18, p. 503; Pierret, 1923, p. 191; Trouessart, 1891, p. 129; Vulpian, 1895, p. 623.
215. NAF 18019, f.P. 83.
216. Darlue, 1755, p. 182; Darlue, 1756, p. 258; Masgana, 1821, p. 17.
217. Loir, 1938, p. 74.

Pasteur did not turn to Roux, who was a physician, but who had, at the time, clear reservations about administering Pasteur's anti-rabies treatment to human beings. Of course, the Girard case had not been encouraging. Moreover, Roux practiced medicine very little or not at all. Grancher, on the other hand, was a pediatric specialist with an active clinical practice. On October 26 and 27, 1885, before the Academy of Sciences and then of Medicine, Pasteur declared: "*Therefore, on July 6 at 8 in the evening, sixty hours after the bites inflicted on July 4, and in the presence of doctors Vulpian and Grancher, we inoculated, under a fold made in the skin of the right hypocondrium of young Meister, half a Pravaz syringe...*"[218]. Grancher gives a slightly different version: "*We* (Vulpian and Grancher) *were of the opinion that M. Pasteur's experiments authorised him to respond to a natural humanitarian impulse and inoculate young Meister.*"[219] Pasteur does not mention Loir, who must have been present, since he had brought Grancher back with him.

Absorbed in the experiment, Pasteur must have been very apprehensive, but everything went well. The last inoculations caused "a convulsion" and reddish marks that were a little worrisome. The final inoculation was made on July 16, 1885, twelve days after the bites, with spinal cord dried for one day. The degree of virulence of the injected matter was verified *a posteriori*, one dose at a time, by inoculating rabbits.

Summer 1885, Brief Visit to Marrault, then Stay in Arbois

Pasteur wasted no time. Young Meister received his last inoculation on July 16, at 11 in the morning. On the back of the page, Pasteur wrote: "*I left for Marrault on July 18; from Marrault to Arbois on July 23. Joseph and his mother insisted on leaving on July 23. The father is impatient to have them back. M. Grancher has written to the City* (Schlestadt) *to Dr. Weber asking him to keep watch on Joseph.*

Up to July 23, day of his departure for his village, Joseph was in perfect health.

July 27, letter from his mother Joseph is in very good health, 23 days after the bites and 11 since his last inoculation on July 16.

August 6, news from Dr. Weber to Mr. Grancher, very good, idem to me from his mother, on August 7 [idem from Joseph on August 7]...

From August 12, very good news about Jospeh Meister [August 17, idem]

September 17 idem idem (75 days after the bites on July 4.)

October 28 all the trepanned rabbits left are given away like new..."[220].

Thus, Pasteur left Paris to visit the Marrault Castle, near Avallon, in Burgundy. Pasteur must have enjoyed visiting his daughter's in-laws. Their mansion was a beautiful, tasteful example of classic architecture. Pasteur no doubt savoured his family's ascension from his parent's modest beginnings in Dole, where he was born, and then in Arbois until his daughter's marriage. The road had not been easy, but after much hard work and many obstacles, success had come at last. In 1885, it was possible to travel the 230-kilometer distance between Paris and Avallon by train, with one or two changes[221]. It was a long trip. This visit had probably been planned long in advance; Pasteur must have been very anxious about the Meister case, and the visit came at an

218. Pasteur, O.C., t. VI, p. 606.
219. Grancher, 1893, p. 680.
220. NAF 18019, f.P. 83 back.
221. Trousset, 1886, p. 29.

inopportune time. Although he was very confident about his treatment, on a personal and human level Pasteur must have been tormented. Once in Avallon, at the Hôtel de la Poste, Pasteur received two telegrams sent the day after his departure. Obviously, he had planned to stop there and spend the night, before continuing on to Marrault. Grancher's telegram, sent on July 19, at 12:30, said: "*All is well. Your little Joseph drinks, eats and sleeps perfectly well. The subcutaneous marks are almost completely gone. My regards to everyone, Grancher.*"[222] The other telegram, from Loir, sent the same day, said: "*The boy is doing very well.*"[223] In Marrault, Pasteur received two telegrams from Grancher, dated July 20 and 22[224]. He did not delay. On the 23rd, he left Marrault for Arbois. He was impatient to be in his country house.

On the 23rd, Grancher sent a telegram to Arbois to say that the Meisters want to return home. Grancher would prefer that Joseph stay a few more days with his uncle, and return home with him on July 31 or August 1[225]. Pasteur had to advise him to let the child leave with his mother. Grancher sent another telegram the same evening: "*Joseph Meister and his mother left this evening and will arrive home tomorrow. Joseph is very well. He drinks, eats and sleeps well, he is growing and gaining weight. The inoculation marks have completely disappeared and the bites on the finger and legs have healed. Let us hope that your attempt will be completely successful.*"[226] Grancher is not altogether reassured. He writes to Dr. Weber, asking him to keep a close watch over young Meister: "Mr. *Pasteur has kindly consented to give this child a preventive treatment that he hopes will be effective... Mr. Pasteur, who asked me to assist him in the treatment he instituted for J. Meister, saw fit that I should write you...*"[227]. Grancher also wrote Pasteur: "*It goes without saying that* Mr. *Weber will not know the actual details... If you have new instructions to give me, dear Master, I am ready to receive them and follow them.*"[228] Joseph Meister was asked to send news every four, then eight and finally fifteen days. On July 29, Grancher wrote Pasteur: "*I will inform you by telegram of those* (news) *I will receive on the critical days of July 30 and 31, and August 1 and 2.*"[229] Grancher and Pasteur must have discussed the days to come; Pasteur could have told Grancher that after August 2 all danger would be over. This lapse of time corresponds to between 26 and 30 days after the bites. And the last virulent injection would have been given 14 to 17 days before. Why this lapse of time? Either because it indicates the peak moment of onset of street rabies after a bite (which is not, in fact, accurate), or because, and this is more likely, it could correspond to the appearance of the first symptoms of treatment-induced rabies, due to the last injections of virulent *spinal cord*. Finally, on August 21, 1885, good news arrived from Alsace, and Grancher wrote Pasteur: "*I am delighted for the boy, for science and for your glory.*"[230] Grancher was clearly relieved.

In May 1884, Pasteur, always eager to try out his procedures, had addressed an appeal not only to individuals bitten by a rabid animal, but also to owners of dogs or bovines likely to become rabid, or even already showing signs of rabies[231]. In July 1885, a

222. NAF 18103, item 400.
223. NAF 18014, item 415.
224. NAF 18013, items 401 & 402.
225. NAF 18013, item 404.
226. NAF 18013, item 404.
227. NAF 18013, item 406.
228. NAF 18013, item 404.
229. NAF 18013, item 407.
230. NAF 18013, item 409.
231. Pasteur, O.C., t. VI, p. 586.

veterinarian in the Seine-Inférieure French administrative division of the territory (present-day Seine-Maritime) notified Pasteur that eighteen bovines belonging to his clients had been bitten by a rabid dog, and requested the benefit of Pasteur's new treatment. Loir was sent to administer the treatment, and none of the animals were infected with rabies[232]. This fact is confirmed, but was the dog really rabid? What is certain is that the animals were not infected with rabies by the "Meister vaccine protocol", albeit the risk was limited with subcutaneous inoculations.

Pasteur never set aside his scientific activities. During young Meister's treatment, and then during his holidays in Arbois, he pursued experiments in Paris: dogs were being immunised with more or less modified "Meister" treatments, and then they were tested with an injection of virulent tissue: "*Rabies Other applications of the new method of vaccination at p. 73, 74, 75, 80 etc. 83 etc.*

July 12, 5 new dogs are inoculated subc. with a syr..." The protocol is six inoculations, one a day, of spinal cord aged 5,4,3,2,1,0 days. "*We stop after these six inoculations. Will they suffice to produce a refractory state?*

*July 27 These 5 dogs are inoculated subc. with 2 syringes of passage spinal cord (83 passages at p. 68) as well as a new control dog (*a priori*, a strong dose).*

NB We want to know if these 5 dogs are already refractory and can all withstand 2 syringes even if the control dog does not die of rabies, it is certain that all 5 cannot respond the same way unless they be truly refractory due to their 6 inoculations between the 12th and the 17th...

August 3, 1 of the 5 dogs is infected, completely paralysed, lying down (1 word) *all the time. He seems to suffer in his head, touches it with his paws constantly as if to remove something that bothers him.*

Were we wrong to inoculate the 2 syr. As early as the 27th, 10 days after the 6th inoc. It's possible. But it is difficult to admit that the inoculations of the 27th could have produced an effect in 6 days. The experiment on the dogs at p. 86 will be very instructive, I believe the vaccination was insufficient because there was no inoculation of non-virulent spinal cord, nor of long-incubation virulent spinal cord." On August 5, one of the "vaccinated" dogs, subsequently tested, died. On August 21, the control dog that was tested died; therefore, four out of five dogs vaccinated using a very short protocol survived and were sent to Villeneuve with collars 121,122,123,124[233].

• **July 30, 1885**, six new dogs are immunised [spinal cord 10, then 9,8,7,6,5,4,3,2,1,0 days old, on August 9] and then tested at the same time as six controls. The twelve dogs are tested on August 9 "*subc. with 1 syr. 0 day spinal cord (numerous rabbit passages)*". Three control dogs and the twelve immunised dogs withstood the test. Pasteur noted: "*Thus immunity seems to be acquired immediately following the treatment. This is quite remarkable. Sept. 14. Still 3 control dogs out of 6 are in good health - This means 3 out of 6 controls infected with rabies. 1 out of 2 by bites, that is by small qies* (quantities) *We have more cases of rabies, 2 out of 3, 3 out of 5, it is more than 1 out of 2 therefore times ...* (1 word) *rarely one out of two [1/2 = 50/100 // 12/3 = 66.60/100 // 13/5 = 60/100 // 3/4 = 75/100].*"[234] The first injections of a twelve-day treatment can provide protection. This indicates that treatment with nervous tissue that has lost its virulence (stored the longest in dry flask) can, very probably, protect

232. Loir, 1938, p. 75.
233. NAF 18019, f.P. 84.
234. NAF 18019, f.P. 86.

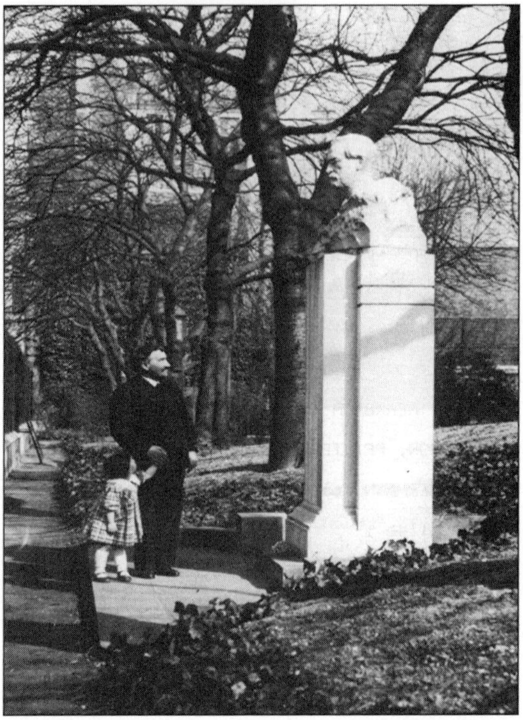

Figure 9. Joseph Meister next to the statue of Louis Pasteur erected before the main entrance of the *Institut Pasteur*. (Photograph kindly provided by André Dubail.)

against a virulent inoculation. The numerical formulas at the end of the paragraph are amusing; Pasteur seems to have been scribbling while he reflected...

• **August 1rst**, an immunisation test is performed on two dogs by trepanation. One survives, the other dies of rabies. Pasteur writes: "*We now have a dog that appears to have been vaccinated by the new method against inoculation by trepanation. This is highly significant for the effectiveness of the method.*"[235]

• **September 3.** "*Small and large quantities.*" The question of dosage has still not been solved[236].

• **September 5, 1885.** Two vaccination trials (see p. 87 and p. 89); in the margin: failure[237].

Once the vaccinations are completed, Pasteur goes back to Paris. He attends the meeting of the Academy of Sciences on October 19[238].

The Second Treatment, October 1885: the Shepherd Jupille

A few days later, Pasteur received a letter from the mayor of Villers-Farlay, a small village near Arbois. A child had been bitten by a rabid dog. Mr. Perrot, the mayor, had met Pasteur some time earlier, and the latter had described his studies on rabies and his hopes for a treatment. A teacher in Villers-Farlay, Mr. Louis Joseph

235. NAF 18019, f.P. 87.
236. NAF 18019, f.P. 90.
237. NAF 18019, f.P. 90.
238. Arch. Acad. Sc., 1B20.

Horiot, gathered documents about Jean-Baptiste Jupille and his struggle with a rabid dog, and presented them on the occasion of a public conference, on December 27, 1922. At the time, witnesses to the incident were still available to be questioned. This communication was published under the title *Horiot Louis Joseph, Louis Pasteur et le berger Jupille*[239]. Six village children guarding animals (cows, if Isenbart's painting is accurate) in a prairie known as "aux Arbues" or "en Chemenot" had been attacked by a dog on October 14, 1885: "*... A large, raw-boned dog, with his fur bristling, his tail between his legs, his eyes crazed and his mouth foaming. The children cried out in their slang 'un tsin feu'* (a mad dog). *When they were face to face with him, the dog left the road and jumped on them.*"[240] The oldest boy, 14-year old Jean-Baptiste Jupille, bravely faced the mad dog to give his friends time to get away. He was able to overpower the animal, stun him and drown him in the Larine, a near-by small river. But he had been cruelly bitten in the process. On December 9, 1888, he recounted: "*I was bitten by a rabid dog on both hands and had several wounds; on my left hand, the thumb nail was thorn off.*"

This account constitutes the content of a letter certified by Gros Félix, mayor of Villers-Farley, on December 1888[241]. Jean-Baptiste's wounds were cauterised with alkali. At the time of the incident, Mr. Perrot, mayor of Villers-Farley, had the foresight to see to it that the body of the dog be recovered. Its autopsy, performed by veterinarians Louvrier and Jacquemin, from Arbois and from Poligny respectively, established that the dog was indeed rabid. Of course, autopsy as a diagnostic procedure has its limitations. Be that as it may, Perrot quickly wrote to Pasteur (October 1885) to inform him of the incident. Pasteur answered promptly, offering to treat the young man. In Paris, Jean-Baptiste Jupille stayed with the family of one of Pasteur's laboratory attendants, Jean Arcony, who lived very close to the *Ecole Normale Supérieure*. Jupille was treated from the 20th to the 29th of October. He received rabid rabbit spinal cord stored in dry flask 15,12,10,9,8,7,6,5,4,3, and 2 days[242], and did not develop rabies. The mayor of Villers-Farley wrote a detailed account of these events[243]. The boy's family received all sorts of advice in the mail, including the description of an infallible rabies remedy containing *Datura stramonium*, distributed freely by the clergy on the recommendation of a former missionary to the kingdoms of Annam and Tonkin, a treatment that was said to have cured over sixty people. Pasteur took the trouble to answer that this remedy was useless.

After the treatment, Jean-Baptiste spent some time with his aunts in Paris. He was rewarded for his bravely by being awarded the Montyon Prize for valour, 1,000 francs (about 3,200 euros) that were deposited in a *Caisse d'épargne* account, as well as lesser prizes awarded by the *Société des victimes du devoir* (Society of the Wounded in the Line of Duty) and by the Rouen Rescuers Society. He also received a letter of congratulations from the students of the Chevreuse primary school (Seine-et-Oise), accompanied by a gift that must have been a book, judging by Jupille's thank-you message; but the fact is that at the time he did not know how to read. He was also nominated honorary member of several rescuers societies (including the Corrèze Society, in central France), and received numerous letters

239. Horiot, 1922 (1995).
240. Horiot, 1922 (1995), p. 29.
241. NAF 18110, item 386.
242. NAF 18019, f.P. 109.
243. NAF 18094, items 92 to 104.

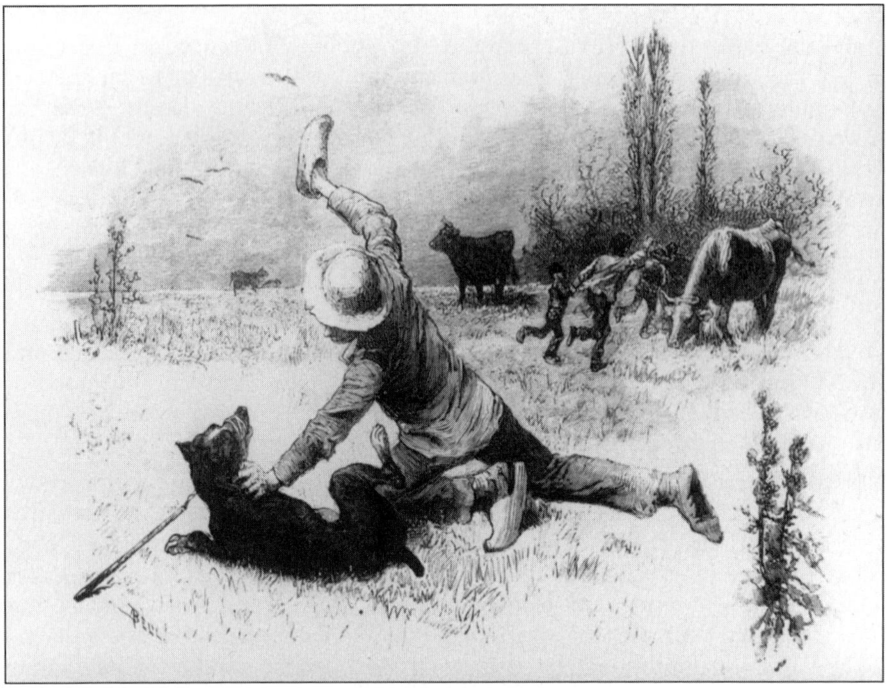

Figure 10. The struggle of the young shepherd Jean-Baptiste Jupille with the mad dog, from the painting by Emile Isenbart. The article accompanying this illustration describes the boy as follows: "*He was a slim boy, taller than average, sun-tanned, with expressive and energetic features.*" The author of the text concludes: "*Today we can affirm that our illustrious countryman has triumphed over the most terrible of diseases, as no one before him or after him has done.*" At the Academy of Sciences, M. Vulpian concluded: "*This new work seals Mr. Pasteur's glory and throws a brilliant light on our country.*" Of course, at the time, proof was still uncertain and questionable, but most people were convinced that the treatment was valid. (*L'Illustration*, n° 2228, November 7, 1885.)

that, based on Pasteur's letters to the mayor of the township, did not incite him to progress in his reading abilities. The "Jupille case" was widely circulated in the press. Truffaut, the sculptor, used the theme to compose a bronze group that would be placed before the main building of the *Institut Pasteur*, and then moved to the side of the building after Pasteur's death, so that Pasteur's bust could take its place. Pasteur visited the mayor of Villers-Farley and the Jupille family. He asked for a photograph of the place where the boy struggled with the rabid dog. A Dole photographer took the picture, and later the landscape painter Emile Isenbart from Besançon created a painting depicting the scene. The hero of the story became a caretaker at the *Institut Pasteur*; from his lodgings, he could look out on his own standing statue, reminiscent of St. Michael's struggle with the dragon! Jean-Baptiste Jupille was the son of a railroad employee who after losing an arm in an accident, while he was off duty, was dismissed and was left without a pension. For this family with six children, the situation would have been desperate had not the good mayor Perrot given the man employment as rural warden. Jean-Baptiste was hired as cowherd by a farmer, before becoming concierge at the *Institut Pasteur*; one of his brothers found employment at the *Institut Pasteur* in Cairo. The mayor of

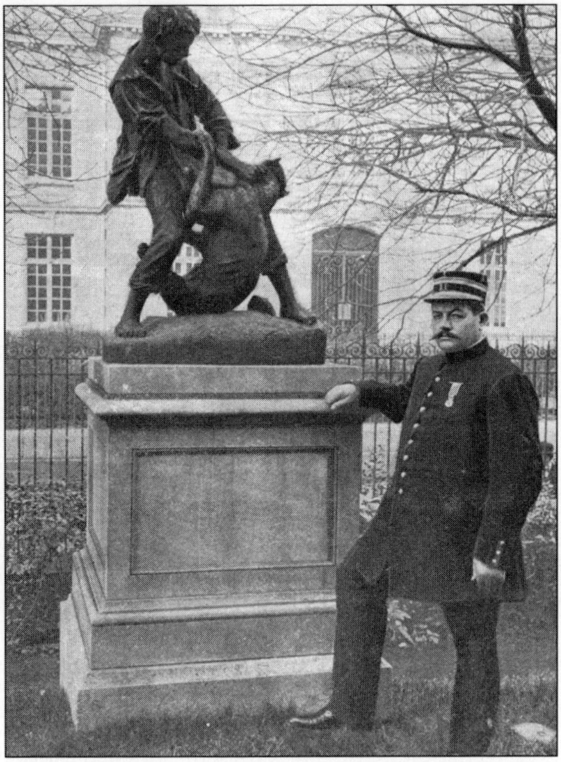

Figure 11. Guardian of his own statue! In the gardens of the *Institut Pasteur*, Mr. Jupille, concierge of the institution, poses before the statue that shows him as a young prairie lad overpowering a rabid dog. (*L'Illustration européenne*, n° 47, November 23, 1913.)

Villers-Farley's summary of the story is noteworthy: "*The result of these events was that, thanks to Mr. Pasteur, Jupille J-B can say unequivocally that the best day of his life, the happiest for himself and for his family, through its consequences, is the day when he was bitten by a rabid dog. J.P.*"[244]

First Official Reports

Pasteur presented his results to the Academy of Sciences during the October 26, 1885 meeting: "*A method of preventing rabies after bites*", by Mr. L. Pasteur[245]. He described his new "Meister" method; he cited "*a large number of dogs*" witnessed by the members of the Rabies Commission, but who received different treatment protocols, and not at all the treatment given to young Meister. Pasteur presented several possible interpretations of his results, explaining that he still hesitated between "attenuation" and "small quantities". However, he was clearly not fully aware of his daring when he made the leap from dogs to a human being: "*Thus, on the last days, I inoculated Joseph Meister with the most virulent rabies virus... Once a state of immunity is attained, it is safe to inoculate the most virulent virus in any quantity. It has always seemed to me that this had for sole effect to consolidate the refractory state to rabies. Therefore, Joseph Meister not only avoided the rabies that his bites could have provoked, but also the rabies that I inoculated to test the immunity induced by the treatment, a rabies more virulent than that caused by*

244. NAF 18094, item 103.
245. Pasteur, O.C., t. VI, p. 603.

stray-dog bites. The final, very virulent inoculation also has the advantage of putting an end to the apprehensions concerning the consequences of the bites."[246] Galtier's immunisation results in sheep and Pasteur's results in dogs showed that there were differences between species. Pasteur was definitely audacious. Despite everything, the scientist's apprehensions must have persisted longer than those of the child, who did not know what was at stake. Little Joseph's mother probably had blind faith in Pasteur. Understandably, Pasteur and Grancher were no doubt the two people who suffered the greatest anxiety.

The Anti-Rabies Pasteurian Treatment Becomes Universal

Pasteur's successes quickly became the subject of commentaries that spread through the entire scientific world. Their impact was impressive. For some years, the classic treatment for rabies had been cauterisation, now people "*went to Pasteur*". Veterinarian Thierry, from Beaune, stated unequivocally: "*If there is doubt in his mind* (the veterinarian), *if the animal has bitten people or animals, he must assume that the disease is present... Without any risk, the bitten individuals can be cauterised and given anti-rabies vaccinations... When dealing with rabies, the greatest caution must be recommended.*"[247] Later, as confidence grew, Pasteurian treatment completely replaced frightening and painful treatments by cauterisation.

The news spread quickly: "*Then, from all points of the civilised world, arrived a procession of unfortunate individuals bitten by a dog suspected of rabies, and haunted by the dread of the terrible disease...*"[248]. The first treatment was given on July 6, 1885; the second on October 20, 1885, the 100th on December 15, 1885, the 200th on February 15, 1886, the 688th on April 15, 1886... At the *Ecole Normale Supérieure* inoculations were administered in the master's office; Grancher was inoculating the stored rabbit spinal cord prepared by Viala. This matter was (potentially) dangerous to handle. One day, Grancher pricked himself with a contaminated syringe. Pasteur told him to give himself the treatment, and Grancher accepted immediately. Loir told Roux about it; the latter expressed doubts about the necessity of the operation. Loir recounts: "*I told him* (Grancher): '*Monsieur, you are not going to have the inoculation? We still don't know what effects this treatment can have on humans.' He* (Grancher) *replied dryly: 'Do you think, young man, that I would do this work every morning if I was not sure of the method?'* Pasteur also asked to be vaccinated. Grancher refused, because at that time Pasteur was no longer handling dangerous material. Eugène Viala and Adrien Loir were both vaccinated[249]. This incident is probably true, although the precision of the details cannot be ascertained.

At the end of Register 13, Pasteur keeps count of foreign patients who received the treatment: "*English: 2; Algerians: 5; German: 1; 8 foreigners out of 47*" people treated[250]. Very soon, Pasteur'laboratory at the *Ecole Normale Supérieure* became overcrowded. Pasteur had a small building erected in the courtyard of the annex at 14 Vauquelin Street. Crowds of bitten individuals filled the premises constantly. In 1887, Suzor portrayed the vaccination sessions vividly. Four rooms were dedicated to inoculations. The largest was a waiting room where ladies could stand behind a screen (for reasons of modesty), to uncover a small area (about 2.5 cm^2) of their hypochondrium (upper

246. Pasteur, O.C., t. VI, p. 607.
247. Thierry, 1897, p. 710.
248. Desplats, 1886, p. 5.
249. Loir, 1938, p. 77.
250. NAF 18019.

lateral portion of the abdomen). The second room was the secretarial office where personal information about patients was collected. One of the two remaining rooms was used to inoculate, while the other served to treat bites and wounds under Mr. Terrillon's supervision. The names and particular characteristics of each patient were recorded in registers. In the inoculation room, Dr. Roux performed the injections, seated. On occasion, it was Pr. Grancher himself who inoculated. Suzor considers him to have a hierarchical status superior to that of Roux, a point of view not shared within the Pasteur group, where everyone is a colleague like the others. Mr. Viala is standing at the side, before a small table holding the wooden boxes containing the complete series of conical vials filled with virus preparations, two or three syringes and an alcohol lamp heating a small pot of water containing calcium chloride, to elevate its boiling temperature. In the boiling water, there is a tube of ordinary oil at a temperature of about 100° C. At 10 o'clock the patients arrive and are carefully identified, particularly new patients. The secretary fills lists of patients according to their stage of treatment. Pasteur was not adverse to registering new patients himself on occasion. At 11 o'clock the inoculations begin with those who are receiving the first injection, with the most attenuated virus. Two people assist the inoculator: Mr. Viala fills the syringe through the sheet of paper covering the virus vials of the number of days appropriate for the patient. The needle is plunged into the hot oil and handed to the inoculator, who injects a more or less high dose depending on the patient's weight. Because the same syringe is used for all the patients, the most virulent virus is injected last. Syphilitic patients have a separate syringe, reserved just for them[251]. The second assistant, whose role is not specified by Suzor, must be the person standing behind the patients to prevent a sudden movement at the moment of inoculation. Desplats explains that the

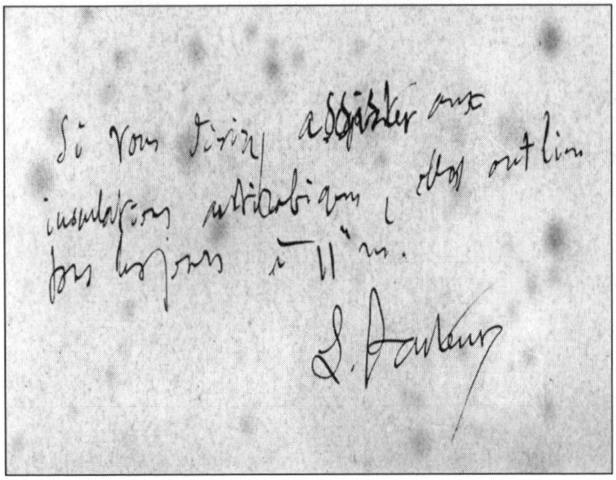

Figure 12. Pasteur never forgot to publicise his work. On a portrait of himself, made from the photograph taken by Pierre Petit and published in the *Journal de la Meunerie* (Journal of the flour trade), he wrote in his own hand: "*If you wish to attend the anti-rabies inoculations, they are given every day at 11 o'clock. L. Pasteur.*" Pasteur, delighted with the wide distribution of his treatment, is said to have greeted visitors with pleasure. Of course, the office used at the time to inoculate was very small. When inoculations were transferred to the building erected for this purpose in the courtyard of the former Rollin College on Vauquelin Street, conditions improved. (Author's document.)

251. Suzor, 1887, p. 183.

bitten individuals who could not come to be inoculated received the treatment from an assistant who went to give them the injections in their hospital beds, with or without Pasteur[252]. The Pasteur laboratory was not prepared to receive so many patients. The situation soon became overwhelming, especially since patients were dispersed. Pasteur notified Eugène Viala: "A *Russian forgotten at Hôtel Dieu Hospital. Prepare a 12-day tube of spinal cord*"[253].

Later, after the inauguration of the *Institut Pasteur*, the rabies inoculation Unit moved into the *Institut*. "*The room where patients wait to see the doctor is a large hall paved with flagstones, with high windows letting in the light, furnished simply with wooden benches and a large table; on the walls, photographs of the* Institut Pasteur *in Rio de Janeiro, maps and large posters with the following information: 'The* Institut Pasteur *was established and is funded by public subscriptions. Anti-rabies treatment is free. Donations and gifts from persons treated can be made at the Accounting Office between ten o'clock and noon. All bitten individuals must bathe on the day of their visit and every two or three days during the treatment. Persons under treatment are informed that no innkeeper is authorised to claim to*

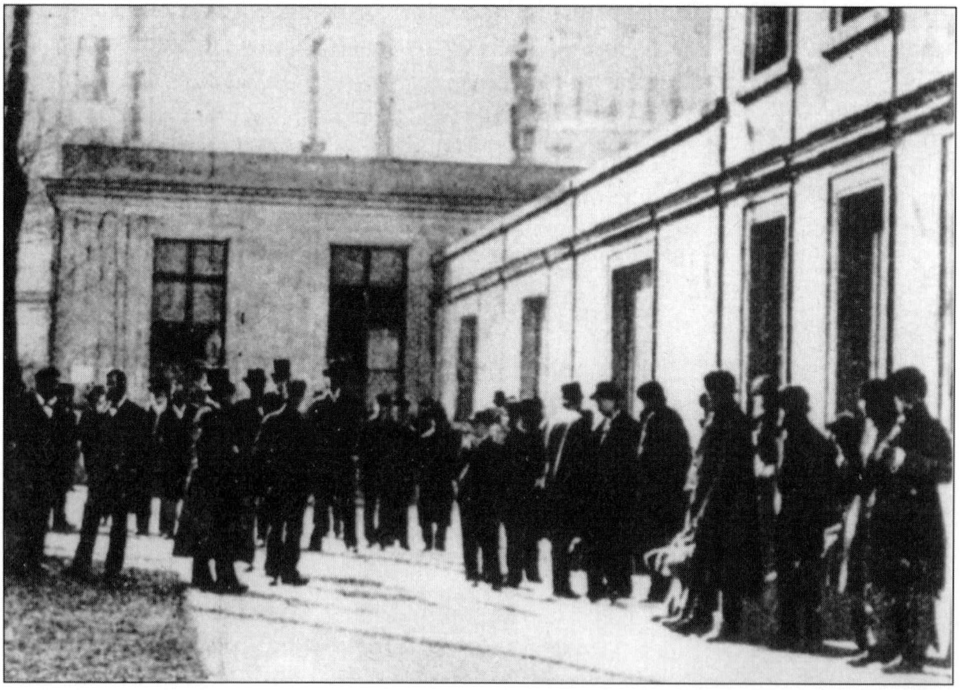

Figure 13. "Bitten" Russians and visitors waiting for the vaccination session to start, in front of the laboratory. Laboratory buildings as they were when Pasteur left the *Ecole Normale Supérieure* to the new *Institut Pasteur*. From right to left: the first pavilion assigned to Pasteur in 1857 or 1858. The wing connecting the pavilion with the big laboratory. The first window is that of the room added in 1862, the rest was built at the same time as the laboratory. At the same level, the window on the left is that of Pasteur's office; at the right, a door leading to the exterior. [Centenial Commemoration of Pasteur's Birth by the City of Paris (*Commémoration du centenaire de Pasteur par la Ville de Paris*, 1924, p35.)]

252. Desplats, 1886, p. 5.
253. NAF 18094, item 2.

be charged by the Institut Pasteur *with housing bitten persons. No hotel is subsidies by the* Institut Pasteur'." *La Nature* published a complete layout of the rabies treatment Unit when the Institute was inaugurated. Headed by Dr. Grancher, the Unit was composed, clockwise, of the hall, a waiting room for people in treatment, registration room, inoculation room, fainting (sic) room, operating rooms, toilets, dressing rooms and archives[254]. This influx of country dwellers and foreigners attracted a number of more or less shady opportunists. A category of "*rabies merchants*" emerged, offering second-rate lodgings and board to the unlucky patients who were receiving the Pasteur treatment[255].

Soon, Grancher, professor of pediatric practice at the Faculty of Medicine, acquired two young assistants: Pr. Charcot's student Chantemesse and Pr. Bouchard's student Charrin. Dr. Terrillon, Grancher's classmate, treated the patient's wounds. In 1889,

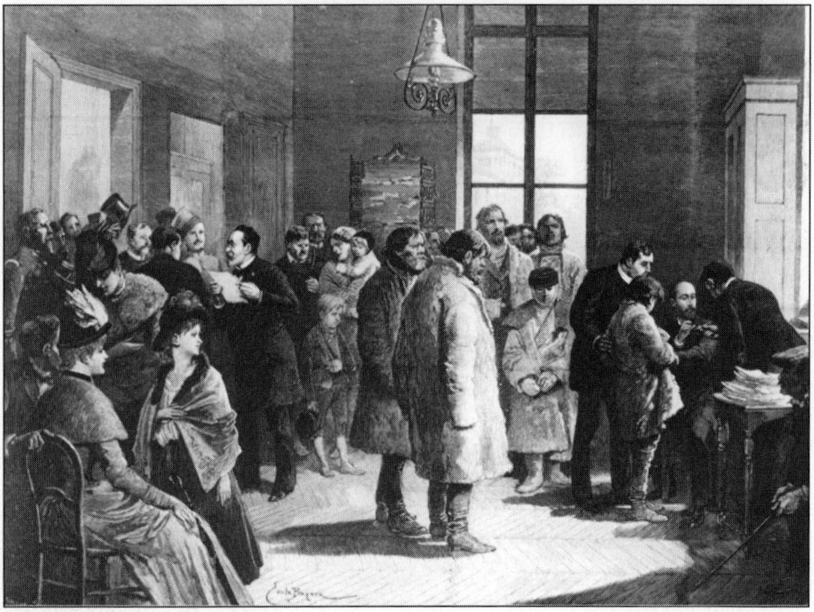

Figure 14. "***Rabies vaccine. Inoculation session at Mr. Pasteur's laboratory, based on the sketch for Emile Boyard's painting... Each morning, a little before 11, the small laboratory at the*** **Ecole normale** ***starts to fill with people. The patients wait in the first room that serves as an antechamber; they are inoculated in Mr. Pasteur's office. The latter stands near the door, holding a list, and calls the patients one by one, by categories, depending on the virulence of the virus they are to receive. Dr. Grancher... asks each person when his treatment started, so that he can decide the order in which patients will be treated, and the vaccine each person should be given... In less than an hour, over a hundred people are vaccinated. And what diversity in this crowd... Over there, a whole colony of Russians from Smolensk... Other Russians have just arrived from the Moscow area... people from Finland; then, at random Spahis, an Arab, a policeman, a combat engineer, a boarder guard, a hurdy-gurdy player, a country postman, some Belgians, some Portuguese, people from the Basque region, Americans, some charming English women bitten when they unknowingly stroked a rabid dog, little children in their mother's arms. Rich and poor, big and small, here everyone is equal.***" **(C. Talansier *in L'Illustration*, n° 2250, April 10, 1886.)**

254. Tissandier, 1888, p. 402.
255. Lemaistre, 1896, p. 208.

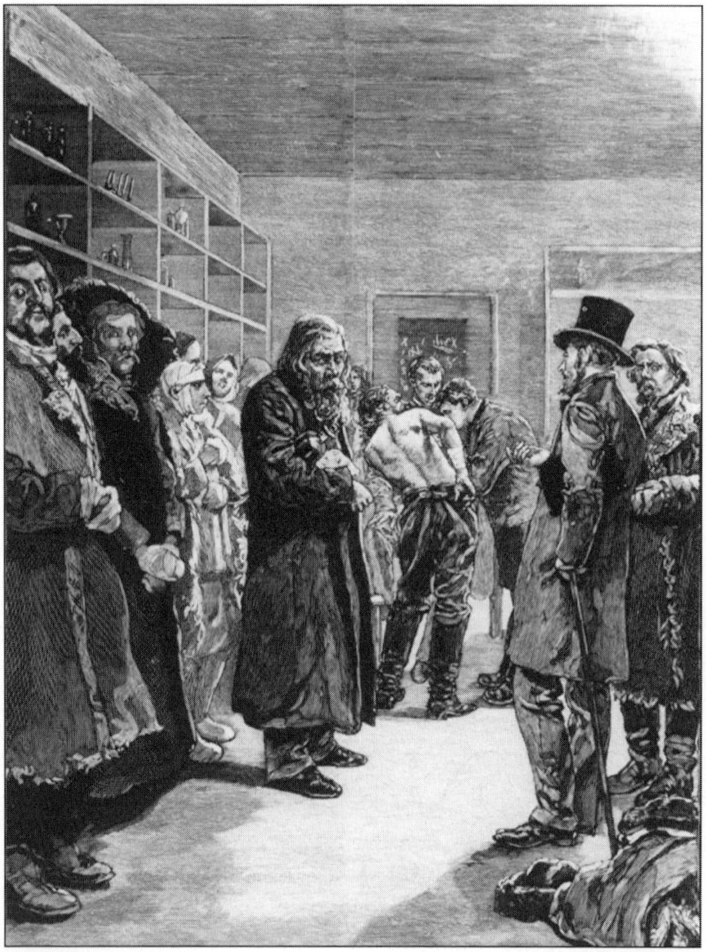

Figure 15. *"Russians from Beloï (village near Smolensk) in the antichamber of Pasteur's office at the* Ecole Normale Supérieure*; painted from life by M. Marc-Aurèle." Le Monde illustré,* March 27, 1886.

Grancher was heading a complete team: Drs Chantemesse and Charrin (inoculations), Terrillon and Prengrueber (wound treatment), students Germond and Perdrix (patient history and archives). All of them were destined to have a brilliant future. "Microby" soon to be called "microbiology", had proven its worth. The team also included two laboratory assistants, Eugène Viala (whom Pasteur trusted completely) and Jean Arcony. All these people were at the service of rabies vaccinations twice a day, including Sundays and holidays. The work comprised spinal cord preparation as well: buying the rabbits and looking after them, inoculations, taking spinal cord samples, storage in dry flasks... Pasteur, anxious to maintain his assistants in good health, ordered that the teams rotate every three months[256]. It was important to look after his group, and especially to avoid mistakes, which must not have been easy. Fortunately, there

256. Rameau, 1889, p. 34.

were the registers. Salaries were modest, the highest being 6,000 francs and the others between 1,200 and 3,000 francs. Pasteur and Grancher had no remunerations. Pasteur, Chamberland and Roux donated the gains from anthrax vaccinations to the Institute[257].

Diversity of Immunisation Protocols

To understand the great diversity of Pasteur's anti-rabies vaccination protocols, his "immunological" concepts must be kept in mind. These concepts kept changing over time, but remained far removed from reality as we know it today. Pasteur's series of injections varied, and not always in a way that can be clearly understood. For the chicken cholera, anthrax and erysipelas vaccines, Pasteur considered his exhaustion theory as the perfect foundation.

On January 29, 1985, while attending a meeting of the Académie française, Pasteur wrote this curious note to himself and later pasted it in his laboratory notebook: "*I cannot conceal any of my ideas from those who work with me, but I would have liked to keep to myself a little longer the ideas that I will present the experiments that will test them are already on the way... I am inclined to think that the figuration of the rabies virus must be accompanied by a matter that, when absorbed into the nervous system, makes it unsuitable for the culture of the microbe particle. This explains vaccinal immunity. If this is so, the theory could well have very wide applications. It would be a gigantic discovery.*"[258] Pasteur has doubts about his exhaustion theory because the immunity he obtains with his rabies vaccine is not accompanied by any signs of the disease. He is looking for another explanation. Pr. Hannoun comments on the above note in these terms: "*These few lines contain the foundations of a new discipline that would develop extensively around Pasteur and after him, particularly with* Metchnikoff*: immunology. The figuration of the rabies virus is the virus particle, the virion, which Pasteur has never seen and that would not be described specifically as being bullet-shaped until 1960. The 'matter' accompanying the virus consists of what we call today surface antigens, antigenic glycoproteins, that is, able to provoke the appearance of antibodies and other forms of immunity. Antigens 'are absorbed' by the nervous system and even by the whole system, rendering it indeed unsuitable to the culture of the virus thanks to the mechanisms better known today as humoral and cellular immunity.*"[259] This interpretation is rather idealistic; the truth of such things is always subjective. In a note in his "*Letter on rabies*" written in Bordighera on December 27, 1886, intended for the first issue of the "*Annales de l'Institut Pasteur*", Pasteur himself says: "*Let us not lose sight of the very original and so fruitful theory of Mr. Metchnikoff. If a vaccinal substance in fact exists, could it be in dead microbes?*"[260] Pasteur reflected on this new concept, which had not occurred to him, on January 29, 1885. The chemist in him found it very attractive. He considered with great interest Roux and Chamberland's work[261] on protection induced by dead substances[262]. His ideas on immunity continued to evolve. In June 1887, the British commission charged with evaluating the usefulness of the Pasteurian treatment wrote in its report: "Mr. *Pasteur believes that the virus of rabies is a living-organism, and that, like some others, it produces in the tissues it invades an excretory*

257. Rameau, 1889, p. 35.
258. NAF 18019, f.P. 9.
259. Hannoun, 1995, p. 156.
260. Pasteur, O.C., t. VI, p. 645.
261. Roux, 1887, p. 561.
262. Roux, 1887, p. 567.

substance by which, when present in sufficient quantity, its own development and increase are checked, as are those of the yeast ferment by the alcohol produced in the vinous fermentation. In accordance with this theory, he thinks that the spinal cords of animals that have died of rabies contain both the virus and this excretory substance, which, practically, may be deemed its antidote. He believes therefore that the injections of an emulsion from such spinal cords into the systems of animals bitten or inoculated with the virus of rabies, the antidote may be able, during the period of incubation, to arrest and prevent the fatal influence of the virus. But, in order to avoid the possibility of injecting a still potent virus, Mr. Pasteur holds that the virus in the spinal cord must be weakened by drying the cord in a pure and dry atmosphere at the temperature of 20° C.; in which the efficiency of the antidote may be reduced to a much lesser extent than the potency of the virus. By such drying this potency may be so reduced that an emulsion of the dried spinal cord may be injected without any risk of producing rabies; and this risk is no measure increased by the daily injections of emulsions from cords dried during a gradually less number of days, and which, though more virulent than those first used, still contain a larger proportion of the antidote than of the virus."[263] This theory led Pasteur to increase injections, at times probably excessively, believing them to be harmless.

Pasteur must not have had total faith in his own theory, since he accepted Metchnikoff's cellular theories, and later Behring's humoral theories, rather easily, although they were opposed to each-other by their respective advocates, and were very different from his own previous concepts.

As far as rabies was concerned, Pasteur knew only that rabbit spinal cord dried for one day is virulent, and that cord dried for fourteen days is no longer virulent (if the drying temperature is adequate). At first, he believed the "virus" became attenuated, but quickly abandoned this idea. His notion of a "*vaccinating matter associated with the virus*" led him to multiply the injections of rabbit cord, and therefore of vaccinating matter. This matter was supposed to kill the living "virus" in the bitten individual. From the start, Bouchard has doubts about this procedure. "*Why give a succession of inoculations with increasingly more virulent cord? Why not use only the fourteen-day cord, the one that is no longer virulent but still vaccinates, which has what is useful and no longer contains what could be dangerous? The practice of inoculation against rabies after a bite has remained unchanged because it has proven effective. The new theory* (that of vaccinating matter) *will no doubt make it possible to introduce a simpler, more rational and safer method in animals, and then apply it to human beings. In the meanwhile, loyalty to the old ways of doing persists.*"[264] Bouchard was not an opponent of Pasteur's; one of his assistants worked in Pasteur's rabies Unit.

Very quickly applied to humans, this new method led to obvious experimentation with the injection protocols. At the end of his treatment, young Meister received an inoculation with one-day spinal cord. Jupille's last injection contained two-day cord. Subsequent patients were inoculated with cord dried for at least three, four or often five days[265]. "*As for Mr. Pasteur, after his October 26 communication crowds of people from all regions of France and all parts of the world came to see him... he worried about accidents and eliminated treatment with the most virulent cord samples... However, after three out the nineteen Russians from Smolensk died, he made an exception for the sixteen*

263. Paget *in* Pasteur, O.C., vol. VI, p. 882.
264. Bouchard, 1889, p. 170.
265. NAF 18019.

survivors, several of whom had bites to the face. All of them received the most intensive treatment, that is, a series of successive spinal cord inoculations, ending with first-day cord."[266] On March 13, nineteen wounded Russians, bitten by a wolf on March 1, 1886 and cauterised six hours later with nitric acid, arrived in Paris[267]. "A *number of them presented deep wounds, irregular and jugged, incompletely treated, to the head, the face, the lips, the neck, the hands.*"[268] Four men and one woman were admitted to the Hôtel-Dieu Hospital and treated there. The others were given rooms at the Gay-Lussac Hotel, and were charged 4.5 francs a day for board, paid by the Pasteur Laboratory[269]. Another bitten patient, Emile Monestier, receiving treatments at the Pasteur laboratory at that time, recounts his first meeting with these unfortunate people: "*Standing, hatless, barely daring to move, they survey their surroundings with shy, surprised glances. Wearing high leather or cloth boots and the national sheepskin, a kind of fur-lined coat smelling of wild animals and suet, they involuntarily bring to mind barbarians of ancient times.*"[270] Their countrymen living in Paris, Baron Mohrenheim, ambassador of Russia, among them, came to their aid. They received intensive treatment with repeated injections, but "*aside from some double-dose injections, the three series of inoculations were only the repetition of the first, which was given according to the protocol for 'dog bites'*"[271]. Unfortunately, three of the Russians died of rabies, in the midst of terrible suffering, as was usually the case[272]. The wolf had certainly been rabid. All authors agreed that without treatment there was a mortality rate of six to eight out of ten cases, after rabid wolf bites. This percentage had probably decreased because cauterisation had been performed, but the severity of these poor peasants' wounds did not bode well for them. After treatment, the sixteen surviving Russians returned home safe and sound.

A second group of Russians composed of nine peasants from Wladimir, bitten on March 25, 1886, cauterised six hours later with nitric acid, arrived in Paris on April 8, with Dr. Vicknevsky who had treated them in Russia. In their case, Pasteur used the "wolf bite" treatment for the first time. Three injections a day, with a double dose (except the two-day and three-day cord) of spinal cord dried from fourteen to two days. Unfortunately, three patients died of rabies, one of them at the end of the treatment, causing the group to leave; a second patient died during the return voyage, and the third a few days after their arrival in Russia. One third of the treatments failed... But these were wolf bites, treated fifteen days later... James concluded: "*Obviously, in this situation Mr. Pasteur handles his virus like a tamer handles his animals.*"[273] Yes... but the so-called intensive treatments were the least well-established and barely tested in animals.

The arrival of all the "bitten", especially the exotic ones, must have disturbed the neighbourhood. A leaflet dated April 10, 1886 describes the treatment of the nine Russians from Wladimir, three from Denza, seven from Orle[274], and on April 14, the

266. Grancher *in* Pasteur, O.C., t. VI, p. 770.
267. CT., 1886, p. 212.
268. Cornil, 1890, t. 2, p. 537.
269. CT., 1886, p. 212.
270. Monestier, 1886, p. 198.
271. James, 1886, p. 49.
272. James, 1886, p. 50.
273. James, 1886, p. 50.
274. NAF 18094, item 5.

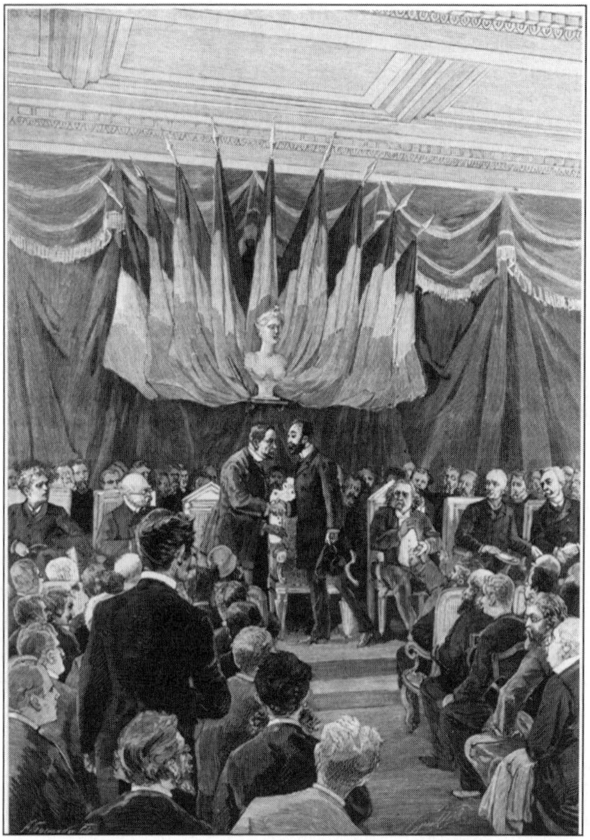

Figure 16. Official inauguration of the *Institut Pasteur*, on November 14, 1888. (Drawing from life by Mr. Guilliod, published in *L'Univers illustré*, n° 1757, Nov. 24, 1888.) The ceremony took place in the old library and was attended by the president of the Republic, Mr. Carnot; Mr. Pasteur and many famous men including Mr. Chauveau, Mr. Ricord, Mr. Poubelle... Grancher and Duclaux were granted the title of Officer, and Mr. Chantemesse was made a Knight of the "*Légion d'Honneur*".

same patients plus ten from Wilna[275]. Léo Claretie, an *Ecole normale* graduate, recounts: "*Among the first client were five moujiks lacerated by wolves. All along Gay-Lussac Street, in the morning they could be seen making their way to the laboratory in fur hats, red jackets tied with a belts, wide trousers made of black velvet and disappearing into big boots. Their heads and their hands were bound in compresses... For a few days, at first, they caused quite a stir in the neighbourhood, provoking both curiosity and unease. Rabies sufferers, like lepers, are kept at a distance. Little by little, people got used to them...*"[276]. The account sounds authentic, but none of the actual groups were composed of five people, unless these five were just a segment of a group.

The diversity of Pasteurian anti-rabies treatments is surprising. The different protocols and dosages can be confusing. On April 7, 1887, Grancher showed Pasteur the draft of a letter in which he described, for Victor Horsley, secretary of the British Committee,

275. NAF 18094, item 7.
276. Verdunoy, 1922, p. 131.

charged with assessing the effectiveness of Pasteurian anti-rabies treatments, the treatments employed at the time:

- **Simple treatment:** a sequence of inoculations of crushed dried cord, from J1 (day 1 of treatment), 14-day cord (14 days in dry flask) to J10, 5-day cord;
- In **case** of **bites** to the face, treatment is repeated 3 or 4 times.
- **Treatment for wolf bites:** J1: 14, 13 and 12-day cord; J2: 11, 10 and 9-day cord; J3: 8 and 7-day cord; J4: 6 and 5-day cord; J5: 4 and 3-day cord; J6: 2-day cord; J7: 1-day cord; J8: 6 and 5-day cord; J9: 4 and 3-day cord; J10: 2 day cord; J11: 1-day cord.

However, in December, finding the virulence of rabbit cord to be much less attenuated, Pasteur returned to five-day cord as the maximum[277]. On April 13, 1887, Grancher considers that fatalities caused by the treatment could have occurred before it was noticed that cord virulence attenuation was a much slower process in winter; but he refused to admit that the death of Gaffi (a bitten patient treated) led to the use of 5-day cord as a maximum (as Pasteur must have recommended in a letter to Grancher). Grancher even adds that he sees this as being "*more perilous and less precise*."[278]

In 1888, the Larousse Dictionary listed three types of treatment, depending on the seriousness of the bites; these treatments were simplified compared to the ones defined by Grancher a few months earlier. Injection of one-day cord, the last injection given to young Meister, had disappeared almost entirely...

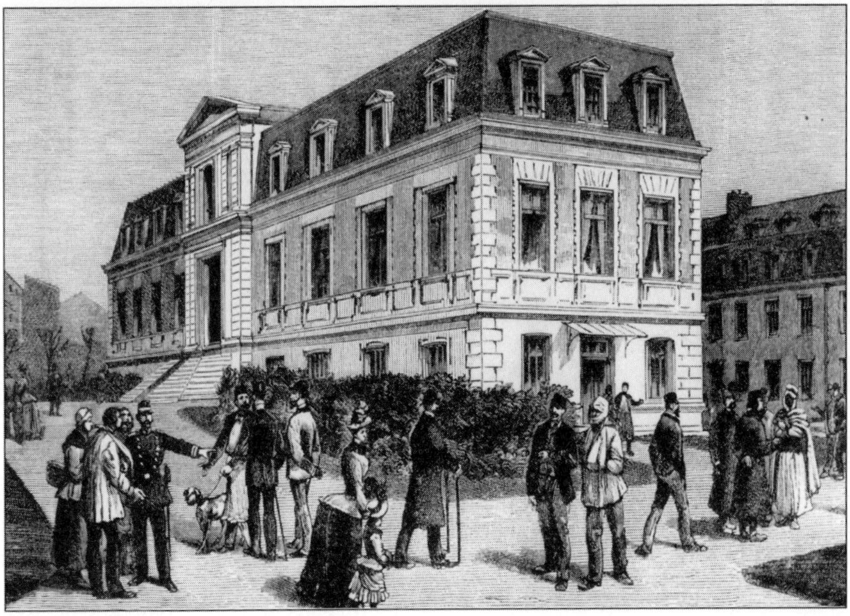

Figure 17. The new *Institut Pasteur*, built on market gardening land, located on Dutot Street, has just opened its doors. The "bitten" arrive in great numbers. Some wear dressings, others do not. A guard or a soldier (wearing a weapon on one side) shows new arrivals where to proceed. One person is seen in conversation with a member of the personnel (long apron and skullcap) who is holding a dog on a leash... (*L'Ami du Foyer illustré*, n° 50, October 10, 1895.)

277. NAF 18103, items 471-473.
278. NAF 18103, item 476.

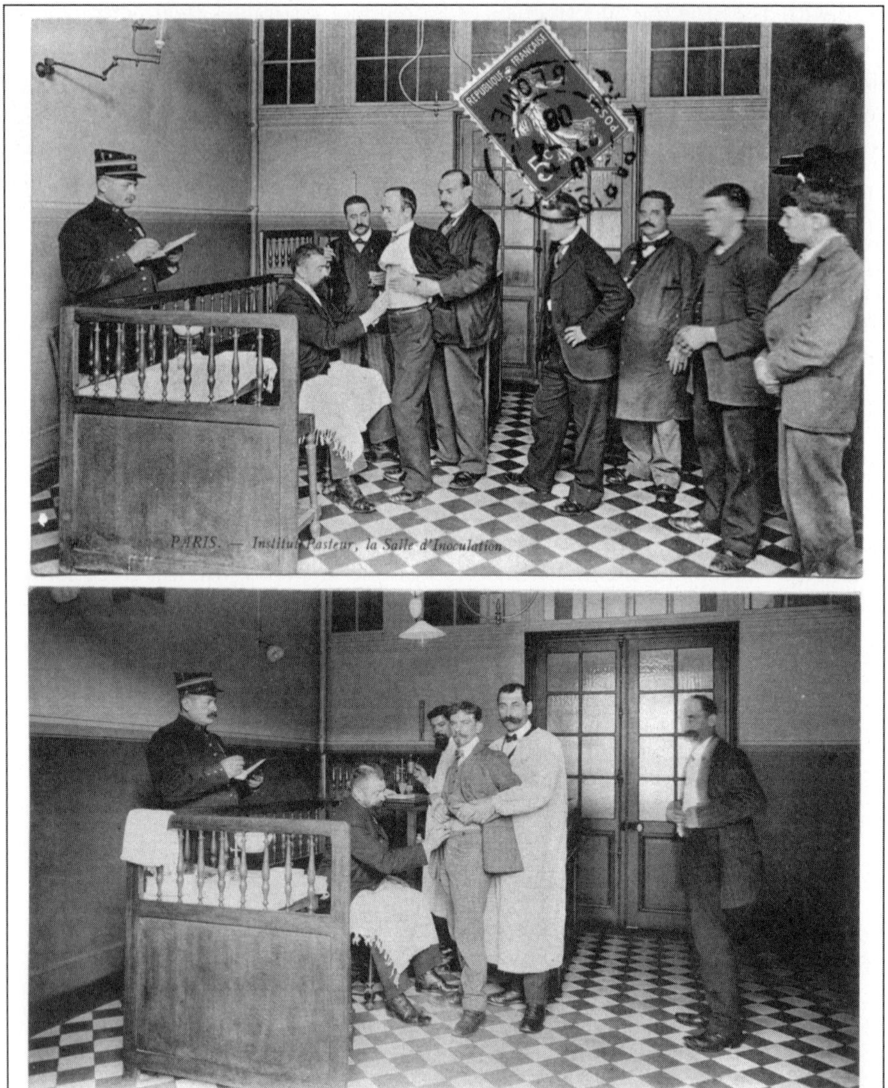

Figure 18. Two postcards showing the inoculation room at the *Institut Pasteur*, on Dutot Street (now Dr. Roux Street). A lapse of time of several years has not changed the picture, except for the lighting and the guard's moustache! Above, gas lighting; below, electric lights... but the gas fixtures are still in place. After all, around 1893-1894, competition between gas and electricity was fierce. Inoculations are given in the hypocondrium. The procedure remains the same: the patient uncovers an area of skin, an assistant holds the patients hands, in case he makes a sudden movement. The guard, (J.B. Jupille?) surveys the scene. The enterprise is serious. A preparator (Eugène Viala above?) is responsible for filling the syringes with the right inoculum. Because the syringes can leak, the person (here, probably Dr. Chaillou) who inoculates covers his pant legs with a towel. Syringes are being filled in the background. A patient waits. He moved as the photograph was taken, he must have been nervous, quite understandably.

The Grand Larousse of the XIX century specified that "*ladies too nervous to accept being treated in public have the option of retiring to a private room...*"[279].

The simple protocol, the most classical, was now well defined. But in difficult cases like multiple bites to the face or to the hands, or wolf or cat bites, the Pasteurians had no clear answers for countering the progression of the virus. There still appeared to be variations in particular cases. "*He* (a young man 20 years old) *received two injections a day of anti-rabies vaccine for one month, followed by one injection a day for 3 weeks.*"[280] The hypotheses (immunological) used by Pasteurians were based on mistaken considerations, but who was going to condemn them? In 1909, twenty years later, treatment protocols used at the *Institut Pasteur* had become standardised, but they were still based on a scale of seriousness of possible contamination[281], not necessarily a good criterion.

One factor of variability is the weight of the inoculated rabbits. To remedy this problem, "*Hogyès replaced dried cord with diluted fixed virus, given that according to Pasteur drying out does not change the quality of the virus, but only its quantity*"[282]. After conducting an experiment on seventy dogs, Hogyès used the dilution method to vaccinate the personnel of the *Institut Pasteur* in Budapest, and then bitten patients. The treatments were identical to those used by Pasteurians in Paris, but the virus was normal (viral strain adapted to rabbits, called fixed) and dilution was between 1 per 10,000 and 1 per 100*.

Ferran in Barcelona used fresh cord to immunise humans. He wrote: "*Massive inoculations of fresh pulp from rabid dogs do not always kill rabbits, just as fresh pulp from rabbits with rabies, used to inoculate massively, kills neither humans nor dogs, but does kill rabbits.*"[283] His method relied on the use of large quantities of unmodified fixed virus; he called it "superintensive vaccination method"[284]. Between May 1887 and December 1895, in his microbiology laboratory in Barcelona, Ferran used his anti-rabies vaccination to inoculate 1,792 individuals, with ten fatalities[285], which is a very good result. Bareggi's results (five fatalities using Ferran's method) are often praised in comparison[286], although the two techniques might have differed somewhat.

The notion that the fixed rabies virus was safe eventually became an accepted idea: "*We* (Marie, 1909) *also believe that the fixed virus used in laboratories, and particularly in the laboratory of the Paris* Institut Pasteur, *has lost its pathogenic power for humans, or at least that its injection into the cellular subcutaneous tissue of the abdominal region can be performed without any risk. But this might not be true if the point of injection was a site particularly rich in nerve endings, such as the fingertips.*"[287] After a series of fixed virus inoculations to dogs, Remlinger from the Constantinople Imperial Bacteriology Institute concluded: "*We believe that it is possible to make an argument for the adaptation of the fixed virus to the system of the rabbit, and for its limited risk for other animals, and*

* Not so different of the Pasteur small quantities.

279. Larousse, 1888, 2e Suppl., p. 1758.
280. Marciguey, 1893, p. 445.
281. Marie, 1909, p. 277.
282. Marie, 1909, p. 281.
283. NAF 18094, items 187 to 195.
284. RoA, 1974 (?), p. 387.
285. Gillet, 1904, p. 612.
286. Cornil, 1890, t. 2, p. 547.
287. Marie, 1909, p. 293.

particularly man."[288] A German author by the name of Citron agrees[289]. Charles Nicolle, after performing a series of one hundred passages of the Pasteurian rabies virus on dogs, during which the virus never reverted to its original characteristics, added: "*It is logical to think that the discovery of the anti-rabies vaccination method is due to a fortunate and hidden mutation*"[290], that is, a fortuitous event, and not to a gradual adaptation of the virus to the rabbit. When exactly did the rabies virus of the *Institut Pasteur* lose all or part of its pathogenic power for humans, when inoculated at the doses and in the conditions used by this Institute? The question is interesting*. But a note written by Pasteur on September 10, 1886 introduces some uncertainty into the matter of the rabbit-adapted viruses, at least in the first years of their use: "*Eugène* (his technician). *This Sept. 10, 1886 A new series of rabbits must always be in preparation - Therefore take a dog with street-dog rabies (that died biting and furious) inoculate two rabbits with its cord and carry on like this in successive passages. We will call them: rabbits, 3rd series. L.P.*"[291] This note shows that Pasteur was worried about something. But what... losing his fixed virus strain, or an unforeseen modification of its properties?

In 1941, Andrée Tétry repeated Pasteur's experiments: rabbit marrow stored in a double-headed flask to dry out. She explained: "*Several factors come into play (drafts, potash, thickness of the marrow, temperature, time).*"[292] Spinal cord thickness is designated as a disruptive parameter in reference to Russian rabbits, smaller than those sold out at "les Halles" in Paris. Pasteur noted: "*Roux believes that our 3-day cords from large rabbits are just as virulent as those from the smaller Russian rabbits.*"[293] Similarly, temperature is an important factor that Pasteur had already identified. Tétry elaborated in these terms: "*In a Mariotte flask, proteolysis of the rabic rabbit spinal cord is intense at the start; then it becomes attenuated due to the drying out of the cord; when the latter is completely dry, proteolysis is no longer present. Virulence attenuation is parallel to autolysis; it is a factor of the degree of freedom allowed ferments that are only active in humid milieu... The consensus is that after rabbit-to-rabbit passages the virus acquires greater sensibility to desiccation; in fact; it is more sensitive to the action of proteolytic ferments...*"[294]. Interestingly, Tétry did not quote Nicolle, who believed in a random event, a mutation. And then there were all those who believed that the rabbit-adapted virus was no longer infectious when inoculated subcutaneously and in reasonable doses... Possibly, and even probably, several mechanisms exerted concerted action: adaptation of the virus to the rabbit species, with possible mutation(s), proteolysis and/or virus inactivation linked to the treatment and to the method of inoculation... In any case, Tétry's conclusions are not far from those of Pasteur himself, as she wrote on June 18, 1885: "*Therefore air does not attenuate during dry-flask storage. It gradually destroys virulence, but the virulence still present is full virulence.*"[295]

In addition to Pasteur's hesitation concerning the clinical aspects of these treatments, their improvised character must be remembered. The unexpected arrival of crowds of

* The progressive and slow adaptation of "street rabies virus" to the rabbit did not seem linked to its toxicity for humans.

288. Remlinger, 1904, p. 414.
289. Citron, 1912, p. 28.
290. Nicolle, 1933, p. 187.
291. NAF 18094, item 41.
292. Tétry, 1941, p. 386.
293. NAF 18103, item 421.
294. Tétry, 1941, p. 386.
295. NAF 18019, f.P. 73 & back.

bitten people to Pasteur's laboratory must have caused some panic... At the Saint Hubert sanctuary, named after the Saint who cures rabies, the crowds must have been similar, but there was no need for all the preparations associated with the rabies virus.

The archives of the French *Bibliothèque nationale* contain numerous lists of patients to be treated, carefully assembled on small files[296]. Lost among all these documents, some of Pasteur's notes to Eugène Vialla are disconcerting. "*Eugène-Madame Fanny de Dayer will come at 4 o'clock or before to take a rabbit inoculated with passage virus (in her presence). Give her one of the small cages. L.P. this May 14.*"[297] "*Eugène, July 21, 1886, never give an inoculated rabbit without having the person fill out a card with his name, address, the name of the laboratory where the rabbit is taken. L.P.*"[298] These were, of course, rabbits inoculated with the fixed rabies virus... Pasteur also wrote in his notes: "*August 20, 1886. Marius Bouvier did indeed die of rabies (if there was no mistake in the labels) (or a fallen rabbit put back in a different cage) (sic).*"[299] It is clear that Pasteur and the Rabies Unit are overwhelmed with demand; Pasteur knows it and seems nonplussed.

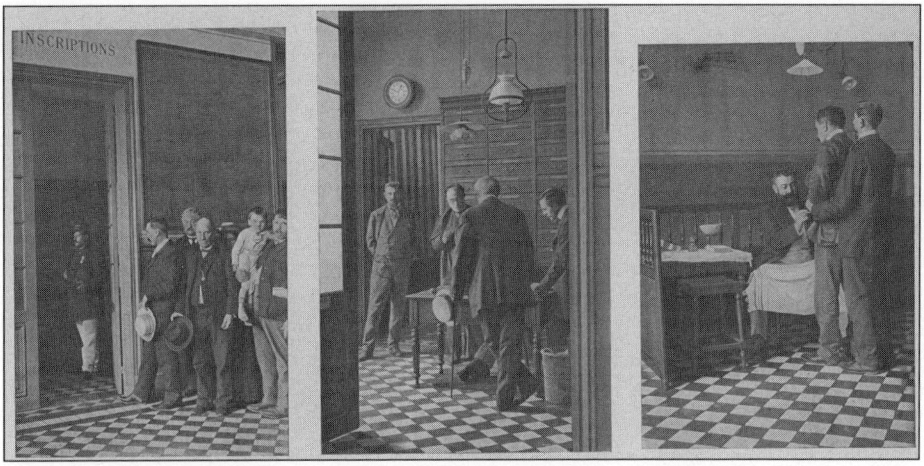

Figure 19. Treatment of bitten patients at the Paris *Institut Pasteur*. From left to right: "*Bitten patients wait in a room until they see a doctor and explain the circumstances in which they were wounded. In the registration room, bitten patients provide all the information needed to decide what their treatment should be. Dr. Chaillou inoculates the vaccinal fluid under the skin, in the flank of the patient.*" (Charpentier, 1909)[300].

Effectiveness of Pasteur's Anti-Rabies Treatment

How could Pasteurian treatment provide a cure? Rabies is an infectious disease whose average incubation period is long, between one and two months, sometimes more. Therefore, the infected system, when treated by Pasteur, had time to trigger an immune response before the onset of rabies. Rabic virus inoculations with attenuated virulence adapted to humans or small quantities were given subcutaneously in poorly innervated

296. NAF 18094.
297. NAF 18094, item 19.
298. NAF 18094, item 27.
299. NAF 18020, f.P. 10.
300. Charpentier, 1909, p. 311.

tissues. But why was it that virus inoculated by bites did not provide the same protection? It is possible that certain people who suffered bites, and who were not treated, protected themselves from the rabies virus, with no external help, by producing an immune response rapidly.

Was Pasteur's method effective? *A priori*, the answer is yes. The investigation conducted by an official British commission (James Paget, Chairman; T. Lauder Brunton, George Fleming, Joseph Lister, Richard Quain, Henry E. Roscoe, J. Burdon, Sanderson; and Victor Horsley, Secretary appointed on April 12, 1886) concluded, in June 1887: "*From the evidence of all these facts, we think it certain that the inoculations practiced by Mr. Pasteur on persons bitten by rabid animals have prevented the occurrence of hydrophobia in a large proportion of those who, if they had not been so inoculated, would have died of that disease. And we believe that the value of this discovery will be found much greater than can be estimated by its present utility, for it shows that it may become possible to avert by inoculation, even after infection, other diseases besides hydrophobia. Some have, indeed, thought it possible to avert small-pox by vaccinating those very recently exposed to its infection; but the evidence of this is, at best, inconclusive; and Mr. Pasteur's may justly be deemed the first proved method of overtaking and suppressing by inoculation a process of specific infection. His researches have also added very largely to the knowledge of the pathology of hydrophobia and have supplied what is of the highest practical value, namely, a sure means of determining whether an animal, which has died under suspicion of rabies, were really affected with that disease or not.*"[301]

This report had considerable impact on Pasteur's work; its contents were widely disseminated and commented[302]. Nevertheless, from the start of anti-rabies vaccinations, doubts about their effectiveness existed. There was no precise count of persons bitten and infected with rabies; the number of people who arrived to Pasteur's laboratory was not at all representative of the probable number of those bitten by rabid dogs or wolves. Finally, a certain number of individuals bitten by aggressive animals must have rushed to Pasteur's laboratory as a precaution or to be able to brag about withstanding the Pasteurian procedure. What percentage of these people was infected? It is impossible to know exactly. Vulpian's somewhat childish enthusiasm caused him to present statistics showing that between July 1885 and 1887, 3,852 inoculations were given, and 54 deaths occurred, the equivalent of 1.4%. Given that the generally accepted mortality rate was 20%, Vulpian concluded that 770 people should have died, and that, therefore, 716 people were saved from a horrible death by Pasteur's treatment. Even at the time, these statistics were not taken at face value by observers favourable to Pasteur, who remained lucid. "*Therefore, I agree with all the arguments advanced by those who accuse Vulpian of exaggeration.*"[303] Grancher was also a little startled: "*Such a flood of bitten patients was a little surprising, but we had to admit that the numbers of people bitten and of people dying of rabies were much greater than we initially believed. Many cases of rabies were misdiagnosed daily by physicians because all the clinical forms the disease could take, and particularly the paralytic form, were unknown.*"[304] This argument was not necessarily valid, because lack of awareness of the clinical forms of rabies would not have influenced the number of bitten people, but the idea must have set Grancher's mind at ease.

301. Horsley *in* Pasteur, O.C., t. VI, p. 870.

302. Anonyme, 1887, p. 94; Figuier, 1888a, p. 397.

303. Bouchard, 1889, p. 172.

304. Grancher, 1893, p. 680.

The *Institut Pasteur* sorted out high-risk patients from individuals at lower risk. Those who received inoculations were divided into three groups: A, B and C[305]. Patients in the Pasteurian group A were those who had been bitten by truly rabid animals. Patients were included in this group when there was irrefutable proof (symptomatic rabies in the animal which inflicted the bite), or experimental proof (inoculation of brain matter from the biting animal to experimental animals that became rabid). Out of the 273 persons included in group A, 4 died, so that the mortality rate was 1.36%. Group B was composed of people who were simply required to present a certificate recommending that they be treated. Bouchard had reservations about this: "*But I also know that physicians and veterinarians are less strict about delivering certificates that will obtain entrance to the* Institut Pasteur."[306] The cautionary principle was being applied to this group that was by far the largest: 2,175 cases and 28 deaths, that is, a 1.28% mortality rate. Nocard disagreed with Bouchard's argument: "*We could cite several cases of mortality that occurred after the veterinarians consulted reassured the individuals concerned with impardonable carelessness...*"[307]. Lastly, group C includes all persons who were bitten by animals likely to have rabies: 552 cases, with 2 deaths, that is, a mortality rate of 0.36%. Clearly, only group A could be taken into account for the purpose of establishing reasonable statistics. This group shows treatment effectiveness to be almost certain. If the analysis is deepened, to take into account the location of the bites, to the face, to the hands, or on the contrary, through boots or clothing, statistics are still clearly in favour of Pasteurian treatment. Among those with bites to the face in groups A and B, the mortality rate was 4.58%. Finally, among 199 victims of wolf bites, mortality was 16%. Renault and Mesnil's statistics concerning untreated cases showed respective mortality rates of 66% (254 subjects in the study) and 65% (300 bitten subjects in the study). Other studies produced results showing up to 80% mortality rate in these cases. Pasteurian treatment seemed to be effective[308], even when it first started and even taking into account its somewhat varied and hazardous protocols.

Reaction of Contemporaries

Overall, the Pasteurian method was given a good reception. But certain reservations were expressed. The December 20, 1885 issue of *L'Illustré pour tous, choix de bonnes lectures* described in very warm and benevolent terms the official ceremony where the Montyon Prize was awarded to Jupille. "*Jupille was acclaimed; but* Mr. *Pasteur even more so, and with good reason... Such moments only happen once in a lifetime. He was overwhelmed with all this glory and, crying like a child, hiding his face in his hands...*"[309]. But in the same issue of the same newspaper, two pages later, an anonymous article was taking up Jules Guérin's arguments claiming that Pasteur's experimental rabies might not be "true" rabies; Pasteur was merely experimenting in his laboratory: "*It is therefore theoretical rabies treated with theoretical remedies.*" The anonymous author continues, in 1885: "*There is much uncertainty in all this. It is probable, in short, - and certainly what we should wish for, - that* Mr. *Pasteur has had, in his search for the truth about the rabies microbe, a sublime intuition of this truth... but the fact is that nothing is certain yet concerning this altogether experimental treatment presented before the Academy. What seems more helpful*

305. Pasteur, O.C., t. VI, p. 860.
306. Bouchard, 1889, p. 172.
307. Nocard, 1896, p. 757.
308. Bouchard, 1889, p. 175.
309. L.G, 1885, p. 249.

is to make the pilgrimage to Saint Hubert. A few years ago we have shown how effective the protection of this great saint is to those who invoke his intervention and submit to the traditional treatment."[310]

This can seem very surprising. But the pilgrimage to Saint Hubert[311] is not so different from recourse to alternative medicine today. But as long as these practices do not replace real treatment and are not financial frauds, they are acceptable; they offer reassurance to those who believe in them.

On December 21, 1885, children from Newark (near New York), bitten by a rabid dog, arrived in Paris to be treated by Pasteur, thanks to public funds raised by the *New York Herald Tribune*. The story is interesting. The children were accompanied by Dr. Frank Billings, a famous veterinarian. Another passenger on the ship bringing the young Americans to France was Dr. Biggs, sent by the Carnegie Laboratory of the Bellevue Hospital Medical College (New York) (the first American laboratory created to study bacteriology) to observe Pasteurian anti-rabies treatment. Biggs was still a young man. He later described his visits to Pasteur's laboratory, on the occasion of the hundred-year anniversary of the scientist's birth. He recounted the numerous visits he made to Ulm Street, and he spoke particularly of the members of the British Hydrophobia Commission. Biggs described Pasteur as being affected by his hemiplegia, pale, always serious and silent, speaking little but personally seeing each new arrival who wanted to be treated, and being considerate to these patients. At first, Biggs was a fervent supporter of the Pasteurian treatment. But as Pasteur became the object of attacks from every side, a year later Biggs was much more reserved, going so far as to express a negative opinion. His doubts were to disappear in the coming years, and his initial faith in the method returned. As to the Newark children, there is no certainty that they were infected with rabies by a supposedly rabid dog. Two children bitten by the same dog did not go to Paris, and several other dogs bitten by the same animal did not develop rabies[312]. But what can be certain in cases like these? The children who were treated left in good health. They "*fell prey to a Barnum* (circus) *that exhibited them in public*"[313].

On November 2, 1886, the number of people who had been treated in Paris reached 2,490; 1,726 were from France and Algeria, 80 were from England, 52 from the Austro-Hungarian Empire, 9 from Germany, 57 from Belgium, 10 from Spain, 10 from Greece, 14 from Holland, 157 from Italy, 691 from Russia, 18 from the United States, 3 from Brazil. It is clear that what established the value of Pasteurian treatment was the cumulation of results obtained.

In the March 1895 issue of the *Chicago Clinical Review*, Mr. Lagario published the results of 366 Pasteurian anti-rabies treatments, administered in that city between July 2, 1890 and December 31, 1894. Among those vaccinated, 123 people had been bitten by animals that were in fact rabid. In 160 cases, diagnosis was based on clinical signs, and in the remaining 83 cases, on very suspicious signs. Out of the 366 persons treated, 2 died, giving a mortality rate of 0.54%[314].

Such statistics, established in or outside of France, speak very clearly.

310. Anonyme, 1885a, p. 251.
311. Bazin, 2007, p. 104.
312. Winslow, 1929, p. 71.
313. Cartaz, 1886, p. 214.
314. Anonyme, 1895b, p. 478.

Failures and Reactions they Provoked

Outside of France, resistance to all Pasteurian vaccines crystallized in German-speaking countries around Koch, and most German bacteriologists and their students. Thus, in 1887, Flügge was not a supporter of Pasteurian vaccines: "... *Pasteur undertook preventive inoculation in humans, after bites inflicted by allegedly rabid dogs... Hundreds of people have been treated by this method in Pasteur's laboratory. Some of them died of rabies. In the case of some fatalities that occurred after the preventive treatment, certain suspicions can arise... In the final analysis, neither the rabies vaccine nor the other inoculations presently in use do not constitute an ideal method of prevention of infectious diseases.*"[315] His French translator, one of his former students, Dr. Henrijean of the University of Liège (Belgium), added several notes like the following to the original text: "*AL- in the wake of the work of V. Frische of Vienna, which showed his method to be ineffective, Pasteur changed his procedure... This procedure, like the initial one, was put into practice too quickly. It is based on incomplete experiments whose results are presented only in part.*"[316] Henrijean gave no reference.

A movement of opposition against Pasteur existed in France as well. There were failures, such as the case of little Louise Pelletier. On November 9, 1885, a 10-year old girl arrived in Mr. Pasteur's Laboratory, thirty-seven days after she had been bitten. Pasteur hesitated to treat after this length of time, but he gave in to the parent's entreaties. Very quickly, the state of the child worsened and she died on December 6. Did she die of street rabies or as a result of the treatment? "*After trepanation, a small quantity of brain matter from the child was aspirated and then inoculated by trepanation to two rabbits that developed paralytic rabies eighteen days later. After these rabbits died, their medulla oblongata was inoculated to two other rabbits that developed rabies fifteen days later. This proved without a doubt that the young Pelletier girl's rabies came from the dog bite, since if she had died from rabies caused by the fixed virus injected, the inoculated rabbits would have died in seven days at the most.*"[317] Pierret provides no reference for the different timings.

Toward the end of 1886, Grancher wrote: "*Storm clouds were slowly gathering. At the Academy of Medicine, which would soon resound with battle crises, Mr. Pasteur's friends were silent and although most of the academicians were still sympathetic, they were becoming defiant. At the Faculty where I had been teaching for two years, I sometimes overheard strange comments. One day, as I was about to enter the examination room to look for a file and I heard one of my colleagues shouting: 'Yes, Pasteur is an assassin! He does not cure rabies; he gives it!' I went in and the group composed of five professors dispersed without saying a word to me. Another day, one of my colleagues stopped me and asked ironically if the recently collected funds for the Rabies Institute* (original name of the Institut Pasteur, well before its opening) *so were not being too quickly depleted by the indemnities due to the victims of the Pasteurian treatment.*"[318]

The death of a 12-year old child named Rouyer, on November 26, 1886, was a very trying event for the Pasteur team. According to Loir's account, the poor child had been bitten by a stray dog on *Filles du Calvaire* Street, on October 8, 1886. He received his first Pasteurian treatment on October 20. On November 23, one of his playmates hit him with his fist, the blow landing on the child's side; he died three days later, on October 26. His father filed a complaint with police authorities, because the State physician

315. Flügge, 1887, p. 581.
316. Henrijean, 1887, p. 581.
317. Pierret, 1923, p. 198.
318. Grancher, 1893, p. 680.

refused to issue a burial permit. It was Roux who heard the news: "A *few days after the Master's departure* (for Bordighera, where he was going to rest), *we were advised that a child treated for rabies had died. Roux learned of it and told me to go to the child's home...*"[319]. Complications arose. The police superintendent who received the complaint accompanied Loir to the office of the Prosecutor, who asked Loir to choose a pathologist. Brouardel, famous in the field, was designated to perform the autopsy; Grancher and Loir were authorised to attend. Loir was going to ask for the *medulla oblongata*, to inoculate it to two rabbits. The next day, on November 28, all concerned gathered together, in the presence of two somewhat intimidating figures, municipal council Rueff and Georges Clemenceau, both of them physicians. Loir described the scene in these terms: "*Rueff the municipal Council, and the little doctor in the black frock coat constituted the adverse party, whose interests were represented by a formidable opponent, Dr. Georges Clemenceau. He was known to be a fervent defender of heterogeny. His 1865 thesis, written under the supervision of Charles Robin, was entitled 'On the Generation of Anatomical Elements'.*"[320] But in fact, Clemenceau (French politician nicknamed "*Le Tigre*" (The Tiger), who would play an important role in the Allied victory in the First World War) was not such a fierce adversary at that time; having never obtained the title of house doctor ("*interne*"), he was definitely not equal to Brouardel. At that time, and in this situation, he was still only a "paper tiger"... Rueff was the attending physician. Brouardel arrived, performed the autopsy and gave Loir the *medulla oblongata*, that the latter placed in a jar. Brouardel declared that the child's death was caused by uremia. The *medulla oblongata* was used to inoculate two rabbits by trepanation... "*a few days later...*"[321]. Loir does not give a specific date; Maurice Vallery-Radot would write: "*About two weeks later*", without providing a source for this indication[322]. The rabbits became paralysed; the Pasteurians were greatly distressed! Loir was sent urgently to Italy, where Pasteur was resting, because the master had taken the vaccination registers with him. But this did not make much difference. Loir writes: "*I took one of the rabbits, placed his front legs on the edge of the cage and saw that he could not pull himself up. He was paralysed and so, the child had had rabies. Probably the dog bite had done its work, despite the treatment. I went to tell Roux, who was still in bed* (Roux was living in a very small room, in Pasteur's laboratory). *He came down quickly* (sic), *saw for himself that the rabbits were paralysed and told me to go and get Grancher right away.*"[323] The child had most probably died of rabies. But which rabies, street rabies or laboratory rabies, that is, transmitted by the virus adapted to rabbits, used in the treatment?

Galtier, an expert on rabbit rabies, wrote: "A *rabbit that develops rabies* (street rabies) *appears at first despondent and dejected... From the start, very pronounced weakness is observed... Paralysis, which can be said to set in suddenly, or which appears shortly after the initial weakness, usually starts in the renal region and the hind legs, gradually progressing and taking over...*"[324]. In his doctoral thesis in medicine, Roux observed: "*In rabbits, whatever the means of infection, rabies is always paralytic.*"[325] In 1883, he cited only two exceptions that occurred in the course of Pasteur's laboratory experiments. Paralytic rabies in rabbits is not necessarily laboratory rabies.

319. Loir, 1938, p. 83.
320. Loir, 1938, p. 84.
321. Loir, 1938, p. 85.
322. Vallery-Radot *in* Rosset, 1985, p. 87.
323. Loir, 1938, p. 85.
324. Galtier, 1880, p. 761.
325. Roux, 1883, p. 26.

It is interesting to note the opinion of another witness to these events. Grancher wrote on November 27, 1886 to Pasteur, regarding the Rouyer case: "*The bad news first. Little Rouvière* (sic), *58 Bretagne St., 10-12 years old, I think, bitten in September and treated in October, died last night. Roux advised me by telephone as soon as he learned of it... Thursday the child took to his bed and he died Friday - with the symptoms of ascending paralysis, ending in medullary paralysis. We will have the autopsy and the experimental test will determine, in the absence of visible lesions, the true cause of death. If, as I fear, this child succumbed to medullary rabies, we must gradually sort out here, as with the case of Schmitt and others no doubt, the part imputable in this accident to the very particular sensibility of the nervous system seen in alcoholics, in those with hereditary tuberculosis of the brain, etc. Therefore, let us record the facts to put them to good use later, and continue with a cool head.*"[326]

Grancher's subsequent letters to Pasteur, dated December 7 and 9, and January 3 and 6, no longer mention the Rouyer case... Grancher speaks of the Barregi problem and of Milano (see Ferran's method of anti-rabies vaccination), of the attacks of Fisch from Vienna, of the Réveillac case, but not a word about Rouyer[327].

The rabbits inoculated with little Rouyer's tissues died of rabies, but the existing data makes it difficult to say whether it was street rabies or laboratory rabies. Paralysis of the rear legs is not a sign of laboratory rabies in rabbits. The incubation period, the lapse of time before the onset of paralysis in the two rabbits, probably provided an indication, but this data is not mentioned by Loir, or by Grancher. The Rouyer case could have been an obvious failure of the Pasteur treatment. It could have been sufficient to cause concern among the members of the Pasteur team, especially since legal action was taken. But there was a crucial difference between the failure of a treatment undertaken late or very late and inoculation of fatal laboratory rabies. According to Loir, Brouardel asked Roux for advice, since the latter was the head of the laboratory in Pasteur's absence. Roux promised to look after vaccinations personally in the future.

The protocols needed to be more clearly defined. Brouardel established uremia as the cause of death; he absolved Pasteur and Grancher, the inoculator, of responsibility. On January 11, 1887, at the Academy of Medicine, Brouardel declared that Roux had informed him that the two rabbits inoculated with *medulla oblongata* tissue from the Rouyer boy were still in good health on January 9, forty-two days after the inoculations[328]. It's Brouardel's or Roux's word against that of Loir. The latter does not indicate that the rabbits died within the period recognized as specific to laboratory rabies. On the contrary, Loir wrote: "*Probably the dog bite had done its work, despite the treatment.*"[329] Once again, Loir's version is different than all the others, but the details he provides make it difficult to refute his testimony outright, although there is no indication of the latency period.

Still according to Loir, Pasteur remained very calm when he learned of the boy's death. But two letters Pasteur wrote to Grancher, on December 1 and on December 4, 1886, show great distress, as well as little (or no) concern about his anti-rabies protocols. He relies on data sent by Gameleïa, but not on data he recorded himself[330]. As he wrote in a letter dated December 27, 1886, "*I no longer want (and cannot) go on working alone,*

326. NAF 18103, item 419.
327. NAF 18103, items 421-429.
328. Brouardel, 1887, p. 43.
329. Loir, 1938, p. 85.
330. Pasteur, Cor., t. 4, pp. 124 & 125.

and want to provoke studies..."[331]. Finally, some letters from René Vallery-Radot to Grancher give the impression that the boy's death could have been caused by the Pasteur treatment, based on incubation periods of the rabies inoculated to the rabbits using the tissues of the Rouyer boy. On December 20, 1886, Vallery-Radot wrote Grancher: "*My very dear friend, your letter of this morning gave M. Pasteur some reassurance. He truly needed it since yesterday, he had fallen silent. He was so pale and sad that we feared for him and shared his distress. You who not only know how to hold yourself in check, but also how to restore balance in others, be they great or simple, you have the gift of finding just the right words to say in painful situations, as I had guessed when you wrote me two weeks ago* (that is, in early December) *to weigh fairly the causes keeping you in Paris, and that you must have even more pressing reasons not to stay away. All the weight is on your shoulders, but what a heavy burden and how often M. Pasteur blames himself for letting you carry it! His gratitude and ours are almost equal to your devotion...*"[332]. Then, in a letter dated December 30: "*Thank-you for your letter in which I read between the lines all that I had surmised* (sic). *The thing that will make you forget for a moment, or rather for a long while, your troubles and your worries, is that M. Pasteur is truly better...*"[333]. These lines are more suggestive of a dramatic event than a mere incident, confirming a well-intentioned cover-up... but nothing is certain.

Grancher wrote to Lutaud, the editor-in-chief of *the Journal de Médecine de Paris*, to protest the content of an article published by that paper. On April 8, 1887, Grancher proclaimed "*Rouyer: Did not die of rabies. Experimental proof was obtained by unsuccessful inoculation of the child's* medulla oblongata."[334] This was a new version of the facts: no rabies present in Rouyer... Still, real doubt persisted... and in any case, one failure would not have discredited the method.

The Réveillac case also created a stir. This 20-year old man was bitten by the dog of his employer. The animal, declared rabid by a veterinarian, was killed. The next day, young Réveillac went to see a pharmacist to be cauterised. The pharmacist sent him to see Pasteur; Réveillac did so the following day. He received a total of nineteen inoculations[335]. On December 12, 1886, he developed pain at the vaccine injection sites, but felt too weak to return to Vauquelin Street. His condition worsened and he died on Thursday, December 14. On January 4, 1887, Peter triumphantly brought this case before the Academy of Medicine. Dujardin-Beaumetz, supported by Brouardel, replied that the case was not at all clear, and could be interpreted differently. Chauveau pointed out that if the subject died of rabies, which was not proven, this only meant that the Pasteurian treatment had been ineffective. It would not be the first time that a medical treatment failed. In January 1887, Pasteur was to write, in this regard: "*We have had failures with the simple and with the intensive vaccination, and we will have more... Mr. Pasteur's method would not be human, but divine, if it was not subject to this law.*"[336] This attitude was wise. Pasteur adopted it two years after the introduction of his rabies treatments, around 1887, in the midst of much turmoil and upon incitement from his medical entourage.

Peter was to announce, raising a great hue and cry, the deaths from rabies of Louis-Victor Jansen from Dunkerk, Bernard Soudini from Constantine, Léopold Née from Arras,

331. Pasteur, Cor., t. 4, p. 134.
332. NAF 18110, item 91.
333. NAF 18110, item 97.
334. NAF 18110, item 373.
335. Pasteur, O.C., t. VI, p. 769.
336. Pasteur, O.C., t. VI, p. 769.

Goffi from London and Wilde from Rotterdam, then of Amédée Gérard from Boran and the gentleman L. de Gourgeon. Peter insisted: "*In the meanwhile, there is insufficient scientific basis for the introduction, in humans, of a preventive treatment of rabies after a bite.*"[337] This statement is not untrue, but many medical practices have been, and still are, without scientific basis. Be that as it may, the failures of the anti-rabies Pasteurian treatment were made known in the medical and popular press. Thus, Desguin described

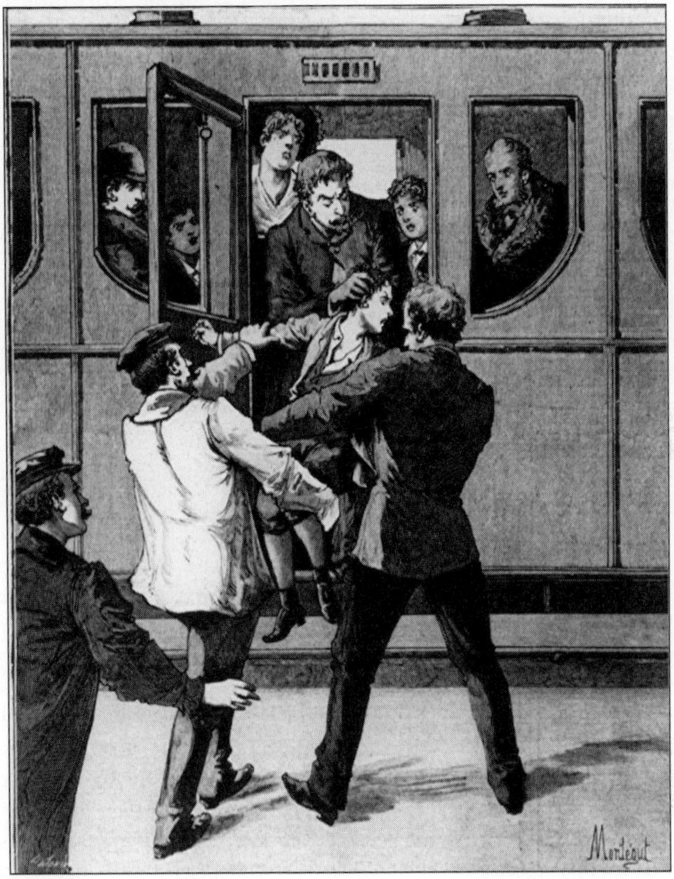

Figure 20. Child with rabies. Print by Montégut. Henri Rochefort's *l'Instransigeant illustré*, n° 122, Thursday, January 12, 1893, informed its readers: "*On December 31, at ten forty-five, the Paris train was arriving to the Bordeaux station bringing six Portuguese children who had just received at the* Institut Pasteur *on Dutot Street inoculations of the supposed anti-rabies virus. When the train stopped, a man came out of a compartment asking for help to constrain one of the children, 10-year old José-Joachim Almeida. The poor child had just woken up, wild-eyed, foaming at the mouth, seized with a sudden fit of madness, and was screaming uncontrollably. Rabies had just broken out. The station employees came to the aid of the unfortunate father. They succeeded in wrapping him in a large blanket and tying him up... but he soon succumbed to the disease. Two days earlier he had left the* Institut Pasteur *with an exeat, that is, a certificate of recovery...*". Of course, no information is provided about the circumstances of the accident. Political journalist Henri Rochefort was one of Pasteur's declared opponents.

337. Peter *in* Pasteur, O. C., t. VI, p. 807.

a case of death from rabies of a bitten man treated by Pasteur, in an article published three years after the bite and the treatment. The dog that inflicted the bite had been identified and had died of rabies. Pasteur acknowledged the case in a letter and specified that the treatment (around March 1887) had not been strong enough, and that "intensive" treatment would have been preferable, given that the bite was to the chin[338].

The national press (here, *l'Univers illustré*) did not always take Pasteur's side. In January 1886, after giving an accurate description of the Pasteurian anti-rabies method, Dr. Decaisne wrote: "*The future, and a near future at that, will reveal for all to see the inanity, not to say the danger, of your* (Pasteur's) *inoculations, each time that you will find yourself in the presence of a person who not only has been bitten, but is on the verge of developing rabies, as was the case with the Pelletier girl, who died recently of the disease in the midst of terrible suffering, a few days after your inoculations intended to save her.*"[339] Pasteurian treatment can only exert its effect in the incubation phase of the disease. Once clinical signs appear, it is without effect... Therefore, this attack was unjustified!

Pasteur's Ethics in the Context of his First Rabies Treatment

The anti-rabies vaccination administered to young Meister was Pasteur's first complete attempt to prevent rabies in a human being after a suspicious bite. In order to understand the moral implications of this act, it is important to bring answers to several essential questions.

• **Point 1:** Did Joseph Meister receive a treatment that could have been dangerous for him? The treatment given to Meister was the last immunisation protocol used in dogs before a bite; it came to be called the "*Meister vaccine protocol*". How many dogs had Pasteur treated with this protocol, and with what results? He speaks of fifty: "*Through the application of this* (without any doubt the 'Meister vaccine protocol') *method, I had succeeded in rendering fifty dogs of all ages and all races refractory to rabies, without a single failure when, unexpectedly, three people arriving from Alsace came to my office last Monday, July 6.*"[340] Pasteur often repeated this number - fifty - that he no doubt found preferable to twenty (or at best forty), the number of dogs in the May and June 1885 experiments. His confidence very soon after the end of the treatment was due to the fact that he injected a last, highly virulent dose, at least for rabbits. "*Once immunity is established, it is possible to inoculate safely the most virulent virus, in any quantity. It has always seemed to me that this had no effect other than consolidating the refractory state to rabies. Thus, Joseph Meister has escaped not only the rabies that could have developed as a consequence of his wounds, but also the rabies I inoculated him with to verify treatment-induced immunity, a form of the disease more virulent than street rabies. The very virulent final inoculation also has the advantage of limiting the duration of the worries one can have as to the consequences of a bite. If rabies were to develop, it would appear faster due to a more virulent virus than due to the virus from the bites.*"[341] Pasteur showed lack of caution in putting forth this questionable argument.

This dose had the potential of giving certain rabies to the inoculated dogs, Pasteur would say. But even this statement can be questioned, since the injection was given subcutaneously, with virus adapted to rabbits, which did not always transmit rabies,

338. Desguin, 1889, p. 249; Rommelaere, 1889, p. 251.
339. Decaisne, 1886, p. 39.
340. Pasteur, O.C., t. VI, p. 603.
341. Pasteur, O.C., t. VI, p. 603.

as Pasteur himself admitted. On December 27, 1886, he wrote: "*Any method of inoculation against rabies, except virus inoculations under the dura mater by trepanation, induces at times, and even often, a state refractory to rabies, without any manifestation of attenuated rabic disease.*"[342] Elsewhere, Pasteur also wrote: "*It is true that my fifty dogs were not bitten before I determined their rabies - refractory state, but I knew that this factor should not give me reason to worry, because I had already obtained this refractory state in a great number of dogs after they were bitten. That year, I presented to the members of the rabies Commission this new and important advance.*"[343] Pasteur described this process at the Copenhagen Conference[344], and in the August 4, 1884 report of the Rabies Commission[345].

Sufficient perspective makes it apparent that the classic treatment was perhaps not dangerous at all, or in very small measure. But on July 6, 1885, this fact was not yet known. Later, it came to light that this treatment could, in rare cases, produce immune reaction accidents prejudicial to nervous tissue; but such immune reactions were not identified at that time. When Pasteur had young Meister inoculated, he knew that dogs could be immunised, but he had carried out no actual trials in man, except for two aborted attempts at cure.

It is difficult to arrive at an objective judgement on this issue from our present-day perspective. Pasteur was, in essence, alone; in truth, the same problem arises every time a new therapeutic substance is administered to man, but the risks are minimised... However, when Pasteur inoculated Joseph Meister with virulent spinal cord, especially one-day spinal cord, he was probably exposing the boy to an unnecessary risk. It would have been judicious to conduct a few more immunisation trials with the "Meister vaccine protocol" in dogs and in some other animal species. Some of these should have left out the last, highly virulent injections.

Pasteur was caught unprepared. Vone and Meister arrived unexpectedly, and a decision had to be made without delay. Today, this type of problem is left to Commissions that make arbitrary decisions based on the scientific data available. We can consider Pasteur's protocol dangerous because of the last injections, especially the final one that was probably unnecessary.

• **Point 2:** Was this treatment, administered after a bite, effective? Of course, Pasteur had already treated bitten dogs, but he had always used an immunisation method with rabies virus passed to monkeys or rabbits, and had obtained variable results. In fact, Pasteur had always considered these results in dogs transferable to humans, a supposition which was not certain before being tested... The new method had not been tested... Meister did not develop rabies, if in fact he had been contaminated. However, given the statistics on the results of treatments administered over the years in dozens of centres to hundreds, to thousands of people, it is clear that the treatment was effective, as Pasteur believed (although he could not be certain).

• **Point 3:** Was Meister a potential candidate for this treatment, was the dog that bit him rabid and was the boy contaminated? Pasteur insisted on the fact that young Meister was in great danger, although he had no proof of this. However, there was definitely a risk: the circumstances of the aggression and the German inquest tended

342. Pasteur, O.C., t. VI, p. 636.
343. Pasteur, O.C., t. VI, p. 603.
344. Pasteur, O.C., t. VI, p. 591.
345. Pasteur, O.C., t. VI, p. 753.

to confirm that the dog was rabid. But at the time of the boy's treatment, there was no way to prove that Joseph Meister was contaminated.

The diagnostic technique, consisting of intracranial inoculation, was not accessible to the veterinarian of a small town like Sélestat, who was not specialised in rabies, a rare disease. The description of the first intracranial inoculation was published in 1881 by the Pasteurians. The technique was still an experimental procedure, not used to diagnose the disease outside Pasteur's laboratory. Loir pointed this out at the end of 1886, speaking of the Rouyer child who was autopsied by Brouardel, a case ulterior to those of Meister and Jupille. "*At that time, the laboratory at the* Ecole Normale Supérieure *was the only one performing this type of procedure* (inoculation by trepanation, to rabbits, of nervous tissue from patients killed by rabies)."[346] In fact, a few laboratories, like Galtier's for example, could have performed the test. But Meister was bitten in July 1885. How could the technique have been known and applied in Alsace, under German rule? Did this veterinarian have a trephine to perform the operation? This instrument was not usually part of the instruments of an ordinary veterinarian in private practice. *A priori*, this would have been the first such inoculation he performed. What tissue sample would he have taken and introduced in his experimental animals? Where would these animals have come from? With rabbits, one had to know the technique. How would they have been anesthetised... for surgery to even be possible? Strictly speaking, the head of the Vone's dog would have had to be taken to Paris, but the Pasteurians would have received it forty-eight hours later, in the middle of summer, probably lysed. On the other hand, keeping the suspicious dog alive would have allowed a solid diagnosis. A rabid dog died in a few days. Vone and/or the gendarmes probably did not know this, as we can easily imagine. Given the circumstances of young Meister's accident, there could have been doubt as to actual contamination, but this factor played no role in determining whether the treatment was suitable. The question was whether to treat or not. After clinical onset, rabies was fatal; intervention had to be rapid. Once the first symptoms appeared, it was too late. In 1896, Nocard and Leclainche expressed a definite opinion about experimental diagnosis used to make a treatment decision: "*Finally, treatment must be carried out as quickly as possible; it would be a gross error and evidence of great ignorance to wait for experimental proof before deciding if intervention is opportune...*"[347]. Of course, laboratory diagnosis would have been interesting from a historical perspective. The dogs that attacked Meister and Jupille were already dead when the veterinarians saw them. As for Pasteur, they only had second-hand information. But whether laboratory results would have been positive or negative, they would have arrived too late to influence the decision to treat or not. Clearly, a risk, however small, existed that Meister would contract rabies; therefore, it was perfectly legitimate to give him a reliable treatment.

• **Point 4:** Could the treatment be beneficial to young Meister? The information relative to the dog that inflicted the bites tends to show that he had rabies. Transmission of the disease from the dog to the child was possible. The possibility of transmission after bites to the hands has been established at between 10 and 20%. Clearly, the child had to be treated. Dr. Weber's cauterisation is not likely to have been effective, because it was performed late and was light (no scarring is mentioned in the reports...) as well as incomplete, since the child had fourteen bites. Looking back, it is reasonable

346. Loir, 1938, p. 84.
347. Nocard, 1896, p. 757.

to say that Joseph Meister's treatment would have been beneficial. But at the actual time of treatment, no such certainty existed.

• **Point 5:** Did Joseph Meister or his mother give informed consent? Having made the trip from Steige to Ulm Street, it can be assumed that young Meister's mother had come to seek Pasteur's help for her son. Some witnesses speak of her pleas[348], but this cannot be confirmed.

• **Point 6:** What weight should be given to the advice to treat coming from Vulpian and Grancher? To answer this question, it is best to refer to the accounts of those who witnessed the events.

Suzor (1887), who came from Mauritius to Pasteur's laboratory, sent by the Island's government to study the value of Pasteurian anti-rabies treatment and its application, reproduces Pasteur's official account of events in the laboratory in 1886-87: "*The weekly meeting of the Académie des Sciences was held on that same day, July* 6. *I* (Pasteur) *saw there our colleague Dr. Vulpian, to whom I related what had occurred. Dr. Vulpian, joined by Dr. Grancher, professor at the school of Medicine, kindly consented to come at once and see the state and the number of the wounds of little Joseph Meister. He had been bitten in fourteen different places. The advice of our learned colleague and of Dr. Grancher was, that owing to the depth and number of his wounds, Joseph Meister was exposed to almost certain death from hydrophobia. I* (Pasteur) *then communicated to Dr. Vulpian and Grancher the new results I had obtained in my studies of rabies since the time of my lecture in Copenhagen a year before. The child, being apparently doomed to inevitable death, I resolved, not without feelings of utmost anxiety, as may well be imagined, to apply to him the method of prophylaxis which had never failed me in dogs. My set of fifty dogs, indeed, had not been bitten before they were made refractory to rabies, but that objection had no share in my preoccupations, for I had already, in the course of the other experiments, rendered a large number of dogs refractory after they had been bitten.*"[349]

In 1886, Grancher, who had not been among Pasteur's close associates in the months before the Meister case, commented on Pasteur's work: "*During the first half of 1885, he* (Pasteur) *conducted a series of experiments with increasingly successful results, and finally arriving at the one that served as a basis for human vaccination, I mean the experiment involving 50 dogs, using the following method. Inoculations were given successively, and day by day, to 50 dogs, with more and more virulent cord, starting with fifteen-day cord and ending with fresh cord collected on the day of the autopsy. After this preparation, the 50 dogs proved to be refractory to the most virulent subcutaneous or even intracerebral inoculation; on the other hand, 50 control dogs were infected with rabies in numbers corresponding to the usual ratios for the various modes of inoculation.*"[350] Pasteur did not speak of the fifty control dogs in his laboratory notes. Did he discuss them? Did Grancher examine Pasteur's notebooks in 1886? It is unlikely that he would have, before young Meister's treatment, since he was not working at the *Ecole Normale Supérieure*, although he inoculated bitten patients there. He was repeating what Pasteur told him.

But in 1893, six or seven years later, Grancher wrote: "He (Pasteur) *started his vaccination experiments on dogs before and after infection, by inoculating increasingly more virulent fragments of spinal cord in emulsion, diluted in a little sterilised water. The dogs*

348. P.A, 1936, p. 69.
349. Suzor, 1887, p. 93.
350. Grancher, 1886, p. 33.

treated in this manner, even after bites, even after trepanation and infection, most often recover or better yet, do not develop rabies. They are vaccinated."[351] This perspective is more subtle, qualified by the "*most often*", and no doubt reflects more detailed knowledge of the subject! At this time, Grancher could have had access to Pasteur's notes, since he was inoculating patients at the *Ecole Normale Supérieure*, and Grancher must have discussed the experiments with Roux who was familiar with Pasteur's notebooks.

On March 6, 1886, Cartaz described the situation by speaking of "*about fifty dogs, treated in this manner* (anti-rabies vaccination with rabbit cord stored in "dry flask", containing increasingly more virulent rabies virus), *remained for many months absolutely safe from any inoculation, even the most virulent. The immunity induced in dogs guaranteed success for human cases of rabies, if the victims were treated in time. In man, the rabies incubation period varies between three or four weeks to several months. If, right at the beginning, a series of inoculations of increasing intensity is administered, it becomes possible, before the onset of accidents, to develop in the system a suffusion that will confer to the patient the same immunity as that seen in dogs. Of course, at the stage where there would be symptoms of this disease now only in its second or third day of evolution, the patient can no longer benefit from this treatment. It would be like vaccinating at the height of smallpox infection; prevention has no effect.*"[352] Obviously, Dr. Cartaz misunderstood Pasteur's statements (?): *a priori*, the number of dogs treated with rabbit cord was not fifty, and there was no period of many months before Joseph Meister's treatment.

In 1890, Peuch wrote: "*After 50 dogs were vaccinated by this method without a single failure, and after experiments on a large number of dogs showed that the method made it possible to induce immunity to rabies in them after bites and even after inoculation by trepanation, that is, by an operation that unfailingly transmits rabies, Mr. Pasteur applied his method to human beings* in 1885."[353] Peuch, an expert on rabies, specifies that he understood that the 50 dogs were treated using the so-called dry flask method.

In 1891, Trouessart wrote in a document presented to the Academy of Sciences by Pasteur himself: "*By this method* (dried rabbit cord), *much simpler than the previous method* (virus passed to monkeys), *Mr. Pasteur was able to render fifty dogs refractory to rabies. It was possible to inoculate them with rabies virus subcutaneously, and even by trepanation, without developing the disease. By virtue of these precedents, which established rabies prevention in dogs by inoculation either before or after bites, Mr. Pasteur decided to attempt preventive inoculation, after bites, in man.*"[354]

Vulpian, 1895. "*But although he was convinced by numerous experiments, and above all by the recent ones conducted on a series of fifty dogs, that preventive inoculations, as he was practicing them, never produce rabies...*"[355].

René Vallery-Radot, in 1900, in his book *La Vie de Pasteur*, did not provide any more details, although he probably had Pasteur's notebooks, or had access to them, because they would have been in the possession of Mrs Louis Pasteur, who died on September 23, 1910: "*Pasteur was conducting two parallel series of experiments on 125 dispersed dogs. The first series consisted in producing, by preventive inoculations, dogs refractory to rabies;*

351. Grancher, 1893, p. 673.
352. Cartaz, 1886, p. 213.
353. Peuch, 1890, p. 503.
354. Trouessart, 1891, p. 129.
355. Vulpian, 1895, p. 623.

the second consisted in preventing rabies from developing in bitten and inoculated dogs. Each series included control dogs, as it had the previous year."[356] These were the experiments conducted for the Commission. This passage in Vallery-Radot's book is on the page preceding the beginning of the account of Joseph Meister's arrival to the *Ecole Normale Supérieure*. The author wanted to link these events in the reader's mind, by recounting them one after the other. In addition, he described young Meister's first treatment as follows: "*Vulpian was of the opinion that Pasteur's experiments on dogs were sufficiently conclusive to make it possible to expect the same success in the human pathology. This professor, usually so reserved, even asked why not try the treatment. Was there any other effective treatment against rabies? And if only hot-iron cauterisation had been performed! But what good was carbolic acid cauterisation twelve hours after the accident? Weighing in the balance on the one hand the almost certain danger for the child of dying of rabies, and on the other hand the chances of saving him from death, it was more than a right, it was an obligation for Pasteur to apply the anti-rabies inoculation to young Meister. Dr. Grancher, whom Pasteur wanted to consult as well, was of the same opinion.*"[357] Of course, this version of events is biased, like much of this book.

We cannot be certain to what extent Pasteur had told the absolute truth in the description he was making of his work on rabies to Vulpian and Grancher, at the time when a decision about treating little Meister had to be made. I know of no account of a conversation between Pasteur and Vulpian, or a discussion involving the two of them and Grancher, as Loir indicates[358]. This point remains obscure. Pasteur's notebooks give the impression that the fifty dogs treated by the Meister method never existed. Should this because for indignation? What would Joseph Meister have become without his treatment? The story as we know it leaves room for interpretation...

• **Point 7.** What was the legal context in which Pasteur treated Joseph Meister? Pasteur, who was not a physician, stated several times publicly that he was not practicing illegal medicine, by which he meant that he would not inoculate a human being himself, but would ask a physician to do it, that is, to take responsibility for it: "*Not being a doctor, I will ask a physician to be so kind as to assist me, so that I will not practice illegal medicine...*"[359]. However, in his October 26, 1885 communication, Pasteur wrote: "*Since this child's death seemed inevitable, I decided, not without sharp and cruel quqlms, as you might well imagine, to try on Joseph Meister the method that I had always used successfully with dogs.*" Or: "*Last Tuesday, with the kind assistance of* MM. *Vulpian and Grancher, I had to start treating a young boy of fifteen* (Jean-Baptiste Jupille), *bitten fully six days ago on both hands, in particularly serious circumstances.*"[360] Pasteur took responsibility for the first two complete treatments, but for Meister there was no great risk, since the treatment had taken place in July.

In 1885, pharmaceutical legislation was governed by various texts that "scientific progress", real or not, had clearly made obsolete[361]. In France, at the time of Joseph Meister's treatment, the 1883 edition of the *Codex medicamentorius* was in effect. It was the official version approved by the government and containing all its prescriptions for pharmaceutical preparations to be delivered by pharmacists (article 38 of the law

356. Vallery-Radot, 1900, p. 598.
357. Vallery-Radot, 1900, p. 601.
358. Loir, 1938, p. 74.
359. Pasteur, O.C., t. VII, p. 371.
360. Pasteur, O.C., t. VI, p. 603.
361. Dechambre, 1876, t. 18 première série, p. 260; 1876, t. 3 series 3, p. 371; Littré, 1886, p. 330.

of Germinal, year XI of the French revolutionary calendar - April 1803). This Codex included only substances or preparations to be sold commercially.

On February 25, 1884 Pasteur wrote: "*Is it not possible that human medicine might benefit from the long incubation period of rabies to try to establish in this lapse of time, before the onset of the first rabies symptoms, a refractory state in the bitten subjects?*"[362] And on May 19, 1884: "*Thanks to the duration of the rabies incubation period after bites, I am surely justified in believing that it is altogether possible to determine the refractory state of the subjects before the fatal disease develops following a bite.*"[363] Pasteur obviously considered his treatment preventive of an onset of rabies. In his reports on his first inoculations, Pasteur used many expressions to designate these inoculations: the word "*treatment*" several dozen times, "*a method for the prevention of rabies after a bite*"[364], "*rabies prevention method*" or "*rabies prevention*" or "*the method of rabies prevention*"[365], "*preventive inoculations*"[366]. Obviously, Pasteur thought that he was giving his patients preventive treatment, before the onset of the clinical phase of rabies. Moreover, he knew that once symptomatic, rabies was, *a priori*, incurable, at least in laboratory animals[367] and in man, with traditional treatments.

In 1885, Pastorien antirabies treatment was considered preventive rather than curative by Pasteur, and outside the sphere of approved or secret remedies. It was not governed by the French pharmaceutical legislation of the period. It remained outside its jurisdiction. It seems that rather daring treatments at the time, such as Brown-Sequard glandular extracts, goat blood transfusion to one tuberculosis patient and many others, remained outside the scope of any legislation. The fact remains that in various countries many laboratories were rapidly organised to prepare and administer Pasteurian antirabies treatment, *a priori* without any legal problems. It was clear that in France, as in other countries, a legal void existed in this area. In France, this lack was remedied by a law applying to opotherapy as well as to sera and vaccines, passed in 1895.

It is difficult to guess what would have been the outcome of legal proceedings against Jacques-Joseph Grancher and perhaps Louis Pasteur in case of unfortunate consequences of the Pasteurian antirabies treatment administered to a patient. This almost happened in France when 12-year old Rouyer died on November 26, 1886, but fortunately the case was settled out of Court (*see Rouyer case*). This case would have been governed by the existing legislation.

Louis Pasteur's ethics, at the time of the first antirabies treatments, is a subject to be considered in the context of the times. Today's standards can be applied neither to the man nor to his work. This work can give indications about the positions Pasteur took, if it is viewed in the historical context of the times. Any judgement expressed must consider the value of the treatment, its safety and the circumstances of the trials. The first two attempts (Girard and Julie-Antoinette Poughon) involved persons who, at the time of treatment, were considered by the physicians in charge to present the clinical stage of rabies, with no hope of being cured. Meister and Jupille had been

362. Pasteur, O.C., t. VI, p. 579.
363. Pasteur, O.C., t. VI, p. 586.
364. Pasteur, O.C., t. VI, pp. 612 to 614, 617, 621.
365. Pasteur, O.C., t. VI, pp. 619 and 623.
366. Pasteur, O.C., t. VI, p. 621.
367. Pasteur, O.C., t. VI, p. 575.

badly bitten by dogs with probable, if not certain, rabies. At the time, a legal void existed that left civil responsibility to the treating physician, but Pasteur seems not to have acted against the law.

History has shown Pasteurian antirabies treatment to have been overwhelmingly successful. Pasteur succeeded and we can only be awed and thankful, along with the thousands of people he saved. The moral assessment of the first trials of Pasteur's treatment remains an individual matter, but this assessment must be nuanced.

Pasteur's ethics in regard to the first anti-rabies treatments must be assessed in the context of his time. Pasteur, the man, cannot be adequately judged based on present-day criteria. Moral judgement of Pasteur's first trials of his anti-rabies treatment on human beings is necessarily subjective, but this work can explain Pasteur's attitudes, once they are placed in their proper historical context.

National and International Dissemination of the Method

Very quickly, bitten persons, contaminated or not, came to see Pasteur in great numbers. The most urgent problems had to take priority. It became necessary to open anti-rabies treatment centres abroad, the first in Odessa, then a second in Saint-Petersbourg. Adrien Loir travelled to that city, taking with him a cage containing two rabbits inoculated with rabies virus. In 1888, seven Pasteur Institutes were treating patients infected with rabies in Russia. Between 1886 and 1892, out of 14,369 people vaccinated 256 died, and there were 101 fatalities among the 1,621 people bitten by mad wolves[368], a remarkable result. In New York, a Centre opened on July 4, 1886, thanks to Dr. Mott, who had made the trip to Paris to obtain rabies virus and to be given instructions by Pasteur in person[369]. Calmette was sent to Saigon to organise a vaccine centre. He took with him rabic brains and spinal cords in glycerine. When he arrived, two months later, these organs were still virulent[370]. The Saigon (Hô-chi-Minh City) Pasteur Institute was founded in January 1891. Between May 1, 1893 and May 1, 1894, 49 people were treated there against rabies; 31 of them were Europeans, half of them Dutch from Batavia (Jakarta, Indonesia)[371]. An anti-rabies Institute opened in Marseille on December 9, 1893, approved by Pasteur and receiving an annual subsidy of 10,000 francs (about 32,000 euros) from the City of Marseille. The Institute treated bitten individuals from the South of France, Corsica and Algeria[372]. And the method continued to produce good results.

In 1909, Remlinger published a summary of all the anti-rabies vaccinations performed up to that time, and gave a total of 131,579 people treated, and 549 fatalities, that is, a mortality rate of 0.41%[373]. Between 1886 and 1937, 54,484 people received antirabies treatment in the various Pasteur Institutes: 151 died despite the inoculations; between 1922 and 1939, no fatalities occurred[374]. Even fault-finders will have to admit that the "classic" Pasteurian treatment was at least incapable of transmitting rabies to people who had not, in fact, been contaminated. All these results are very impressive, and it is easy to see why Pasteur is glorified. The impact of such results was, and still is, incalculable!

368. Chronique, 1897, p. 158.
369. Chronique, 1886, p. 142.
370. Nocard, 1892, p. 248; Anonyme, 1895a, p. 316.
371. Anonyme, 1895a, p. 317.
372. Anonyme, 1893, p. 794.
373. Remlinger, 1909, p. 114.
374. Cadilhac, 1939, p. 368.

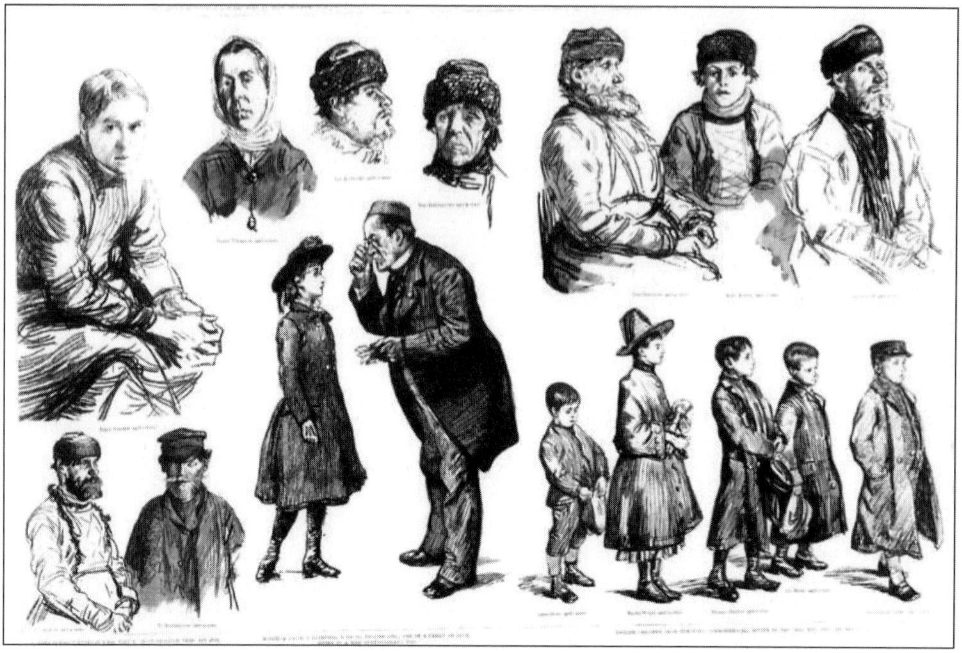

Figure 21. Illustration published in the British newspaper *The Graphic* on April 3, 1886, with the following caption: "*Mr. Pasteur's experiments in Paris for the cure of hydrophobia - The doctor and some of his patients. From left to right, top row: Russian peasants bitten by a mad wolf at Beloi, Smolensk, February 28th. Nikola Vassilev, aged 17 years, Natalie Tchomirov, aged 30 years, Ivan Andronsovsky, aged 50 years, Ivan Demianov, aged 40 years, Andrei Azarow, aged 19 years, Gartchewich, aged 49 years. From left to right, bottom row: Mr. Pasteur examining a young English girl, one of a family of four, bitten by a mad Newfoundland dog. English children from Bradford, Yorshire - All bitten by the same mad dog, January 24th: James Hosty, aged 7 years, Martha Wright, aged 10 years, Thomas Sharkey, aged 8 years, Asa Moore, aged 8 years, Swithenbank Turner, aged 7 years.*"

The fight against rabies was profoundly changed by Pasteur and his work. Adaptation to the new knowledge took various forms. "*In England, in 1886, The Government appointed a Committee to inquire into the Pasteur's method. It reported favourably: and, after a* Mansion House Meeting *on July 1, 1889, Sir James Whitehead presiding, a thank-offering of 40,000 francs was sent to the* Institut Pasteur. *We have to note, that the passing of the muzzling* Act, *and the consequent stamping out of rabies in this island, were largely due to Pasteur's influence.*"[375a] Paget based this on a note written by Sir Victor Horsley, secretary of the Committee: "*The freedom of England from rabies I take to be one of the great achievements of modern science: and we owe it entirely to M. Pasteur… I had the honour of acting as secretary of a committee that was appointed by the Government to inquire into M. Pasteur's treatment; and, when the Committee was in Paris, M. Pasteur said to us, 'Why do you come here to study my method?… You do not require it in England at all. I have proved that this is an infectious disease: all you have to do is to establish a brief quarantine covering the incubation period muzzle all your dogs at the present moment, and in a few years you will be free.'*

375a. Paget, 1914, p. 85.

When the Committee returned and reported to the houses of Parliament, this point, of course, was always before us. - Sir Victor Horsley, Evidence before the Royal Commission of Vivisection, November 13, 1907."[375b]

The Committee also proposed the application of Mr. Pasteur's treatment. In the ten years before 1885, there had been an annual overage of 43 deaths from rabies in England, 8.5 of them in London. At an average transmission rate of 5 percent, there would be 860 people to treat yearly, 170 of them in London[376]. The Committee was officially impartial, but it clearly favoured eradication of the disease, a solution that was in fact implemented thanks to the insular nature of the territory. "*But what Act could muzzle all the pariah-dogs in India, and all the wolves in Russia?*"[377]

The Pasteurian treatment certainly saved a great number of people, but even a small number would have been a considerable success. Eradication of rabies in vector animals was initially the result of measures of hygiene and public health protection, followed by the vaccination of more or less tame or wild animals that constituted reservoirs of virus. Unfortunately, bat rabies still exists in many countries, and has already made human victims. The vaccines available today are unsuitable for these emerging viruses, which have to make the object of new studies.

The Last Stages of Pasteur's Active Scientific Life

From the end of 1885 on, Pasteur deserted, for all intents and purposes, his laboratory, to concentrate on the application of anti-rabies treatments; but he continued to show great interest in these experiments. For instance, he tried treatments administered over very short periods, to prevent rabies from wolf bites.

On August 3, 1886, on one of the little gray cards (about 12 by 8 cm) on which he noted his instructions to Eugène or the names and treatments of current patients, he wrote: "*Written this August 3, 1886 Note for Eugène. 14 at the Pound 20 at Fréjis 6 at Vauquelin 10 at Bourrel Vaccinate 50 new dogs with 14,12,10,8,6,4,2,0 - day cord within 24 hours, giving 50 vaccinated dogs. Take them to Villeneuve at 8 o'clock in the morning, 10 o'clock, 12, 2, 4, 6, 8 o'clock the next day and 10 o'clock. Leave these dogs at Villeneuve.*"[378] The remaining instructions are written on a second card. "*After 6 months, trepanate 2; after 8 months, trepanate 2, after 21 days, trepanate 2; after 12 months, trepanate 2; after 2 months, trepanate 2, after 4 months, trepanate 2; after 6 months, trepanate 2; after 8 months, trepanate 2; after 22 months, trepanate 2; after 12 months, trepanate 2;after 14 months, trepanate 2; after 16 months, trepanate 2; after 18 months, treapnate 2; after 20 months, trepanate 2; after 22 months, trepanate 2; after 24 months, trepanate 2. I have a copy of this card, August 3, 1886. L. P.*"[379]

This experiment was carried out, at least in part, on August 10, 12, 14 and 20. Out of eight dogs, four survived and four died of rabies[380]. The trials of vaccination after trepanation were not always successful. Pasteur never had a reliable and reproducible method of inoculation, less intrusive than intracranial inoculation but more effective than subcutaneous inoculation at random.

375b. Horsley *in* Paget, 1914, p. 85.
376. Horsley *in* Pasteur, O.C., t. VI, p. 870.
377. Paget, 1914, p. 85.
378. NAF 18094, item 28.
379. NAF 18094, item 29.
380. Pasteur, O.C., t. VI, p. 637.

On August 10, 1886, Pasteur was concerned about the safety of his treatments: "*Finally it is imperative to be able to vaccinate with cord passed numerous times, which no longer gives rabies.*"[381]

"*This August 20, 1886. Various comments. To trepanate a new dog with cord from dogs with street rabies, then vaccinate, is one of the most peremptory proofs of the effectiveness of the method when the vaccination is successful. Indeed, it is sometimes successful. See a first successful trial out of two attempts 13th notebook page 87… Roux (this August 20) thinks that virus of cord from current passages between the 118th and 122nd passages might no longer provide protection in humans as it did between the 110th and 115th passages, because in these subc. experiments this virus subjected to very numerous passages no longer gave rabies. I believe that he is wrong.*"[382]

"*September 6, 1886. Trial of vaccination with non virulent cord.*" In a note: "*Total failure.*" "*Vaccination of 4 guinea pigs as follows: one with 6 syringes: cord from August 17, which is 20-day cord… These 4 guinea pigs will be trepanned and inoculated with street rabies virus in ten to twelve days… Therefore no vaccinal matter in the 20, 18, 16, 14-day cord above.*"[383]

In 1887 and 1888, there are summaries of experiments and vaccinations of "dogs with owners". Pasteur also had experiments conducted on chicken cholera contagion among rabbits, in 1888[384].

Pasteur's feverish pace of experimentation ended little by little, but not completely. Thus, a note he wrote on August 5, 1890 indicates: "*Note for* (1 word) *Have n° 123 bitten* (with new control) *on August 1890. Take back the 2 dogs to Villeneuve l'Etang. This August 5, 1890. Sacrifice n° 49, 73, 41, 91, 92. T.*"[385]

Pasteur Today... in the Field of Vaccines

"*It is not possible to measure, or to put into words, the value of Pasteur's work and the range of his influence. All attempts to estimate or explain him are mere foolishness. Genius made his work what it was: and genius is no more the result of circumstances than a play by Shakespeare is the result of a theatre and an audience.*"
Stephen Paget, 1914[386].

"*Pasteur is unique, and not only in his native country. With Newton, Darwin and Einstein, he stands as an immortal scientist… He is part of the Pantheon.*"
W.F. Bynum, 1995[387].

Throughout his life and after his death, Pasteur was crowned with glory but was also the object of severe criticism, which persists still. Scientifically, his work was nearly perfect, but he skipped stages as he saw fit, at the risk of impinging on or even overlooking certain principles...

381. NAF 18020, f.P. 5.
382. NAF 18020, f.P. 9.
383. NAF 18020, f.P. 12.
384. NAF 18020.
385. NAF 18094, item 70.
386. Paget, 1914, p. 1.
387. Bynum, 1995, p. 25.

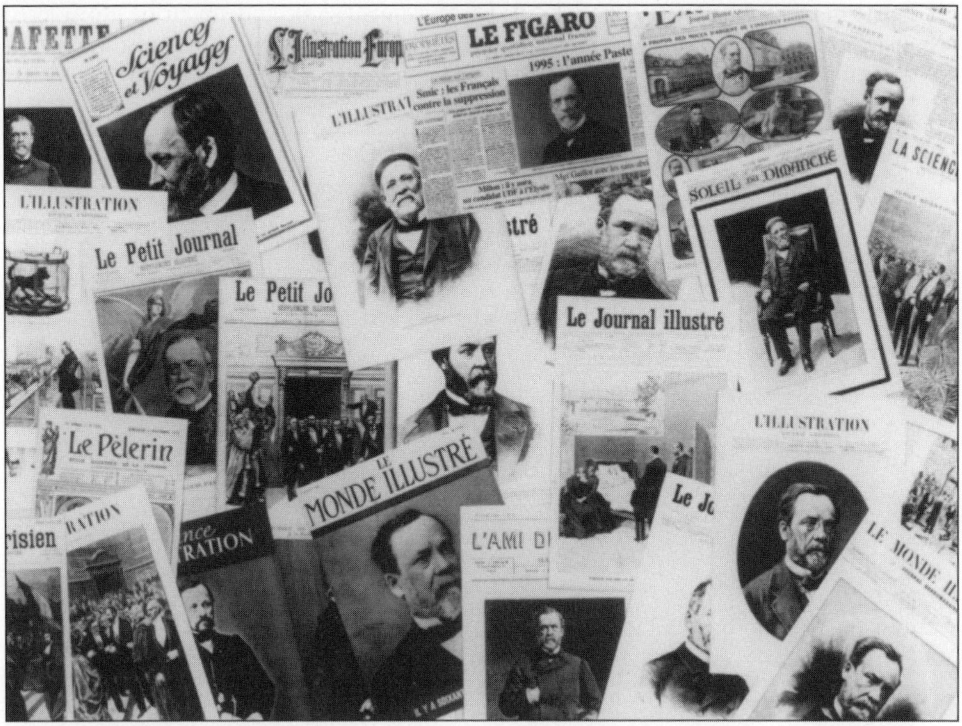

Figure 22. Throughout most of his life, and particularly in the last years and after his death, Pasteur was the object of veritable veneration. He often appeared on the cover of numerous French publications.

Pasteur's invention of "Pasteurian"vaccines makes his contribution to medicine, science and humanity enormous. Of course, his vaccines were still at a primitive stage of development. He probably made a more useful contribution to agricultural economy by discovering the bacterial origin of several animal diseases and the principles of their prophylactic effect than by marketing his vaccine against ruminant anthrax. In truth, the application of his results is not their most important aspect, although the anti-rabies treatment was an undeniable success, and no doubt saved thousands of people from a horrible death. Dr. Léon Moynac wrote in 1887 or 1888, in the Paul Labarthe 2072-page Medical Dictionary for the general public, the following lines: "*Allow me to end this article, already quite long, by submitting a simple question for your consideration. Why is it that* Mr. Pasteur, *instead of concentrating so relentlessly on preventing and healing rabies which, after all, causes no more than 30 deaths per year in France, does not work on applying his method of attenuation and prevention to typhoid fever, which kills over 20,000 Frenchmen per year, or to tuberculosis which, in the same space of time, kills no less than 100,000 of our countrymen! The day he will triumph over one of these terrible afflictions, he will have fully earned this superb title of 'benefactor of humanity'*."[388]

It is difficult to deny the logic of this argument, but scientific results cannot be willed. And is it not true to say that the inventors of vaccines against the plague or tuberculosis

388. Moynac, 1887-1888, p. 849.

are direct heirs of the Pasteurian School? Pasteur pursued an endeavour he considered promising. It is the path of investigation he established that remains his most important contribution.

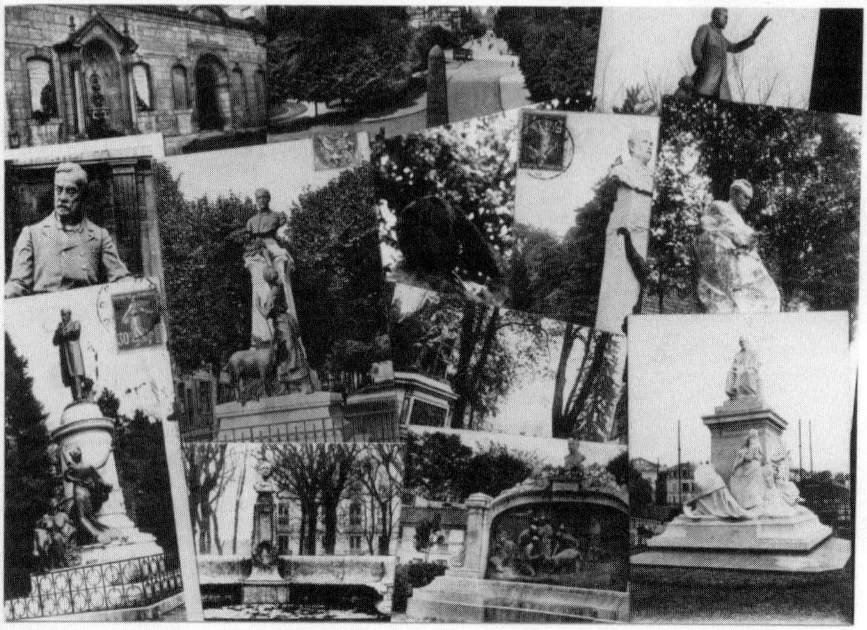

Figure 23. Pasteur was held up as a model to the French (and to the rest of the world) by his country, particularly during the Third Republic. Within a short time, statues of him were erected in all the cities and towns where he had lived and worked. Between 1940 and 1945, some of them were, sad to say, destroyed by being melted down by the "*Groupement industriel de récupération des métaux*" (Industrial Group for the recovery of metal), for the benefit of the German occupational army. Some of these statues survived, like the ones in Dole and Arbois; some were rebuilt, like the one in Chartres, others disappeared... The statues resemble each-other: they pay tribute to Pasteur for his anthrax vaccine, and the later ones commemorate his rabies vaccine.

Pasteur's rabies treatment protocols can be questioned, particularly in terms of the very scanty preliminary studies to which they were subjected before use. In Pasteur's time, there were many treatments administered to patients without too many precautionary measures: syphilisation; Koch's tuberculin; goat blood transfusions against tuberculosis (painting by M. Jules Adler, 1892 Paris Salon, reprinted in *l'Illustration*, in the March 7, 1891 issue (N° 2506); metal transfusion with a static electricity machine, in the *Petit Journal* (Sept. 1, 1901) to treat tuberculosis; and no doubt many others... In comparison, Pasteur's anti-rabies treatment has proved to be effective in the long term, and there seems to be a very small number of fatal accidents associated with it, in a compassionate use setting, real or not... if any certainty can exist in such matters!

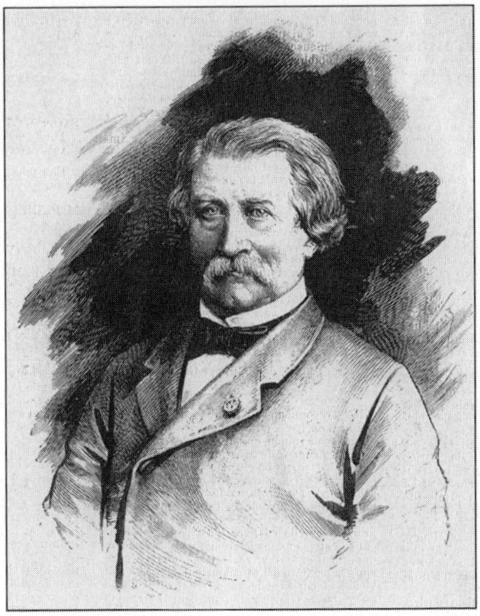

Henry Bouley (1812-1885). President of the Academy of Sciences (Paris); many newspapers devoted an article to him upon his death. Drawing by M. Tradée. Photo: Trachelut-Walkman, published in *La France illustrée*, N° 576, December 12, 1885.

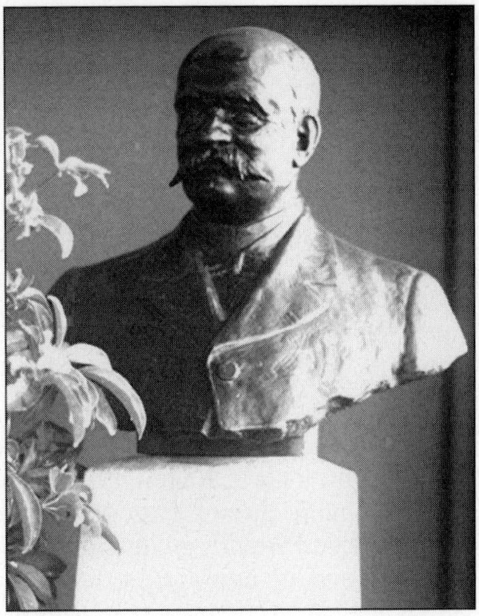

Pierre Galtier (1846-1908). This bust is one of the few representations of this worthy scientist, relentless researcher and forerunner of Pasteur in the fight against rabies. (Photo kindly provided by Dr. G. Chappuis, Mérial.)

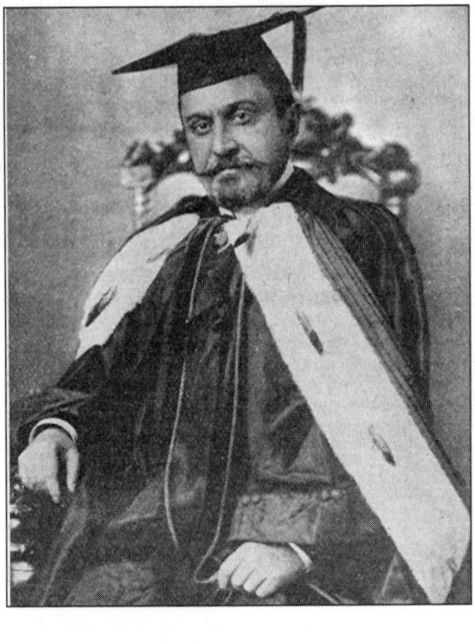

Adrien Loir (1862-1941). Dr. Loir, professor at the University of Montreal. Photograph by J-A Dumas. "*For the first time in 1906, a French professor was given an official teaching position in a Canadian medical Faculty. Dr. Adrien Loir was the person designated to receive this honour.*" This mark of recognition shows the high esteem in which Loir was held. The name of this nephew of Pasteur's, through maternal lineage, is too often associated mostly with the recollections (of questionable accuracy) in his book *A l'ombre de Pasteur* (In Pasteur's shadow). (*Le Supplément du Journal de Voyages*, N° 6017, June 7, 1908.)

Figure 24. Three people close to Pasteur during experiments on the anti-rabies vaccine.

In laboratories, Pasteur's experiments have left their mark: "Pasteur pipettes" are in common use, and pasteurisation has become a process familiar to everyone... Pasteur was a pioneer, as witnessed by the fact that his two contemporaries, competing vaccinators - Ferran and Toussaint - unequivocally declared themselves his disciples and never changed their position. At the very start of anti-rabies vaccinations, numerous establishments were created to implement his method of prevention; they were commonly called "*Institut Pasteur*" or "*Centre antirabique*". In 1910, the British newspaper *Spectator* wrote: "*There are more than sixty Pasteur Institutes...*"[389]. Many of them disappeared when the network of treatment centres was restructured, but this number illustrates that the Pasteurian method and its usefulness were held in high esteem far and wide. But the most concrete expression of this success was the creation of the *Institut Pasteur* in Paris, the mother house of the international network, and of the *Institut Pasteur* in Lille.

Pasteur opened a new path. He did not do it alone; many others contributed to its development. Joubert, Raulin, Perdrix and especially Duclaux, Chamberland and Roux, as well as more distant Pasteurians like Nocard, Yersin, Haffkine, Gameleïa... and others outside Pasteur's group, an entire diaspora disseminated throughout the world, were then and are now part of the great Pasteurian family. Today, the name "Pasteur" can be applied to the man as well as to a community.

This chapter was not intended to defend a myth. Examination of Pasteur's laboratory notes at the *Ecole Normale Supérieure* show the scientist in a decidedly human light and reveal, beyond a few errors and approximations, the quality and determination of his work. The present text attempts to draw a living portrait of the man, and to place his work on the first vaccines in its proper context.

Pasteur has made an immense contribution to medicine, not only through four vaccines, but thanks to the concept of artificial vaccines. Not simply an advance, but a veritable revolution.

He is a benefactor of humanity. His scientific work has to be seen in this perspective. It is an immense, magnificent and exceptional body of work.

The criticisms directed against Pasteur and the vaccines of the last years are for the most part unfounded (and most of all intended to bring credit to their authors). Most of them reveal scientific incompetence and historical ignorance, as well as clear bias*.

As to Pasteur himself, as a personal figure... He still exerts fascination[390], but that is a separate subject... and each perspective is different. The myth surrounding Pasteur has developed for understandably human reasons. He was an example to follow for French children and even for children everywhere. He was a man with universal appeal: he came from humble origins, worked tirelessly and achieved exceptional success. Furthermore, popular opinion credits him with kindness, modesty and humility. For those in power, he was a glorious example to give to the French population in times of adversity; the ideal model for children to follow...

* These critical remarks will be the subject of a separate analysis.

389. Paget, 1914, p. 87.

390. Bazin, 2009.

III
Vaccines Reach Maturity

9
The Arrival of the Classic Vaccines: Heralding in the New Medicine

"With Pasteur, chemistry established its hold on medicine. And this hold was likely to endure."
Emile Duclaux, 1896[1].

In the years following the exceptional work undertaken by Pasteur, Koch and their students, most research in microbiology and immunology focused on the search for new pathogenic agents responsible for major human and animal infectious diseases, as well as on the development of "Pasteurian" vaccines: first-generation vaccines composed of the pathogenic agents themselves, or of the products they secreted. Much later, the field of genetics introduced a new, decisive stage in biology, with the arrival of second-generation vaccines.

The Invention of Dead or Chemical Vaccines: 1884, 1885, 1886...

Between 1884 and 1886, Daniel Salmon and Theobald Smith published a great discovery, that of the first dead vaccine (with killed bacteria), that is, the use of an inert substance to provide immunity. Their work involved an experimental model of purely scientific interest: the immunisation of pigeons against *salmonella*, agent of a swine disease Salmon and Smith called "hog cholera"*[2]. Roux and Chamberland were pursuing the same objective, but they were a little late. Their experimental model was acute septicaemia induced in guinea pigs. This was a good model, because the septic vibrion kills guinea pigs, even at very low doses, within a few hours. The two French scientists were just a step behind the Americans, to whom they gave credit openly in a note: "*Just as we were about to publish, we read in the Annual Report of the United States Department of Agriculture that Mr. Salmon has been able to confer immunity to pigeons against hog cholera by injecting these animals with sterilised cultures of the microbe of this disease.*"[3] But they also claimed credit for themselves, pointing out the superior quality of their results, which they considered more conclusive than those of the scientists one step ahead of them.

---

* "Hog cholera" or classical swine fever.

1. Duclaux, 1896, p. 395.
2. Salmon, 1884-1886.
3. Roux, 1887, p. 563.

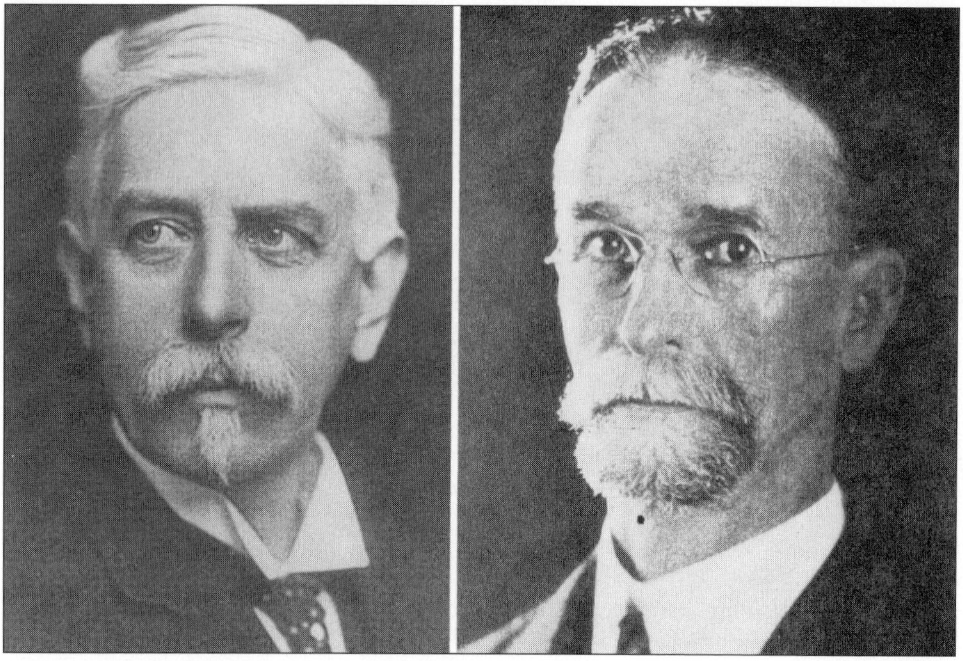

Figure 1. Left: Daniel Elmer Salmon (1850-1914), American veterinarian and microbiologist. He discovered a genus most commonly associated with various types of food poisoning named after him *salmonella*. Right: Theobald Smith (1859-1934), American physician, microbiologist. He showed that Texas cattle fever was spread by ticks, the first proof of the role of arthropods in transmitting human or animal disease (1888-1893). Salmon and Smith demonstrate that the injection of heat-killed bacilli can confer immunity against the disease (chemical vaccine). (Bigger, 1939, plate 11.)

They concluded their article with a long discussion of the obvious advantages of killed organism vaccines, much easier to prepare than attenuated living organism vaccines[4]. In 1880, Pasteur had investigated this possibility of immunisation using killed microbes, but his model, chicken cholera, did not produce immunisation[5]. He had chosen the wrong model, and he did not try again. This failure had reinforced his belief in the theory of "immunisation by exhaustion". He came back to this theory in 1885, after having conceived of a "vaccinating matter". On January 31, 1885, he experimented with a soluble vaccinating matter: anthrax-contaminated blood, heated and then inoculated to guinea pigs that subsequently died of anthrax. Pasteur wrote: "*Experiment to be redone.*"[6] He continued: "*Chicken cholera - Vaccination trial with filtered cultures.*"[7] He filtered a culture and inoculated it to a chicken that survived. But the same chicken did not withstand a virulent test dose, and neither did the control chicken. Pasteur wrote: "*To be tried again. Should filtering take place in the presence of CO2? Air can destroy vaccinating matter.*"[8] Interestingly, Pasteur informed Chamberland of his concept of a vaccinating matter on January 29, 1885. The latter asked him to experiment on anthrax. Pasteur did

4. Roux, 1887, p. 561.
5. Pasteur, O.C., t. VI, p. 303.
6. NAF 18019, f.P. 18.
7. NAF 18019, f.P. 18.
8. NAF 18019, f.P. 19.

not record his answer to this suggestion, but two days later (January 31) he started his own anthrax experiment[9], and soon afterwards (February 7) his experiment on chicken cholera[10]. Both these experiments failed and remained "*to be redone*".

Ferran and Pauli (*see infra*) are considered to be among the first discoverers of killed microbe vaccines. Their letter to the Academy of Sciences, presented at the January 18, 1886 session, described very clearly the process of obtaining immunity against cholera in guinea pigs by inoculating dead bacteria: "*1° Dead coma bacillus conveys a tolerance that imparts resistance to the effects of living coma bacillus, 2° the active principle of the coma bacillus, isolated by known processes, conveys an immunisation that imparts resistance to the effects of the living microbe, and vice-versa.*" A note specifies that "*immunity is in effect an immunisation phenomenon that can be obtained with purely chemical agents...*"[11]. The printed text found in the Reports of the Academy of Sciences (*Comptes rendus de l'Académie des Sciences*) is probably an excerpt reproducing passages from a Note by the authors. Unfortunately, the originals are not (any longer) in the Archives of the Academy of Sciences. The results presented seem valid. The interpretation is mistaken but, at that time, all interpretations were mistaken. Ferran's scientific life was so chaotic that it is difficult to believe all his assertions... Areas of doubt persist. Moreover, he used a living organism vaccine during his anti-cholera vaccination campaign. Ferran also wrote to Pasteur from Tortosa, on August 4, 1888, to establish that he was the first to discover the chemical anti-cholera vaccine[12].

Therefore, Salmon and Smith are considered the discoverers of killed microbe vaccines. Their data is convincing. The practical application of this extension of Pasteurian methods was to lead to the development of killed microbe vaccines against cholera, typhoid fever, plague... a few years later. At that time, attenuated virulence vaccines with living organisms had favour, and serotherapy was emerging.

The Invention of Serotherapy and Its First Application to Diphteria: 1890-1894... Then to Tetanus and Many Other Diseases

The origins of serotherapy seem to be related to the observation that animal species are not susceptible to certain pathogens. But early researchers had no clear idea about the reasons for this type of difference in susceptibility. Some believe it to be species-related, others believe it is a matter of individual difference. In 1877, Maurice Raynaud was searching for "*the vehicle that transmits to the entire economy the principle, whatever it might be, that confers the benefit of immunity for the future*"[13]. He first looked for this principle in the blood of thirty-five children vaccinated against smallpox, on day 1 to 42 after the inoculation. He obtained no reaction by inoculating a drop of blood from healthy subjects. The transfer was too minimal. He then went to the vaccine-producing Chambon Institute in Paris and injected a healthy heifer with 250 grams of blood from a heifer with pustules of Jennerian cowpox, on the sixth day of their evolution. Fourteen days later, the healthy heifer was vaccinated by scarification and... had no reaction. The same batch of cowpox vaccine was

9. NAF 18019, f.P. 18.
10. NAF 18019, f.P. 18.
11. Ferran, 1886, p. 159.
12. NAF 18103, item 256.
13. Raynaud, 1877, p. 453.

used on another control heifer that had the usual eruption. Raynaud advanced several explanations. The first was that the animal was already immunised against cowpox, a phenomenon never observed by Chambon, who had vaccinated over four hundred animals. The second explanation, that "*transfused blood... can... be considered a very powerful vehicle of vaccinal virus*", or, as a third explanation: "*or at least of the principle able to transmit immunity*"[14]. This "principle" bore a remarkable resemblance to circulating antibodies, but Raynaud did not pursue the experiment!

In general, rabbits are very susceptible to *Staphylococcus pyosepticus*. In 1888, Héricourt and Richet inoculated rabbits with dog blood, by intraperitoneal injection. They observed that if the blood came from a healthy dog, the rabbits succumbed to a mortal dose of *S. pyosepticus*; on the other hand, if the blood came from a dog that had received *S. pyosepticus* inoculations a few months earlier, the rabbits survived a mortal dose of this organism[15]. Richet and Héricourt attempted to apply the same method of transferring immunity to tuberculosis, the deadliest disease of that period. On December 6, 1890, in the Verneuil ward of the Hôtel-Dieu Hospital, they injected a tuberculosis sufferer with immune serum, in vain[16]. These two researchers had unwittingly chanced upon a disease with cell-mediated immunity, whose serum component is practically nonexistent. Chance plays an important role in science!

Nineteenth century physicians had noted that diphtheria killed either by asphyxia or by a sort of general poisoning. The disease affected mainly children between the ages of 2 and 7, but could also attack adults. For instance, it is believed that George Washington, the first American president, died of diphtheria at the age of 68! The infectious nature of the disease was contested, and its origin was unknown. The croup (laryngeal diphtheria) was devastating for small children; in Paris, it was the primary cause of epidemic mortality: 1,800 to 2,000 deaths per year.

Diphteria can take several clinical forms, more or less severe. In severe forms, disease progression is very rapid, between three and seven days on average. Greyish or whitish pseudomembranes develop in the mucosa of the upper respiratory tract. Their adherence to the throat mucosa can be so strong, and they can extend over such a large area, that air passages can be completely blocked, causing very serious breathing problems and even death by suffocation in extreme cases. At the time, two treatments existed: one was rather ineffective drug therapy, and the other was heroic surgical intervention. In order to prevent suffocation, the physician attempted to burn the pseudomembranes with silver nitrate, caustic agents or even a hot iron! Sometimes, a metal tube was introduced into the larynx, to enable air passage in the back of the throat: this was called "intubation". The last-resort procedure was tracheotomy, consisting of opening the trachea and inserting a canula to re-establish the passage of air between the breathing passages and the exterior. This last-chance surgery had been proposed in France by Bretonneau, who after seven trials succeeded in saving one child. Out of his first seventeen attempts, five were successful[17]. In 1885, average results were about two deaths out of three patients undergoing the surgery!

In 1889, Roux and Yersin discovered the toxin secreted by the diphtheria bacillus, also known as Klebs-Loeffler bacillus. In 1890, Behring and Kitasato demonstrated that the

14. Raynaud, 1877, p. 456.
15. Héricourt, 1888, p. 748.
16. Rostand, 1962, p. 81.
17. Bretonneau, 1859, p. 229.

immunity of laboratory animals, acquired through repeated injections of small doses of diphtheria toxins, more or less denatured, was due to substances contained in their serum[18]. Behring first treated a patient in Berlin, at the Charité Hospital, in 1891. Unfortunately, the first attempts to use serum from animals immunised against the diphtheria toxin were not very conclusive. Roux and Yersin continued their study of diphtheria toxin and succeeded in purifying large quantities thanks to the new "Chamberland filter". As a result, in 1892 Roux and his friends, Nocard and Vaillard, were able to immunise horses in Alfort. Martin and Chaillou, physicians specialised in diphtheria, agreed to test this animal serum in humans. Trials started at the Enfants-Malades Hospital. At the same time, at the Trousseau Hospital, the classic treatments were still being used, for lack of antiserum. At the Enfants-Malades, the mortality rate fell from 51% to 24%, while at Trousseau it remained constant, at 60%. At the Budapest Hygiene Conference in 1894, Roux revealed his brilliant results; it was "*the occasion for the triumph of our countryman and promoter of this method, Behring from Berlin*"[19]. In 1899, Roux wrote in his presentation of titles and studies: "*Each day we appreciate more and more the discovery of Mr. Behring and Mr. Kitasato. Our own role consisted only of having proven clearly enough the excellence of the new treatment so that it could spread practically without impediment.*"[20] All chauvinism is absent from these comments. Roux always paid tribute to Behring and his work, insisting that the credit for anti-diphtheria serotherapy was rightfully his. Dr. Apert's testimony supports this well-deserved tribute: "*When I was a young external physician at the Enfants-Malades Hospital in 1891, the diphtheria ward was full of dying patients; the few survivors remained weak for months, suffering from anemia, albuminuria and paralysis. When I came back as on-staff physician in 1895 to this same hospital, where the serotherapeutic method had just been introduced, it was with great joy and amazement that I noted the transformation: children recovering in a few days, pink-complexioned convalescents, hale and full of cheer.*"[21] Serotherapy was to be used widely to fight the two forms of diphtheria, croup and toxaemia. In Great Britain, the use of anti-diphteria serotherapy was applied rapidly: "*Case-mortality diphtheria in children under fifteen at the Eastern Hospital: not treated with serum (Jan. 1, 1893 - Oct. 22, 1894) 797 cases and 310 deaths, mortality percentage 38.8; treated with serum (Oct. 23 - Nov. 27, 1896) 72 cases and 15 deaths, mortality percentage 20.8.*" In the appendix of their book, these authors wrote in 1896: "*The report* (based on 2,182 cases treated in 1895 and 3,042 non treated cases in 1894) *of the Medical Superintendants of the Fever Hospital of the Metropolitan Asylums Board on the use of antitoxic serum, is finished by 'We are further of the opinion that in antitoxic serum we possess a remedy of distinctly greater value in the treatment of diphteria than any other with which we are acquainted'.*"[22] Statistical figures concerning a large number of sick children were those published by the American Pediatric Society, in 1897; they comprised results obtained in 116 cities in 15 different states: "*After eliminating incomplete observations, the investigation includes 5,794 cases, with 713 deaths, giving a mortality rate of 12.3 percent. If we eliminate 218 cases of children already dying at the time of injection or who died in the first twenty-four hours, we have 5,576 cases left, with a mortality of 8.8 percent.*"[23] In 1907,

18. Behring, 1890a & b, p. 1113 & 1145.
19. Cartaz, 1894, p. 282.
20. Roux, 1899, p. 28.
21. Apert, 1922, p. 7.
22. Goodall, 1896, pp. 162 & 356.
23. Sevestre, 1897, p. 647.

the *Institut Pasteur* was to donate 60,142 doses (10 centigrams each, that is, 600 litres in all!) of anti-diphtheria serum to hospitals in France and to a lesser extent abroad[24]. Quality control measures were already being applied, using the health of the horses and the cleanliness of the sera serving to neutralise diphtheria toxin. Depending on the patient's weight, 5 to 40 centilitres of serum were administered. Before 1894, out of the 12,700,000 residents of French cities with over 5,000 inhabitants, there were 6,000 to 7,000 annual deaths from diphtheria. After this date, thanks to serotherapy, mortality figures fell to 1,500 - 2,200 cases, with no noticeable reduction in prevalence, that is, in the number of cases recorded in a given population.

Starting in 1901, 34,350 prophylactic rather than therapeutic inoculations were administered to prevent small epidemics. Results were satisfactory, but the protection obtained was of short duration, lasting only two to three weeks.[25]

One of the disadvantages of the serotherapy practiced at the time was the fact that it conferred a massive supply of animal-source serum proteins to the inoculated patients. The latter were immunised against horse serum and, theoretically, could no longer benefit from this type of preventive or therapeutic treatment. Therefore, starting in 1898, the *Institut Pasteur* serum was heated to 56° C four consecutive times at two-day intervals, allowing part of the useless proteins to be precipitated, and thus considerably reducing seric accidents[26]. Actually, such accidents were rare, even counting only the most minor, and serious cases of anaphylaxis were almost nonexistent[27]. A definitive solution to the problem of diphtheria prevention would only be provided by the advent of vaccination (*see infra*).

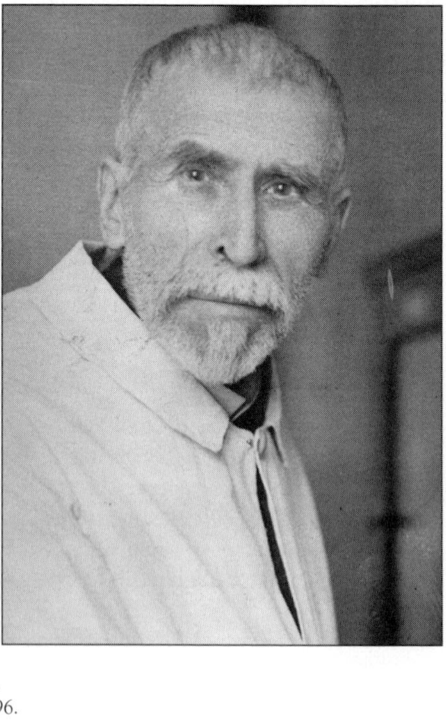

Figure 2. Emile Roux (1853-1933), photographed in his office a few weeks prior to his death. Emile Roux combined the qualities of a relentless researcher with those of a just and compassionate man. (Photo provided by Wide World Photos, Paris.) (Author's document.)

24. Conseil supérieur d'hygiène publique de France, 1908, p. 696.
25. Moizard, 1901, p. 568.
26. Moizard, 1901, p. 568.
27. Lucas-Championnière, 1914, p. 215.

In 1897, the *Institut Pasteur* in Garches produced animal sera against diphtheria and the plague[28]. At the end of the nineteenth century, small plague epidemics occurred in Europe, including the one in Porto in 1899. Two teams were sent there: Ferran from Barcelona, and Calmette, with Salimbeni, from the *Institut Pasteur*. The epidemic was stopped quite rapidly thanks to the anti-plague sera produced by the *Institut Pasteur*. However, these sera caused rather significant side effects after their injection[29].

Many institutes dedicated to immune sera against human and animal diseases, for human and veterinary use, were created; among them, Berhingwerke in Germany (1904), Burroughs Wellcome & Co in London, and the Mérieux Institute in France.

Classic serotherapy, using sera from animals immunised against a pathogenic agent or a toxin, or sera from recovering animals, served to combat numerous diseases. It was while he was immunising horses to produce anti-diphtheria sera that Ramon discovered adjuvant substances in immunity[30]. Until the discovery of chemotherapy and antibiotherapy, prevention and treatment with immune serum were the only effective means of fighting infectious diseases. Examples abound; they include anti-tetanus serotherapy that saved thousands of wounded men in the First World War.

The Priority: an Anti-Cholera Vaccine. Ferran, Haffkine: 1884, 1892...

"*The most terrible and dreaded scourge of humanity is doubtlessly the cholera-morbus, one of these deadly epidemics that decimate urban and rural populations, spreading terror throughout entire nations and, at the same time, stifling all impulses of humanity and philanthropy that elevate civilised societies.*" Baron Larrey, 1831[31].

Cholera, the terrible disease that swept through Europe and North America in successive waves throughout the nineteenth century, left death and destruction in its wake. The first major epidemic broke out in 1831 (Poland, Prussia, Austria, England...) and in 1832 (France, Sweden, Norway...), reaching Canada (June 1832) and the United States (July 1832); the second started in 1845 in Europe and in North America in 1848; the third swept through Europe in 1854; the fourth in 1865 and 1866. The United States was severely affected once again in 1873; the last cholera epidemic occurred in France in 1884 and spread to Italy and Spain[32]. Depending on the epidemic, the average mortality rate was between 10 to 25 deaths for a thousand inhabitants, and reached 200 out of one thousand in Küscamp in 1859 (3,000 fatalities for 15,000 inhabitants). Among those who caught the disease, mortality rates often reached 50% and more[33]. During the 1832 epidemic, Seine Department statistics showed 18,402 deaths from cholera out of a total population of 759,349 inhabitants, that is, 2.42%[34]. Cholera still exists today. It infects 5 to 7 million people in the world and causes about 100,000 deaths per year[35].

28. Tiburce, 1897, p. 524.
29. Metchnikoff, 1901, p. 509.
30. Ramon, 1925a, p. 506; Glenny, see this chapter.
31. Larrey, 1831, p. 5.
32. Daremberg, 1892; Creighton, 1894; Surgeon General's office, 1875; Ernst, 1886, p. 218.
33. Lacroix, 1855, p. 163.
34. Commission, 1834, p. 49 and Table 54; Laveran *in* Dechambre, 1874, t. 16, p. 796.
35. Kirkpatrick, 2003, p. 369.

Cholera morbus or summer Cholera was the common or popular name of an acute gastroenteritis that could take two forms: sporadic or epidemic.

• **Sporadic cholera**, also called "simple, European or British cholera", was more or less endemic in Western Europe, and relatively unthreatening. It(s) pathogenic agent(s) is (where) hard to identify because symptoms are variable and often benign.

• **Epidemic or Asiatic cholera** came from India and its neighbouring regions. The description of the symptoms of this terrible disease is horrifying: "*This last disease* (the terribly fatal disorder called Asiatic, malignant or epidemic cholera) *seems to have been known in India for centuries, and to have its natural home or headquarter in the delta of the Ganges... Very frequently when cholera prevails diarrhoea also does so, and an epidemic of cholera is frequently ushered in by an unusual prevalence of the other malady* (the British cholera). *In point of fact in a case of ordinary, though by no means of maximum, intensity the disease is ushered in by an attack of diarrhoea. This may last a longer or a shorter period, but speedily the matters passed by the bowel alter in character. They assume a peculiar flocculent or rice water character. Vomiting, too, comes on, the fluid being thin and colourless. Then follow severe cramps, especially of the abdominal muscles and legs, which become like rigid cord. The flow of urine ceases, breathing and circulation are so much impaired that the body becomes icy cold on the surface, the tongue is cold, and so even is the breath. The lips are blue and shrivelled, the face pinched, the voice is hardly audible, the very eye-balls are flattened. This is called the cold or algid stage of the disease. The condition may go on getting worse till the heart stop, the patient being quite conscious to the end.*"[36] Fortunately, a certain percentage of cholera patients escaped suffocation and death. Until Koch's discoveries, sporadic and Asiatic cholera were not easily distinguished from each-other.

The Royal Academy of Medicine (Paris) published an excellent report in 1831, a few months before the start of the first epidemic that broke out in France. "*The Academy, fully convinced of the vast importance of its commission, has neglected nothing that could elevate it to the utmost height of its duties.*"[37] Its message remains reassuring: "*Blessed with a most advantageous geographical position, a serene sky, temperate climate, fruitful soil and a happy distribution of territorial property, with industrious habits, instruction pretty generally distributed and, consequently, with a public and private hygiene which leaves but little to be desired, the French have reason to hope that they will be preserved from the visitation of this scourge.*"[38] This learned assembly was far too optimistic. Reality was not going to live up to its illusions. The Academy's report ended with very good advice and wise recommendations in case of an outbreak. These soon proved to be inadequate in the face of the extreme brutality of events.

A little before the middle of the nineteenth century, the Englishman Snow was probably the first to notice the correlation between the distribution and consumption of polluted water and cholera epidemics, at a time when the contagious nature of this disease was only acknowledged by a minority. Snow led enquiries throughout Great Britain to learn more about the circumstances in which the various epidemics broke out, city by city, village by village. In 1832, during the cholera epidemic in London, he studied very closely the incidence of cholera cases. A particularly terrible epidemic, focused on Broad Street in London, killed 500

36. Haydn, 1874, p. 73.
37. Keraudren, 1832, p. 234.
38. Keraudren, 1832, p. 186.

people in ten days. Snow discovered that most of the dead were users of a water pump located on that street. He concluded that the water from the pump was poisoned by infiltrations from a septic hole or a faulty, contaminated sewer. He was able to persuade the local authorities, "*and once the neighbourhood committee was convinced to remove the pump, the epidemic stopped immediately*"[39]. History has focused on this removal of the pump, which conferred glory on Snow (at least posthumously). Apparently, the cholera stopped suddenly after this action. But reality was less glorious. It would have been too simple for this gesture alone to completely stop a cholera epidemic[40]. Snow had to lead a long-lasting battle to make it clear that there was a relation between the feces of cholera sufferers and the contamination of healthy population, through drinking water. Snow had considerable influence on the means to be used to combat cholera: distribution of drinking water and hygienic methods of wastewater and solid waste disposal. In 1866, Burrall described Snow's theory and added: "*Cholera is pathologically a disease exclusively of the alimentary canal. The primary change is in the alimentary canal, and is always caused by the introduction into it of a specific poison. The poison itself is exclusively contained in the intestinal excreta of the infected person; that is, in the vomit or dejections.*"[41] There is no reference to a pathogenic organism, a theory that was to emerge in the following years. And yet, long before, in 1688, Redi had published his work on insect generation: "*Having considered these things, I began to believe that all worms found in meat were derived directly from the droppings of flies, and not from putrefaction of the meat...*"[42a]. Spontaneous generation theory, dismantled by Pasteur in the 1860s, survived for several more years in regard to pathogenic agents. It took a few more years for the idea of poison to be transformed into that of germs that have the power to multiply. Snow's thesis on this subject earned him a well-deserved 30,000 French-franc prize (at least 96,000 euros) awarded by the *Institut de France*.

At the start of the nineteenth century, physicians started to compensate the loss of fluids, through blood or diarrhea, seen in cholera sufferers, by giving them liquids, enemas or intravenous injections of purified water, or of water with acetic acid or with blood. "*If the reader remembers what we said about the changes produced in the blood and the chemical composition of excreted matters, he will easily understand how, as soon as* Mr. O'Shaugnessy's *analysis was published, practitioners had the idea of trying to remedy the losses through blood by administering saline substances. It seems that, by instinct or by some other means, the peasants in some regions of Russia had discovered a treatment of this type as early as 1830. We even witnessed some attempts using kitchen salt, made by* Mr. *Searle in Warsaw in 1831; but it was not until 1832 that physicians, guided by chemical analysis, perfected this method, and it was in Scotland that the first attempts were carried out. Doctor Thomas Latta, practitioner at Leith (Scotland), imagined first administering in enemas, and having the patient drink a saline infusion, a kind of artificial serum, more or less analogous to that found in the blood; but because this procedure did not succeed in stopping the vomiting, he proceeded to use injections into the veinous system. The successes he obtained at once attracted much attention and these experiments were repeated in Edimburg, Glasgow and a number of other cities in*

39. Hare, 1954, p. 129; Snow, 1849.
40. Newman, 1932, p. 220.
41. Burrall, 1866, p. 51.
42a. Redi, 1688 (1909), p. 33.

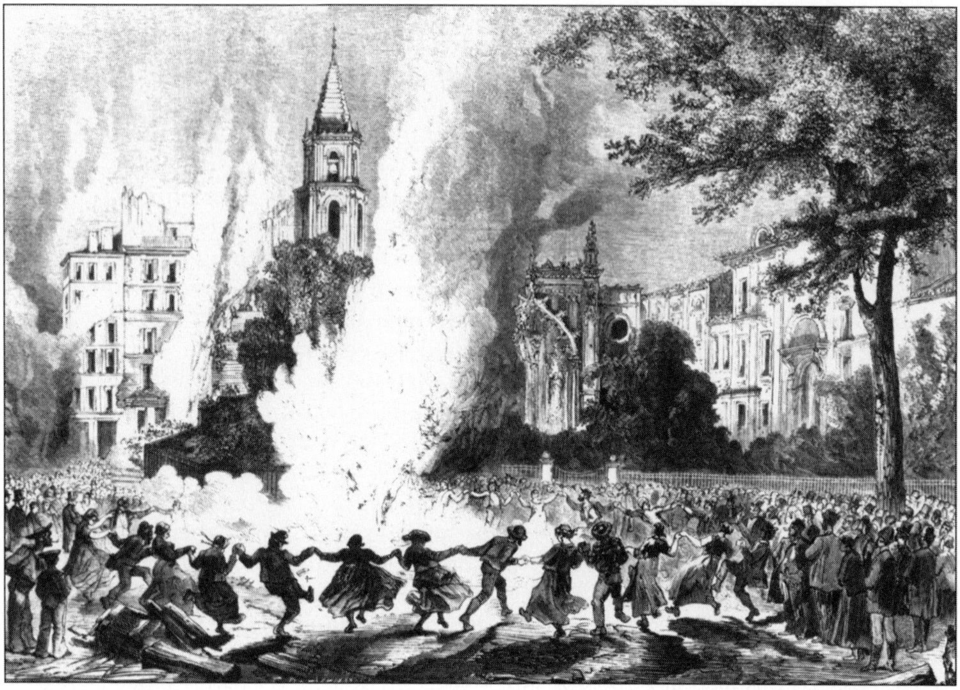

Figure 3. In 1865, germ theory was not yet known and neither was the coma bacillus. In Marseille, as in many other cities and countries, people attempted to drive away cholera *miasomata* by lighting great fires meant to purify the air, and danced around them. "*The cholera, represented by mannequins, was burned in all quarters in the midst of sniggering from the crowd that defied the scourge by dancing the farandole. But... the young people started to throw rockets and sparklers, and several serious accidents were caused by snakes and fire crackers: the police had to forbid the fires and the fireworks to prevent the city from being set on fire.*" (Le Monde *illustré*, n° 443, October 7, 1865.)

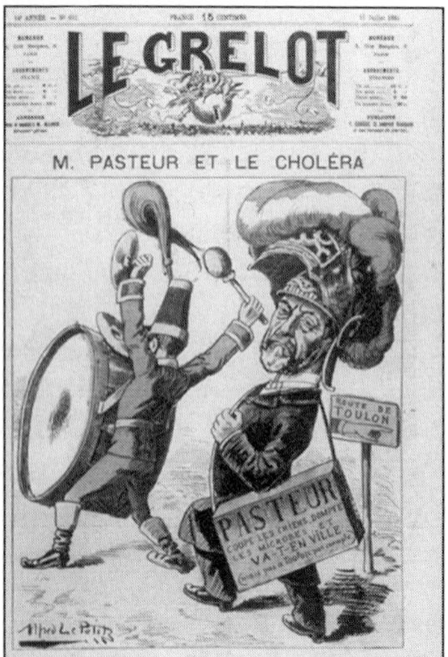

Figure 4. "Mr. *Pasteur and cholera.*" On the bag carried by Pasteur, the following inscription can be read: "*Pasteur cuts dogs, tames germs and GOES TO TOWN (but not to Toulon).*" Pasteur prevents rabies in the "bitten" but does nothing about the cholera raging in Toulon (France). Pasteur was the object of severe criticism throughout his life. *Le Grelot* is not wrong: cholera is much more dangerous than rabies. (*Le Grelot*, July 13, 1884.)

England, in the manner and with the results described below. The composition of the injected fluid was not always the same. In general, three large balls of common salt (sodium hydrochloride) and a grain of sodium carbonate were dissolved in five to six litres of water. This concentration of saline substances, somewhat stronger than that used at first by Mr. Latta, resembles the one adopted by most experimenters. Some of them added a little albumin, to no advantage whatever. This mixture must be injected in a short time, ounce by ounce, into a vein of the arm, which will be treated with the greatest care and properly bound, to prevent phlebitis... The proper temperature to be used is normal blood temperature (110 to 112 degrees Fahrenheit. Mr. Latta). As to the quantity that should be injected, this is what is difficult to determine. In a number of cases a few pounds had been enough; in other cases, much more was needed. Doctor Lewins once injected a quantity of 33 pounds in 52 hours, with total success."[42b] A certain Dr. Herman used the same treatment successfully in 1830, but the details are not known. In 1884, in Paris, Geroges Hayem used this treatment routinely, and achieved good results[43]. Later, Rogers proposed intra-abdominal administration of hypertonic saline solutions[44]. This was a treatment based on facts from the field of chemistry, which was remarkable for the period in question. On the other hand, a multitude of remedies, as plentiful as they were useless, filled the pages of medical and popular newspapers, often motivated by undisguised commercial interests. Charlatans were plentiful, then as now.

Developing a vaccine was a cherished ambition for many, but it was not an easy dream to achieve. Pasteur was blamed for focusing on rabies rather than on cholera. The July 13, 1884 *Le Grelot* published a caricature that was typical of this sarcastic attitude. In fact, Pasteur had taken the initiative of organising the expedition to Egypt, where Thuillier died of cholera. This must have been a painful memory for Pasteur. In 1884, during a cholera epidemic, he sent two of his students, Roux and Straus, to Toulon. They returned discouraged. And Yet Koch himself observed again his coma bacillus in Toulon[45]. Pasteur and Roux did not cease their work on cholera. Written records show that on November 10, 1884 they went to take samples of water suspected of being contaminated, at the hospice on Breteuil Avenue, and that they found what could perhaps be a coma bacillus in it. "*I went with M. Roux to take water from the tap located outside, at the foot of the 3 or 4 steps leading to the kitchen. The supervisor asserts that this water comes from the Ourcq* (very polluted). *On Saturday, Nov. 15, we went again to take some water, but this time we were told that an employee from the Water Department had come to inspect the water distribution taps and had said that the tap mentioned above carries only water from the Vanne* (in principle, not polluted), *and that water from the Ourcq only feeds the laundry room, where we went to collect about fifteen litres...*". Pasteur (and Roux?) succeeded in cultivating a microorganism, and "*interestingly, this organism cannot be cultivated, or only very slowly, on gelatine. This clearly distinguishes it from Koch's and from Eberth's bacilli.*"[46] Very likely, this was not the coma bacillus discovered by Koch in 1883.

42b. Dalmas, 1834, t. 7, p. 451.

43. Langlois *in* Berthelot, 1885-1892, vol. 11, p. 216.

44. Rogers, 1909, p. 29.

45. Figuier, 1885, p. 378.

46. NAF 1018, f.P. 132.

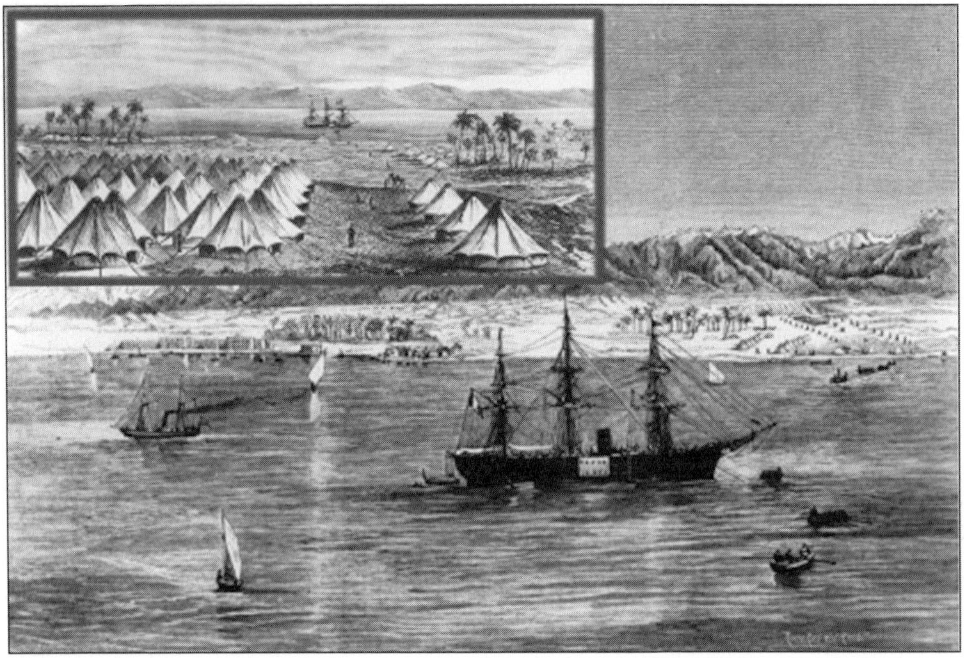

Figure 5. Europe, and particularly France, dread a new cholera epidemic. The ship "*La Corrèze*", with cholera on board, under quarantine in the Red Sea (Drawing by Mr. Scott, based on the sketch by M.F.L. published in *Le Monde illustré*, n° 1068, on September 29, 1877). "*Quarantine of* La Corrèze *in the Djebel-Tor colony (Red Sea): view of the Djebel-Tor deck and of* La Corrèze." Tents in the sleeping area (*L'Illustration*, n° 1806, October 6, 1877.) *La Corrèze*, a ship transporting troops, from Saigon, with 830 people on board, soon had three deaths from cholera. The ship was forbidden to enter the port of Singapour. By the time it arrived in Suez, thirty-two deaths from cholera had occurred, but the epidemic seemed to be over. The International Health Commission, responsible for the application of the Treaty of Constantinople, assisted by an Egyptian infantry company, imposed a forty-day quarantine for the eight hundred passengers of the ship; fifteen days were actually respected. Passengers could leave the ship between 6 in the evening and 6 in the morning, under the supervision of the army. In the main illustration, on the right, rowboats are seen heading toward (or leaving) a landing point. Two lines of troops are positioned between this point and the tents in the sleeping area. The tents to the left of the landing point are those of the Egyptian military and of the health officials. The *Monde illustré* comments: "*This operation should be enough to reassure us if we did not have numerous examples provided by reputable physicians showing that cholera is not contagious.*" Much time was needed before the contagious nature of cholera was acknowledged by everyone. The Djabel-Tor isolation colony lent its name to the Vibrio el Tor, also called *Vibrio cholerae* Serogroup 01 Biotype El Tor, or Serogroup 0139 (not yet discovered at the time of these events). *La Corrèze* arrived in Toulon on September 21, 1877, apparently free of its cholera bacilli.

In 1884, the municipality of Barcelona[47] or the Academy of Barcelona[48] entrusted the Catalan physician Jaime Ferran with an official mission: he was to go to France to study the cholera epidemic that was in full swing there. This physician from Tortosa, a small town south of Barcelona, had a great interest in microbiology, but possessed only meagre means. He was selected for the mission from among other applicants

47. Anonyme, 1924, p. 883.
48. Respaut, 1885, p. 52.

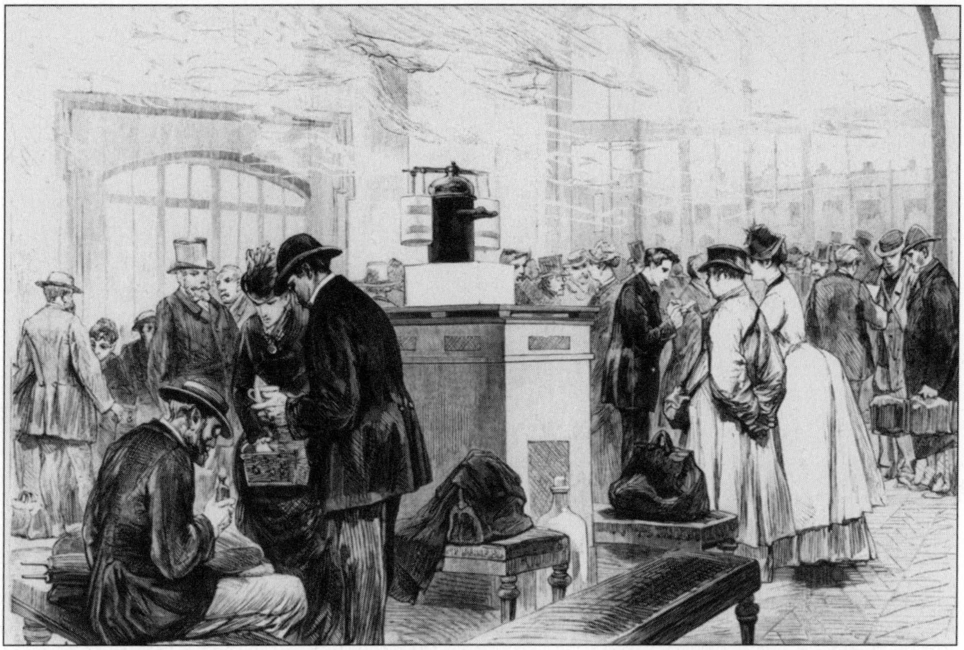

Figure 6. In France, the last cholera epidemic occurred in 1884. The bacillus was known. The contagious nature of the infection was most often acknowledged. Disinfection was compulsory. Here, disinfection measures taken at the "*Gare de Lyon*" train station, with passengers arriving from Toulon and Marseille. Drawing from nature by M.A. Lançon: "*Passengers… enter for half an hour a special disinfection room sprinkled constantly with sodium phenate in great quantities, and in which apparatus containing nitrous sulphuric acid crystals has been placed. During this time, their names and addresses are recorded so that their state of health can be surveyed over the next few days.*" Of course, this process of disinfection had no clear effect whatever; but the recording of names and addresses constituted a remarkable advance. (*L'Illustration*, n° 2159, July 12, 1884.)

subjected to a qualifying examination. He set off with his faithful companion and friend, the chemist Inocente Pauli. In Marseille, they went to see two local physicians, Drs Nicati and Rietsh, working in their Pharo Palace laboratory, provided by the office of Marseille Hospices in 1884. These two researchers were studying the cholera bacillus. Koch had visited them on his way back from Toulon. "*We are grateful to the famous bacteriologist for the kindness with which he showed us his coma bacillus and gave us verbal explanations that were not published until several weeks later; at the time, the coma bacillus was only known through reports from Egypt and India.*"[49] In France, these two researchers were pioneers. In July 1885, they published a note on the attenuation of the cholera bacillus by cultivation in broth or in gelatin culture medium, at an average temperature of 20° to 25° C[50].

While they were in Marseille, the two Catalan visitors were introduced to the coma bacillus in Rietsh and Nicati's laboratory, learned to cultivate it (and try to attenuate it, like Nicati and Rietsh?). They also travelled to Toulon and then to Naples, where

49. Nicati, 1886, p. 1.
50. Nicati, 1885, p. 186.

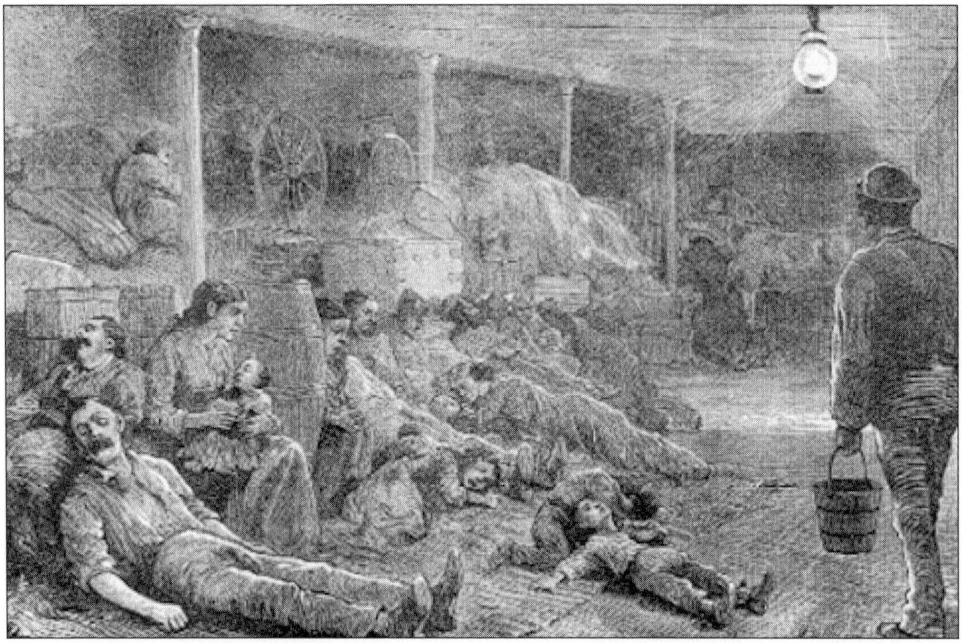

Figure 7. ***"During the American epidemic of 1873... During the month of May, in that year, the disease was first brought northward along the line of the Mississippi River... It is among the desk passengers of a stream-river that infectious diseases, cholera especially, is conveyed from point to point..."*** **(Surgeon-General's Office, 1875, p. 52.)**

cholera was raging. On their way back, Spanish officials subjected them to a ten-day quarantine, which did not stop the two ambassadors from keeping their precious cholera bacillus culture alive, and taking it with them to Spain. Back in Tortosa, Ferran and his friend, assisted by a lawyer named Pasqual, a professor of obstetrics and a young physician, continued their work. They found new morphological forms of the cholera bacillus, whose virulence they tested on guinea pigs. Being injected in advance with diluted cholera bacillus culture subcutaneously allowed these animals to resist subsequently to a test dose that was fatal to non immunised animals. Ferran published this finding in the December 1884 issue of *El siglo medico*. The special morphology bacillus was named *Perinospora ferrani* by Ferran's friends, in his honour. He was given official recognition by a special Commission of the Royal Academy of Barcelona[51]. Encouraged by this result, Ferran inoculated the cholera bacillus to himself, under the skin, in his abdomen. He suffered some unpleasant side effects, but quickly recovered.

About thirty of Ferran's friends had themselves vaccinated. On December 9, 1884, Ferran sent the following telegram (probably in Spanish) to the King of Spain and several ministers including Albert Bosh y Fastegueras, General Director of Health, to Romero Robledo, Minister of the Interior, to the mayor of Barcelona and to some celebrated medical figures: "*New morphological faces* (sic) *of the cholera microbe have been discovered. The problem of cholera transmission to animals, and of their vaccination, has been solved. Man is resistant to the vaccination. Pauli and I are vaccinated. Ferran.*"[52] In

51. Rochard, 1888, p. 491.
52. Respaut, 1885, p. 62.

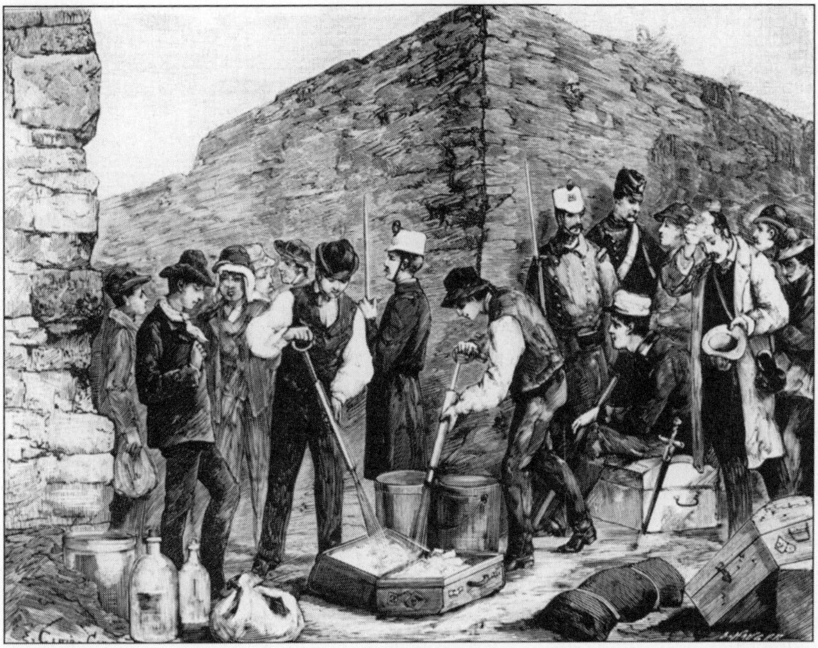

Figure 8. "*Luggage disinfection at the Latta isolation colony, based on a sketch by* Mr. Clair-Guyot, *special correspondent to* L'Illustration." There is a cholera epidemic in France, Italians protect themselves, in a rather disorderly manner... (*L'Illustration*, n° 2160, July 12, 1884.)

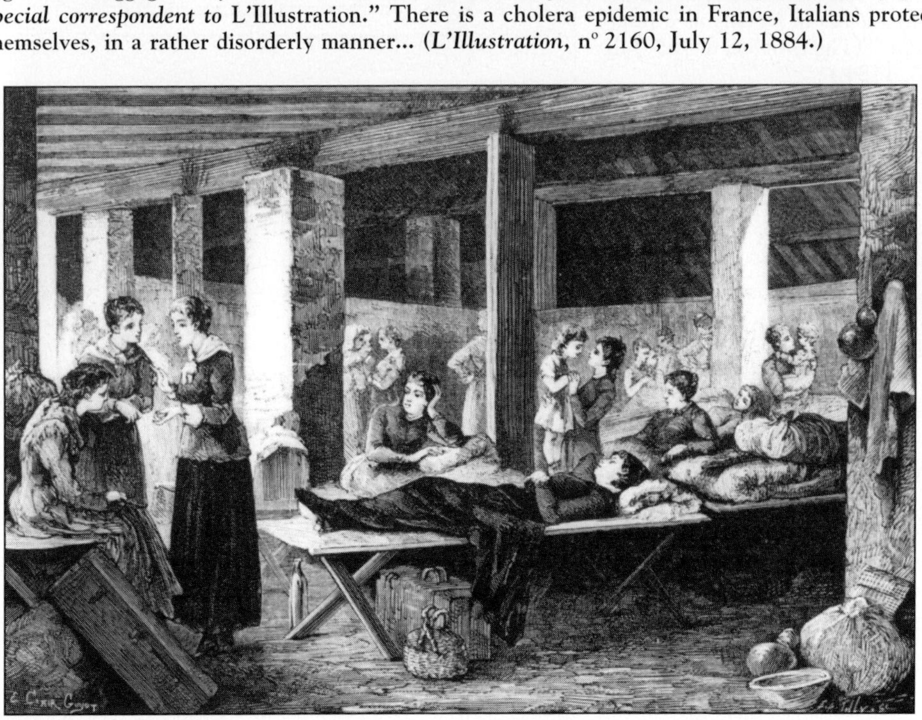

Figure 9. "The *cholera in France. Patients in the Latta isolation hospice (Franco-Italian border), based on the sketch by* Mr. Clair-Guyot, *special correspondent for* L'Illustration." The women's dormitory, shared by a number of children as well. (*L'Illustration*, n° 2161, July 26, 1884.)

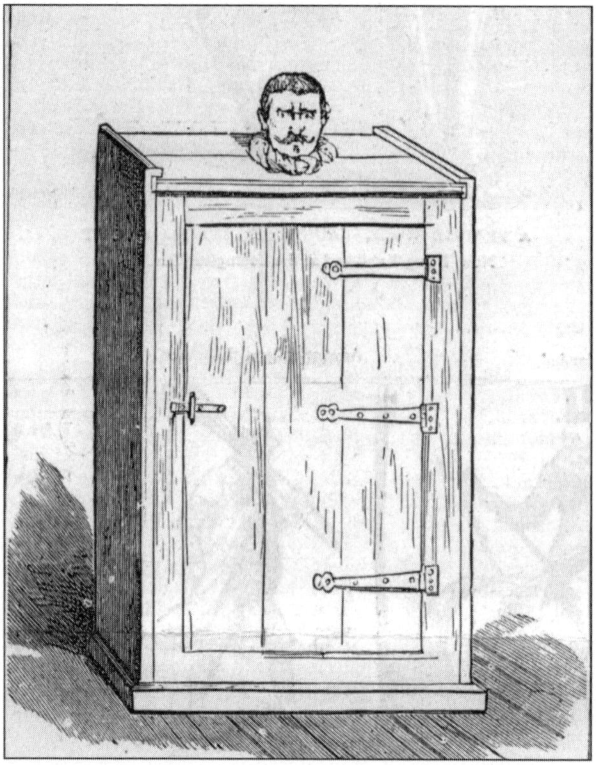

Figure 10. Individual disinfection, having no effect whatever, since cholera bacilli are present mainly in the digestive system of patients... "*A cholera fumigating box in Geneva; according to another correspondent, Mr. Thomas Howie, still more stringent precautions are adopted. The suspected person is placed in a box which is about six feet high, and in which he stands upright, with only his head outside, a towel being wrapped round his neck. The process occupies from three to four minutes, and the disinfectants used are chloride of lime and carbolic acid. The top piece of the box is made to slide in, and is removed when the process is completed by simply pulling outwards. While the sliding board is being removed the towel comes in handily as a respirator.*" (The Graphic, n° 765, July 26, 1184.)

fact, Ferran was presenting special morphologies of the coma bacillus: spirilla, oogons, spherical cocci, spirilla with spores, fusiform bacilli with or without filaments... Drawings of all these "faces" of the coma bacillus can be found in various scientific publications[53] and even in *L'Illustration* of July 25, 1885[54], reprinted from an issue of *Revista de Ciencias medicas (Barcelona)*, 1885, an. XI, n° 1. In an article published in the June 25, 1885 issue of *La Nature*, Dr. Cartaz reviews Ferran's work favourably. He explains to his readers the transformations of the coma bacilli into spirilla or oogons, then into granulations or spindle-shaped bodies... He asserts: "*So far the facts support Dr. Ferran's conclusions. We must wait for the findings of various Commissions of Enquiry to draw definite conclusions on this question. But even if his vaccine was to fail being recognized as authentic or legitimate, as we say of the Jennerian vaccine, we would have to be grateful to the experimenter for having found the means to appease populations living in terror of the very word cholera.*"[55] Cartaz was a wise man. Looking after the patient's morale is always useful. A short article by Dr. Respaut, published in the July 25, 1885 issue of *Illustration*, speaks very positively: "*And this is the man whom in our country we so dismissively called a charlatan and a slight-of-hand artist...*"[56]. To support his statements, the author, who had taken the trouble to go to Spain, cites the population of Alcira, half of which (not clearly identified) was vaccinated between May 1 and June 30. Among the

53. Van Ermengem, 1885.
54. Respaut, 1885, p. 52.
55. Cartaz, 1885, p. 58.
56. Respaut, 1885, p. 62.

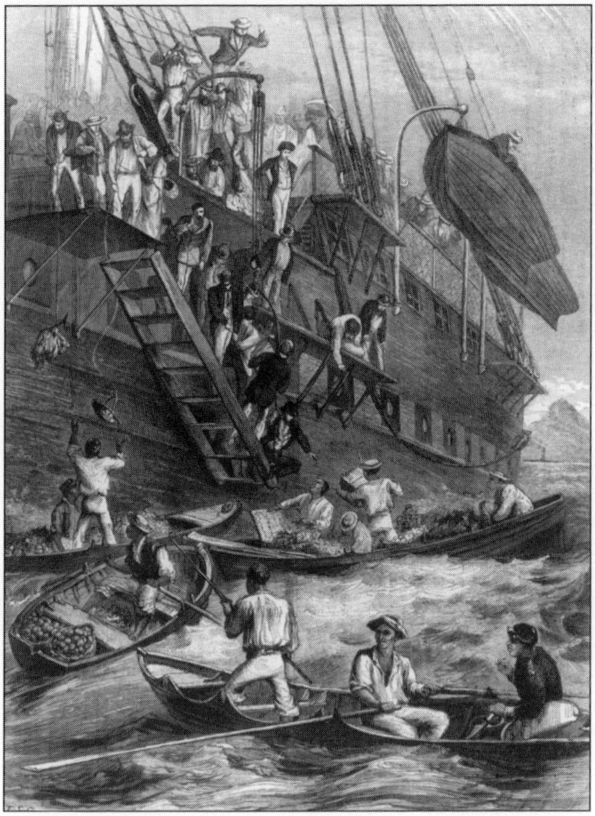

Figure 11. Toward 1880, quarantine against cholera was instituted just about everywhere in the world. "*Quarantine - Ships and fruit vendors.*" The sanitary barrier does not seem very tight in Saint-Vincent, in the Lesser Antilles. Passengers can buy oranges, pineapples, bananas, avocados and guavas that the island inhabitants come to sell them. There is obvious contact between the quarantined travellers and the vendors. (*Journal des voyages*, August 22, 1880.)

unvaccinated, there were 148 fatalities, and only 13 among those who were vaccinated. It is suspected that these data may be biased. *Le Journal illustré* of August 2, 1885 published a portrait of Ferran on its cover, but the accompanying article expressed clear reservations. Its author might have lacked accurate information, since he located Ferran's work in Madrid[57]. Overall, Ferran's findings were looked upon with favour by the advocates of germ theory. On the other hand, opponents of germ theory rejected his vaccinations, just like Pasteur's: "*Once again, we do not hesitate to proclaim ourselves among the most fervent admirers of Mr. Pasteur's wonderful work, but we oppose with all our might the introduction of microbian theories into human medicine. If they were to ultimately again recognition, we would soon inoculate for any reason and against all diseases, from cholera to the simple cold, without asking ourselves what mixtures all these more or less authentic, more or less attenuated viruses, like Ferran's, can produce in our system. But we are firmly convinced that we will soon see the demise of this parasitic pathology that "taking the effect for the cause", as it has been said, underestimates the vital spontaneity of superior organisms, having come to admit only the vital spontaneity of inferior organisms. After a brief moment of triumph, it will crumble under the weight of its failures and excesses.*"[58] Decaisne, who is quoted above, was a professor at the Museum of natural History (Paris).

57. Anonyme, 1885e, p. 254.
58. Decaisne, 1885, p. 455.

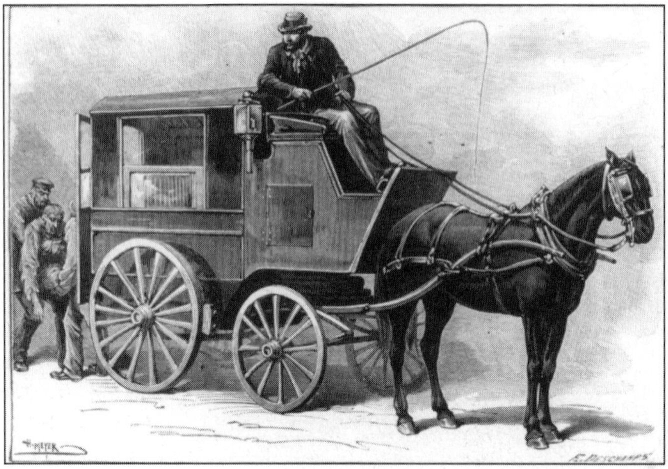

Figure 12. A municipal vehicle designed for the transport of cholera sufferers, based on a drawing by Henri Meyer. "*As soon as the cholera made its appearance in France, public health officials took the most stringent preventive measures... The prefecture of police had already prepared the vehicles that had been used to transport the sick to hospitals during previous epidemics... These vehicles resembled little railway cars: they were painted black and their interior was set up so that the patient could be seated or lie prone, depending on the severity of his condition.*" (*Le Journal illustré*, n° 47, November 23, 1884.)

Ferran's success with vaccination, and his recognition by the Royal Academy of Barcelona, might be due to the special forms of the coma bacillus. Trouessart describes in detail the polymorphism of the "*Bacillus Komma*" which "*lengthens, forms flexuous filaments, then swells at one of its extremities until it reaches the size of a red blood cell, thus becoming an oogon filled with protoplasma. A transparent envelope (periplasma) forms around the oogon, which then becomes spherical... showing that the cholera microbe belongs to a much higher category of bacteria than the one in which this microbe had been classified so far..., a microbe M. Ferran calls Peronospora Barcimonae, but which his friends insisted on calling, after its discoverer, Peronospora Ferrani.*"[59] These initial discoveries were well-received. Van Ermengem, in Brussels, received samples from Ferran and was able to reproduce some of his results. His report, sent to the Belgian Minister of the Interior on November 3, 1884, was detailed and contained 13 illustrations; it was 358–pages long. *A priori*, it is a very serious document. The text ends with a list of those who first attempted to vaccinate human beings (Ferran himself, Pauli, Amalio Gimeno, Colvé and Garini) against cholera by using pure coma bacillus cultures[60]. Ferran's work did not arouse any animosity; it was greeted with admiration for the most part, Ferran's boldness being the only cause for reservation. His first publications, in Spanish, in 1885, were greeted with interest in his own country as well as abroad.

But Koch, a very rigorous observer, could not believe these claims. Ferran's beautiful descriptions were soon torn to shreds by him and by other experimenters who did not find any of the successive forms of a cycle of a cholera bacillus. A little later, Ferran himself admitted that he no longer had specimens of these special forms. This might explain the incipient doubt that greeted his subsequent publications.

59. Trouessart, 1886, p. 193.
60. Van Ermengem, 1885, note C.

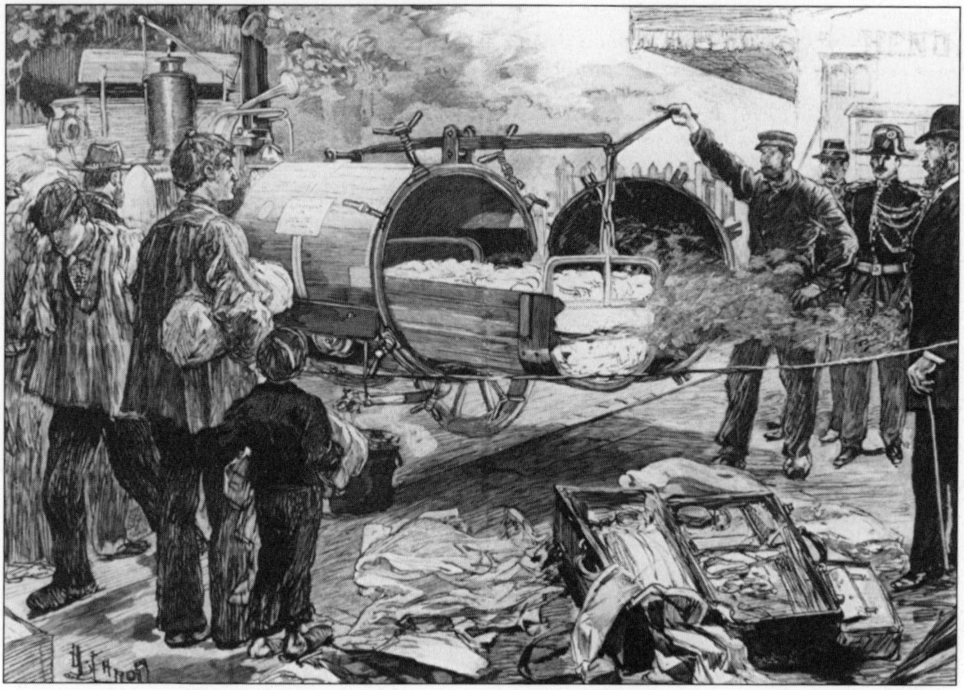

Figure 13. Cholera in Spain: disinfection of travellers' luggage at Hendaye train station. Drawing from nature by Mr. Lanos, special correspondent from *L'Illustration*. Because there had been sporadic cases of cholera in Spain in 1890, French health authorities introduced luggage sterilisation for passengers coming from that country. Use of "*a Geneste Herscher steriliser, based on the scientifically proven principle that steam under pressure, at a temperature of 110-115° operating for fifteen minutes, destroys all living things*." The article does not specify if all luggage was sterilised, or only clothing... The chaos reigning in the crowds raised doubts about the effectiveness of these measures. Although the technique is excellent, its application leaves much to be desired. (*L'Illustration*, n° 2470, June 28, 1890.)

Ferran began to be known and to overshadow Pasteur's work, although he considered himself a disciple of Pasteur. In July and August 1885, in France alone, *Le Monde illustré*, *L'Illustration*, *L'Univers illustré*, *Journal illustré*, *Le Voleur*, *Série illustrée* and *La France illustrée*, among other weekly publications, published long illustrated articles on Ferran's vaccinations. The daily papers no doubt also published articles concerning him. Dr. Amalio Gimeno, therapy professor at the Faculty of Medicine of Valencia, (whom Ferran had vaccinated), and professor of Medicine Candela advised the governor of the province to call in Ferran to put an end to the epidemic in Jativa. Ferran set off to vaccinate in the province of Valancia. The year 1885 was catastrophic in Spain. Out of a population of 16 million, there were 338,685 cases of cholera, and 119,620 fatalities. Braving the danger, Ferran vaccinated the inhabitants of Alcira and Algemesi, that is, over 20,000 people. But in most cases the inoculation was followed by painful effects. After the injection of eight drops of fresh cholera bacillus culture in the arm, "*four to five hours after the injection, the vaccinated person feels a rather intense pain in his arm, followed by a sensation of unwellness and muscle pains. Fever and violent chills appear ten to twelve days after the inoculation; the pulse is accelerated, the temperature*

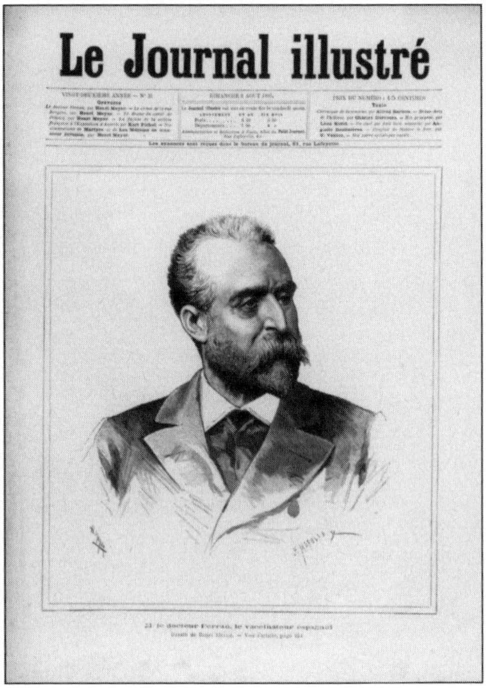

Figure 14. Dr. Jaime Ferran (1851-1929), "*the Spanish vaccinator*". Drawing by Henri Meyer. Ferran is an imposing figure. He has already vaccinated about 5,000 people against cholera, while Pasteur has only vaccinated young Meister... and not officially, at that. The article accompanying this portrait seems ambivalent. It asks for proof of the effectiveness of Ferran's vaccine. At the same time, it brings to light the impact of Spanish vaccines on the French population: "*In the meantime, while we wait for him to provide proof, we publish his portrait because of the great interest he has solicited.*" (*Le Journal illustré*, n° 31, August 2, 1885.)

reaches 39°, 40°. Then abundant sweating begins, there is nausea and the fever breaks within twenty-four hours; only some pain and swelling of the arm remains. This illness is obviously not anything like even a light attack of cholera; and yet at times some of its symptoms are present: vomiting, cold sweats, light diarrhea; in fact, these are more likely to be septicaemia or toxic poisoning accidents. Dr. Ferran believes that in order to be fully protected, a second vaccination must be performed."[61] At the same time, the Brouardel enquiry notes that the sequels of the Ferran inoculation are rather light. The Larousse dictionary[62] specifies: "*The after-effects* (of Ferran's anti-cholera vaccination) *are usually insignificant, but on some occasions phlegmons* (inflammation infiltrating the tissues and possibly resulting in an abscess) *of the arm have occurred.*" It is hard to know what to think; reports are contradictory. Ferran himself insists on the sequels of his cholerisation (vaccination): "*... We have come to be able to see a general picture, whose resemblance with that of true cholera cannot be denied; spotted chills; lipothymic state; general fatigue; cramps; vomiting; heavy head; cold and viscous sweats; more frequent stools than usual, without the onset of true choleric diarrhea.*"[63] Ferran is obviously thinking of the benign illness that accompanies smallpox vaccinations or Pasteur's vaccinations against chicken cholera and anthrax. As recommended by the authors who described these vaccinations, Ferran administered a single injection, followed or not by a booster shot. Apert had described a series of three injections[64]. But all this was nothing compared to the fear of cholera that obsessed candidates to Ferran's vaccination.

61. Cartaz, 1885, p. 58.
62. Larousse, 1888, p. 821.
63. Ferran, 1885a, p. 959.
64. Apert, 1922, p. 172.

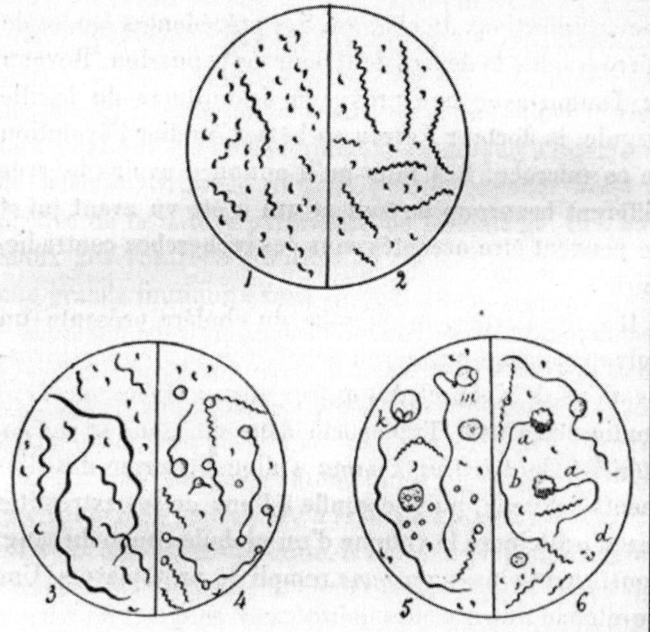

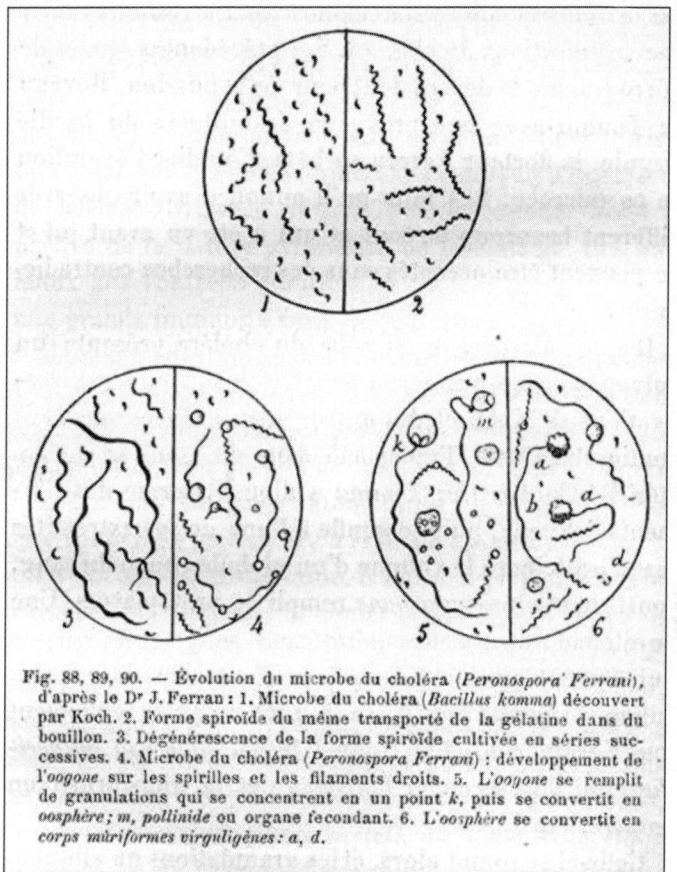

Fig. 88, 89, 90. — Évolution du microbe du choléra (*Peronospora Ferrani*), d'après le Dr J. Ferran : 1. Microbe du choléra (*Bacillus komma*) découvert par Koch. 2. Forme spiroïde du même transporté de la gélatine dans du bouillon. 3. Dégénérescence de la forme spiroïde cultivée en séries successives. 4. Microbe du choléra (*Peronospora Ferrani*) : développement de l'*oogone* sur les spirilles et les filaments droits. 5. L'*oogone* se remplit de granulations qui se concentrent en un point *k*, puis se convertit en *oosphère ; m, pollinide* ou organe fecondant. 6. L'*oosphère* se convertit en *corps mûriformes virguligènes : a, d.*

Figure 15. "Evolution of the *cholera* microbe (*Peronospora Ferrani*), according to Dr. J. Ferran." (From E. L. Trouessart, *Les Microbes, les ferments et les moisissures*, 1886. Figures 88, 89 and 90, page 194). The second edition (1891) reproduces the same figure (page 181), with a change in the first sentence, which reads: "*Evolution of the supposed cholera microbe...*" In the intervening years, some doubt has seeped into the minds of Ferran's readers.

In Spain, the medical milieu was swept up in the controversy. Stormy debates took place at *the Instituto Medico Valenciano* and at the *Ateneo of Madrid*. It seems that opponents sent messages to external medical authorities. The Academy of Sciences in Paris apparently received a dispatch from the Academy of Medicine and Surgery of Valencia (Spain) (*Instituto Medico Valenciano*) asking it to wait for the results of an enquiry requested by the *Instituto*. The first Commission appointed by the Royal Academy of Medicine of Madrid, headed by Franscisco Alonso Y Rubio, gave a rather favourable opinion of the procedure. But despite everything, no doubt responding to pressure from various sources, the Minister of the Interior, Romero Robledo, decided to forbid Ferran to continue his vaccination campaign. According to other sources, the Minister ordered him to vaccinate in person only, and in the presence of a government representative, which Ferran refused. He immediately started to fight back. On June 1885, he wrote to Pasteur in French: "*... my preventive cholerisation experiments... Because the new anti-cholera vaccination should be seen as a small ring detached* *from your great halo, I assumed that you would not consider it unworthy to support a discovery whose rightful godfather you are, in a manner of speaking, so that this support might lend me the energy necessary to vanquish the obstacles that ignorance and envy place in the way of the spread of the inoculation... Following an order from the Minister of the interior, an order based on mistaken and slanderous information, the anti-cholera inoculation has been forbidden.*"[65]

Ferran was seeking Pasteur's help against the order of the Spanish minister. In his letter, he also stated that an official commission was studying the results of his vaccinations. The convenient replacement of R. Robledo by Canovas del Castillo as minister allowed Ferran to once again carry out vaccinations as he saw fit[66]. In fact, although the effectiveness of this vaccination was difficult to assess, at the time its safety was not questioned. As for Pasteur, he apparently did not answer Ferran's letter.

In Europe, public opinion was impassioned about this debate, because cholera inspired great dread. Official delegations abounded. In France, the special commission of the advisory Committee on Public Hygiene, in charge of cholera-related problems, recommended sending a scientific mission to Spain. The president of this commission presented his request to the Minister of Commerce and Health. The latter had already entrusted such a mission to Dr. Paul Gibier, assistant naturalist at the Museum, working in Mr. Bouley's pathology laboratory. Bouley was the president of the Academy of Sciences, who had made the request. However, the minister hastened to defer to the recommendation of the Advisory Committee, and sent a second delegation. He named Roux, from Pasteur's team, Joachim Albarran and the inevitable Brouardel to be part of the delegation. Roux declined, in favour of Dr. Charrin, laboratory director at the Faculty of Medicine[67]. Roux's refusal was justified either by the fact that he was part of the Pasteur laboratory, or by the fact that his previous investigations (in Egypt and Toulon) on the subject could have caused him to be biased.

Albarran, who was interning in the Paris hospital network, spoke Spanish, which was his native language. He was born in Cuba, had studied medicine in Havana, in Barcelona, and finally in Paris, where in 1884 he graduated in first place when he took entrance examination for a housemanship[68]. This was obvious proof of his great competence in medicine.

Albarran was also a competent bacteriologist, which was very useful for the work of the mission. It seems that on certain occasions he listened to conversations in Spanish without revealing his knowledge of the language: acting as a spy, as it were... The mission had a letter of introduction from Pasteur himself, asking for permission, for the members of the mission or for him, to examine Ferran's work. Pasteur's letter, dated June 26, 1885, is open-minded: "*Some people mock you, others are hostile, and many are very appreciative... The first thing that must be made clear is whether you prevent cholera in those you inoculate. The question of the attenuated virus and of vaccinations is still so mysterious that no one has the right to condemn you based on preconceived ideas and on conclusions drawn in advance. Only the facts should be considered to make a judgement of your method.*"[69] Pasteur is open to novelty and his attitude is altogether fair.

65. NAF 18103, item 252.
66. Respaut, 1885, p. 62.
67. Rochard, 1888, p. 493.
68. Dupont, 1999, p. 8.
69. Pasteur, O.C., t. VI, p. 545.

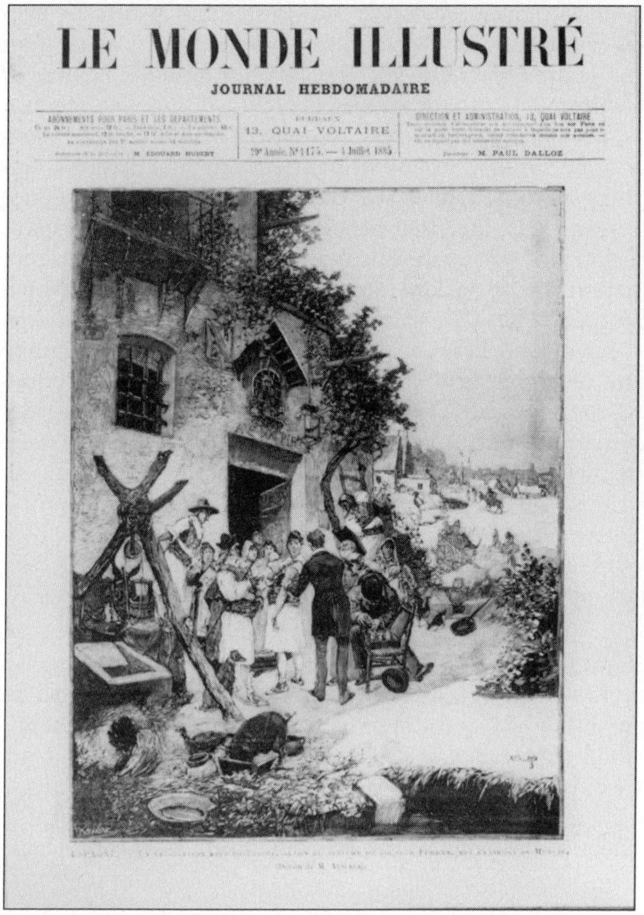

Figure 16. *"The anti-cholera vaccination, as Dr. Ferran practiced it, in the Murcia area (Spain)."* Based on a drawing by Mr. Atalaya. In this country setting, the vaccinator's (probably Ferran himself) hat is at the foot of the chair that serves as a table. A crowd of curious onlookers is present. The animals seem to pursue their peaceful existence undisturbed. It is possible that this illustration encouraged Pasteur to inoculate the young Meister, since it was published a few days prior to Joseph Meister's arrival to Paris. At that time, Ferran had already vaccinated 4,700 people against cholera, while Pasteur had vaccinated none. In addition, this magazine had a very wide readership in France. (*Le Monde illustré*, July 4, 1885.) The same illustration can be found in *Harper Weekly*, August 1885, p. 491.

On June 27, 1885, Brouardel, Charrin and Albarran left Paris to see Ferran, who gave them a rather unfriendly reception, refusing to reveal his method of preparation, or even to let a sample of his vaccine leave his laboratory. He offered to sell his procedure to the delegation. It must be said, in his defence, that the title of the French minister who sent the delegation was Minister of Commerce, and only secondarily Minister of Health! This mission, headed by Brouardel, is often said to have been sent by the *Institut Pasteur*[70], which is not the case.

Ferran also informed the delegation that the preparations of special morphology forms of the coma bacillus, which he had described, no longer existed because he had not kept them. Yet a few months earlier they were the basis for his success.

When he returned to Paris, Brouardel made a presentation at the Academy of Medicine[71]. His polite speech was full of moderation and fairness, but reflected the deep disapproval of the members of the mission. Dr. Ferran's laboratory was poorly equipped. His only equipment consisted of two microscopes with a maximum field diameter of

70. Jonas, 1960, p. 245; Lutzker, 1987, p. 366; Sack *in* Plotkin, 1994, p. 635, or 1999, p. 639.
71. Brouardel, 1885, p. 902.

700 to 800, a wooden incubator without a regulator, and no staining agents for bacteriology... Brouardel's mission witnessed the vaccination of about twenty nuns from the hospice of the "Little Sisters of the Poor". The vaccine, brought from the laboratory in a vial inadequately closed with a wad of cotton, was poured into a coffee cup not previously sterilized by a flame, provided by the sisters. No asepsis measures were taken during the inoculations. The same syringe, not sterilised between inoculations, was used for all of them. The syringe was filled quickly and the air trapped in it was not let out before the injection. Ferran vaccinated four people per minute, that is, he gave eight 1cc injections (each person was vaccinated in both arms). There was no pre-inoculation exam. The vaccination cost 5 to 12.50 francs (about 16 to 40 euros), which was a considerable sum at the time. The daily earnings of a Parisian manual worker, for ten hours of work, would have been between 5 francs for a mason's assistant to 9 francs for a carpenter[72]. The next day, the delegation made sure that no serious accidents had occurred among the inoculated nuns, and tried to correct the statistics given by the defenders of the method. But in vain, for at that time no statistics were credible. This is not hard to believe: populations were not subjected to census, inoculated persons received no certificates with the dates of vaccinations, and the control population was not representative. It is likely that because of the speed with which people were vaccinated, it would have been difficult to record the names and addresses of the vaccinated. The illustrations of the period do not show any scenes of registration, nor of payment[73].

According to a rumour circulating at the time, Ferran had been able to stamp out an 1885 cholera epidemic in five days, which seems hard to believe. Immunity cannot be obtained so quickly. But Ferran did provide a list of some vaccinated persons, including physicians, showing that he had confidence in his "vaccine". However, he did not present the results of these vaccinations. At the time, it would have been difficult, if not impossible, to provide such results. Ferran answered Pasteur's letter, in Spanish; in his answer, he expressed clear resentment at the account given by the Brouardel mission[74].

The process used to produce Ferran's anti-cholera vaccine is clearly described in his letter to the Academy of Sciences, dated March 31, 1885 and presented during the April 13, 1885 session[75], before the departure of the Brouardel mission. Ferran inoculated virulent cultures subcutaneously, without special preparation of the coma bacillus: "*That is, a coma bacillus culture whose seed comes from colonies that have developed ('évolutionné') on plates… Maximum virulence is obtained by seeding in very nutritious broth… with incubation (at 37°) lasting just the time needed for the broth to become cloudy… Effects of the microbe in man… From these facts, so clear and so easy to reproduce, we can rightfully conclude that: 1° Cholerisation is possible in man as it is in guinea pigs, by means of hypodermic injection 2° Protection conferred by cholerisation is obtained by injections of progressive doses or virulence; I remain at the disposal of the Academy to reproduce before it the experiments I have just described. Names of persons who have been cholerised (38 names are given)*."[76]

72. Anonyme, 1885d, p. 671.
73. Rochard, 1888, p. 493; Trouessard, 1891, p. 182; Larousse, 1888, p. 821; "illustrated" papers already quoted.
74. NAF 18103, item 258-262.
75. Ferran, 1885a, p. 959.
76. Ferran, 1885a, p. 959.

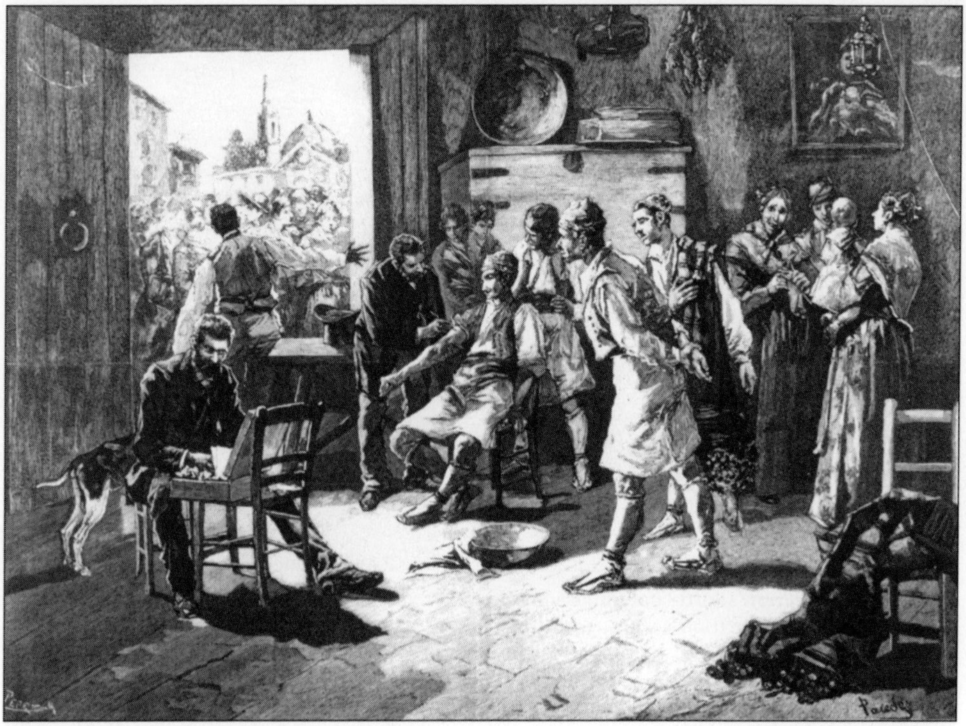

Figure 17. Double page in *La France illustrée* (August 8, 1885), entitled: "*The cholera in Spain: Dr. Ferran's vaccination*". Drawing by Mr. Paredes, engraving by Mr. Pérez. The scene is interesting, for the crowd is gathered at the door to look, or to be vaccinated. On the floor, a towel is lying near a basin.

Ferran's vaccine was composed of normal cholera bacillus cultures, probably more or less contaminated by other bacilli. In his note to the Academy of Sciences (Paris), read at the July 13, 1885 session, and written, therefore, around July 1 (taking as reference his March 31 letter read at the Academy of Sciences April 13, 1885 session), Ferran describes his method once again: "... *The culture* (of the coma bacillus) *with the highest virulence was perfectly well tolerated by man; I added that a second dose equal to the first did not produce general symptoms, although it had the same virulence as the first and I concluded that the first inoculation confers immunity that creates better resistance to the second... Obtaining immunity to cholera is both very simple and harmless. The vaccine is nothing other than a pure culture of the coma microbe of the Asian cholera, in very nutritious broth; the degree of virulence is directly related, to a certain point, to the nutritive quality of the milieu. In other circumstances, exposure to air increases the intensity of the culture. The best vaccine is the most virulent, that is, that which produces the greatest number of cases of experimental cholera among those inoculated. The dose I use at all ages, starting at 2 years, is 1 cc in each arm. The symptoms that develop, although they can be very intense, do not require treatment... The microbe does not reproduce in cellular tissue and its prophylactic action is due to a sort of acclimatisation or familiarity of the system with the spreading of the active substance introduced by the microbe.*"[77]

77. Ferran, 1885b, p. 147.

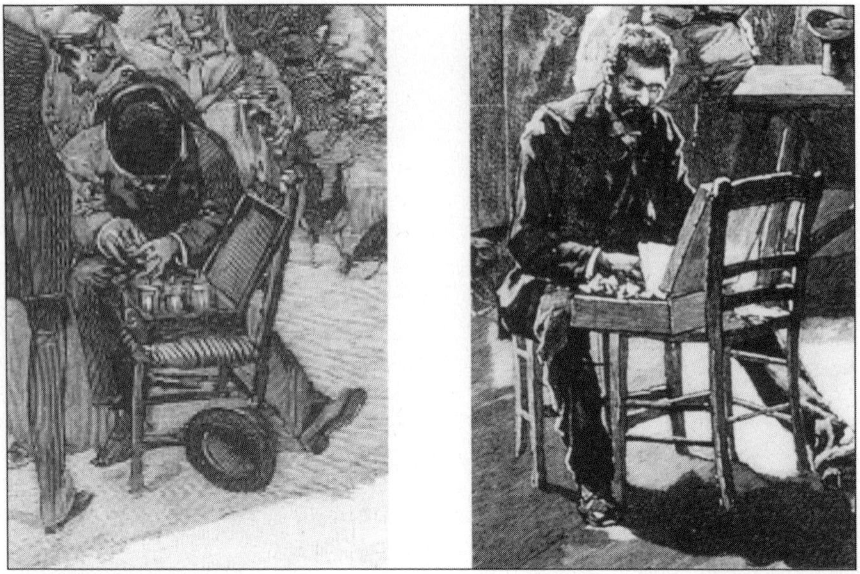

Figure 18. Dr. Ferran's anti-cholera vaccinations. These two illustrations, published one month apart, show two vaccination scenes, with the Ferran vaccine being transported in the same way: a kind of case or box placed on a chair during the procedure. An assistant is seated beside the inoculator and fills the syringe or syringes used by Ferran, or assists him in some way. The two vaccination sessions are depicted similarly, making it likely that they are true reflections of the actual scenes. Unfortunately, asepsis measures seem rudimentary, if they exist at all. (Left: *Le Monde illustré*, July 4, 1885; right: *La France illustrée*, August 8, 1885.)

This text was reproduced in Figuier's "*L'Année scientifique et industrielle*" (1885, published in 1886). Figuier wants to know why the very official French commission, sent by the Minister of Commerce to see Ferran, asked him to reveal the secret of his method of immunisation against cholera. In fact, there was no secret[78], but only a multitude of information communicated by Ferran, part of which was fact and the rest fancy. The July 13, 1885 presentation which describes in detail the method of preparation of his vaccine must have been written during the stay of Brouardel's mission in Spain. The mission had left Paris on June 27, 1885! Clearly, there was no affinity, and above all no agreement, between Brouardel's mission and Ferran, despite Abarran's presence!

It seems that Ferran had no equipment for the preparation of his vaccine. He prepared it on the spot and extemporaneously. On August 3, 1885, Ferran sent another letter[79] to the Academy of Sciences, promising statistics, following an official request from the Bréant award commission for official vaccination statistics[80]. The Academy answered, through Vulpian, that it regrets "*that M. Ferran did not understand the intention of the note inserted in the last report of the Academy. The commission had not asked for M. Ferran's statistics, but for the official statistics gathered by the Spanish authorities. It is to be hoped that on a question like cholera, which is of such vital importance to Humanity as a whole, the Spanish government would make it a point of honour to fully enlighten all nations on the*

78. Figuier, 1886, p. 333.
79. Ferran, 1885c, p. 367.
80. Gosselin, 1885, p. 227.

value of Mr. *Ferran's vaccinations.*"[81] No one had asked as much of Pasteur. There were never any official statistics given by the French government on anti-rabies treatments, nor any official declarations from the Academy of Sciences or of Medicine. There were only unofficial statistics gathered at the request of various authorities. Of course, Pasteur's vaccinations were not comparable to Ferran's. The first were properly identified on the premises of Pasteur laboratories, the second produced hastily in large quantities, at any location across the country.

Ferran sent several more notes to the Academy of Sciences, in 1888[82] and over the following years.

His results were analysed by many commissions, particularly those of the Academies of Medicine of Barcelona and Madrid, of France, Belgium, Portugal and Italy. There were also Italian, Russian, Brazilian and American observers. They all made the trip to Spain. The British commission stated that Ferran's cultures did not contain coma bacillus (cholera bacillus), a fact the commission did not consider very important because they believed that the bacillus, discovered by Koch, was not the direct cause of cholera... Van Ermengem, an excellent bacteriologist, appointed by the Belgian government to study the value of Ferran's vaccinations "*returned from his mission to Valencia with the impression that the pratical value of this preventive method had not all been demonstrated by the statistics cited by its advocates*"[83]. Van Ermengem had changed his mind since 1885, when he had written a cautious but rather favourable initial report. Gibier, the first French envoy, and van Ermengem, the Belgian envoy, co-authored and published a study in which they state not having been able to confirm Ferran's results in guinea pigs, using material from the latter's laboratory[84]. Nicati and Rietsch were also unable to obtain preventive immunity against a test dose of coma bacillus administered in the stomach by subcutaneous injection to guinea pigs[85]. Reports were all negative or hostile, with two exceptions: those of the Portuguese and American commissions which were late-comers and might have judged the results with greater perspective[86]. The report of the American commission was written by Shakespeare, its President, who expressed regret that most of the opinions submitted were based on those of the French mission headed by Brouardel. The first statistics concerning Ferran's vaccinations were certainly without value, since they were gathered by his followers, who were not neutral enough to conduct an impartial enquiry. Later, at the time of the second official Spanish commission, the data appears to have been gathered by government delegates, and verified.

Later, Ferran's statistics for twenty-two cities showed: 104,561 subjects not inoculated, of whom 8,046 developed cholera, which caused 3,512 deaths; and 30,491 inoculated subjects, with 387 cases of cholera and 104 deaths[87]. These results seem accurate, at least according to Bornside[88], who analysed them carefully. The unresolved difficulty is the impossibility of comparing two groups of individuals considered separately, and therefore not really comparable since they were not subjected to the same conditions

81. Vulpian, 1885, p. 367.
82. Ferran, 1888, pp. 454 & 645.
83. van Ermengem, 1908, t. 2, p. 20.
84. Gibier, 1885, p. 470.
85. Nicati, 1886, p. 76.
86. Bornside, 1981, p. 516; Roy, 1886, p. 173.
87. Sternberg, 1895, p. 122.
88. Bornside, 1981, p. 529.

of contagion. Netter admitted that Ferran's results were perhaps accurate, since animals inoculated in an identical manner were found to have specific antibodies[89]. No other details are available. It is somewhat surprising that Ferran did not use his official statistics, favourable to his vaccinations, if indeed they existed, to support his numerous applications for the Bréant award. There is a contradiction between Shakespeare's declarations and Ferran's writings on the subject of his own results.

Ferran seems to have had a talent fort turning everyone against him. A long article by Chauveau on Ferran's work starts as follows: "*I know as well as anyone the reasons that make microbiologists fail to grant their confidence to* Mr. *Ferran: his fanciful tergiversations on the evolution of the coma bacillus, the assertions and the theories he extrapolates from his experiments on animals, the thoroughly unscientific reasons that impelled him to allege that he possessed a secret process of cholera virus attenuation.*"[90] Ferran might have drawn on previous texts which showed, to all intents and purposes, the harmless effects of injecting his vaccine of cholera bacillus cultures to animals and even to man[91]. Still, the effectiveness of the hypodermic inoculation was not proven. He took the risk of experimenting on human beings, and on himself first of all. His method resembled "variolation" more than "vaccination", because the bacilli were natural (wild). This does not diminish his merit for having been the first person to attempt protecting human beings from cholera. With the exception of smallpox vaccinations, he was also the instigator of the first large-scale human vaccination campaign. He vaccinated 4,700 people in the Murcia region, in 1885, with no ensuing fatalities[92]. In Spain, Ferran was the object of veritable worship; many people insisted on being inoculated by him and no one else... It is difficult to evaluate his work more explicitly, but it is certain that it deserves consideration.

In time, the epidemic abated and finally ended, as was expected. Then, the Cambrils affair created a stir. The note in the "*Union médicale*" that describes this episode is a little lengthy, but interesting: "*The Diaro de Tarragona published the following excerpt from the local Cambrils paper of September 5, 1,885. Cambrils is a small sea-side town located between Tortosa and Tarragona, 20 kilometres from this city. We are presenting a literal translation of this article: 'before any inoculations were undertaken in Cambrils, there had been no case of cholera, or even a suspected case, in the upper city; in the seaside area, there were only ten to twelve convalescent patients. Since the day when inoculations started until today, these are the names of persons suffering from cholera, as declared by the physician who treated them:*

Inoculated deceased... (4 names are given).

Not inoculated, deceased... (9 names are given).

Persons who had to be amputated of one or both arms to stop the gangrene... (9 names are given). *To this list must be added two other persons who were told they would have surgery the next day, and the persons who are confined to bed as a result of the inoculation... Given these deplorable accidents, the panic that has taken hold of the inhabitants is indescribable, especially among the inoculated. Today, the Ferran method no longer has its passionate advocates who so admired him and accompanied him in his campaign.' The physicians who read, in Brouardel, Charrin and Albarran's reports, in Van Ermengen's and Gibier's reports,*

89. Netter, 1903, t. VI, p. 778.
90. Chauveau, 1885, p. 353.
91. Desnos, 1867, t. 7, p. 380; Bochefontaine, 1885, p. 1148.
92. Anonyme, 1885c, p. 478.

the description of the procedures employed by Mr. Ferran to practice his inoculations, were surprised that the absence of any precautions did not produce accidental infection, septicaemia, etc.

Today, the Cambrils disaster justifies their worries. The paper gives little information on the number of inoculated persons, or on the date when the accidents started, but it reports that gangrene required that nine of those who were inoculated be amputated of one or both arms...

The Academy of Madrid was right to say, in one of the conclusions at the end of its report on Mr. Ferran's inoculations, that it has not been demonstrated that they are without danger."[93]

In 1888, three years after this publication, Rochard described this accident once again[94]. He did not contribute any news facts, but did not deny any of the facts three years later! A rather dark stain on Ferran's career... that neither Shakespeare, nor Ferran biographers like Bornside, mention. The accuracy of this tragic episode is somewhat doubtful. A more in-depth study would be needed to verify the truth of this information. If these events are true, they are apparently due to a septic accident. This does not discredit the value of Ferran's vaccinations, but rather his working conditions.

Flügge, a good microbiologist at that period, but opposed to Pasteur's ideas, did not take Ferran's anti-cholera vaccine seriously at all: "*The preventive inoculations given in Spain by Ferran, with so-called attenuated bacilli, are, according to this author's own data and to the reports concerning them, completely without any experimental or statistical basis and therefore cannot make the subject of any serious discussion.*"[95]

Ferran was one of the many candidates for the Bréant award of the Academy of Sciences (Paris). Bréant made an endowment to the Academy of Sciences and instituted an award of 100,000 French francs (at least 320,000 euros) "*to the person who has found a means of treating Asian cholera, or who has discovered the causes of this terrible blight*". Thinking that the award would not be granted before some time, Bréant asked that the interest on the capital, 5,000 French francs (about 16,000 euros) per year be awarded to a person who has contributed to the advancement of science on the question of the cholera, or more generally, the question of infectious diseases. This endowment, or the prizes ensuing from it, incited much writing and prompted much greed. When a new cholera epidemic broke out in 1884, the Academy of Sciences received 240 letters and numerous reports within a few weeks, all of them of little interest[96].

Ferran tried desperately to win the Bréant award, as early as March 1885. The successive commissions charged with granting this award displayed more and more questionable attitudes. In 1865, they had attributed 2,500 francs (about 8,000 euros) to Davaine for his discovery of the presence of anthrax bacteridium in the blood of ruminants with anthrax, and an award of 4,000 francs to Mr. Grimaud de Caux who had gone to Marseille to study cholera "*at the height of the epidemic.*"[97] Between 1880 and 1895, the Academy of Sciences awarded prizes (but never the 100,000 francs prize, which was unique), rewards, honourable mentions, support, or nothing at all... particularly to Koch, the discoverer of the cholera vibrion in 1883, and to Ferran, the first vaccinator (variolator) against cholera[98].

93. Anonyme, 1885b, p. 553.
94. Rochard, 1888, p. 494.
95. Flügge, 1887, p. 323.
96. Vulpian, 1884, p. 175.
97. Andral, 1866, p. 538.
98. Secrétaires perpétuels, 1900, p. 1539.

The Russian Gamaleïa sent a communication to the Academy of Sciences (of Paris), that was read by Pasteur on August 20, 1885[99]. In Odessa, after a few months of training at Pasteur's laboratory at the *Ecole Normale Supérieure*, Gamaleïa had made repeated passages of cholera vibrions in pigeons. This strain of cholera vibrions had then acquired very high virulence for this species. By cultivating it in nutritious broth heated to 120° C for twenty minutes to kill microbes, Gamaleïa obtained a vaccinating preparation. To protect a guinea pig or a pigeon, two or three doses had to be administered. This was a sterile vaccine, also called "chemical". Gamaleïa intended to continue his studies in man. His work provoked much commentary[100]. The Gamaleïa vaccine was very similar to one proposed by Ferran, who accused the Russian of plagiarism. The latter's dead microbe vaccine appears not to have gone past the experimental stage. With Pasteur's unwavering support, Gamaleïa obtained a Bréant award (annual arrears) before Ferran. This was to be the only reward for his work. On September 17, 1888, Grancher wrote to Pasteur on the subject of the Gamalaïa "vaccine". "*... The other, the dangerous great masses, believe in a new vaccine* (against cholera), *and if tomorrow cholera breaks out in Marseille, they will ask you for the vaccination. Can you provide it? And if not, do you think that the public will make Gamalaïa pay for its disappointment? I am therefore taking the liberty to write you, dear Master, what everyone in Paris and Houlgate thinks but does not dare to tell you. I will go ever further...*"[101]. Grancher is no longer the young lad he was in 1885. He shares his point of view: Pasteur supports Gamaleïa's vaccine too openly, although the vaccine is experimental. But at this stage, Pasteur no longer has enough energy to continue the work that allowed him to discover and produce his previous vaccines... Gameleïa was suspected of having cultivated the bacillus of a fowl gastroenteritis, rather than *Vibrio cholerae*[102]. This might be true... or not.

Ferran complained to Pasteur. In a letter dated August 21, 1888, he protested the Academy of Sciences' decision to award the Bréant prize to Gamaleïa (arrears, in fact): "*As your proposal seems to indicate a total forgetting on your part of our experiments and our right to priority, I beseech you, in the name of justice...*"[103]. Ferran was very disgruntled... and with good reason.

Pasteur, *a priori*, remained quite indifferent to all this fuss. As was his habit, he supported blindly those close to him and was not interested in those who were far.

As for the arrears, that is, the interest generated by the investment of the capital of the Bréant prize, they were shared by Mr. Vaillard and Mr. Dopter on the one hand, and Mr. Ferran on the other hand, in 1907. Roux was the author of the report concerning this decision. The report was cautious: "*To his interesting description, Mr. Ferran added the list of the works he has published since 1884 on the cholera microbe...*" Roux then described Ferran's work and "*... without making a judgement of the preventive value of this prophylactic procedure* (his method of preventing cholera in human beings), *the Bréant award commission considers that Mr. Ferran has contributed greatly to the advancement of our knowledge about cholera; it awards him half* (of the annual interest) *of the Bréant prize.*"[104] Roux and the members of this commission showed proof of wisdom and honesty by writing this report, as did the Academy of Sciences by adopting its

99. Gamalaïa, 1888, p. 432.
100. Anonyme, 1888a, p. 230; Cornil, 1890, t. 2, p. 205; Daremberg, 1892, p. 35; Figuier, 1889, p. 398.
101. NAF 18103, f. 479.
102. Lutzer, 1987, p. 366.
103. NAF 18103, item 257.
104. Roux, 1907, p. 1030.

conclusions. It is clear that Ferran was a very patient man. Bréant made many people dream and satisfied the ambition of some. Unfortunately, no one won the great prize...

When the 1885 epidemic ended, Ferran retired to Tortosa; it was there that he was persuaded to be the founder of the municipal laboratory of Barcelona, for the prevention of rabies after a bite, using the Pasteurian method. Ferran was a very charismatic man. He had aroused the enthusiasm of the crowds when he campaigned for cholera prevention. He was a man endowed with an exceptional personality. And what rhetoric! Such fanciful inventions to speak of real discoveries... Finally, Ferran wrote a great deal, too much to always be taken seriously. And he did not hold back on extravagant compliments. *Le Temps* published a letter (the issue is not specified) written by Ferran, and reprinted in an unidentified paper: "*The two greatest men humanity has known were Christ, who brought it redemption, and Pasteur who gave us the laws that should lead to our physical redemption.*"[105] For once, he made no reference to himself. He was showing some modesty.

Ferran's texts were all criticized and refuted, one after the other. Soon they deserved no more than a mention, until they gradually disappeared[106].

The Russian Haffkine started to work on cholera at the *Institut Pasteur* in Paris in 1889. Following the Pasteurian model, he developed, from fixed virulence bacteria, a vaccine to be given in two increasing-virulence injections. Their side effects were powerful: "*Local and general reactions are very intense.*"[107] Haffkine presented his first findings, made on himself and three other people, to the "*Société de Biologie*" (Society of Biology) on July 30, 1892, then in *The Lancet*[108]. Haffkine's vaccine, tested on fifty confident people[109], proved to be interesting but did not convince everyone.

Ferran again protested vigorously against Haffkine and his vaccines, repeating that they were only replicas of his own work[110]. This reproach was unfounded, since the conditions for the preparation of the Haffkine vaccine were much better established than those of Ferran's vaccine.

Catastrophic events often solicit exceptional behaviour. In 1892, an American journalist, Mr. Stanhope, editor at the *New York Herald*, had himself inoculated with the Haffkine vaccine, at the *Ecole Normale Supérieure* (*sic*, this detail is strange, because the *Institut Pasteur* was inaugurated on November 14, 1888). In fact, not everyone moved to Dutot Street right after the inauguration.

Duclaux continued to work for some time on Lhomond Street[111]. Stanhope, vaccinated with a product that was still very experimental, left for Hamburg, a focal centre for cholera at that time. He obtained permission to eat and sleep in the cholera patient's room at the Epperdorff Hospital, to sleep in the bed of a patient who had died of cholera, between two patients, at the height of the epidemic, to look after patients without taking the recommended precautions, and to drink the water of the Elbe that was said to have caused the first infections... On September 26, 1892, he wrote: "*I left ward F. where I had just spent eight days among the dying and the dead... I had tears in my*

105. NAF 18092, item 372.
106. Cornil, 1890, t. 2, p. 205.
107. Apert, 1922, p. 172.
108. Haffkine, 1892, p. 740; Haffkine, 1893, p. 316.
109. NAF 18092, item 334.
110. Ferran, 1892, p. 771.
111. Duclaux (Mary), 1906, p. 203.

eyes when I closed the great wooden door of the ward behind me and, if no one had been looking, I would have hidden my head in my hands and would have cried like a woman..."[112]. Perhaps a little condescending for the so-called weaker sex, but the sentiments are those of a courageous man! Unfortunately, as the "*Magasin pittoresque*" of that era points out, one example does not mean much[113]. Some individuals seemed to be refractory to cholera. Statistics on a large number of people were to show that Haffkine's vaccines provided protection, but that the induced immunity was temporary.

In December 1892, Beauval described the daily anti-cholera vaccinations administered at the *Institut Pasteur* by Haffkine or his colleagues; the description was even accompanied by an illustration. But Beauval expressed considerable reserve as to its as yet unproven value, except for the Stanhope case[114]. The method had to be tried on a high-risk population.

In 1892 or 1893, Haffkine solicited first the Russian government which, worried about the controversy surrounding Ferran's vaccine, as well as about a disaster associated with vaccinations against sheep anthrax in southern Russia[115], declined his

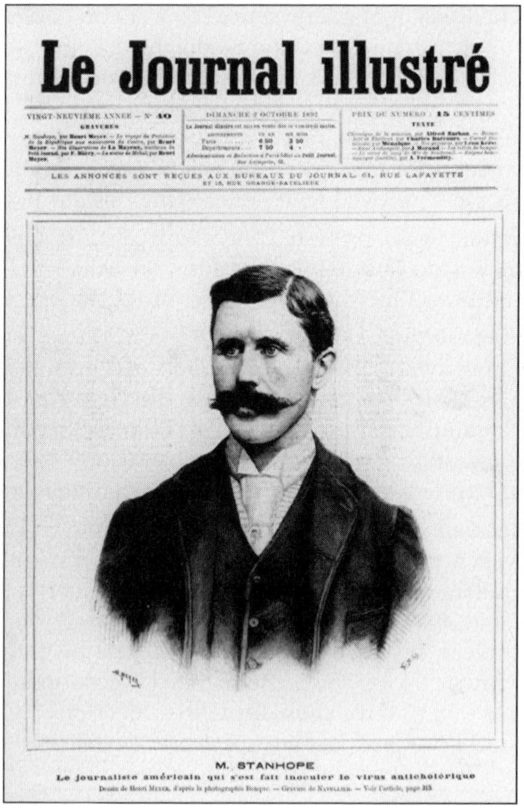

Figure 19. "Mr. *Stanhope, the American journalist inoculated with the cholera vaccine.*" This journalist was inoculated with the cholera vaccine by Haffkine before travelling to Hamburg where a terrible cholera epidemic was raging. There, he went into a hospital that cared for cholera victims, and ignored all the precautions recommended to avoid infection. He did not contract the disease and became an excellent publicity for the Haffkine vaccine. (Drawing by Henri Meyer, after a photograph by Benque, engraving by Navellier. *Le Journal illustré*, n° 40, October 2, 1892.)

112. Anonyme, 1892a, p. 315.
113. Anonyme, 1892b, p. 43.
114. Beauval, 1892, p. 26.
115. Haffkine, 1895b, p. 1541.

offer to try this new vaccine. Haffkine then turned to Great Britain. He visited the persons most likely to help him with his project. At the end of January 1893, he carried out a demonstration at the Army Medical School, located in Netley (Hampshire, England), in the presence of Wright and Bruce[116], and he gave a lecture (lecture delivered by Dr. Ruffer using a translation of Haffkine's text (since Haffkine spoke English poorly at the time), before the Royal College of Physicians and Surgeons in London[117]. A descriptive text (probably the same one) was sent by Haffkine from London on January 29, 1893 to Pasteur[118], who received it on February 8. Haffkine developed two types of vaccine from cholera bacillus with exalted virulence by successive passages to between twenty to thirty guinea pigs. One type of vaccine was inactivated by carbolic acid and by heat, a procedure Haffkine himself did not recommend, and the other was a living vaccine. In the latter case, a first injection used a strain highly attenuated by re-inoculation in *in vitro* cultures, and a second injection used a fixed strain with exalted virulence. There was a problem connected with this strain, which in *in vitro* culture only maintained its exalted virulence for about ten days. Therefore, it had to be passed successively to three or four guinea pigs, for it to recover its maximum virulence[119], which must have considerably increased the difficulty of preparing this vaccine. Haffkine was greeted warmly by Joseph Lister, by Dr.Turner from Guy's Hospital, by Wright (cf first vaccine against typhoid fever) and by Bruce[120].

Convinced by a letter of recommendation from the British government, India accepted the experiment. On April 12, 1893, Haffkine wrote to Pasteur as soon as he arrived in India. From his lodgings in Bombay, where he met with complete indifference on the part of the local medical milieu, on March 5 he wrote to several high-ranking officials in Agra, a secular focal centre for cholera. He found solid support in the person of Mr. E. H. Hankin, the Chemical examiner and bacteriologist with the government of Agra. Haffkine was probably in awe at the sight of the Taj Mahal and the Red Fort, but distressed by the misery he saw in the living conditions of the population. The location had been well chosen. Europeans as well as native Indians dreaded the cholera. "*Fifteen physicians and superior officers immediately volunteered to be the first ones subjected to the procedure, in order to serve as an example and motivate the natives. The wives followed their husbands, and offered children to be vaccinated, in order to inspire confidence in a benevolent procedure, in the population they governed. The general of the brigade, not daring to personally take the initiative of introducing the vaccination among the soldiers under his command, volunteered to be inoculated first. All of them recommended the vaccination to their servants and their families, and the impetus was given.*"[121] Two thirds of the subjects were vaccinated with Haffkine's living whole vaccine, using two injections, and one third received a single injection. Each time, subjects to be vaccinated were chosen among populations where there were unvaccinated control groups. Haffkine administered 70,000 doses of vaccine to 42,179 persons, 31,056 of them Indians, persuaded with no need to exert any pressure on them. Haffkine's report tends to prove that his vaccine was effective, but his conclusions

116. Wright, 1893, p. 227.
117. Haffkine, 1893, p. 316.
118. NAF 18092, items 334 to 355.
119. Wright, 1893, p. 227.
120. NAF 18104, f.P. 52.
121. NAF 18104, f.P. 45.

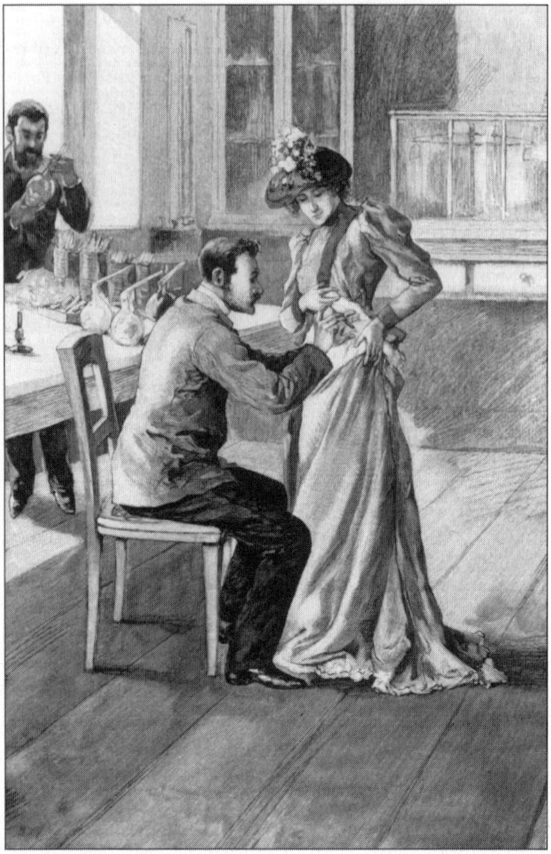

Figure 20. Haffkine's anti-cholera inoculation. (*La Science illustrée*, n° 262, December 3, 1892.) The author of the article which comments the illustration is very cautious in his remarks: "*The vaccination protects those who receive it from hypodermic injection of cholera but, despite Stanhope's experience, we cannot affirm that it protects from intestinal cholera.*"[122] The vaccine is a suspension of inactivated coma bacillus, or coma bacillus with attenuated virulence. At the end of January 1893, Wright and Bruce described Haffkine's technique as follows: "*For injecting the vaccine Mr. Haffkine employs a very simple form of hypodermic syringe, which is provided with a caoutchouc or elder pith piston (Malassez's or Strauss-Collin's syringe). This is taken to pieces and placed in boiling water for some minutes before use. Before transferring the contents of the vaccine tube to the hypodermic syringe, the tube is carefully tapped with the fingernail to dislodge any sediment which may be clinging to the walls of the tube. One of the closed ends is then heated in a flame to sterilize it, and the tip is broken off with a sterile forceps... The vaccines are to be introduced into the hypodermic tissue, not into the depth of the muscles. The seat of election for the vaccination is under the skin of the flank halfway between the crest of the ileum and the lowest rib. The inoculation of the first vaccine is made from three to five days before the inoculation of the second vaccine. When the first vaccine is inoculated into the right flank, the left flank is to be chosen for the inoculation of the second vaccine.*"[123] Technically, this injection is very similar to that used at the *Institut Pasteur* for rabies. The sterilisation of the instrument used in the procedure is noteworthy, although there is no indication of disinfecting measures prior to the injection.

122. Beauval, 1892, p. 26.
123. Wright, 1893, p. 230.

express certain reservations. Protection against cholera was rather short-lived, but it was genuine[124].

Koch's comments on Haffkine's report were very favourable: "*I* (Haffkine) *was most happy to learn that, for Prof. Koch, the demonstration was already complete; that he believes the protective power of the method to be established finally by the observations collected in India up to now; that further perfections and simplifications may be possible, but that the main questions at issue, the chief part of the problem, is solved by the facts recorded in the above report*"[125]. Haffkine also points out that the protection conferred by anti-sera is very brief, and that the use of serotherapy should be limited to patients already infected with cholera. He addressed an enquiry on this subject to Prof. Pfeiffer in Berlin, who provided him with a description of his experiment and a supply of antitoxic serum. But Haffkine adds: "*On the day I came back from India I found Pasteur lying on his death-bed. Whatever might have been his appreciation of the work, I have only one desire, that the whole of the honour that may come from my efforts should be referred to his sacred memory.*"[126] Obviously, the ties between Haffkine and Pasteur's team at the Institute were not as close. He turned to Pfeiffer and mentioned Pasteur's criticism (unspecified) of his work. Upon the death of Pasteur, who had given extravagant support to Gamaleïa's work, competition between Yersin and Haffkine in terms of their work on the plague became heated... Roux was to be the rapporteur of the Bréant award commission of the Academy of Sciences, for 1907. The commission proposed granting a 4,000-franc (about 12,800 euros) prize to Haffkine for his "*work on vaccination against cholera and Bubonic plague*"; the proposal was accepted by the Academy of Sciences. Roux praised Haffkine for his painstaking work and efforts to develop his vaccine against cholera. But he expressed reservations about the vaccine itself, whose preventive virtues were hard to assess. On the other hand, he praised Haffkine unreservedly for his vaccine against the plague[127].

Another interesting incident in the fight against cholera consisted in an unexpected suggestion submitted by Ferran: "*I do not hesitate to say that the most practical method to quickly confer immunity to a whole population is to infect the drinking water with large quantities of attenuated coma bacillus culture. This would result in the sudden occurrence, from among all the inhabitants, of one or two cases of diarrhoea-type stool, followed by a light reaction and temporary fatigue, symptoms that we* (Ferran and his friends) *experienced by drinking our cultures.*"[128] Chauveau spoke immediately after Ferran's note was read. First, he congratulated Ferran for having initiated vaccination against cholera; then, he expressed complete disapproval of the rapid procedure of collective vaccination proposed by Ferran. Chauveau saw it as an illegal and dangerous practice[129]. In addition, Ferran's vaccine was probably a more or less pure culture of cholera bacillus, without any attenuation. Results could have been disastrous. It was strange to propose the use of such a method. Ferran's subcutaneous vaccine was perhaps effective... but given orally in uncontrolled doses - the natural means of contamination -, it could have been dangerous.

Ferran and Haffkine's vaccines (used in India) were living microbe vaccines, but Haffkine makes a more precise distinction: "*It is the difference between vaccination and*

124. Haffkine, 1895a, p. 1555; Haffkine, 1895b, p. 1541; Enriquez, 1909, t. 1, p. 1306; Gautier, 1896, p. 193; Netter, 1903, t. VI, p. 778.
125. Haffkine, 1895b, p. 1541.
126. Haffkine, 1895a, p. 1555.
127. Roux, 1909, p. 1258.
128. Ferran, 1892, p. 771.
129. Chauveau, 1892, p. 773.

variolation that distinguishes the method which I have applied in India from that tried in Spain by Dr. Jaime Ferran in 1885. Ferran's operations consisted in inoculating vibrios collected from cholera patients. The method employed in India consisted in inoculating a vaccine worked out following the proceedings of Jenner and Pasteur."[130] In 1896, Kolle introduced a vaccine composed of cholera vibrios killed by heat, to which phenol was added as an agent of conservation; this vaccine was very similar to one of Haffkine's. The *Institut Pasteur* was to produce a vaccine containing 4 billion vibrios killed by being exposed to a temperature of 56° C for thirty minutes[131]. Even today, anti-cholera vaccines only confer relative immunity lasting a short time.

The mortality still associated with cholera is mainly due to lack of appropriate preventive measures. Cholera eradication is above all a problem of hygiene: access to clean drinking water, proper treatment of wastewater, decontamination of infected objects and personal hygiene are sufficient to avoid cholera epidemics. But fulfilling these requirements is expensive!

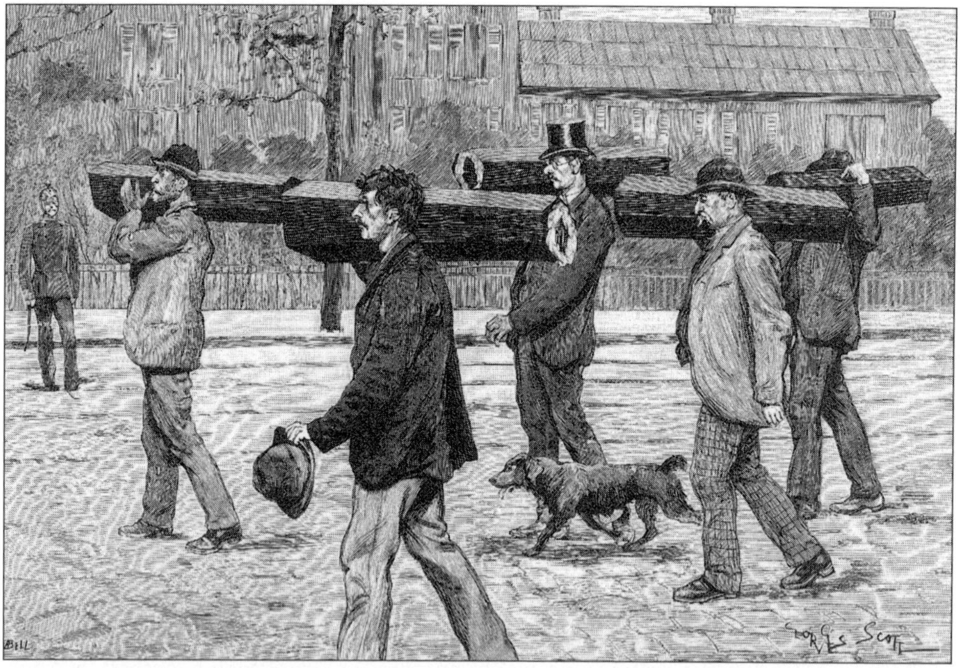

Figure 21. The cholera in Hamburg. Convoy of conscripted carriers, carrying children's caskets (based on a drawing by Max Kuchel). These employees of the emergency services advance toward the cemetary with their dreary load. (*L'Illustration*, September 17, 1892.)

The First Killed Microbe Vaccine "Marketed": Anti-Typhoid Fever Vaccine - 1887, 1896...

Typhoid fever, caused by Eberth's bacillus (*Salmonella typhi*) discovered in 1880, is an acute systemic febrile disease. The disease was almost always present at that time.

130. Haffkine, 1895b, p. 1541.
131. Violle, 1928, p. 388.

"*The illness that it* (Elberth's bacillus) *provokes does not break out suddenly: most often it drags on at length before breaking out outright. This incubation period can last two or three weeks, and its premonitory signs are very insidious: the sufferer feels fatigued, loses his appetite, is unable to work, experiences light headaches, chills and quite often nosebleeds as well. After this initial period, the characteristic symptoms come on: the headaches intensify to the point of making rest impossible; fatigue becomes prostration and sometimes even stupor. All this gives the patient's face a particular appearance that doctors call 'typhic character', easily recognizable by an experienced eye... It is one of the diseases associated with the most serious and diverse complications: nervous, pulmonary (pneumonia, pleurisy) and intestinal complications (perforated intestine, haemorrhage); circulatory system complications (heart and blood vessel problems), etc.*"[132] It was a serious disease, especially in adults, 10 to 20% of whom could die of it. The disease was just as dreadful when it recurred...

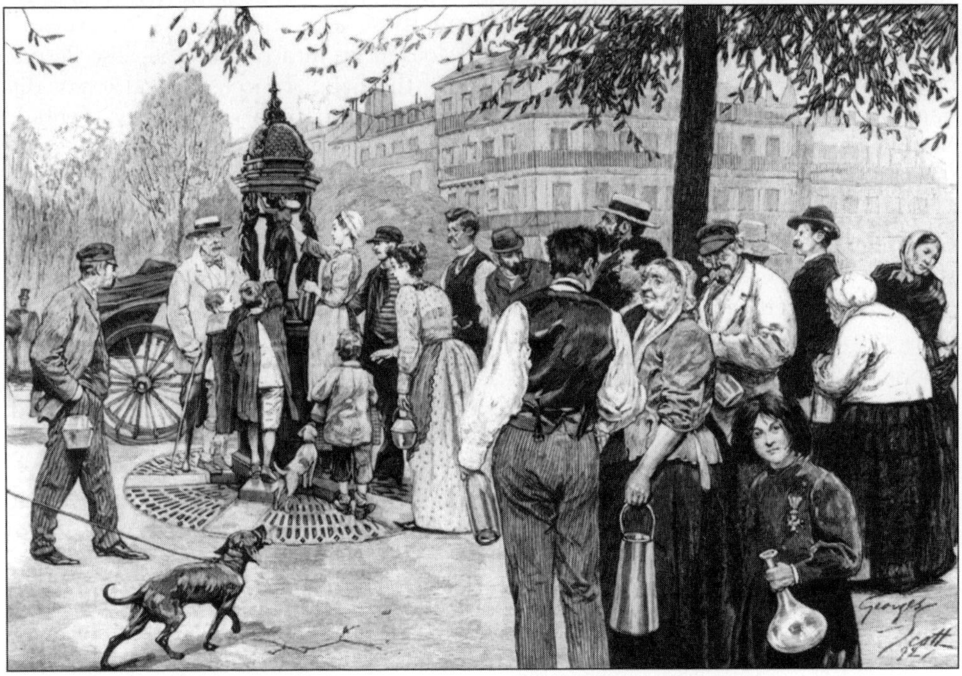

Figure 22. Paris 1892! "*Distribution of the water of the Seine - A public fountain giving spring water, in the Ternes neighbourhood.*" The article accompanying this illustration states that "*the substitution of spring water for the water of the Seine, which takes place once a year in every Paris arrondissement in turn, is also the occasion for interesting street scenes, animated and pictoresque. This one, at the corner of Wagram and Ternes Avenues, is a good illustration...*". The water (a thin trickle unable to provide drinking water for a whole arrondissement) of this Wallace fountain (named after the British philanthropist who made a gift of about fifty of these pretty little fountains to Parisians) is diverted from the neighbouring arrondissement whose spring water was not replaced. Parisians came to get their drinking water... The water of the Seine (or from the Ourcq canal) was not filtered. (*L'Illustration*, n° 2577, July 16, 1892.)

132. Haibe, 1914, p. 80.

At the beginning of the 20th century in France, there were 30,000 cases per year, and 4,000 fatalities. Mortality due to typhoid fever decreased with better hygiene and, above all, with the distribution of clean water. In Paris, the percentages of fatalities due to typhoid fever out of 1,000 deaths decreased regularly, dropping from 0.22 in 1891-1895 to 0.13 in 1911[133]. Epidemics were greatly exacerbated by wars. During the Spanish-American War (1898), there were 20,738 cases of typhoid fever among American troops, with 1,580 deaths out of a total of 107,973 men enlisted, while direct and indirect losses in combat due to wounds added up to 243 deaths, that is, seven times less[134].

Typhoid fever is contracted by swallowing infectious germs which then multiply in the intestines, if the subject is receptive and not immunised. The contaminated water in drinks is one of the main sources of infection. Some cured patients can be healthy carriers of bacilli and become foci of infection. The case of Mary Mallone is a classic example. Still called "typhoid Mary", this woman was a healthy carrier of Eberth's bacillus, and unknowingly spread death among those who ate the food she prepared as a restaurant employee. She ended her life locked up in a hospital because despite repeated warnings she remained unconscious of the harm she caused, and it was difficult, if not impossible, to control her. According to Hansen and Freney, Typhoid Mary made fifty-one victims, three of whom died[135].

In 1896, Achard and Bensaude described bacilli they called paratyphic, but the reality of their existence was contested. In 1900 they were rediscovered by Schottmüller at Hamburg. Kayser classified them as A and B. Their existence was only fully accepted after the epidemics that raged during the First World War among troops vaccinated only against Eberth's bacillus[136].

In 1887-1888, Chantemesse and Widal demonstrated that it was possible to immunise laboratory animals with Eberth's bacilli killed by heat (100° C), but these preparations were only weakly immunogenic. Almost at the same time, Wright on the one hand, and Kolle and Pfeiffer on the other hand, prepared anti-typhoid vaccines and demonstrated the possibility of immunising with dead salmonella. On September 19, 1896, Wright reported in the *Lancet* that he had applied Haffkine's technique of anti-cholera vaccination (dead typhoid bacilli)[137]. Wright did not present the results of his vaccinations. In this publication, he focused primarily on coagulation problems, the subject of his studies at the time.

On November 12, 1896, Koller and Pfeiffer published the results of inoculations given to two men with a dead vaccine, whose side effects were described as violent. Serum from these subjects proved to be bactericidal and to cluster Eberth's bacilli. On January 30, 1897, Wright published a study on the inoculation of eighteen patients (sixteen volunteers plus Wright and Semple) with a preparation of salmonella killed by heat. The vaccine was standardised by inoculation to guinea pigs of doses chosen based on their protective effects. The side effects produced in the inoculated subjects included fever, vomiting, headaches... Wright and Semple's article begins: "Mr. *Haffkine suggested more than twelve months ago to one of us that the method of vaccination*

133. Georgel, 1917, p. 18.
134. Zinsser, 1918, p. 484.
135. Hansen, 2002, p. 36.
136. Achard, 1929, p. 11.
137. Wright, 1896, p. 807.

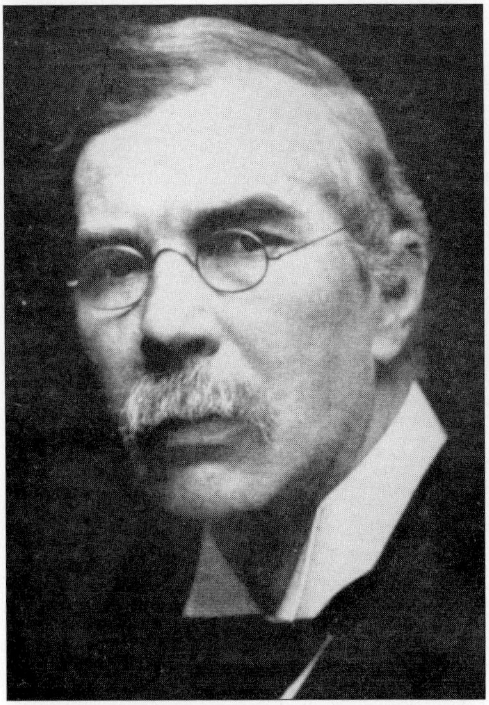

Figure 23. Almroth Wright (1861-1947), then Professor of Pathology at the Royal Army Medical College of Netley, who developed and promoted the anti-typhoid vaccine.

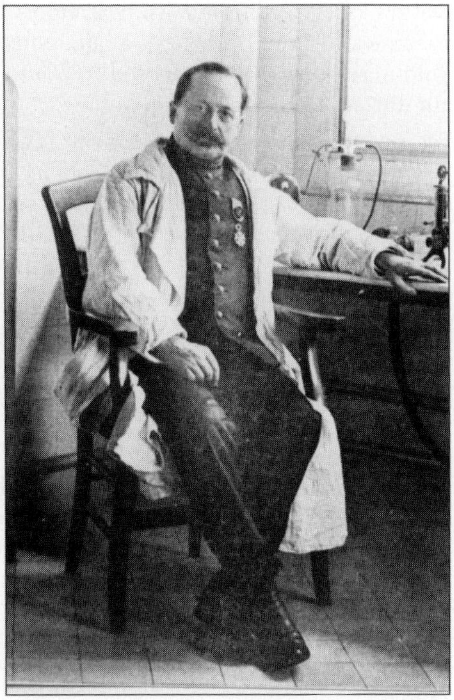

Figure 24. Hyacinthe Vincent (1862-1950). Military physician who developed, with Wright, Pfeiffer, Kolle and Chantemesse, the antityphoid vaccination. As early as 1910, in his Val-de-Grâce laboratory in Paris, he started to vaccinate military personnel with a vaccine killed by ether. This vaccination, which would become compulsory in the French army, has practically eliminated all cases of typhoid fever. (*L'Illustration*, n° 3671, July 5, 1913.)

shown to be so effective in fighting cholera epidemics in India could, mutatis mutandis, be applied as well to typhoid fever prevention."[138] As Wright and Semple specify, the idea and the technique for an anti-typhoid vaccine came from Haffkine, who developed it at the *Institut Pasteur* in Paris. In fact, they use the typically Pasteurian term "vaccination" to speak of this procedure, rather than the term "immunisation" used by Anglo-Saxons.

The first trials on volunteers from the British army in India, in Malta, in Egypt, in Jamaica and in South Africa showed real effectiveness, reducing morbidity and mortality by at least half compared to controls[139]. However, the side effects of this vaccine were so violent that the British Parliament took control of the matter after a campaign conducted by medical papers, and forbade its use. Finally, vaccination with Wright's vaccine was taken up again eighteen months later, on the recommendation of the

138. Wright, 1897, p. 256.
139. Anonyme, 1902b, p. 15; Citron, 1912, p. 31.

Royal College of Physicians, in London[140]. During the Boer war, Wright's anti-typhoid vaccine was used on a large scale, with an observed mortality rate of 16.6% in non immunised persons, as opposed to 8% in vaccinated subjects. But these statistical data are not always considered reliable...

Priority for this discovery was the object of bitter disputes for years[141]. Wright and Semple wrote: "*Our first vaccinations against typhoid were undertaken in the months of July and August of last year* (1896). *These vaccinations were put on record by one of us in the* Lancet *on September 19th 1896, in a paper which dealt primarily with the question of serous haemorrhage. A reprint of this paper was sent among others to Prof. Pfeiffer. Nearly two months after the date of this paper Prof. Pfeiffer published, in conjunction with Dr. Kolle, a paper on Two cases of Typhoid vaccination. The method of inoculation which these authors have adopted, is exactly similar to the one that we had previously adopted. Like our own method, it was based upon the methods which have been so successfully employed by Mr. Haffkine in his anticholera inoculations.*"[142]

It is very difficult to take sides in such a conflict, without new evidence. But it is rare for scientists to go so far as to call others plagiarists as openly as Wright does speaking of Pfeiffer and Kolle. However, the priority of use of vaccines containing dead microbes to immunise human subjects seems clearly ascribable to Haffkine, even if he made little use of the "dead" version of his anticholera vaccine. In the same period, Haffkine developed with Yersin, Calmette and Borrel his dead-microbe vaccine against animal plague, at the *Institut Pasteur*, and used it later in human beings in Bombay. Of course, Ferran's poorly described anti-cholera vaccine cannot be counted.

France was clearly behind in terms of protection for civilians and military personnel. In 1910, Lucas-Championnière expressed regret that vaccination was not practiced at least for troops going to the colonies, since results obtained by the British and German health services were very favourable, given that Pfeiffer and Kolle's vaccine was probably better than Wright's. Antityphoid vaccines did not provide total protection, but they considerably reduced morbidity (percentage of people infected within a period of time) and mortality due to typhoid fever in troops on the battlefield[143].

It was the military health services that started large-scale vaccination. Chantemesse immunised navy personnel with a vaccine killed by heat, similar to Wright's. Vincent immunised the personal of the metropolitan army with a vaccine killed by ether. In 1915, Widal added paratyphoid bacilli A and B to the antityphoid vaccine. Morbidity and mortality decreased rapidly thanks to this combined vaccine. Between 1914 and 1915, there were 105,000 cases of typhoid in the French Army, and 14,000 deaths. Once vaccinations were started, the number of casualties dropped to 12,000 deaths in 1916, 1660 in 1917 and 665 in 1918[144], although the troops' conditions of hygiene had not really improved. Very quickly, this vaccination was used on a large scale in the British, American and Japanese armies. In 1914, Lumière and Chevrotier took up Courmont and Rochaix's work and developed an "antityphocolic vaccine",

140. Achard, 1929, p. 98; Anonymous, 1905, p. 1453.
141. Sansonetti, 1996, p. 212.
142. Wright, 1897, p. 256.
143. Lucas-Championnière, 1910, p. 22.
144. Lépine, 1975, p. 39.

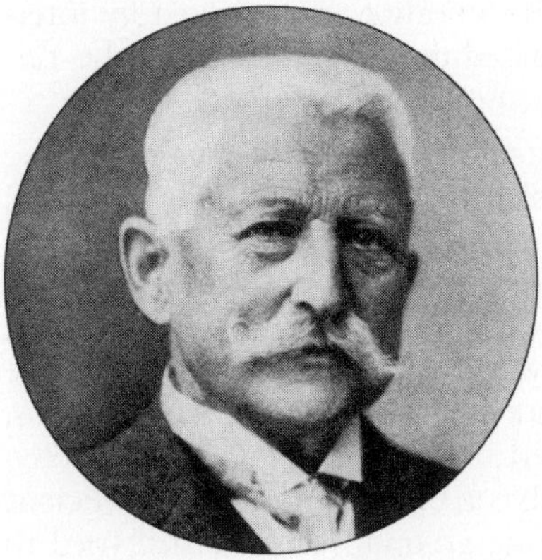

Figure 25. Richard Pfeiffer (1858-1945) who developed an efficient anti-typhoid vaccine. (Bulloch, 1938.)

administered orally in coated capsules resistant to gastric juices. This vaccine proved completely harmless in animals and later in man. In 1917, 250,000 people had already been immunised using this dead vaccine[145]. A lysate of Eberth's bacillus, without a bacterial body, was also proposed by Vincent[146], but it was apparently rarely used.

Unfortunately, fatal accidents were reported after antityphoid vaccinations. They were extremely rare, but did occur. Their causes were unknown. Ramon and Boivin reduced the number of germs per vaccine dose, and exposed them to formalin after heating them for 1 hour and 15 minutes to 56° C. A triple vaccine, adding tetanic and diphtheria anatoxins to the typhoid vaccine, was then heated to 54° C for 45 minutes. Side effects were considerably reduced in children and adults, but were still real[147]. Sometimes, the paratyphic C bacillus was added to the other germs. Despite everything, antityphoid vaccinations had undesirable side effects: local pain, light temporary fever[148]. Rest was recommended after the vaccination.

The protection conferred by vaccination was effective for troops on the battlefield and for tourists who travelled to regions at risk. A vaccine called TAB, for typhoid and paratyphoid A and B, composed of bacilli killed by heat and acetone is still used today. An attenuated living vaccine has been proposed, but its effectiveness is uncertain. A vaccine with a capsular component containing the Vi antigen, which confers protection and provokes little reaction (having few or no undesirable effects) is being developed.

In 1916, Le Moignic and Pinoy wrapped typhus bacilli in a fatty substance (lanolin, vaseline), creating a "lipovaccine". This technique has been widely used for other vaccines[149].

The Plague

At about the same time, a tentative solution was found for another disease. During a plague epidemic in Hong-Kong in 1894, Yersin discovered the bacillus of the disease, *Yersinia pestis*. A long dispute opposed Yersin and the francophone scientists on one side, to the Anglo-Japanese researchers on the other side, who felt that the discovery

145. Georgel, 1917, p. 65.
146. Bouquet, 1912, p. 420.
147. Joannon, 1941, p. 482.
148. Boivin, 1947, p. 348.
149. Le Moignic, 1916, p. 201; Bordet, 1939, p. 109.

of this bacillus should be attributed to Kitasato. This conflict was resolved by international committees of nomenclature, which designated the bacillus to be of the *Yersinia* genus, and the plague bacillus to be *Yersinia pestis*.

What is certain is that Haffkine, with his colleagues from the *Institut Pasteur*, Yersin (who returned from Indochina for this purpose in April 1895 with a plague bacillus culture), Calmette and Borrel, immunised animals with a dead plague vaccine. Haffkine prepared a vaccine intended to immunise human beings in Bombay[150]. Used in India, it gave excellent results. It was a vaccine made of bacteria killed by exposure to 70° C heat for one hour, after a long period of culture of five to six weeks[151]. However, Haffkine was impeded by the measures of hygiene promoted by British health authorities: search for infected persons, transport to hospitals, families expelled and interned in tent camps outside the city, disinfection of houses... These health measures, effective in Great Britain but insufficient in this situation, did not stop the plague from gaining ground. Haffkine still tried to vaccinate, without much success. He was more successful in Damaun, a Portuguese possession in India, where he was able to vaccinate 2,177 inhabitants out of a total of 8,230. According to Haffkine, mortality in the vaccinated population was 1.6%, while in the non vaccinated population it was 24.6%. Commissions travelled to India to judge the effects of Haffkine's vaccinations. The most prestigious of these commissions, composed of Koch and Gaffky, decided in favour of Haffkine's anti-plague vaccine[152].

Back in his Nha Trang Institute in Indochina, Yersin was preparing anti-plague serum, but his local production was of poor quality... Fortunately, he received eighty vials of anti-plague serum from the *Institut Pasteur* in Paris. He inoculated his first patient, suffering from acute plague, in Canton. The patient recovered. In Amoy, Yersin injected his serum to a number of patients, and saved twenty-one out of twenty-three[153]. He proposed that one or two Pasteur Institutes be founded in China. To accomplish this, he returned to France to find financial support. This is when the municipality of Bombay, where the plague was raging, appealed for his help. In 1897, Yersin stopped in Bombay with seven hundred doses of serum, but the serum was not of very good quality and the patients he was to treat were dying... Results were disappointing. In addition, Yersin found himself competing with Haffkine, who had arrived in Bombay to vaccinate with his "lymph". His vaccine was very similar to that developed on animals at the *Institut Pasteur*, where Haffkine had spent some time. The vaccine had undergone little testing on animals before being used in human beings. In a subsequent report, Yersin wrote that the safety of Haffkine's lymph was not certain, and that the immunity conferred lasts ten to fifteen days, just as long as that conferred by the anti-plague serum. Clearly, no ties of friendship were established between Haffkine and Yersin. The latter returned to Nha Trang in July 1897.

Yersin's anti-plague serum continued to interest public opinion. Every time a plague epidemic broke out, newspaper articles were dedicated to it, boosting the readers'confidence. The *Institut Pasteur* Annex could "*supply 3,000 vials a day*", a figure which seems rather high[154].

150. Lutzker, 1987, p. 366.
151. Anonymous, 1899, p. 35; Haffkine, 1897, p. 1461 (Haffkine claimed to be from the *Institut Pasteur*. He did not have a real laboratory at that time.
152. Metchnikoff, 1901, p. 509.
153. Roux, 1897, p. 91.
154. XXX, 1899, p. 654.

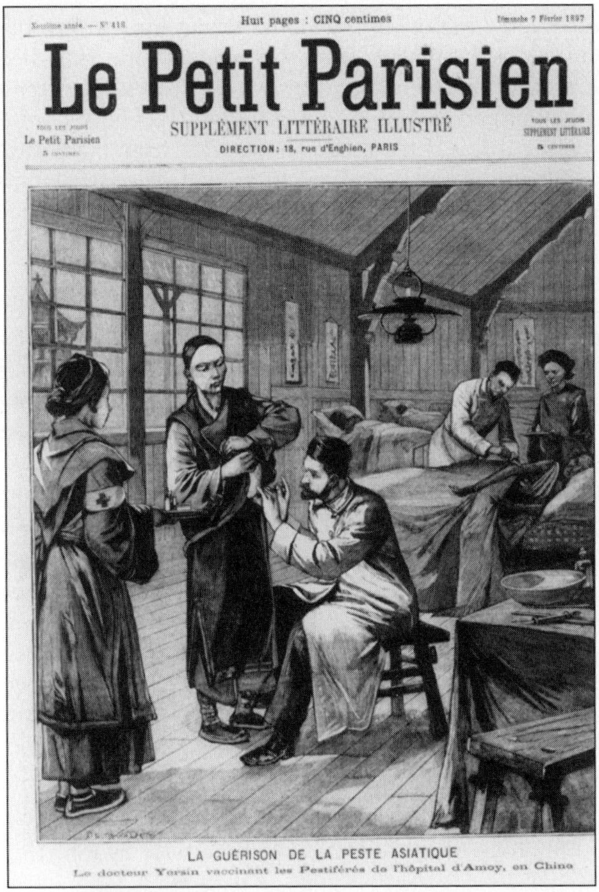

Figure 26. Alexandre Yersin (1863-1943) discovered the plague bacillus, *Yersinia pestis*. Here, Yersin uses anti-plague serum from the *Institut Pasteur*, because his local production is of poor quality, to inoculate a plague sufferer in Amoy (China). Out of the twenty-three patients he inoculated, twenty-one recovered. (*Le Petit Parisien*, February 7, 1897.)

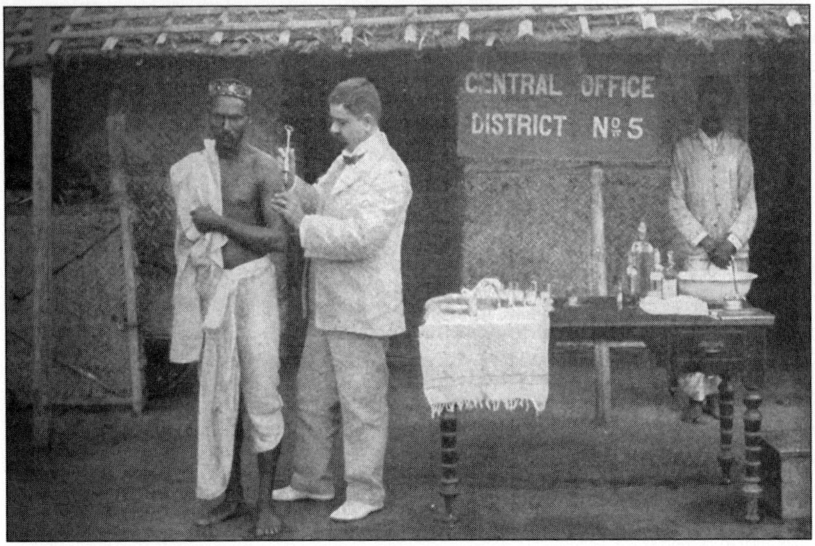

Figure 27. Example of Haffkine's anti-plague vaccination, in Bombay. (*La Science illustrée*, 1903.)

Unfortunately, a serious accident disrupted the use of the Haffkine vaccine. In October 1902, nineteen people vaccinated against the plague, from the same vaccine vial, died of tetanus in Mulkowal. Haffkine was held responsible and was very distressed. After a lengthy inquest, he was absolved of all responsibility. A vial of vaccine had been contaminated by tetanus bacilli spores, while it was being used. The vaccine from Haffkine's laboratory was properly prepared. Only its use had been improper: a vial soiled by clumps of earth had been used to immunise. His old laboratory now bears the name Haffkine.

Exanthematic Typhus

Exanthematic typhus has given rise to serious epidemics all over the world, especially among populations living in deplorable hygiene conditions. The disease is caused by Rickettsia transmitted to man by fleas. The man who made this discovery, Charles Nicolle, won the Nobel prize in 1928. The disastrous retreat of Napoleon's Great army from Russia can be imputed in part to typhus. Rickettsiae, named after the American doctor Howard Taylor Ricketts who died while studying it, only multiply in living organisms, making it problematic to transform them into vaccines.

1931-1933. The first vaccine was developed by Rudolf Weigl (1883-1957) by inoculating fleas anally, one by one, and extracting their intestines after 8 days, crushing them in carbolic water and dosing them. About a hundred fleas were needed to produce a dose of vaccine. The procedure was used at the *Institut Pasteur* in Tunis, and was practiced in 1935 in Peking, as witnessed and recounted by Ella Maillart, who crossed China from Peking to Cashmere. She specifies that missionaries were immunised against exanthematic typhus by Weigl's method, used by a Dr. Tchang of Fujen University. Three injections were given, with 4 to 5 milliard germs[155].

1937. American microbiologist Hans Zinsser (1878-1940) developed a killed vaccine from rikettsiae grown in the peritoneal cavity of rats[156].

1937. Zinsser, Fitzpatrick and Wei improved the production of Rikettsiae by infecting chick or mouse embryo tissues[157].

1940. Fortunately, another, easier mode of vaccine production was developed by Paul Durand (1886-1960) and Paul Giroud (1898-1989) by infecting rabbits intratracheally. After four to five days, their lungs were extracted and crushed. The pulp was mixed with carbolic water, inactivating the Rickettsiae. Three successive injections were needed, and a booster dose a year later, to obtain immunity with most vaccines.

But in 1940, Dunham wrote: "*The whole question of immunization, both active and passive, is still in the experimental stage.*"[158]

Sero-Vaccination 1895-1896...

The use of serotherapy considerably reduced mortality due to diphtheria, but did not eliminate it. In addition, its use was limited by adverse reactions to the foreign proteins in the inoculated organisms. Therefore, what was needed was to develop a safe vaccine conferring satisfactory lasting immunity.

155. Weigl, 1933, p. 315; Maillart, 1937, p. 19.
156. Dunham, 1940, p. 860.
157. Dunham, 1940, p. 860.
158. Dunham, 1940, p. 860.

In 1890, Behring and Kitasato described in clear terms the immunisation of mice with a mix of tetanus toxin and rabbit serum immunised against tetanus toxin and left in contact for 24 hours at room temperature. They did not report any precipitate, but observed only neutralisation of the clinical effects of the toxin[159].

According to Park, Babes was the first to use a mixture of diphtheric toxin and neutralising serum to immunise animals, in 1895. Park provides no reference and points out that he himself obtained the same result in 1896[160]. Kolle and Turner are believed to have employed mixtures of virulent blood from contaminated animals and serum from recovering animals to immunise against cattle plague, before 1898. This method is sometimes called "simultaneous vaccination" or "sero-infection"[161]. Behring and Wernicke apparently immunised animals with mixtures of diphtheric toxin and antitoxin. Inoculating a mixture of fixed rabies virus and anti-rabies serum confers reliable immunity to rabbits or guinea pigs[162]. Zinsser quotes Schattenfroh and Grassberger who, while studying blackleg in 1904, are thought to be the first to have used a mixture of toxin and immune serum to confer protection to animals[163]. The ground was prepared for the large-scale use of this method. Between 1896 and 1903 (?), Park successfully immunised guinea pigs using diphtheric toxin and antitoxin mixtures; the animals withstood doses equivalent to 400 times, then 10,000 times the mortal dose. Park undertook to immunise guinea pigs and horses with hyperneutralised toxins. In 1905, Theobald Smith, who was studying the duration of immunity obtained using this immunisation method in guinea pigs, found that this period exceeded two years[164]. The ground had been prepared for von Behring who, in 1913, was the first to attempt immunising a child, and later a small group of people, using this procedure. Hans and Summer then vaccinated 4,300 children in the Magdebourg region, where diphtheria was endemic. Finally, in New York, Park immunised 33,000 children without serious difficulty[165]. The procedure was effective but laborious. A more practical method had to be found.

At the same time, Glenny was deploring the fact that nothing was being done in Great Britain in this field. "*English physicians in charge of schools, institutions and infectious disease hospitals have apparently been too busy up to the present to be able to investigate these two methods. In America, the Shick reactions that have been carried out number many tens of thousands, and thousands of active immunisations have been done.*"[166] The two methods in question were, on the one hand, the use of Schick's test to measure immunity to diphtheria*, and on the other hand, active immunisation through a mixture of diphtheria toxin and of specific immune serum. Glenny is bitter...

He has already inoculated himself with a mixture of diphtheric toxin and antitoxin, which had the effect of elevating his diphtheric antitoxin seric values[167]. He was

* The Shick test consists of injecting into the derm a small quantity of diphtheric toxin that provokes (positive result) or does not provoke (negative result) a small inflammation. A negative test shows that the individual is immunised against diphtheric toxin.

159. Behring, 1890a, p. 1113.
160. Park, 1922, p. 1584.
161. Metchnikoff, 1901, p. 488.
162. Remlinger, 1904, p. 414.
163. Zinsser, 1918, p. 460.
164. Park, 1922, p. 1584.
165. Park, 1922, p. 1584; Renault, 1939, p. 3.
166. Glenny, 1921a, p. 1236.
167. Glenny, 1921b, p. 176.

perhaps the sole volunteer in this experiment... Fortunately, in 1923 he was able to congratulate himself for the fact that in England about some hundred children had been immunised by O'Brien, Eagleton and Okell[168] by injections of the toxin-antitoxin mixture[169]. Sero-vaccination was going to be used on occasion up until the Second World War.

Auto-vaccines and Vaccinotherapy: 1902...

For a long time, vaccines made of a single or several dead infectious agents prepared from laboratory microbial strains were called "stock-vaccines". In contrast, "auto-vaccines" were prepared from cultures of the one or several particular microbes infecting a patient, and were used in that patient's treatment[170]. The idea was to select the actual microbe causing an infectious disease and then use it to vaccinate.

Sir Almroth Wright is the father of auto vaccines in vaccinology, as well as the father of vaccinotherapy. In 1902, while studying staphylococcus infections of the skin, he had the idea of producing curative vaccines from dead cultures of the staphylococcus in question. Encouraged by his initial results, Wright applied his method to numerous micro-organisms: streptococci, pneumococi, collibacilli, gonococci... His laboratory at the Saint Mary's Hospital in London quickly became a vaccinotherapy Unit; this made him express the following rather exaggerated opinion (if we take it as the whole truth): "*The physician of the future will be an immuniser.*"[171] After several months spent in Wright's Unit, Dr. Renaud-Badet described the techniques used there: harvesting from a furuncle or a whitlow... then seeding a culture medium, culture in an incubator, homogeneisation and sterilisation, bacillus count (by comparison with the red blood cells of a sample of fresh blood whose red blood-cell count is estimated *a priori* at 5 million per cubic millimetre – a procedure called Wright-Leishmann), dilution of the dead bacillus preparation to obtain, for each cubic centimetre of vaccine in phials, 200 million bacterial bodies for staphylococci, 5 to 10 million for streptococi, etc. This auto vaccine is injected subcutaneously after disinfecting the skin: doses and booster shots depended on microbial species. Furunculosis, acne, sycosis (hair follicle disease), staphylococcosis, tonsillitis, stomatitis, alveolar pyorrhoea, osteomyelitis, puerperal infection, orchiepdidymitis, blennorrhoeic rheumatism, prostatitis, metrititis, pleurisy and fibrinous or purulent endocarditis, arthritis, enteritis, choleriform diarrhea, appendicitis, angiocholitis, peritonitis, bronchopneumonia, meningitis, etc., and all bacterial diseases (or suspected to be bacterial) were likely to be treated by vaccinotherapy, even infections like typhoid fever or dysentery[172]. Animals also benefited from Wright's vaccinotherapy with auto vaccines. A variation of these methods consisted of "pyotherapy", practiced by "*injecting under the skin or in a vein a pyovaccine made from pus processed in alcohol or ether*"[173].

Wright and Douglas demonstrated that body fluids could modify bacteria and render them apt to be assimilated by phagocytes. He called this phenomenon opsonisation,

168. Glenny, 1923a, p. 19.
169. O'Brien, 1923, p. 29.
170. Fleming, 1934, p. 252.
171. Wright, quoted by Renaud-Badet, 1913.
172. Renaud-Badet, 1913.
173. Clément, 1927, p. 21.

and the elements involved opsonins. Almost ten years earlier, in 1895, the experimental situation had been described by Denys and Leclef of the Faculty of Medicine of the Catholic University of Louvain: these two authors, who were studying *in vitro*, then *in vivo*, the degree of protection of rabbits immunised or not against streptococci, described their observations as follows: "*The leukocyte of a new rabbit, dipped into the serum of a vaccinated rabbit, acquires a new power over the streptococcus. In ordinary serum, the leukocyte only exerts a slight phagocyting activity on the streptococcus, sometimes barely perceptible, which allows the microbe to multiply rapidly; but in the serum of an immunised animal, it integrates and kills the organisms with considerable intensity...*"[174]. Many authors attribute this discovery to Denys and Leclef[175], with reason, although some disagree! But explaining this phenomenon was to be Wright's work; Wright became a major pioneer of opsonisation, and he devoted a considerable portion of his research to it. He eventually created a predictive test of patients' immunity to the bacteria that besiege them. His first project consisted in developing an *in vitro* test that provided him with an index of opsonising power: after exposing the whole blood of a patient to bacteria, he counted the number of bacteria ingested by a certain number of neutrophilic polymorphonuclear leukocytes (cells capable of phagocytosis) in specific conditions. Thus, he was able to obtain a figure he could compare with others that were obtained with the blood of normal (uncontaminated) individuals[176]. Wright used this test to check the effect of auto vaccinations on his patients. His method, at a time when there were practically no other means of fighting bacterial infections, remained in vogue for about thirty years. These testing procedures are sometimes still used by practitioners of alternative medicine. However, their home-made character has caused them to be prohibited in many countries. Their value is still subject to controversy.

From Toxins to Anatoxins/Toxoids: Ramon, Glenny: 1923...

Two diseases had long been known to be due to the action of exotoxins, that is, toxins excreted by pathogenic bacteria: diphtheria and tetanus. Shortly after they were discovered, the toxins secreted by diphtheria and tetanus bacteria were used by Behring and Kitasato to induce protection against these two diseases. However, even when very low initial doses were gradually increased subsequently, it was not easy to obtain a suitable degree of immunity, because the animals died from the effects of the toxin before being immunised. Various procedures were tried to reduce toxin harmfulness. For instance, they were mixed with chemicals able to neutralise their toxicity, such as iodine trichloride, for 16 hours[177]. These techniques were not very practical, because they were difficult to control: sometimes, the toxins were too denatured and no longer induced immunity. Other times, they were still too toxic and killed the animal they were intended to immunise!

Two researchers, Frenchman Gaston Ramon and Englishman Alexander-Thomas Glenny, achieved good results almost at the same time. Both of them were immunising horses to produce antidiphteric sera, and obtained atoxic diphtheria toxin that was still immunogenic, more or less by chance, but also thanks to a good sense of observation. While testing a batch of diphtheria toxin, Glenny noted that it was not very toxic for

174. Denys, 1895, p. 197.
175. Fraser, 1914, p. 11; Bordet, 1920, p. 232; Bordet, 1972, p. 55.
176. Wright, 1903-4, p. 357; Wright, 1904, p. 128.
177. Behring, 1890b, p. 1145.

guinea pigs inoculated during titration. Despite this, he tried to use this very low toxicity toxin to immunise animals intended to produce antidiphteric serum. The toxin still had immunogenic properties. Glenny remembered that this toxin had been stored in a large container, too big to be sterilized in his autoclave. Instead, it had been disinfected with formalin. This modified toxin was given the name "toxoid"[178]. The word "toxoid" had already been proposed by the great German scientist Ehrlich in the description of his side-chain theory. "*The toxin molecule has at least two groups: a combining or haptophore, and a poisoning or toxophore group. A toxin which has lost its poisonous property, its toxophore group, is spoken of as a toxoid.*"[179] Such a toxin has lost its toxicity but retains its attachment to antitoxin properties. Ehrlich had found a means to obtain such molecules by letting the toxins age, or by heating them to 50° C. According to Bordet, in 1929 Glenny and Hopkins "*had noted the attenuating action of this substance* (formalin)", and Eisler and Löwenstein "*recognized that formalin renders tetanus toxin inoffensive, while preserving its immunising power*"[180]. Ramon wrote: "*Let us recall that Löwenstein (and his associates), who recommended the use of tetanus toxin treated with formalin at the start of immunisation of horses used as serum producers, assert that diphtheric serum does not lend itself well to the action of formalin.*"[181] The value of formalin as an antiseptic had been shown by Ramon during his studies at the Alfort Veterinary School in 1907: "*... a thimbleful of formalin in a litre of milk was enough to prevent the milk from turning, without affecting its taste or consistency.*"[182] These early experiments now seem rather remote.

In 1921, Glenny and Südmersen described very briefly the immune responses obtained after inoculation with toxoids: "*The action of certain chemical agents is to destroy the lethal power without altering appreciably the antigenic value of a toxin... The toxin (*diphtheria toxin*) used in this experiment had originally an m. l. d. (*minimum lethal dose*) of 0.005 c.c.; ... The toxin was changed into 'toxoid' by treatment with formalin rendering the product atoxic, so that 5 c.c. would not kill.*"[183a] These authors take up Ehrlich's term "toxoid" correctly, in its wider sense. However, the title of the paragraph is: "*3) Toxin rich in 'toxoid' may produce high immunity*". The "*may produce*" indicates that there is no certainty associated with using "toxoid" in human immunisation and the authors specify: "*It will be noticed that in all cases the second injection was not tolerated so well as the first or subsequent ones [see statement 1,* which reads: '*An increase in susceptibility after an injection of toxin altered to toxoid or in combination with antitoxin is also seen in tables iii and iv'].*" The twenty-four page article contains essentially the characteristics of primary and secondary responses and only a few lines concerning this phenomenon: toxins altered into toxoids. Glenny only describes his initial fortuitous discovery, whose characteristics he does not yet control. This experiment was apparently conducted in 1921 (before Ramon's), but it contributed almost nothing new.

However, Glenny and Hopkins' article, received on August 8, 1923, thanked doctors O'Brien, Eagleton and Okell "*for the information that a mixture of modified toxin and antitoxin has given exceptionally promising results when employed for human immunisation*"[183b].

178. Parish, 1965, p. 141.
179. Morrey, 1921, p. 261.
180. Bordet, 1939, p. 26.
181. Ramon, 1924b, p. 1436.
182. Bressou, 1970.
183a. Glenny, 1921b, p. 184.
183b. Glenny, 1923b, p. 283.

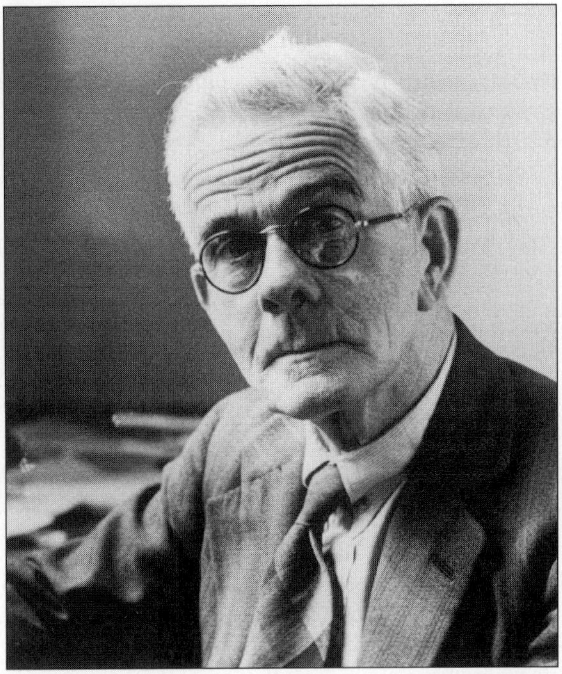

Figure 28. "*Portrait of Alexander Thomas Glenny.*" He contributed to immunization against diphteria, a dreaded disease, worked on primary or secondary immune responses and introduced the alun-precipitated antigens in vaccines. (Reproduced with permission of the Wellcome Institute Library, London.)

This article contained the description of one or several human immunisations, but with a mixture of modified diphtheria toxin (*toxoid*) and a small quantity of antiserum. The article does not mention the exclusive use of pure diphtheria *toxoid* as antidiphtherial vaccine, but suggests a future use for it: "*The use of modified toxin in toxin-antitoxin mixtures for human use enables a far greater number of binding units, i. e. a greater specific antigenic strength, to be presented without any increase in specific toxicity... This would constitute a marked advance in the prevention of diphtheria... The use of modified toxin, however, reduces the amount of serum necessary in a mixture, because such modified toxin need not be fully neutralized; only sufficient antitoxin need be added to reduce the residual toxicity below a certain level...*"[184]. On August 8, 1923, Glenny had not yet immunised a human being with his pure diphtheria toxoid: "*The modification of toxin used in the experiments recorded in this paper was prepared by adding 0.1 per cent formalin to diphtheria toxin and exposing it for 4 weeks at a temperature of 37° C before removing to the cold room.*"[185] He understood the concrete clinical interest of his discovery, but had not yet considered its use in man: "*It may be possible shortly to use toxin so modified* (toxoid) *that it will be completely non-toxic without the addition of antitoxin.*"[186]

In 1930, Glenny had come to the conclusion that "*it is possible that the most favoured method of human immunization against diphtheria in the near future may be by means of a*

184. Glenny, 1923b, p. 283.
185. Glenny, 1923b, p. 283.
186. Glenny, 1923b, p. 283.

suspension of toxoid precipitated by alun..." (and in a note) "*Since this paper was written, W. H. Park, at the Paris congress of the International Society of Microbiology, reported 100 per cent successful immunization with alun-toxoid in small groups of children.*"[187]

It is difficult to know the precise date when diphtheric toxoid was used, without the cover of specific antiserum, for human immunisation, by Glenny and his associates[188]. But it must have been after August 1923, the year when Ramon started human immunisations using his diphtheric anatoxines at least on himself, but without revealing the result.

A few hundred kilometres away, Ramon, a veterinarian from the *Institut Pasteur*, was studying the flocculating and toxic power of the diphtheria toxins he was producing to immunise horses used as a source of antisera[189]. On June 2, 1923, Ramon described the phenomenon of separating the toxic effect from the flocculating power of diphtheria toxins, raising the question of whether a toxin that lost its toxic power while retaining its flocculating power could still induce immune response[190]. On December 3, 1923, he published his findings that modified toxin (called *anatoxine* for "*ana*": "reverse" in Greek), harmless, with full flocculating power, retains its full immunogenic potential in animals. Ramon also described an inoculation experiment on himself, with no side effects; but he did not indicate whether the inoculation produced an immune response. In addition, he described the possible use of his toxoid in children, and the use of the method of measured denaturation for tetanus toxin[191]. Encouraged by these findings, in January 1924, a few months after Glenny, he published a description of an effective and reproducible technique for inhibiting the toxicity of diphtheria (and tetanus) toxins without making them lose the power to generate antitoxin antibodies in the subject to be immunised: "*As we indicated, we always add, to the toxin we use in our different dosages in vitro, a very small quantity of formaldehyde (1 p. 2000 of the commercial solution at 35-40 p. 100) in order to avoid cultures that would completely prevent the contaminations that are inevitable in the course of manipulations. While doing this, we observed that, although the flocculating power of a toxin treated with formaldehyde and left at room temperature in the laboratory remained intact for several months, its destructive power decreased gradually but rapidly (much more quickly than is the case for a toxin not exposed to formaldehyde), especially if the temperature in the laboratory was a little high; taking advantage of this observation, we increased considerably both the formalin concentration, up to 3-4 p. 1000, and the temperature, up to 40-42°... to obtain an anatoxine with the highest possible number of immunising properties, and to have recourse to the flocculation reaction, particularly to regulate the action of physical and chemical agents.*"[192] On April 22, 1924, Ramon described in detail the procedure he used to obtain his anatoxine by "*the action of heat and of formaldehyde*", specifying the application of the procedure with abrin, a vegetable toxin, and cobra venom. His procedure proved to be reproducible and therefore reliable for several different toxins. His technique consisted of "*4 to 5 per 1000 of the commercial solution* (formalin). *After 5 weeks at incubator temperature (38° to 40°)...*"[193]. To conduct trials on a greater number of subjects, Ramon had to ask for help: "*... To test the safety of his antidiphtheric vaccine, he inoculated himself with*

187. Glenny, 1930, p. 244.
188. Parish, 1965, p. 141.
189. Ramon, 1922, p. 661.
190. Ramon, 1923a, p. 2.
191. Ramon, 1923b, p. 1338.
192. Ramon, 1924a, p. 1.
193. Ramon, 1924b, p. 1436.

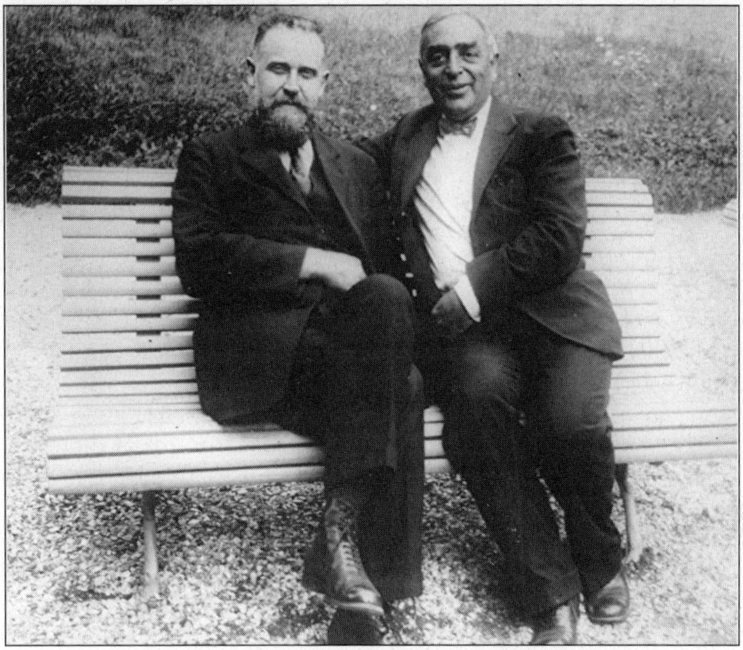

Figure 29. Gaston Ramon (1886-1963), easy to recognize thanks to his full beard, developed diphtherial anatoxine vaccination, after demonstrating that diphtheria toxin, when exposed to the combined effect of a small quantity of formalin and of heat, changes into a harmless derivative which nevertheless retains its full vaccinating power. Later, he introduced the principle of adjuvant substances that stimulate immunity. This photograph shows him with Professor B. Schick from New York, inventor of the test that bears his name, serving to measure immunity against diphtheria. (Photograph Henri Manuel, Paris.) (Author's document.)

a dose of the vaccine; it is not generally known that, to assess its effectiveness, he turned to some of his colleagues, who consented to vaccinate their children and then bring them into contact with diphtheria sufferers or people recovering from diphtheria."[194] In fact, Ramon's technique was rapidly recommended and used in serotherapy (immunisation of horses) and then for human vaccinations. These modified toxins are called *anatoxines* or toxoids. They are still the essential component of antidiphtheric and antitetanic vaccinations. Ramon's work is described in detail, and is reproducible.

One of the first persons to use Ramon's anatoxine was Park, in New York, a foremost international expert in antidiphtheric immunisation.[195] *"In 1924, Zingher and I accepted the superiority of Ramon's anatoxin - or as it is called in this country, the formol toxoid - as compared with toxin-antitoxin. We summed up this superiority by stating that toxoid is 1) more stable, 2) easier to prepare, 3) not dangerous if accidentally frozen, 4) more effective and 5) nonsensitizing. After 1931 administrations of toxoid, in two or three doses, gradually it supplanted the use of toxin-antitoxin both in Europe and in this country."*[196] Ramon's work is presented in detail and is reproducible; above all, its value was demonstrated quickly

194. Bressou, 1970.
195. Park, 1922, p. 1584.
196. Park, 1937, p. 1681.

in human trials. Supremely indifferent to the published work of other authors, Glenny, as well as Ramon, referred almost exclusively to their own previous work.

The Englishmen Fleming and Petrie used the word "*toxoid* (*anatoxine*)" to speak of diphtheria toxin, and used only "*anatoxine*" in connection with tetanus toxin, the exclusive work of Ramon and Zoeller. Fleming and Petrie clearly attribute the discovery of the medical applications of anatoxines to Ramon, although Glenny and Hopkins had first suggested that *toxoids* could be used as antigens in immunisation. Fleming and Petrie wrote, in 1934: "*Although Glenny and Hopkins first suggested the use of toxoid alone as an immunizing agent, it is Ramon and his co-workers in France who have used the method most extensively... Glenny (1931) suggested that the addition of antitoxin may be regarded as a concession to the British conservatism, as any type of toxin-antitoxin mixture was accepted freely, while toxoid alone had little support.*"[197] The first human inoculation of diphtheric anatoxine (pure, without added antiserum) given by Ramon was self-inoculation, but he did not specify if he obtained an immune response[198]. He then inoculated the children of colleagues who accepted to expose them afterwards to diphtheria patients or patients recovering from the disease. Ramon's associates, Darré, G. Loiseau, A. Laffaille, Roubinovitch, Zoeller, immunised children (at least 130) and adults (250 military men) in great numbers before April 29, 1929. Four adults were successfully immunised as early as 1923.[199] These are the only two dates given. The dates of the other immunisations are not specified. In 1939, Loiseau and Laffaille wrote: "*For us, who in November 1923, with H. Darré, performed the first assays of antidiphtheria vaccination using Ramon's anatoxine... Only a few days after G. Ramon communicated his remarkable discovery of diphtheric anatoxine, we attempted, under the direction of L. Martin, to immunise against diphtheria ten patients treated at the Pasteur Hospital, recovering from influenza, diphtheria, scarlet fever, lethargic encephalitis, and one leprosy sufferer. We were already aware of the complete safety of anatoxine for guinea pigs. Before starting these trials, Ramon and one of us had already tested on themselves the safety of the anatoxine...*"[200].

In 1924, other small groups of children were immunised in different places, by other physicians[201].

In 1954, Parish, of the Wellcome Foundation Ltd., wrote in the chapter entitled "*Historical*" of the book on sera and vaccines: "*Antisera, toxoids, vaccines and tuberculins in prophylaxis and treatment: 1923: Glenny, Allen and Hopkins were the first to suggest the use of toxoids in human immunisation. Ramon used toxoids under the name of 'anatoxines' in France.*"[202] This statement is a less than historically accurate shortcut[203]. Parish's book "*History of immunization*" (1965) is interesting but often very partial in its perspective.

In his book on infectious diseases, Bloomfield cites Ramon as the inventor of anatoxines, but does not cite Glenny in connection with toxoids[204]. The Morton Medical Bibliography, edited by Jeremy M. Norman, indirectly attributes the discovery to Ramon, citing none of Glenny's publications[205]. Vitek and Wharton also cite Ramon

197. Fleming, 1934, pp. 429, 435 & 439.
198. Ramon, 1923b, p. 1338.
199. Martin, 1924, pp. 474 & 523.
200. Loiseau, 1939, p. 38.
201. Lereboullet, 1924, p. 1123.
202. Parish, 1954, p. 198.
203. Parish, 1954, p. 198.
204. Bloomfield, 1958, p. 263.
205. Norman, 1991, p. 780.

as the sole inventor of toxoids[206]. Who is to be credited with the discovery of anatoxines (*toxoids*)? Glenny and Ramon both contributed to it. The attenuated toxin concept comes from Glenny and the word *toxoid*, which comes from Erlich, seems to have preceded the term "anatoxine".

The publication of the method of toxoid production seems to be anterior to that of anatoxine, but the specifications are somewhat different. The use of pure anatoxine (without the cover of antidiphtheric antiserum) as a human vaccine against diphtheria seems indeed to be the result of Ramon's work. Glenny seems to have lingered at the theoretical stage, perhaps because he lacked associates ready to try his pure toxoid. He himself seems never to have tested it.

Vaccination with Ramon's anatoxine started in 1923 on a very small number of children, and came into common use around 1928. In France, the vaccination was made compulsory on June 28, 1938; this immediately gave rise to violent protests. A special session of the medical Practice Society (*Société de médecine pratique*), held on January 19, 1939 and attended by about twenty experts on this vaccination, was dedicated to the safety and protective virtue of Ramon's diphtheria anatoxine[207]. The use of vaccines composed of diphtheria anatoxine has now become world-wide. Correctly used, they have saved thousands of people from death. In New York, the death rate due to diphtheria has decreased from 22 to 1 per 100,000 inhabitants between 1922 and 1935, thanks to large-scale use of this vaccination. However, Parish reported some disasters caused by confusion of vials filled with toxins instead of anatoxines, or by anatoxine preparations contaminated during use[208]. The same author reported relatively serious adverse effects in Great Britain after *toxoid* injections. It is difficult to explain the reasons for these differences in results, as compared to those obtained in many other countries.

Tetanus toxin was also modified to become anatoxine, and was used to immunise human beings and animals against tetanus[209]. Toxins of other bacteria, transformed into anatoxines, are included in the composition of some vaccines. For example, the *Bordetella pertussis* toxin, inactivated in acellular antipertussis vaccine either through the chemical action of formaldehyde or of glutardehyde, or genetically by a mutation of its genome, which produces its inactivation[210a]. Sad to say, the future of anatoxines is assured by the great number of infectious diseases caused by exotoxins.

Ramon and Glenny are associated with the discovery of "toxoids/anatoxines". Glenny started to immunise animals used to produce antiserum before Ramon. However, Ramon encouraged, advised and helped clinicians to immunise human beings with his pure anatoxine, as early as 1923, before Glenny. Moreover, he was the first to publish the description of a reliable technique of anatoxine production, as well as numerous convincing results in animals and man. His technique has been used widely the world over.

Ramon also discovered the effect of immunity adjuvants, with tapioca; but Glenny proposed aluminium alun, which is currently the most widely used adjuvant in the world. Ramon and Zoeller proposed the use of "combined vaccines"[210b]. Ramon and

206. Vitek *in* Plotkin, 2008, p. 139.
207. Société de médecine pratique, 1939.
208. Parish, 1965, pp. 151 & 156.
209. Ramon, 1925b, p. 508 & 898; Ramon, 1925c, p. 582; Ramon, 1926b, p. 245.
210a. Rappuoli, 1997, p. 374; Salmaso, 2003, p. 211.
210b. Ramon, 1926a, p. 106.

Glenny have both contributed greatly to the improvement of vaccine development by perfecting the flocculation technique (Ramon) and the analysis of primary and secondary responses (Glenny). These two researchers have provided fundamental data for the development of vaccinology, by working on similar or even identical subjects and obtaining important results. Toxoids/Anatoxines are their common achievement.

Tuberculosis and the Biliated Calmette Guérin Bacillus (BCG): 1922, 1924...

Tuberculosis is a contagious, inoculable disease, common to many species of animals and to man. It is caused by the formation of tubercules in the body, due to the action of tuberculosis mycobacteria. The disease has various clinical forms, depending on the organs involved. A considerable number of people are affected. A third of the world's population are carriers of the tuberculosis bacillus.

It was Villemin who established without a doubt that human tuberculosis was a contagious disease transmitted by an infectious agent[211]. This agent is the microbe *Mycobacterium tuberculosis*, discovered in 1882 by the famous scientist Robert Koch. The microbe is sometimes called "Koch's bacillus" or KB for short. We now know that M. *tuberculosis* belongs to a large family of related bacteria, all of which attack man and animals. Among the best-known, M. *leprae* is responsible for leprosy, and M. *bovis* for bovine tuberculosis.

At the start of the 20th century, tuberculosis became a wide-spread disease in the Western world. Baldwin paints a distressing picture of tuberculosis in Western countries: "*The prevalence of tuberculosis is universal; no other disease is so widespread or produces so much poverty and long continued-distress... From one-seventh to one-tenth of all deaths and an enormous proportion of invalidism are due to it. Kayserling stated at the recent Paris Tuberculosis Congress (1905) that one-third of all deaths and one-half the sickness among adults in Germany can be charged to tuberculosis... The last United States Census (1900) gives a total of 111,059 deaths from consumption, including general tuberculosis, the rate being 109.9 per 1,000 deaths, or about one-ninth of the deaths from all known causes... Occupation and social condition appear to have the most intimate relation to the ratio of mortality. Stonecutters, cigar makers, and plasterers head the list with about half the deaths in these occupations; farmers and persons under the best social conditions have less than one-eighth due to tuberculosis... The economic loss from tuberculosis is enormous even with a low evaluation placed upon an individual life. In the German Empire there were 85,280 deaths in the same year. Estimating the loss of earnings according to Cornet at 600 marks per annum, the sum is 51,168,000 marks... It is safe to say that tuberculosis costs the United States $ 150,000,000 to 200,000,000 yearly...*"[212]. The deplorable living conditions of portions of the population who were coming into the cities to seek work were in part responsible for this. Another contributing factor was the absence of effective antitubercular treatments. Tuberculosis devastated all classes of society, killing workers and their families, as well as members of high society or ladies of the night. There are many consumptives among famous figures and literary characters of the nineteenth and early twentieth centuries. "*Thus, the consumptive has*

211. Villemin, 1868.
212. Baldwin, 1907, p. 137.

the privilege of being better able than others to testify based on his own experience, both personal and social, of the existence of evil... The young consumptive girl seen as the ideal woman in the pre-romantic and romantic eras lived and died exposed to the scrutiny of all."[213] The improvement of hygiene conditions in the population was one of the first changes that had an impact on the situation. In the 1930s, despite considerable progress, the situation remained difficult: " *The disease is widely spread zoologically. In Animal- In the domestic animals tuberculosis is a common disease, particularly in cattle... In Man-Tuberculosis is his most universal scourge, well deserving the epithet bestowed upon it by Bunyan, 'captain of the men of death'. Probably about one-eighth of all deaths are due to it. In England and Wales there were 35,818 deaths from all forms of tuberculosis in 1931. In the United States it is responsible for about 8 per cent of all deaths. The rate of registration areas was 201.9 per 100,000 in 1900 and in 48 states 55.2 in 1936. In the United States tuberculosis as a cause of death has dropped from first to seventh place. Practically everywhere in the civilized world, there has been a reduction in the death rate, the most encouraging feature of the modern sanitation.*"[214] Still, in France in 1930 tuberculosis killed another 65,703 people[215]. Improvement of hygiene conditions was one of the first useful measures against the disease.

Before the First World War, French health authorities took few measures against tuberculosis. A few rare initiatives stood out. The Academy of Medicine was concerned about the extent of the problem. Reports were written: Villemin (1889), Jaccoud (1896), Grancher (1898) defined the future aspects of prevention and proposed that a commission (the Permanent Commission of Tuberculosis Prevention) be created to study it. Then, on the recommendation of Waldeck-Rousseau, parliamentarians created an extra-parliamentary commission charged with looking for practical means of fighting the spread of tuberculosis. Despite all this, the 1902 law on the protection of public health stipulated that reporting tuberculosis was optional. These were very inadequate measures in the face of such a serious scourge. Calmette opened a first dispensary called Emile-Roux, in Lille, in February 1901. He also introduced home visits. These measures were successful. Two more dispensaries opened in Lyon and in Paris a few years later[216]. But these were isolated initiatives and more time would be needed before relatively effective country-wide measures would be implemented.

During the First World War, the situation in France became deplorable. The country was lagging seriously behind as far as infectious diseases and hygiene were concerned. Some progress had been made, but much remained to be done. Conditions in the trenches, the return from Germany of consumptive prisoners of war (through Switzerland), the expulsion of civilians from their homes, the material and moral difficulties of a major segment of the population, produced a constant increase in the number of cases. The French government started to structure the fight against tuberculosis. "Selection Centres" to identify consumptive soldiers, and "health stations", the precursors of "public sanatoriums", were created, to treat tuberculosis sufferers, and above all to provide them with information about prevention, before they were sent home. A "Central Committee of Assistance to Consumptive Veterans" was established. Assistance committees were created in most departments.

213. Guillaume, 1986, p. 21.
214. Osler, 1938, p. 186.
215. Brouardel, 1934, p. 9.
216. Brouardel, 1934, p. 127.

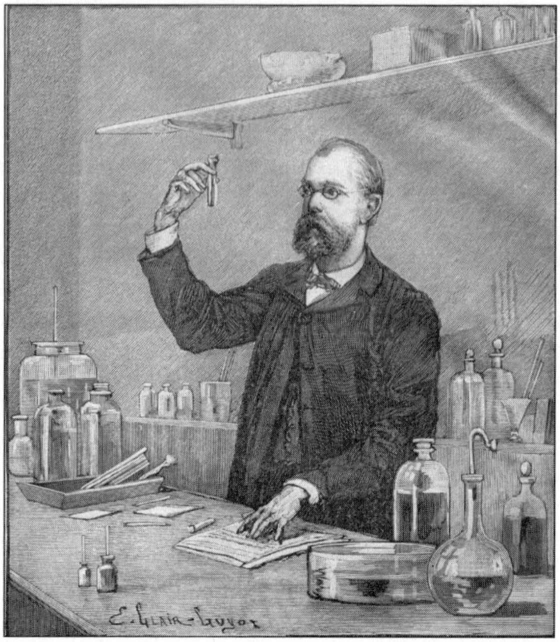

Figure 30. Robert Koch in his laboratory. The revelation of an anti-tuberculosis treatment had wide repercussions. The news gave renewed hope to thousands of families. The discovery was made by Koch, a scientist of immense stature. Numerous newspapers published his portrait: "*One of the most deadly diseases, which causes the greatest devastation in society, is no doubt tuberculous phthisis or tuberculosis. Prof. R. Koch of Berlin, discoverer of the tuberculosis bacillus, has just discovered a sure remedy for this terrible affliction. Where will this discovery lead? No one can say yet with certainty, since the method employed by the German physician has not yet been made public.*" (*Le Petit Parisien*, n° 94, November 23, 1890.)

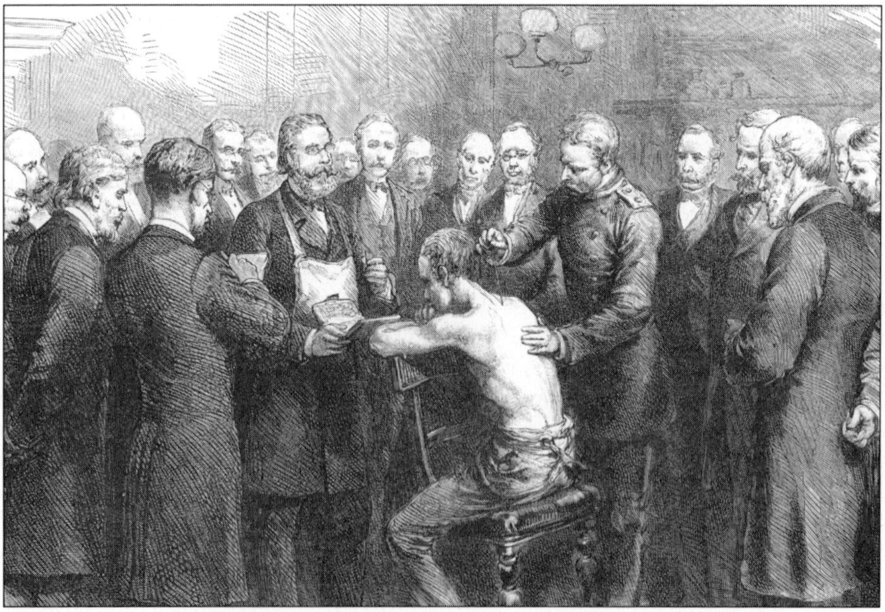

Figure 31. "*Tuberculosis treatment at the Royal Hospital of Berlin: inoculation practiced by Pr. Pfühl, major surgeon and Robert Koch's son-in-law, using his curious syringe, which had to be held vertically.*" Dr. Koch's lymph inspired great hope in Western countries. The secret of its production became subject to debate. Opinions were divided. (*L'Univers illustré*, December 13, 1890.)

In 1917, the Rockefeller Foundation sent to France a four-person delegation headed by Herman Biggs, a recognized expert in the fight against tuberculosis. After some misadventures, the delegation arrived in France to be received by… Adrien Loir (Pasteur's nephew), Director of the Havre Office of Hygiene (*Bureau d'hygiène du Havre*) since 1908. Biggs and his colleagues had to set up "*a committee entrusted with assisting the fight against tuberculosis, whose objectives included: 1° organising a model dispensary and visiting-nurse service in the 20th arrondissement of Paris and in Eure-et-Loir; 2° creating special courses for doctors and visiting health workers; 3° encouraging the creation of antitubercular dispensaries in every region of France; 4° maintaining a public information campaign.*" The Commission completed its mission, very productive for the French, at the end of 1922[217]. The "*Comité central d'assistance aux anciens militaires tuberculeux*" became the National Committee of Protection against Tuberculosis ("*Comité national de défense contre la tuberculose*"). A law passed in 1916 made it compulsory to set up "Antitubercular Dispensaries" on the model of that created by Calmette in Lille. In 1919, another law established sanitariums and then "preventoriums" in each French department. In 1932, France had 777 dispensaries, 60 sanatoriums and 15,000 beds for consumptives[218]. A major publicity campaign was launched. Educational post cards were printed and distributed, the sale of antitubercular stamps started in 1925, etc.

Tuberculosis transmission is essentially airborne, from person to person; that is, a person with a so-called "open case" (having tubercular lesions in direct contact with the exterior) can excrete bacilli into their environment. Pulmonary lesions in particular can lead to the expulsion of small droplets of Koch's bacillus containing fluid. The primary infection often goes unnoticed for long periods of time. Unfortunately, it can be reactivated, to become active tuberculosis. The causes of reactivation are usually unrelated to the Koch's bacillus (KB) organism; they can include immunodepression related to a virus such as that of AIDS. Many other factors such as malnutrition, fatigue, etc. can also contribute to this reactivation. At this stage, the disease develops through the formation of a granuloma enclosing a KB colony and a large number of the patient's cells. Surrounding tissues are destroyed by the association of the microbes with products in the surrounding tissues. As a result "caseous material" will appear. Soon, the tubercule will become fragile and break. Now, tuberculosis bacilli scatter throughout the body, carried by the blood. The disease can then progress toward a fatal outcome, with a multiplication of foci of infection. Tuberculosis symptoms depend on the location of the disease: the lungs, the bones, the intestines, the urogenital apparatus, the meninges, etc. The latter form was still fatal until the 1950s.

Transmission of bovine tuberculosis to man through milk or meat was, of course, an extremely serious problem. Edmond Nocard, Theobald Smith and others rapidly confirmed the transmissibility of bovine tuberculosis to man. In July 1901, at the London conference on tuberculosis, Robert Koch opposed this idea. A long controversy followed, each side using more or less scientific articles as ammunition[219]. The possibility of tuberculosis transmission from bovines to humans was finally accepted by all. This meant that it was absolutely necessary to control bovines and their products: sterilise cow milk and remove contaminated meat from commercial distribution, or sterilise

217. R.M., 1922, p. 17; Grellet, 1983, p. 170.
218. Brouardel, 1934, pp. 149 & 175.
219. Diffloth, 1902, p. 88.

them. Finally, combating bovine tuberculosis led to the hope that the animal disease could be eradicated, along with its transmission to man. Very quickly, Denmark started to screen for bovines reacting to the tuberculin test, and proceeded to slaughter them; their value was reimbursed by the State[220].

The mechanisms conferring immunity against tuberculosis bacilli and other related bacilli are still only partly understood. They form the prototype of cell-mediated immunity, that is, immunity related to physiological properties of cells. This type of immunity can be transmitted among laboratory animals of the same inbred strain (like between identical twins) by living cells and nothing else. What we know about immunity against tuberculosis bacilli started with Koch's phenomenon, discovered in 1891. When a guinea pig is infected using a small dose of tuberculosis bacilli, the inoculation wound heals quickly, then opens again a few days later, to become a small ulcer which endures until the death of the animal. But, if after four to six weeks, the same animal is inoculated again with tuberculosis bacillus, the site of injection takes on a blackish colour, necrosis sets in and the scab disappears. A superficial ulcer remains, which closes in a short time. The tuberculosis bacillus behaves very differently in each of these two cases, depending whether it was inoculated to a healthy animal or one already infected.

First, attempts were made to obtain immunity against tuberculosis bacilli by killing them and extracting some of their components, using the rudimentary means available at the time. These extracts were used for purposes of prevention or treatment. The

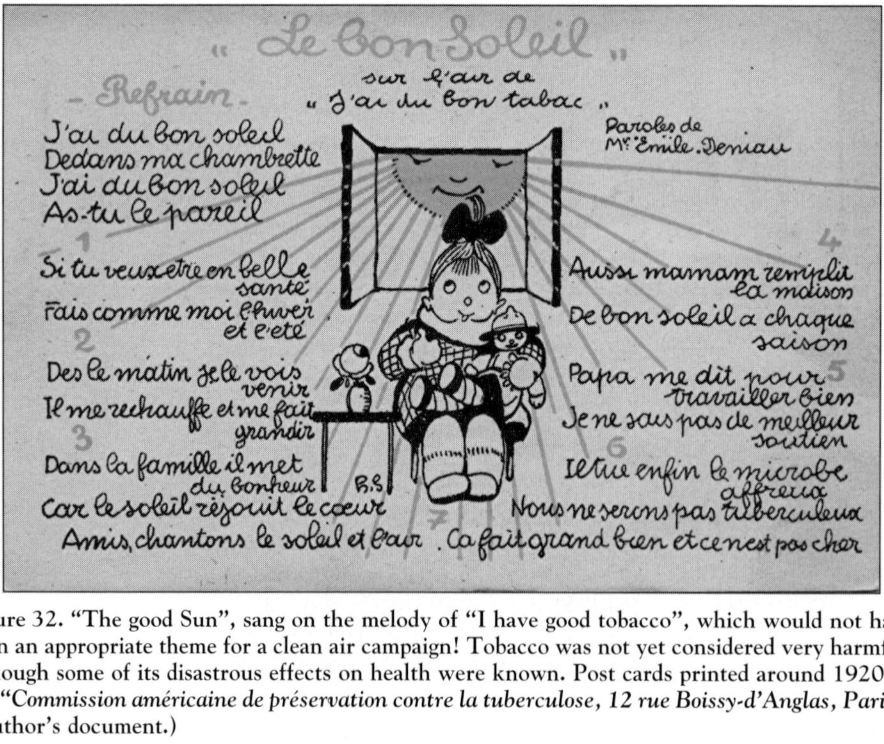

Figure 32. "The good Sun", sang on the melody of "I have good tobacco", which would not have been an appropriate theme for a clean air campaign! Tobacco was not yet considered very harmful, although some of its disastrous effects on health were known. Post cards printed around 1920 by the "*Commission américaine de préservation contre la tuberculose, 12 rue Boissy-d'Anglas, Paris.*" (Author's document.)

220. Diffloth, 1902, p. 88.

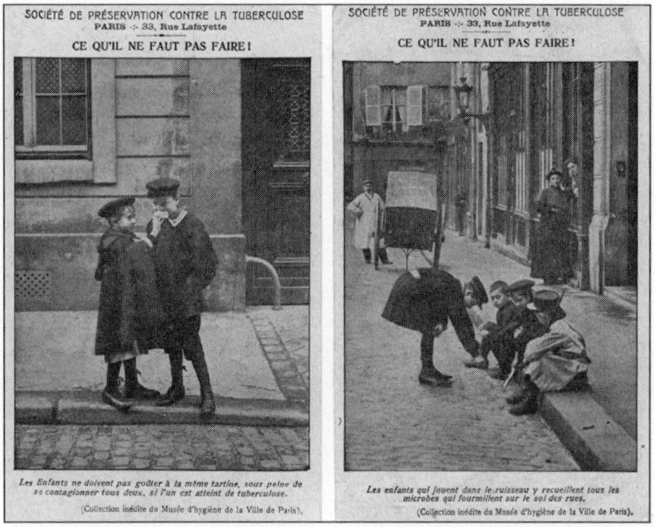

Figure 33. Examples of post cards published by the "*Société de préservation contre la tuberculose*", Paris – 33, rue Lafayette. "WHAT NOT TO DO!" Left: "*Children should not share the same slices of buttered bread to avoid the risk that both catch the infection if one has tuberculosis.*" Right: "*Children who play in street runnels pick up all the germs that cover the ground of the streets.*" These cards are part of the "Original Collection of the Hygiene Museum of the City of Paris" (*Collection inédite du Musée d'hygiène de la ville de Paris*). On the other side of the cards, the inscription reads: "*Do not spit on the ground. Boil your milk. Tuberculosis kills 150,000 people each year. It is avoidable; it can be cured.*" (Author's document.)

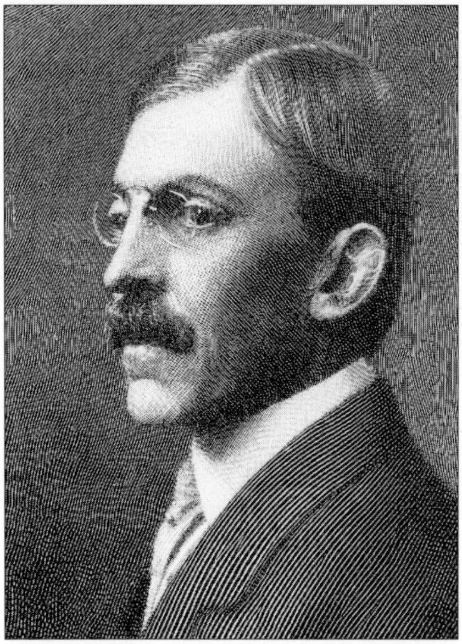

Figure 34. Hermann H. Biggs, physician and statesman in charge of public health. He played an essential role in the fight against tuberculosis in France, during the latter part of the 1914-1918 war and in the postwar years. France owes him and the Rockefeller Foundation an enormous debt of gratitude. (Winslow, 1929, fly-leaf.)

first tuberculosis bacillus extract, developed by Koch himself, was called "tuberculin" or "Koch's lymph", and was the subject of violent controversy for several reasons. Initially, Koch's official announcement at the inaugural session of the International Conference of Medical Sciences in Berlin, on August 4, 1890, that he had discovered a method of curing animals of tuberculosis, and that he was going to try it in man, brought great hope to the Western world. Koch was an internationally recognized expert in the field of infectious diseases. He was extremely respected. The popular press seized on the subject and pressured Koch into saying more than he intended. Comments were at first full of praise. "*And if Koch does not yet disclose his latest secret, it is because, wisely obstinate, stubbornly scientific, he leaves no iota to error or chance... He* (Koch) *is no longer experimenting, he is healing: thus, he is obliged to wait for his cures to be perfect, absolute and remain constant. The day when his last patient will be well...*"[221]. In 1890, *Le Journal illustré* informed its readers: "*The news of the great discovery that holds everyone's attention today... It is possible that the remedy for tuberculosis, whose secret is so well kept...*"[222]. The exact nature of this miraculous substance was kept secret by Koch himself. What followed proved to be disappointing: "*Unfortunately, we soon noticed that Koch's lymph was far from giving the results so exuberantly promised, despite the excessive price at which it was sold. In any case, R. Koch insisted on keeping his remedy secret, and it was not until the following year, when Roux and Nocard were able to prepare it in France, that he decided to reveal how he prepared it.*"[223] Pasteur had been much blamed for hiding the nature of his anthrax vaccine, used in the Pouilly-le-Fort experiment. In fact, patents obtained at that time offered little or no protection from imitators, and the competition reigning between researchers like Pasteur and Koch did not prompt them to reveal the secrets concerning the composition and production of their inventions. They were constantly worried about being "overtaken" by competitors, or worse, of seeing their work repeated incorrectly and refuted. Examples abound: Pasteur's anthrax vaccine and the Turin Veterinary School, Frisch's bad experiences with Pasteurian rabies vaccines, or certain uses of Koch's tuberculin...

Injection of Koch's tuberculin sometimes produced very violent reactions, with expansion of tubercular lesions and appearance of nephritis[224]. Koch's bacillus extracts could also produce more or less extended necrosis depending on the injected dose. Sometimes, results were unfortunate... and included casualties. Koch was severely disparaged. Tuberculin was given the nickname "*la Kockine*", a play on words: in French, "coquin" means "mischievous" as in "playful", but also as in "causing mischief"[225]. Despite this, when used with discernment, it retained a place in the treatment of some forms of tuberculosis until the Second World War. It found its usefulness in the diagnosis of tuberculosis: the famous "tuberculin reaction" test, which made it possible, as well as in Koch himself and his colleague Wassermann, an impending attack of tuberculosis. This method was initially developed in veterinary medicine, to remove animals with tuberculosis from bovine herds[226]; its use in human medicine followed. The same principle was applied for diagnosing other diseases such as glanders (mallein test), brucellosis (brucella test), etc.

221. Hacks, 1890, p. 415.
222. Anonyme, 1890b, p. 378.
223. Laumonier, 1921, p. 443.
224. Littré, 1908, p. 1738.
225. Anonyme, 1902a, p. 385.
226. Nocard, 1896, p. 541; Apert, 1922, p. 191.

Numerous authors - Nocard, Arloing, Grancher, H. Martin, Héricourt, Richer, Smith, Ferran, Shiga, Friedmann Rappin and many others - then proceeded to attempt the immunisation of laboratory animals against tuberculosis bacilli. Calmette lists the experiments of antituberculosis vaccination using bacterial extracts, killed bacilli and sixteen different methods involving bacilli whose virulence had been attenuated by aging, by chemical agents or by repeated passages on animals, or involving bird bacilli or inferior vertebrate bacilli[227]. These dozens (hundreds?) of experiments were rather unsuccessful. The first encouraging results were obtained by von Behring, who used KB cultured for six years in the laboratory, then vacuum dried, to immunise calves. Behring was using human bacilli: "*The human bacillus vaccinates bovine species... Behring used the expression Jennerisation of bovines.*"[228] Baptised "bovovaccine", this discovery raised great hope. Large-scale experiments in Berlin and in Melun (began in 1904, not surprisingly at the suggestion of Rossignol, the man who had initiated the Pasteurian experiments at Pouilly-le-Fort, with scientific assistance from Vallée) unfortunately showed that while antitubercular immunity could be achieved with bovovaccine, this immunity was brief and imperfect. In addition, there was a real danger for the researchers, since the bacilli were of human origin and of very variable virulence[229]. Another vaccine, developed by Koch and named "Tauruman", also made using living human tuberculosis bacilli with attenuated virulence, was placed on the market[230]. Ferran used a tuberculosis bacillus derived from Koch's bacillus, which had apparently undergone a sudden transformation: "*The alpha bacteria, with which he prepares his vaccine, seems to prevent the development of tuberculosis bacillus.*"[231] Calmette, with material received from Ferran himself, was not able to reproduce his results[232]. All these experiments were abandoned for lack of reliable results.

In 1920, Calmette concluded that "*a bacterial infection that remains localised can confer the system a particular state of intolerance to new infections. This is a form of immunity lending the ability to eliminate bacilli as foreign bodies that phagocytes and cellular digestive juices are unable to destroy. This elimination occurs either through normal excretion of solid residues of bodily fluids (biliary ducts, intestine, mucous membrane excretions), or through suppuration and tissue necrosis, leading to the formation of cold caverns or abscesses which finally open to the exterior*"[233]. This explanation reflects the state of knowledge of that period. However, the state of intolerance to tuberculosis bacilli (Koch's phenomenon) was quite well known. This state only persists if it is nourished by a focus of tuberculosis bacilli. Contamination by virulent Koch bacilli can lead to true tuberculosis. Calmette reports: "*Following the observations I made with C. Guérin on the subject of modifications seen in cultured tuberculosis bacilli during their passage through the digestive tube, we noted that the bacillus can be cultured perfectly on a potato or agar medium, saturated with pure glycerinated bile at 5 per 100, and that after a certain number of successive reseedings on this medium the bacillus acquires very particular physiological characteristics. The appearance of the cultures closely resembles that of the malleus bacillus* (Glanders, contagious disease

227. L.M., 1910a, p. 720; L.M, 1910b, p. 12; Calmette, 1920, p. 567; 1922, p. 579; 1936, p. 838; Vallée, 1920, p. 288.
228. Burnet, 1908, p. 67.
229. Burnet, 1908, p. 67.
230. Citron, 1912, p. 29.
231. Honoré, 1924, p. 16.
232. Calmette, 1936, p. 866.
233. Calmette, 1920, p. 567.

of horses, transmissible to man), *and their virulence gradually decreases, to the point that after 70 passages on biliated medium, a young bovine withstands very well a 100-milligram intravenous injection, while 3 milligrams of the same strain of bacillus simultaneously cultivated on glycerinated ordinary potato medium gives bovines of the same age acute granulic tuberculosis, fatal in 28 to 35 days.*"[234] The experiment started on January 8, 1908, with a strain of tuberculosis bacillus isolated by Nocard, taken from a tubercular bovine mastitis. This strain was cultured on pieces of potato cooked in 5% glycerinated beef bile, with resowing every fifteen days. After 230 successive cultures (about ten years), Calmette and Guérin observed that these bacilli were no longer able to infect guinea pigs or rabbits, even at high doses. The experiments continued on young bovines and monkeys. The strain was called BCG for Bilié Calmette Guérin, now Bacillus Calmette Guérin. The BCG creates one or several foci of tuberculosis bacillus capable of maintaining the state of protective hypersensitivity, but because the Koch bacilli are of attenuated virulence, these foci cannot cause tuberculosis. But they can be eliminated by immunological defences, and leave the vaccinated person without protection. Hypersensitivity not maintained by a focus of tuberculosis bacilli (wild or attenuated) decreases quite rapidly and then disappears.

Calmette and Guérin studied the efficiency and duration of the immunity conferred by their strain of bacillus with modified virulence, and the possibility of its use to protect bovines, and therefore to prevent transmission to man. Animal tuberculosis affected a high percentage of the livestock of European countries. In Paris and in suburban communities, in 1908, tuberculosis in dairy cows existed on over 30% of farms. The situation was probably similar in the other European countries and in America[235]. At that time, bovine tuberculosis was both a serious medical problem because of its possible transmission to man and especially to children, through dairy cows, and a considerable rural economic problem because of the slaughter of animals with tuberculosis and the destruction of their carcasses.

In 1920, Calmette ended the chapter of his book on active antitubercular immunity, entitled "Bacillary Infection and Tuberculosis in Human and Animals", as follows: "*I venture to add that I do not find it improbable that one day we will be able to propose its use* (a similar strain of tuberculosis bacillus, with a human origin bacillus) *for the vaccination of young children. With this objective in mind, we are preparing a human origin bacillus which, after being cultured in a long series of passages in human bile medium first, then in beef bile medium, has lost its tuberculogenic properties for guinea pigs and monkeys. Tuberculosis patients withstand quite high doses with no adverse effects, either by intravenous injection or by ingestion...*"[236]. The text is not very explicit as to the species of "tuberculosis patients", who could be monkeys but also human beings with tuberculosis (?). But the BCG (this acronym initially designated "Bilié Calmette-Guérin" rather than "Bacillus Calmette-Guérin", as it generally does today) was originally a vaccine intended for bovines. Calmette and Guérin were preparing another strain for human immunisation.

Hygiene conditions were often still deplorable in the 1920s. In Paris, statistics reported a mortality rate of 24% due to tuberculosis in children born in families infected with this disease. Dr. Weill-Hallé, Paris hospital physician and Director of the "*Ecole de*

234. Calmette, 1920, p. 595.
235. Vallée, 1920, p. 9.
236. Calmette, 1920, p. 597, 1922, p. 610.

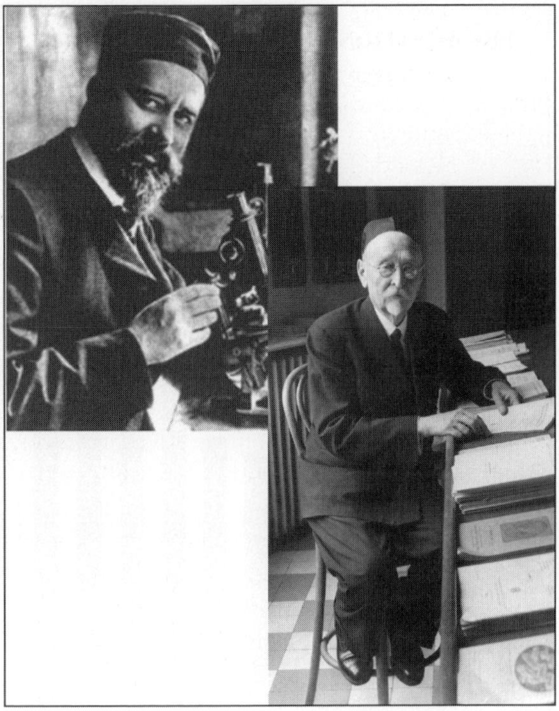

Figure 35. Left: "*Albert Calmette, assistant director of the* Institut Pasteur". He was a great Pasteurian, with outstanding merit in serotherapy, vaccinology and social hygiene. (*Sciences et voyages*, n° 196, May 31, 1923). Right: Camille Guérin at his work table. *Paris-Match* dedicated a long and very elogious article to him. "*A chair, books and a folding bed compose 'Monsieur' Guérin's furnishings. He lives at the* Institut Pasteur *in the old laboratory of Calmette, his master, whose name is still linked to his own. Famous throughout the world, he is largely unknown in France.*" (*Paris-Match*, n° 224, July 4-11, 1953.)

Puériculture de la Faculté de Médecine de Paris" (Pediatric School of the Paris Faculty of Medicine), and Dr. Turpin were very interested in the results obtained in cattle by Calmette and Guérin, as well as in the experiments on many species of monkeys, including chimpanzees, conducted by Prof. Wilbert, Director of the *Institut Pasteur* of Kindia in French Guinea[237]. They proposed that Calmette and Guérin conduct an experiment on infants with very high risk of contracting tuberculosis. They had no means of saving them from almost inevitable death. Calmette and Guérin hesitated for a long time, and finally accepted, honestly thinking that their attenuated bovine strain was not dangerous for humans. The first human trials started in the summer of 1922, in the maternity ward of the Charité Hospital. The first child chosen, dangerously close to death, had been born of a mother who died of tuberculosis shortly after the child's birth. Dr. Weill-Hallé and Turpin took the responsibility of giving him the BCG vaccine, and he grew up in good health! Several children were vaccinated in this way with BCG, with their parents'consent. After a rather long interruption intended to provide the perspective needed to judge the effects of these initial trials, the experiments began again at the start of 1924. The BCG was administered orally at 2 milligram doses in a little warm milk, half an hour before breast feeding on days 3, 5 and 7, or 5, 7 and 9 of life. "*Out of the 217 children of this first series of trials, 178 were maintained under medical control and after 18 months 9 fatalities were recorded, that is, 5 percent, a figure inferior to the normal. All surviving children presented normal development, and none of them manifested digestive problems or changes in their state of health,*

237. A.B., 1925, p. 563.

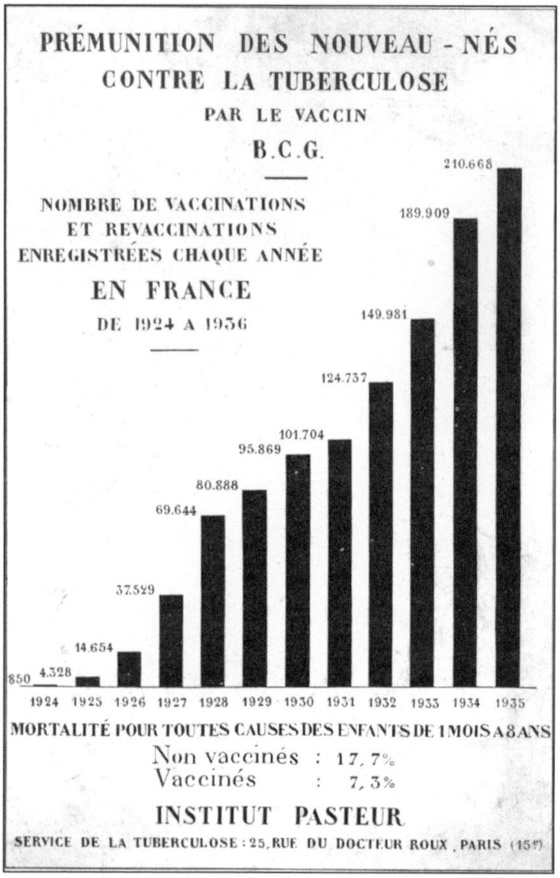

Figure 36. The Tuberculosis Service of the *Institut Pasteur* published post cards indicating the number of vaccinations and revaccinations with BCG registered each year in France. This card provides the data for the period between 1924 and 1935. The objective was to circulate evidence of the safety of this vaccination, and to gain its acceptance by a great majority of the population.

following this vaccination."[238] Doses of BCG prepared at the *Institut Pasteur* were made available to doctors starting on July 1, 1924[239]. Based on data from 204 dispensaries and doctor's offices, among children born and raised in a bacilliferous environment, out of a total of 4,854 non vaccinated children born in 1925, 1926 and 1927, the mortality rate was 15.9%, but only reached 3.4% among the 2,368 vaccinated children of the same age[240]. Given the good results obtained, the pertinent government authorities accepted to bring the trials to other centres and hospitals. The *Institut Pasteur* gave BCG bacillus cultures to the interested foreign centres[241]. In 1927, trials took place in France, Italy, Greece, Rumania, Algeria, Indochina and the Ukraine[242].

In 1928, the Society of Nations organised a conference on the BCG in Paris, where it was solemnly declared that this vaccine was without danger for humans and animals, and that in fact the virulence of this strain had been attenuated in a stable manner. In 1932, Calmette was able to state: "*Now that there are over a million children vaccinated*

238. Laumonier, 1925, p. 686.
239. Berthelot, 1927, p. 404.
240. Calmette, 1936, p. 958.
241. Honoré, 1927, p. 383.
242. Berthelot, 1927, p. 404.

with BCG in the world, 423,000 of them in France (on March 1, 1932), 220,000 in Indochina, 100,000 in Rumania, 20,000 in Spain, 15,000 in Uruguay, etc."[243]

The BCG was also used to check bovine tuberculosis. But a problem soon arose: how to distinguish animals infected with wild bacillus from those that were immunised with BCG? A tuberculin intradermic injection (into the skin to provoke a local reaction), in all species including man, produces a delayed hypersensitivity reaction when the subject is sensitive to Koch's bacillus. This local reaction consists of slight pain, heat, swelling and redness (the "dolor, calor, tumor, rubor" of the Ancients). In bovines, the reaction indicates that the animal has been in contact with the tuberculosis bacillus, but which one? Since it was impossible to distinguish a bovine vaccinated with BCG from an animal with tuberculosis, the use of this vaccine in veterinary medicine was prohibited starting in the 1950s. Because bovine tuberculosis is almost eradicated, any animal reacting positively to an intradermic tuberculin test is slaughtered, in conformity with veterinary public health regulations.

The number of BCG vaccinations rose rapidly in France: 104,000 in 1931, 124,000 in 1932[244]. The BCG was used in humans in very numerous countries. Its effectiveness was demonstrated in most trials, but unfortunately not in all. Today, when BCG is administered at birth or shortly after, it greatly reduces (80% for serious forms, 50% for other forms) infantile tuberculosis. However, the BCG has only little or no effect on pulmonary tuberculosis forms in adults[245]. Every year about two million people still die of tuberculosis caused by tuberculous bacilla strains multiresistant to antibiotics.

Thanks to the programs of the World Health Organisation, about a hundred million children are vaccinated each year, and four billion people have already received BCG: a brilliant career for a vaccine originally intended for veterinary use! The vaccine is effective in children at risk for tuberculosis contamination. Much work is being done to improve the BCG[246] or to find it a possible successor. Most likely, these efforts will lead to a new antitubercular vaccine, safe even in immunodepressed patients, and conferring protection at any age against present-day tuberculosis bacillus strains.

Conjugated Vaccines: 1931...

Some pathogenic bacteria have a capsule composed of complex sugars called polysaccharids. Studies have shown that these sugars are the target of protective mechanisms in organisms. Therefore, what was needed was to create a vaccine composed of these sugars that are polymers, that is, sets of units composed of a number of sugar molecules in the chemical sense of the term. Unfortunately, these sugars are not very antigenic, especially in infants younger than 2 years, who most need to be protected against bacteria. In addition, the responses of the immune system to these sugars consist essentially in the production of short half-life antibodies. Therefore, these responses are short or even absent, with little memory. They protect the vaccinated persons inadequately. These pathogenic agents are of the type *Haemophilus influenzae*, which can cause severe meningitis, sometimes fatal in children and, more rarely, in adults. There are six different types of *Haemophilus influenzae*; type B is the one responsible for most

243. Calmette, 1932, p. 13.
244. Laporte, 1934, pp. 6 & 12.
245. Gicquel, 1999, p. 53.
246. McShane, 2004, p. 1240; Hawkridge 2011, p. 46; Thaiss, 2010, p. 209; Hoft, 2008, p. 164.

infections: epiglottitis, septicemias, septic arthritis, pericarditis, pneumonias... The specific *Haemophilus influenza* type B polysaccharid has been identified and analysed; it is immunogenic but only induces "incomplete" immune responses that provide little protection.

We must go back to much earlier studies to understand how this problem was solved. There are many small molecules that cannot induce an immune response when injected into an organism. In 1929, Landsteiner demonstrated that it was possible to synthesise antibodies able to distinguish these molecules by bringing them together (coupling them) with larger molecules that are immunogenic by themselves (carrier proteins). Thanks to these antibodies, it became possible to identify most (?) very small molecules called haptens[247]. Very quickly, this fundamental discovery was applied by Goebel and Avery[248]. They coupled the polysaccharids of type III pneumococus with horse serum proteins and were thus able to induce in rabbits, antibodies able to precipitate type III capsular polysaccharides, to agglutinate type III pneumococci and to protect mice from a fatal infection caused by these same bacteria. Modern vaccines against pneumococci and meningococci are produced in this manner. The sugars of these bacteria are cut, then purified, leaving only the portions of interest. The most frequently employed carrier proteins are the anatoxins of tetanus, diphtheria, cholera or whooping cough bacilli... whose use is authorised in human medicine. It is also possible to use bacteria proteins. The vaccinated person develops an immune response which includes both anatoxin and bacterial sugars. There are various modes of sugar-protein coupling, and each laboratory producer has his own technique. Moreover, the method of final "coupling" purification is also particular. All these techniques must be authorized by the proper regulation authorities.

247. Landsteiner, 1929, p. 407.
248. Goebel, 1931, p. 431; Avery, 1931, p. 437.

IV
The Modern Era

10
Industrialisation of Vaccine Production

Following the initial success obtained with smallpox vaccine and Pasteurian vaccines, the need for vaccine production on a larger scale became apparent. Most bacteria could be grown in a medium relatively easy to determine and to create. The only problem remaining was to change the quantity from millilitres to litres. In contrast, filterable viruses, agents of many diseases such as smallpox, rabies, yellow fever or foot-and-mouth disease spread by contaminating animals susceptible to a specific virus: bovines to variola or foot-and-mouth disease, rabbits to rabies, monkeys and mice to yellow fever... One almost unsolvable problem remained: parasites...

The First Mass Cultures: Bacteria, 1884...

The first mass bacterial cultures, those of ovine anthrax, were apparently developed by Auguste Chauveau, professor and director of the National Veterinary School in Lyon.

Henry Toussaint was the first to develop an ovine anthrax vaccine (see chapter 6). When his health forced Toussaint to abandon his research, Chauveau continued his work. As early as 1882, he took an interest in the application of the Toussaint vaccine on a large scale[1]. In 1884, Chauveau published "*Of the preparation in large quantities of cultures attenuated by rapid heating... a culture process making it possible to prepare in one step and in the same reservoir the quantity of virus necessary to practice, on four to eight thousand sheep, the double preventive inoculation.*"[2] Chauveau's procedure generated spores that fix and transmit well the attenuation imparted to them. "*The modified procedure involves four consecutive stages: first, a drop of anthrax-infected blood is cultivated in a flask of light broth, at 42.5° (Figure 1). After about twenty hours, the culture presents beautiful asporogenic mycelian filaments. The second step consists of reducing the virulence of these filaments by placing the culture in an incubator at 47 degrees. The next step is to expose the culture to eugenesic temperature (35-37 degrees)... and to wait for bacilliar growth to produce spores; this will take about 5 to 7 days... the fourth step consists of subjecting the sporulated cultures to + 80 degrees (82° C or 84° C) for an hour and a half... (Figure 2)*". This process produces spores with modified virulence, whose germination develops mycelia with the same

1. Chauveau, 1882, p. 337; Chauveau, 1883c, p. 1242.
2. Chauveau, 1884a, p. 73; Chauveau, 1884b, p. 126.

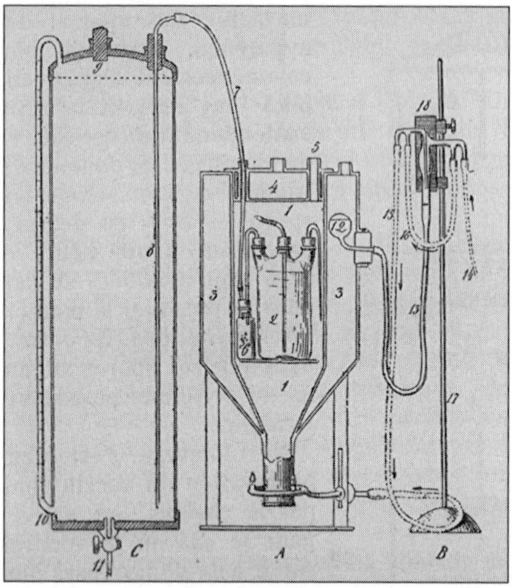

Figure 1. "*Cross sectional view of the position of the thermostat and the vacuum for large cultures. A, Thermostat (often called 'incubator') composed of a modified Arsonval incubator* (known for its precise functioning); *B, Temperature Regulator...; C, Aspirator... 2, Interior of thermostat containing 1 large culture bottle* (2 or 4 litres for 1,600 or 3,200 culture medium)". Thanks to even water flow from reservoir C, which creates a vacuum above the liquid in the culture bottle, and to regular filtered air entering through the central tube, air constantly bubbles in the culture[3].

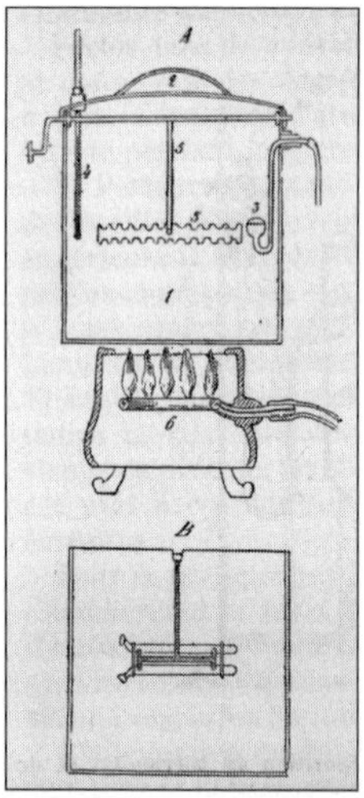

Figure 2. To obtain modified cultures sporulated to the desired degree, the culture in the large bottle is distributed into sterilised 10 ml tubes. These tubes, that are apparently identical to those used by Pasteur and Chamberland (Figure 4, chapter 6) are the ones in which the culture is sent to users. "*Diagram showing a cross-section of the position of the culture heating apparatus in water* (at 84° C for the first vaccine; at 82° C for the second vaccine). A, overview: 1, interior of pot... 3, reservoir (temperature) *regulator not shown* (See figure 1) 5, *virus tube suspension apparatus...*; B, *view in profile of suspension apparatus showing the coupling, two by two, of the virus tubes.*"[4]

3. Arloing, 1891, p. 317.
4. Arloing, 1891, p. 317.

virulence[5a]. Chauveau's 1884 publications, and those of Arloing in 1891, indicate that several techniques of ruminant anthrax vaccine preparation were distributed quickly after those developed by Toussaint and Pasteur.

Bacteria and fungus culture techniques made an enormous step forward with the production of antibiotics and many other substances (vaccines, hormones...), thanks to biotechnology.

Virus Production: a Difficult Problem

Parasitic antigens can confer true protective immunity. But most parasites have reproductive cycles that include one or several hosts. Storing and reproducing parasites in the desired quantity can prove to be very difficult. One of the first (the first?) anti-parasitic vaccines was developed against *Dictyocaulus viviparus* and *Dictyocaulus filaria*, lungworms infecting cattle and sheep/goats respectively. The only nematode vaccine currently in widespread use is made from the radiation-attenuated larvae of these parasites produced in living animals[5b]. Vaccines against the major human[5c] and animal parasites[5d] are at the clinical trial stage of development, thanks to genetic engineering which now makes it possible to produce parasitic antigens.

Filterable viruses have long been multiplied by inoculation to susceptible animals: for instance, cow-pox virus to cows, rabies virus in rabbits, mouse brain to cultivate the Hantaan virus or yellow fever virus to mice (intracerebrally)[6].

This methodology had the great disadvantage of producing viral preparations contaminated with bacteria, when the "culture" was made on the skin (cow-pox/vaccine) or in the mucosa (foot-and-mouth disease) of the animal, etc. Sometimes, viruses could also contaminate the vaccine (cow-pox and foot-and-mouth disease virus; see chapter 3). It was impossible to purify the virus using the preparation techniques available at the time. The vaccines obtained were mixtures of animal tissue antigens and virus (Pasteur's anti-rabies vaccine). Virus multiplication attempts *in ovo* and later *in vitro* started at the beginning of the 20th century. It is difficult to identify their author(s) and to distinguish those who produced the first cell or tissue cultures from those who used them to multiply viruses. Virus titration, after *in ovo* or *in vitro* culture, was conducted by infecting susceptible animals, a method whose results were hard to interpret... Had the virus simply survived or had it multiplied in the culture process? Little by little, results improved. Steinhardt and his associates were probably among the first to have cultured a virus successfully; it was the cow-pox virus, cultured on small pieces of rabbit or guinea pig cornea using the "hanging drops" technique. Their results were convincing: three successive resowings followed by re-inoculation to the rabbit[7]. At about the same time, Levaditi, who used a very similar technique, obtained positive re-inoculation of poliomyelitis virus in a monkey, after five resowings of infected spinal ganglion cells[8]. Despite everything, it might have been argued that simple dilution of

5a. Arloing, 1891, p. 318.
5b. Jarrett, 1959, p. 522.
5c. Girard, 2007, p. 1567; Girard, 2008, p. 3969; Hotez *in* Plotkin, 2008, p. 1295.
5d. Tellam *in* Pastoret, 1997, p. 470.
6. Theiler, 1930a, p. 367; Theiler, 1930b, p. 249; French, 1999, p. 728.
7. Steinhardt, 1913, p. 294; Steinhardt, 1914, p. 87.
8. Levaditi, 1913, p. 202; Levaditi, 1938, p. 572.

the initial inoculum would suffice! Many other experiments conducted subsequently made it possible to control cultures of numerous viruses *in vitro*. But these achievements led to limited virus production which, nevertheless, held the promise of eventually providing cow-pox virus preparations uncontaminated by bacteria[9a].

The nature of cells developed in culture became an important subject of enquiry. The discovery of a carcinogenic virus in hamsters, in cultures of cells that produced certain vaccines against poliomyelitis, came as a shock. Urgent measures had to be taken to stop this contamination. Animal cell cultures stored for one passage only (called "primary cultures") were abandoned in favour of semi-continuous or continuous cultures. In the case of the latter, cells in culture divide indefinitely provided that they are maintained in adequate conditions. The safety of a cell line can be checked as optimally as the available technical possibilities allow, and in any case much better than the safety of primary cultures.

A major advance was achieved when antibiotics, first penicillin and then others, made it possible to avoid most bacterial contaminations of cell cultures. Another obstacle was eliminated thanks to the development of artificial culture mediums with more or less well-defined composition. One of the first culture mediums, still in use today, was the "199" developed by the Canadian firm Connaught. Finally, the manufacture of large capacity culture containers was very important.

In Ovo Virus Cultures, 1936, 1940...

Embryonated egg culture constituted a transitional stage between *in vivo* and *in vitro* virus production. The influenza virus was one of the first to be produced using this technique.

Borrel was the first to produce a pathogenic agent by culture in embryonated chicken egg, in 1907. He inoculated *Spirillum gallinarum* in this "medium" and noticed a proliferation of this organism[9b]. In 1931, Woodruff and Goodpasture cultured fowl-pox on the chorio-allantoid membrane of chick embryo[10]. In 1933, the same authors used the technique again to culture cow-pox virus successfully[11]. This method of culture, favourable to the multiplication of numerous viruses, was a decisive stage in the development of several viral vaccines.

The Influenza Vaccine

Influenza is probably a very ancient disease. Some say that Hippocrates described it, but others disagree. According to Ginctrac, the first known epidemic occurred in 1580. It raged across Europe and perhaps in Asia and Africa[12]. The name *influenza* comes from the Italian. In 1884, there was still controversy about its contagious nature. "*In 1860, when the influenza was rampant in Dijon, Dr. Blanc made the following observations on the contagion. Called to an isolated farm 6 kilometres from Dijon on March 26, he recognized the symptoms of influenza in a 12-year old child. Up until then, no one had been ill on the farm. The sick child had gone to Dijon two days earlier*

9a. Maitland, 1930, p. 119.
9b. Levaditi, 1945, p. 14.
10. Woodruff, 1931, p. 209.
11. Levaditi, 1945, p. 14.
12. Gintrac, 1872, t. 16, p. 728.

to visit relatives whose children had the flu; five days later Mr. Blanc was called to the farm again for another child in the same family, presenting the same symptoms. He was the fourth person in the household to suffer from influenza since March 16; two servants on the farm had fallen ill at the same time."[13] This observation made Blanc think of a contagion and of a two or three-day incubation period, which was correct. The most dreadful epidemic of the so-called "Spanish flu" occurred in 1918-1919, in three successive waves, killing about 20 million people world-wide, including 549,000 in the United States[14]. In France, epidemics considered "normal" can result in highly variable mortality. Thus, the 1957 and 1960 epidemics produced 11,899 and 12,323 victims respectively, the 1961 and 1964 epidemics 2,471 and 2,447, and finally the 1969-1970 epidemic, the most severe, was responsible for 18,000 deaths, 80% of them among elderly persons over 65[15]. Influenza is particularly dangerous for children and the elderly. But certain influenza viruses such as the A (H1N1) 2009, can attack adults in good health.

Influenza is an epidemic disease characterised by acute inflammation of the nasal, pharyngeal and bronchial mucosa, and by generalised symptoms: fever, headache, muscle aches. As the disease progresses, the patient experiences weakness, intense respiratory problems and high fever. The disease occurs in the winter season. Once the virus disappears, organic complications can appear: pulmonary, coronary, renal... Bacterial super-infections are common. For a person in good health, the disease is most often unpleasant but benign.

Influenza viruses are classified into three types - A, B and C - based on antigenic differences in the internal proteins of the virion. Antigenic variations of surface proteins have been studied in depth for influenza A, which has two glycoproteins: haemagglutinin (H) and neuraminidase (N). To date, sixteen H subgroups and nine N subgroups have been identified (all of them observed in viruses infecting aquatic birds. There are few cross reactions between the subgroups, but variations have been observed in the isolates of each subgroup. Each influenza A isolate is designated by the infected species (except human), the location of isolation, the isolate number and the year of isolation, with the H and N subgroups in parantheses; for example: A/swine/Iowa/15/30 (H1N1).

In man, a constant evolution of infecting viruses is observed: new strains appear and others disappear. Different viruses often circulate at the same time (during the winter of 2002-2003: H1N1, H1N2, H3N2 and influenza B). In humans, each pandemic is characterised by the appearance of a new subgroup: 1918 H1N1; 1957 H2N2 (Asian flu), 1968 H3N2 (Hong-Kong flu); 1976 H1N1 (Russian flu, suspected by several authors to be a virus "escaped" from a laboratory); 2001 H1N2. The 1997 Hong Kong chicken flu (eighteen cases recorded in humans) was caused by a H5N1 virus, still active and feared. The aviary influenza epidemic in Holland and in Belgium in 2003 was caused by a H7N7 virus. As for influenza B that apparently only infects man, the H and N antigens show much less variation, and there are no subgroups. Influenza C has only one surface glycoprotein. It infects man and pigs.

During the influenza epidemic of 1889-1892, the "*Haemophilus influenzae*" bacillus was presented by Pfeiffer as the causal organism of influenza. But, at the time of

13. Brochin, 1884, series 4, t. 10, p. 735.
14. Douglas, 1979, p. 1135.
15. G.C., 1960, p. 45; Quid, 1980, p. 488.

the pandemic in 1918-1919, this influenza bacillus was suspected not to be the real agent of that disease. Also, in 1918, Koen first recognized a disease in swine which was so similar to human influenza in its high infectivity, symptomatology and pathology that he concluded that the two diseases were the same. However, Shope, in 1931-1932, proved that swine influenza was caused by the combined action of a filterable virus and an organism very like Pfeiffer's bacillus, which he named *Haemophilus influenza suis*. The virus was caused a mild and transient illness that easily passed unnoticed but provided solid immunity against the natural disease. Shope's work was a model to reinvestigate the human influenza agent. At the start of the 1930s, Smith and his associates, from the National Institute for Medical Research in London, after numerous failed studies on various animal species available to them, observed that the ferret, an animal highly susceptible to dog distemper, was sensible to intranasal inoculation of a filtrate of throat and nose washings from influenza patients. The disease was transmitted even by simple contact among ferrets... A few years later, Francis, in the USA and Smith in England, with their respective associates, transmitted the virus to mice[16]. Then, in 1935, Burnet and Smith separately cultured the flu virus on the chorio-allantoid membrane of embryonated eggs[17]. Finally, between 1936 and 1941, Smith, Hoyle and Fairbrother, Lush and Burnet, as well as Burnet, cultured *in vitro* influenza viruses in embryonary chick tissue[18]. In that same period, Burnet carried out seventy successive passages on embryonated eggs, of a flu virus adapted to the ferret and the mouse. His article ended as follows: "*It seems likely that the development of a virus strain highly pathogenic for the embryonated egg will provide an experimental method of some interest for academic research, and perhaps as a source of virus for any type of human vaccine that might be developed in the future.*"[19] These were prophetic words...

In 1936, Smith developed a vaccine from infected ferret spinal cord. The virus was inactived with formol. Smith tried the vaccine on himself, and then on seventy volunteers from the army, separated into two equal groups. In the vaccinated group, the seric flu antibody values increased, showing response to the vaccine. "Unfortunately" no epidemic broke out to provide the natural evidence necessary to evaluate the protective effect of the vaccine[20]. The following year, in 1937, Chenoweth and Stokes, of the United States, inoculated an influenza virus to eight hundred mentally ill men. This "vaccine" was a mouse lung infiltrate containing the wild living virus. It was administered parenterally, thus producing no generalised infection[21]. It was in fact a sort of "variolation". The effectiveness of the vaccination was judged to be adequate, based on the resistance of those vaccinated to the influenza that subsequently broke out in the region. At about the same time, Francis and Magill reached the same conclusions. Injecting the influenza virus to man subcutaneously or intradermally did not transmit the infection and suggested a specific protection[22].

16. Renaud, 2005, p. 163; Smith, 1937b, p. 112; Williams, 1994, p. 388.
17. Levaditi, 1938, p. 1143.
18. Kilbourne, 1996a, p. 187.
19. Burnet, 1936, p. 282.
20. Smith, 1937b, p. 112.
21. Kilbourne, 1996b, p. 183.
22. Francis, 1937, p. 251.

In the 1940s, another phenomenon came to light: the antigenic variability of the flu virus as a cause for the lack of effect of a batch of vaccine against a particular influenza epidemic. Some of the students in a school were vaccinated against the flu. Four months later, all the students, vaccinated or not, were exposed to a natural flu epidemic in similar conditions, and... were infected in about the same percentage[23]. This inconclusive vaccinal trial underscored the extreme antigenic variability of the influenza virus. Better understanding of this variability made it possible to establish a complicated but effective system. The World Health Organisation, thanks to a world-wide surveillance network, looks for mutated strains of the influenza virus during annual epidemics. The World Organization for Animal Health (or International Office of Epizootics) receives and distributes information from different countries about equine influenza. An expert committee chooses the strains most likely to occur the following year, to vaccinate against human influenza. Pharmaceutical companies adapt these strains to production on embryonated eggs. Since the 1970s, they have made use of the natural tendency of the flu virus to "reassort". This natural process is used by culturing, in parallel, ("co-culturing") the new strains and a virus (A/Puerto Rico/8/34 (H1N1) well adapted to culture in eggs. The desired strain or strains is (are) selected and produced in eggs or sometimes in cells for new vaccines[24].

These viruses are then collected and purified by ultracentrifugation within a few days[25]. The first widely distributed vaccines were marketed at the end of the 1960s. They were produced on embryonated eggs, their viruses were inactivated using a detergent, and they contained the major antigens of the flu virus: hemagglutinins and neuraminidases. This type of vaccine is still widely used.

The yellow fever vaccine is another example of a vaccine produced in vast quantities on embryonated eggs. This vaccine will be the subject of the next chapter.

The First Industrial *In Vitro* Viruses Produced in Cell Culture, 1951...

Foot-and-Mouth Disease Vaccine

Foot-and-mouth disease, a disease of ruminants and suidae, to name only the most classical domestic animals (in fact, all domestic and wild cloven-hoofed ungulates), was and still is a dread disease. Its enzootic character was a cause of despair for our ancestors. The disease starts with a primary vesicle, followed by virus dissemination and the appearance of numerous characteristic vesicles located in the mouth and in interdigital spaces, that is, between the hooves. The animal has fever and chills; it stops eating and milk production decreases; it salivates because swallowing the saliva is painful; it has difficulty walking because vesicles swell its hooves. Vesicles can also appear on its teats, preventing normal milking. Cicatrisation of the wounds occurs between the eight and tenth day. The disease is of long duration and the convalescent animal cannot return to its normal state for many months. Serious after-effects like mastitis can occur. In itself, foot-and-mouth disease is a benign disease that rarely kills, and kills only fragile animals like the young, but its economic consequences are serious; not surprisingly, cattle breeders dread it, with good reason. The reason for describing

23. Taylor, 1949, p. 171.
24. Webby, 2003, p. 1519.
25. Kilbourne *in* Plotkin, 1999, p. 531; Matthews, 1996, p. 189.

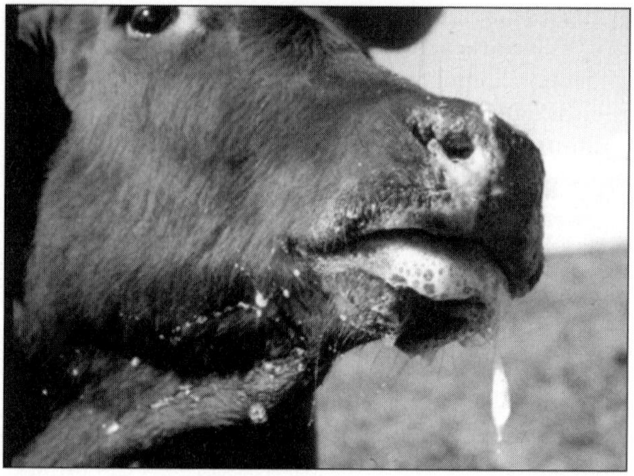

Figure 3. Bovine with foot-and-mouth disease. This infectious disease, caused by a virus, can affect all cloven-hoofed animals. Its main symptom consists of more or less numerous vesicles, often located in the mouth and in interdigital spaces. Foot-and-mouth disease is dreaded because of its economic consequences.

the development of foot-and-mouth vaccine in detail in a history of vaccinology is that this development constituted a technological revolution that transformed the field.

The disease is caused by a virus discovered by German researchers Löffler and Frösch, at the end of the 19th century. This was a remarkable discovery, because it was the first instance where the etiology of an animal (or human) disease was tied to a filterable virus. It is a very small enterovirus of the picornavirus group. Vallée and Carré revealed the existence of two serotypes of foot-and-mouth disease virus that are distinct enough to require different vaccines. To date, at least seven distinct serotypes have been identified, and at least sixty subtypes. This complicates vaccine development considerably. One favourable element in the fight against this disease is that the virus can be easily inactivated by physical or chemical agents. However, minimal quantities of the virus suffice to infect animals, which then contaminate each-other very easily. This epizootic is even harder to control because contaminated animals are contagious before showing clinical signs of the disease. Some can become healthy carriers and can excrete the virus for long periods of time. Very unexpected cases of contagion have been observed. In 1908, during experiments comparing cowpox/vaccine strains, cowpox virus (theoretically pure) was exported from Japan to the United States. Its inoculation to American calves transmitted cowpox to them, as well as... foot-and-mouth disease, to the experimenter's great surprise! A similar case of transfer of foot-and-mouth virus by cowpox occurred in Norway in 1930[26]. This indicates that foot-and-mouth virus might have been inoculated to great numbers of people by vaccinating them against cowpox. Not a very serious accident in itself, but still regrettable even if the foot-and-mouth virus is little or not at all likely to multiply in man. Reported cases date back to 1863 or even earlier. Diagnostic errors can also exist... because other viruses can produce similar symptoms in man.

Foot-and-mouth disease is probably very ancient in Europe[27]. Very wide-spread epizootics occurred in the 1950s and the early 1960s. In 1952, in France alone, 3,500,000 bovines, 900,000 ovines and 900,000 swine were infected. Revenue losses for farmers

26. Schaper, 1948, p. 215.
27. Blancou, 2003, p. 54.

were enormous[28]. Great Britain was severely affected in 2001, and secondarily Iceland, France and the Netherlands.

In the course of his studies, Löffler had noticed that a first attack of foot-and-mouth disease conferred immunity; a more advanced state of knowledge allowed defence strategies to be created. The inoculation (variolation technique) of foot-and-mouth disease to animals was described with this special warning: "*This procedure is not always well-done.*"[29] The immunity conferred was short-lived, one year at the most; but very early Löffler decided to use it. By mixing foot-and-mouth lymph from sick animals with serum from convalescent animals, he was able to immunise animals[30]. This method of serovaccination was widely used in man against diphtheria. Its application to foot-and-mouth disease in these conditions was very inappropriate. The method parameters were difficult to control in the conditions of practice of rural veterinary medicine. However, protection of animals in certain situations was an important consideration, for instance in case of epizootics or when animals were gathered together at agricultural shows, where the best animals were exposed to the admiration of the public and... to infections.

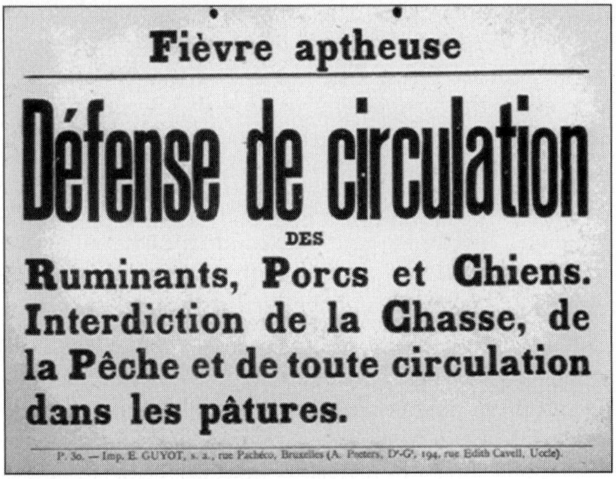

Figure 4. Type of poster frequently seen along European roads, in several languages, during foot-and-mouth disease epizootics... This poster, displayed in Wallonia (Belgium), was printed by the firm A. Guyot of Brussels. Poster text: "*Foot-and-mouth disease. Circulation forbidden to ruminants, pigs and dogs. Hunting, fishing and walking across pastures forbidden.*"

Vaccination with antigen-antibody mixture was difficult to carry out; therefore, it was replaced by serotherapy. The first method used was the hemoprevention proposed by Kitt in 1892. Convalescent bovine blood from an animal having had foot-and-mouth disease was collected. It was immediately citrated to prevent coagulation. Its administration conferred effective protection for ten to fourteen days. This complicated method was used between 1920 and 1940, and up to the 1950s. Departmental hemoprevention centres were created in France[31] and probably elsewhere. Hemoprevention was a rudimentary serotherapy that had the undeniable advantage of being simple, but accidents could happen... since the safety of the serum was not guaranteed. The serovaccination technique was used and even simplified into "hemo-inoculation", combining hemoprevention with aphtisation[32].

28. Claude, 1952, p. 87.
29. Anonyme, 1911, p. 29.
30. De Loverdo, 1898, p. 38; Barrier, 1905, p. 638.
31. Fleckinger, 2004, p. 29.
32. Fleckinger, 2004, p. 29.

Immune serum started to be produced by collecting blood from bovines convalescing after the natural disease or after having been artificially infected; these animals were properly immunised and kept as antiserum donors[33]. The dose to be injected to protect an adult bovine of normal weight for the duration of a show lasting a few days was 200 millilitres! About 300,000 bovines were apparently subjected to this treatment in 1929 alone in Germany[34], a number which seems high. A preventive serotherapy was also introduced at the start of epizootics, along with the slaughter of infected animals[35].

In the years that followed, efforts focused on developing a vaccine. Production of foot-and-mouth disease virus was only possible *in vivo*. Vallée, Carré and Rinjard created the first small-scale vaccine against foot-and-mouth disease by collecting vesicles from infected animals (with natural disease) and using formaldehyde to neutralise the virus obtained[36]. In the absence of vesicles, virulent blood was used, and treated with formaldehyde[37]. In 1938, Waldmann and Köbe brought a considerable improvement to the Vallée vaccine by inoculating foot-and-mouth virus *in vivo* to bovines. In order to keep the cost price reasonable, animals destined to slaughter were used. They were inoculated in the tongue, and a few days later, when the virus had developed on the surface tissues of the tongue, the animals were slaughtered. The tongue mucosa of these animals was collected to serve as sources of virus. The meat of these animals was perfectly suitable for consumption, even the tongues. The foot-and-mouth virus is killed by the spontaneous lactic maturation occurring in the meat within a few hours after death.

The foot-and-mouth virus collected from the tongues was more or less purified and inactivated by formaldehyde. Of course, this procedure was rudimentary, but it was used to immunise millions (?) of animals! And yet, the virulent material provided by a cow could only immunise 170 animals[38]. Many countries used this method of foot-and-mouth vaccine preparation.

In 1938, Waldmann and Köbe improved this method even farther by absorption of the virus on aluminium hydroxide before its inactivation with formaldehyde. The use of absorption on aluminium hydroxide had been proposed by Glenny and his associates as early 1926, to augment immune response after diphtheric toxoid injection in guinea pigs[39]. As a result, the vaccine became much more effective and more economical to produce, because smaller doses of inactivated virus were needed[40]. Some authors attribute the merit of this discovery to the Dane Sven Schmidt[41], who advocated the addition of glycerine before absorption on aluminium hydroxyde[42].

In the Netherlands, Pr. Herman Frenkel was conducting large-scale projects of foot-and-mouth virus production. He had perfected a very original system of foot-and-mouth virus culture, using epithelial tissue from the tongues of slaughtered animals ("still

33. Mérieux, 1988, p. 41.
34. Panisset, 1938, p. 152.
35. Leclainche, 1905, p. 638.
36. Vallée, 1926, p. 326.
37. Verge, 1943, p. 328; Fleckinger, 2004, p. 29.
38. Senet, 1952, p. 351.
39. Glenny, 1926, p. 31.
40. Verge, 1943, p. 330.
41. Schaper, 1948, p. 251.
42. Verge, 1943, p. 332.

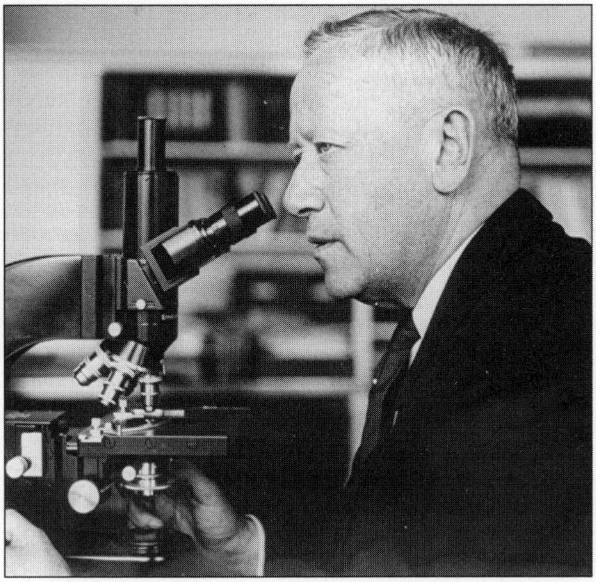

Figure 5. Pr. Herman Frenkel (*State Veterinary Research Institute, Amsterdam*) developed, with very modest means, a system of bovine lingual epithelium culture. Slaughtered bovine tongues were taken from the slaughterhouse. Their epithelia were placed in culture in a suitable medium, in metal vats, then seeded with foot-and-mouth virus which multiplied and provided antigens for the vaccine. (Photograph kindly provided for publication by Pr. Robbert Hans Meloen, Pepscan Systems B.V., Lelystad, Netherlands.)

warm", as his article says), and no longer from living animals[43]. A veritable revolution! But the method was developed with the techniques available at the time, using Roux bottles, that is, glass flasks containing a culture medium measured in millilitres (not in litres) and millions, not billions, of cells. A larger scale production was needed. In 1951, a 60-litre metal vat containing tissue from forty to sixty tongues was ready for use. The material was rudimentary: tongues collected after slaughter were attached to drums and scrubbed by brushes (of the sweeper brush type) under a jet of water. The lingual epithelium was separated from muscle tissue using a cold-cut slicing machine ("Berkel P.14", a deli shop machine), whose blade was sprinkled with Tyrode's solution in order to preserve the life of the collected cells continuously. A good technician could collect the epithelium of four tongues per hour. Stirring (rocking) the tissues in the container was achieved by using a propeller, and aeration was provided by two Chamberland candles. The vat had two windows to allow monitoring of the culture. A strong dose of antibiotics kept bacterial contamination at an acceptable level[44]. This was probably one of the first (the first)? instance(s) of *in vitro* virus culture on a semi-industrial scale, not in the living organism category. A major stage in vaccine production had been entered.

But going to the next stage - the truly industrial stage - was not easy. Part of the technology was borrowed from the advances introduced in the industrial production of antibiotics. But almost all the rest had to be invented: collecting the tongues and their epithelium (external cell layers, the "skin" of the tongue, as it were), placing them in culture in large glass or stainless steel containers (reactors), suitable culture media, seeding them with virus, virus production, its harvesting, its purification, etc. The foot-and-mouth vaccine opened a new era in industrial vaccine production, at the start of the 1950s. This vaccine was the result of extremely fruitful cooperation

43. Frenkel, 1947, p. 155.
44. Frenkel, 1951, p. 187.

between a fundamental research team and industrialists, scientists and economists. The Netherlands was the first country to carry out mass vaccination of its bovine livestock against foot-and-mouth disease, with the Frenkel vaccine[45]. The French firm Mérieux, with the authorisation of the Dutch government and the close cooperation of the inventor, used the Frenkel procedure very successfully to produce its foot-and-mouth vaccine[46]. Some human vaccines benefited greatly from the development of these technologies, particularly the poliomyelitis vaccine.

A few years later, in 1962, Mowat and Chapman discovered that the foot-and-mouth virus of different serotypes multiplied on continuous cell lines called BHK 21 (*Baby hamster kidney fibroblasts: fibroblasts from newborn hamster kidney*), that is, it could multiply indefinitely, with no need to return it to the animal[47]. Capstick and his associates showed that these cultures could be produced in great quantities[48a]. This represented another considerable advance, an unlimited source of virus, and therefore of vaccinating antigens. The next stage consisted in purifying the virus, and then "killing" it (the term "inactivation" is now used, since viruses are not considered living beings) so that it will no longer be infectious. The difficulty with this virus, as with all viruses used in "killed" (inactived) vaccines, is to be able to inactivate the virus without provoking denaturing effects in its components, which must retain their immunising power. All substances likely to inactivate a virus modify its structure to some extent. If denaturation is too great, the virus will no longer induce a protective immune response in the vaccinated person; if denaturation is insufficient, the virus will transmit the disease. Such accidents were sometimes observed with the use of inactivated foot-and-mouth vaccine. At the end of the 1980s, over half of the small foci of foot-and-mouth disease infection in continental Europe, which occasionally emerged, were due to vaccines whose inadequately inactivated viral particles contaminated the inoculated animals. This fact helped the arguments of militant opponents of foot-and-mouth disease vaccination in the European Community.

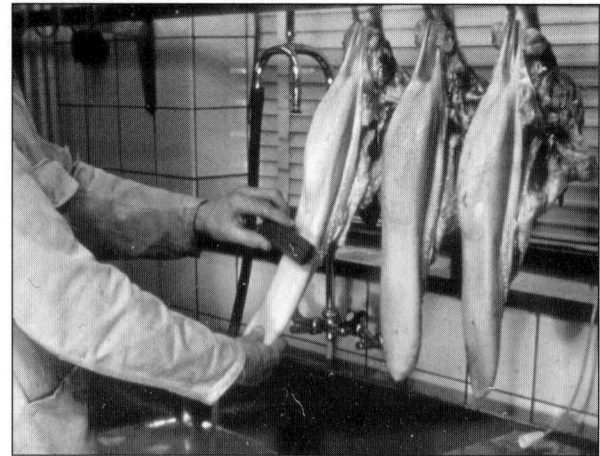

Figure 6. The tongues, taken from freshly slaughtered bovines, are first cleaned by hand... (Photo Rob Meloen.)

45. Salt *in* Pastoret, 1997, p. 641.
46. Mérieux, 1988, p. 80; Mérieux, 1996, p. 8.
47. Mowat, 1962, p. 253.
48a. Capstick, 1965, p. 1135.

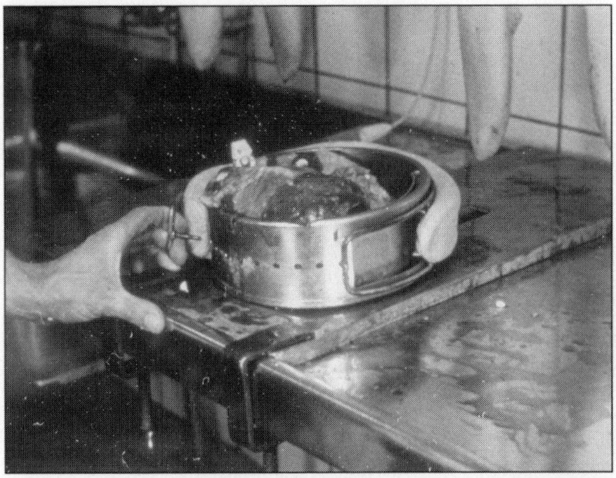

Figure 7. The tongues are attached one by one on and in the revolving drums. The system used to place them leaves the surface of the tongue accessible, to facilitate the next operation... But the muscle mass of the tongue is protected inside the drum. Its commercial value is safeguarded. (Photo Rob Meloen.)

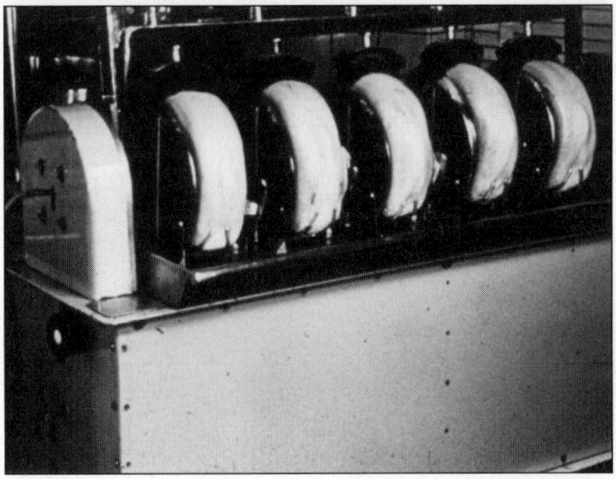

Figure 8. This photograph shows the action of the brushes (at the top of the drums), which clearly scrub the bovine tongues vigorously. (Photo Rob Meloen.)

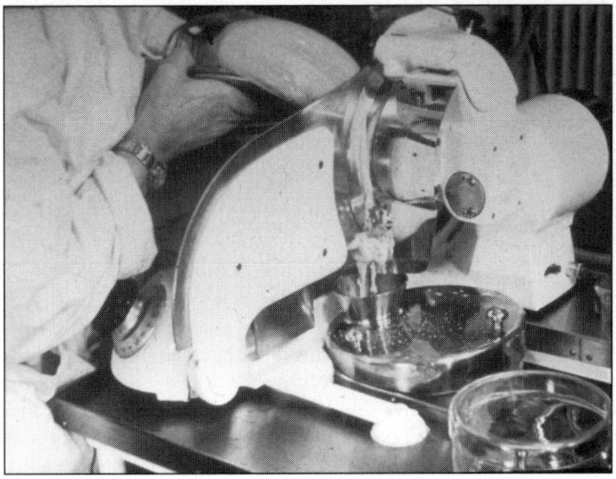

Figure 9. Each tongue, after being brushed, and still held on and in the metal drum, is divested of its epithelium, using a slicer for thin slices of cold cuts. The slicing is done under a trickle of liquid (normal saline or Tyrode solution?) which preserves the good state of the tissues. An experienced technician could remove the epithelium from a tongue in fifteen minutes. The work was painstaking. The pieces of tissue fell into a stainless steel canister. (Photo Rob Meloen.)

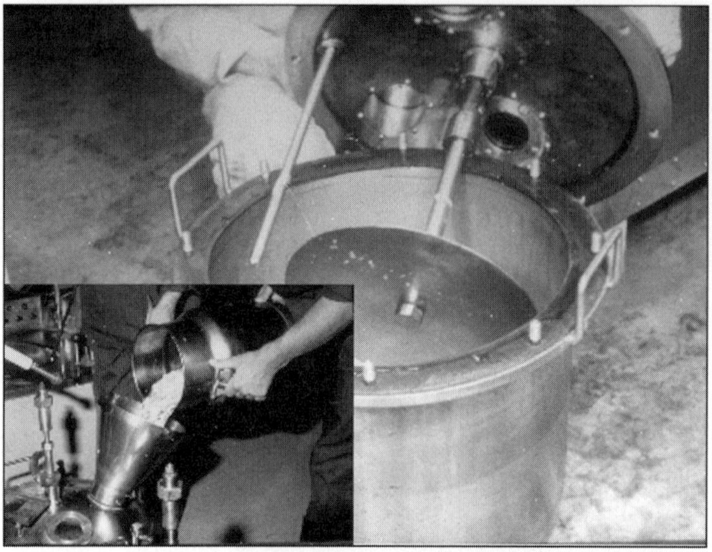

Figure 10. The stainless steel vat is open, showing the propeller which spins slowly, mixing very gently the epithelial and the culture liquid. The rather primitive locking device of the lid on the vat was to be replaced by a more efficient and simpler to use model with a chain, as seen in figures 11 and 12. In insert, thin slices of bovine tongue epithelium are poured from the collection drum into the culture vat, through a large funnel... (Photo Rob Meloen.)

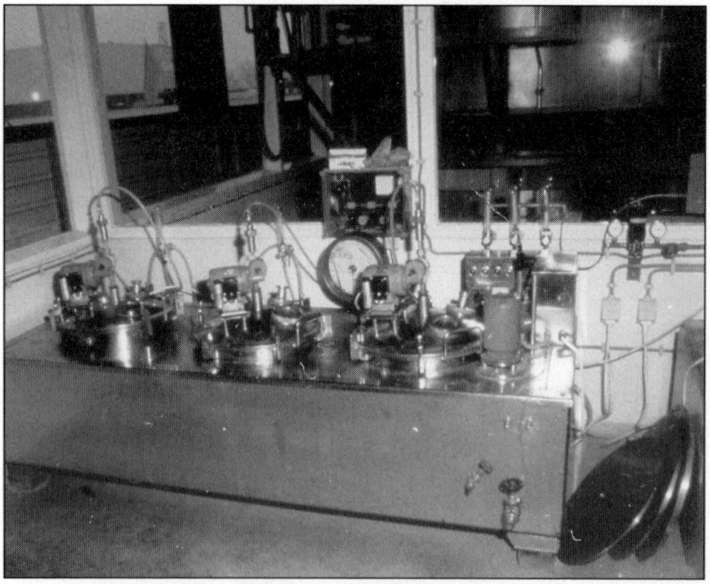

Figure 11. Three stainless steel culture vats can be seen clearly; they are placed in a bath with a thermostat. The lids which can be seen on the counter of the culture vats have been placed to the right of the bath. The main tank has an electric motor that probably rotates a propeller to mix the liquid, which maintains constant temperature for the entire process. Each culture vat has its own motor, rotating the bladeless propeller seen above (the propeller motor movement transmission systems are different at figures 11 and 12). (Photo Rob Meloen.)

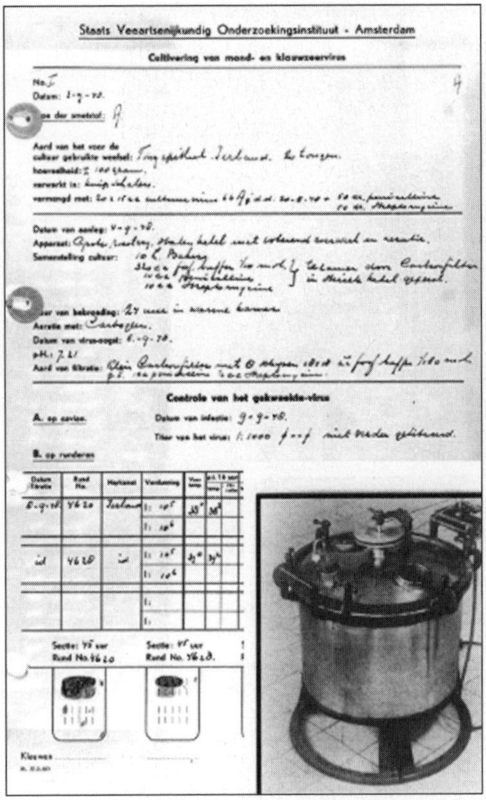
Staats Veeartsenijkundig Onderzoekingsinstituut - Amsterdam

Controle van het gekweekte-virus

Figure 12. Page from Dr. H. Frenkel's laboratory notebook, dated September 3, 1948. The culture: 100 grams of epithelium from twenty bovine tongues in ten litres of culture medium containing penicillin and streptomycin. Titration of the virus harvest is indicated at the bottom of the page bearing the results: it is the titration normally employed at the time, on living bovine tongues, by intradermic injection of dilutions of the culture medium, producing mucosal reactions or not.

Insert: "*Culture vat, showing closed lid with windows, aeration and stirring mechanism, and air vent*". The article specifies that the vat capacity is sixty litres, with a cover firmly attached to the vat by means of brackets held with bolts. Rubber, placed between the vat and the lid, provides a good seal. Two windows make it possible to see inside, by looking through one while the other is lighted. Stirring is provided by a two-magnet system, one propelling, powered by an electric motor, outside, the other propelled, inside. This apparatus is designed to be placed in a double boiler at 37° C. (Frenkel, 1951)[48b]. Frenkel's Dutch team (foot-and-mouth vaccine) was clearly technologically advanced compared to Connaught's American team (poliomyelitis vaccine), particularly since Frenkel's technique was to be that of the future - which was not the case for Connaught's system. This does not apply to the culture media.

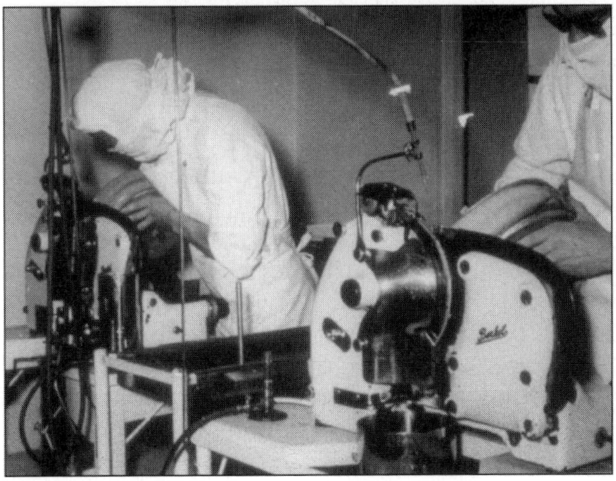

Figure 13. Two technicians at work, at the French Institute of foot-and-mouth disease (*Institut français de la fièvre aphteuse* or IFFA), a few years later. In time, the operators' laboratory wear has improved, but the technique is absolutely unchanged. Note that they work bare-handed, because the task was detailed and the gloves available at the time were unsuitable. (Photo Mérieux Foundation.)

48b. Frenkel, 1951, p. 187.

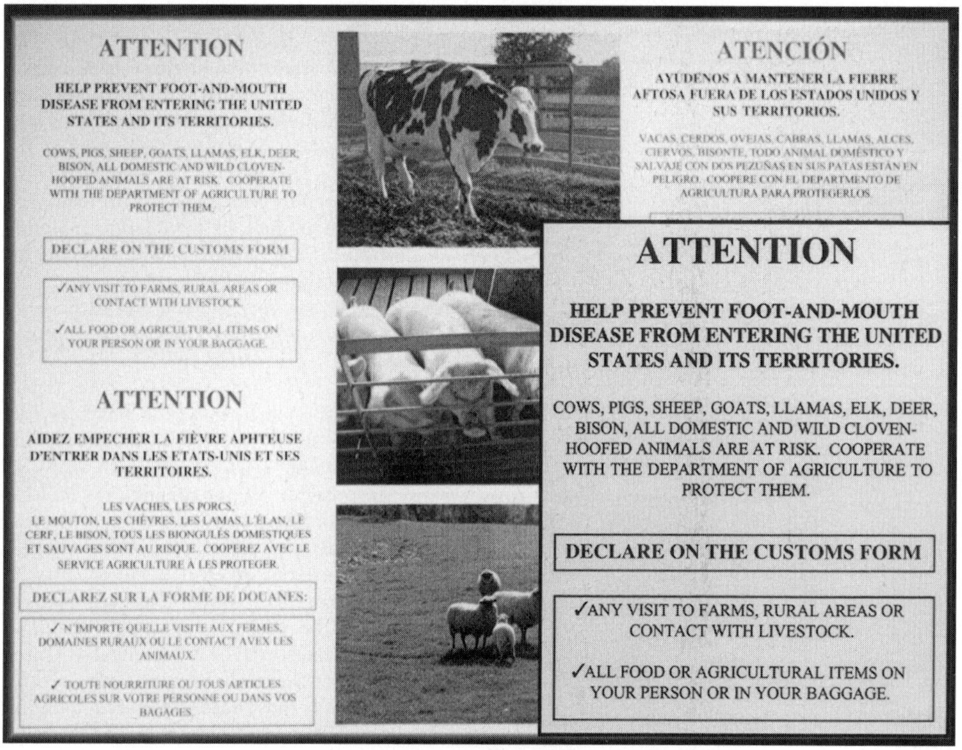

Figure 14. The United States protected itself as best it could against virus importation in general and against the foot-and-mouth virus in particular. All travellers arriving in the country received a form asking them to answer specific questions on this subject. This poster about 46 by 62 centimetres was displayed in the Arrivals hall of the Boston airport in 2001. The text is in four languages: English, French, Spanish and German. (Poster very kindly given to the author in 2002 by an employee of the American Ministry of Agriculture.)

Poliomyelitis Vaccines, Inactivated or Living Virus (1948, 1951), 1954, 1960...

Poliomyelitis (once called "infantile paralysis" or Heine-Medin disease, today most often referred to as "polio") is probably a very old disease. In fact, Egyptian bas-reliefs dating back to about 2000 BC show individuals with atrophied limbs, who could have been victims of poliomyelitis attacks. The disease was identified by the German orthopaedic specialist Jacob van Heine, in 1840. The first epidemic was described by Medin in 1887[49]. At the beginning of the 20th century, its contagious nature was discovered, followed by the discovery that the infectious agent was a virus. Later, in 1949, David Bodian and his associates at Johns Hopking University showed that this virus was of three different serotypes.

Most often, poliomyelitis symptoms resemble those of influenza; they are so light that sufferers do not realize that they have an infectious disease which could be very

49. Milbank, 1932, p. 1.

dangerous. Unfortunately, in about one case out of two hundred or less, probably depending on the age and hereditary traits of the infected subjects, the virus attacks nervous tissue and can cause irreversible paralysis. Thus, in 1949, 58 out of the 275 Esquimaux of the village of Chesterfield on the Hudson Bay in Northern Canada presented paralytic forms of a poliovirus attack, and 14 of them died[50]. This population, which had had no previous contact with this virus, had no immune protection.

Contrary to many other diseases, poliomyelitis is not directly related to hygiene improvement... In regions where the virus is present, most adults are protected against the poliomyelitis virus by repeated natural infections. If the infection occurs very early in the life of the infant, he is protected by the antibodies provided by the mother through the placenta. This is often the case in countries with limited hygiene. This maternal immunity transmitted to the child is effective, but only lasts a few months after birth. In most cases, it allows the child to face the first attack of wild virus with sufficient protection not to risk a serious case of the disease. When the disease occurs later, especially in regions with better hygiene conditions and where the wild virus is rarer, the disease can develop in an individual without immunity in its most serious form.

In the past, only palliative care was available, especially for respiratory paralysis: recourse to the unfortunate "iron lung". This device saved many patients from suffocation. Hospitals were overwhelmed with a growing number of patients; hermetically sealed rooms were built, where patients subjected to artificial respiration were cared for by personnel who could enter through a screen opening.

There are three serotypes of poliomyelitis virus, called 1, 2 and 3, that require different vaccines, one for each type; this obviously makes it more complicated to obtain protection that covers all risks of the disease. Between 1910 and 1930, a great number of assays were conducted in monkeys, using various vaccine preparations. The virus was inactivated by chemical or physical means, attenuated by dilution or neutralised with serum from convalescent or immunised animals[51]. None of these experiments appears to have been conclusive. In 1934, a vaccination attempt was carried out by Willam H. Park and Maurice Brodie of the New York City Health Department Research Laboratory, using a vaccine made from the spinal cord of a monkey infected by poliovirus inactivated by formaldehyde. This trial was reported directly to the popular press, before being published in a scientific journal. The announcement, in a press conference, of scientific news has most often (if not always) been, and still is a bad sign. Two days later, Dr. John A. Kolmer and Miss A. Rule, of the Institute of Cutaneous Research in Philadelphia, announced the successful preparation of another vaccine, also using a suspension of spinal cord from a monkey infected with poliomyelitis virus presumably attenuated by several passages on monkeys, and finally more or less inactivated by treatment with glycerine, sodium ricinoleate, phenyl mercury nitrate at 1/80,000, at 37° C, followed by ten to fourteen days of storage in the refrigerator, at between 12° C and 16° C[52]. It was a "living attenuated vaccine", with a complicated protocol that was referred to in America as a "veritable witch's brew", the product of "kitchen chemistry"[53]. Clearly, the two teams were in competition for the discovery

50. Sabin, 1955c, p. 297.
51. Milbank, 1932, p. 111.
52. Wilson, 1963, p. 47; Paul, 1971, p. 258.
53. Paul, 1971, p. 258.

of the first anti-poliomyelitis vaccine, and were both very careless in their experiments. Brodie had immunised twenty monkeys, and Kolmer forty-two. They quickly went on to man, both in rather objectionable conditions: a few children and adults, probably already immunised. Each team used every means possible to distribute its method, and 20,000 children were vaccinated[54], half with one vaccine, half with the other[55a]. This was a great number of vaccinations for a vaccine that had undergone so little testing! Results were disastrous and were quickly analysed. Leake presented his conclusions cautiously. He studied twelve cases of poliomyelitis that occurred following vaccinations, and concluded: "*Although any one of these cases may have been entirely unconnected with the vaccine, the implication of the series as the whole is clear... Paralytic poliomyelitis was not epidemic in any of these localities at the time of occurrence of these cases if these cases themselves are not included in the count.*"[55b] Twelve cases of paralytic poliomyelitis, six of them fatal, very regrettably occurred after vaccination, in areas where no case of natural poliomyelitis was observed during the same period. An immediate stop to the vaccinations was ordered. This experiment made a lasting and bitter impression.

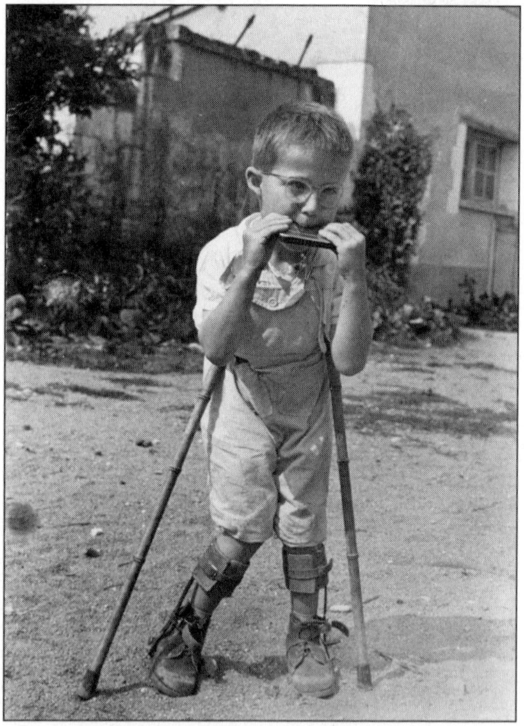

Figure 15. "*Child with harmonica*". Postcard published around 1968-1969, by the French Association of paralysed persons ("*Association des paralysés de France*"). It portrays the suffering of people living with the consequences of a poliomyelitis attack. (Author's document.)

It is disturbing to know that the methods of preparation developed by Kolmer/Rule (inactivated virus vaccine) and by Park/Brodie (in principle, attenuated living virus vaccine) have been examined by other teams, and that their conclusions were unfavourable to both vaccines. In 1936, Levaditi (*Institut Pasteur*, Paris), working with

54. Sabin, 1955c, p. 297.
55a. Paul, 1971, p. 258.
55b. Leake, 1935, p. 2152.

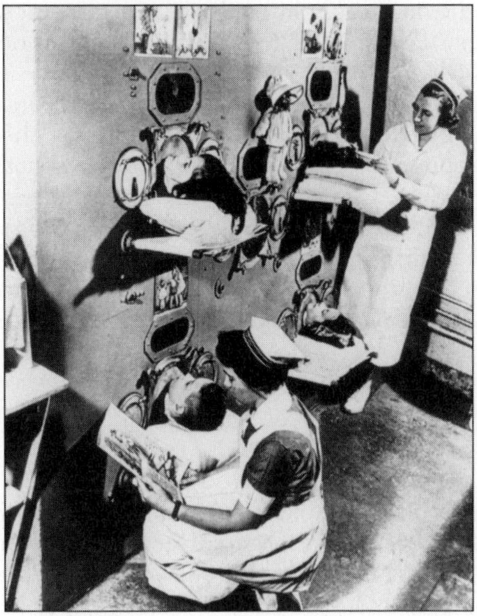

Figure 16. "A *giant iron lung providing simultaneous respiration to four paralysed children.*" In cases of respiratory paralysis, these unfortunate iron lungs made it possible to save many patients from fatal suffocation. (Photo reproduced with the kind authorisation of the WHO.)

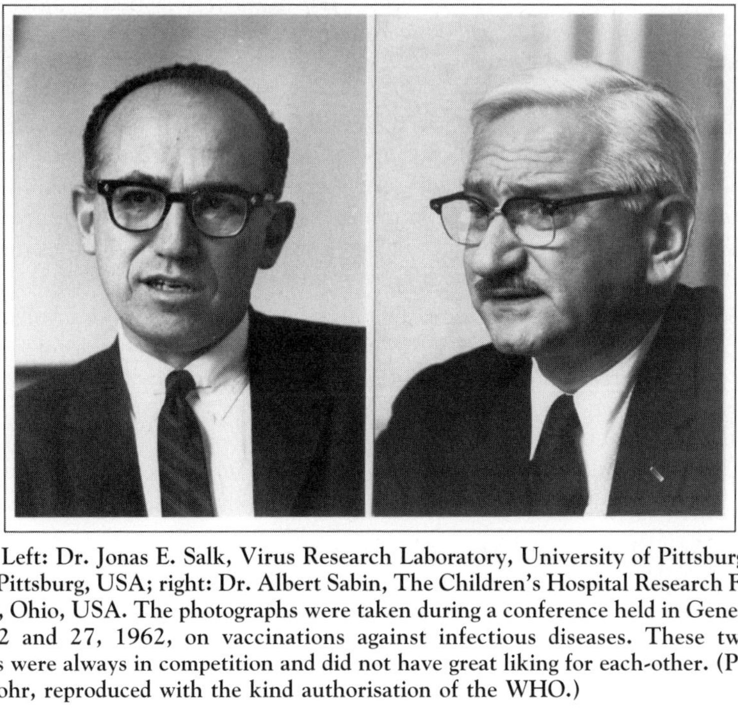

Figure 17. Left: Dr. Jonas E. Salk, Virus Research Laboratory, University of Pittsburg School of Medicine, Pittsburg, USA; right: Dr. Albert Sabin, The Children's Hospital Research Foundation, Cincinnati, Ohio, USA. The photographs were taken during a conference held in Geneva between January 22 and 27, 1962, on vaccinations against infectious diseases. These two eminent researchers were always in competition and did not have great liking for each-other. (Photographs by Jean Mohr, reproduced with the kind authorisation of the WHO.)

Kling and Haber (State Bacteriological Institute in Stockholm) published experimental results showing clearly and unequivocally that Park and Kolmer's vaccines offered no guarantee of safety[56]. Similarly, in 1936 Olitsky and Cox of the Rockefeller Institute published a text suggesting that the Kolmer and Brodie vaccines could transmit paralytic poliomyelitis to monkeys, and *a priori* offered little or no protection against this disease[57]. Parish expressed a less one-sided opinion on the value of these two vaccinations, implying that they could have been valid, that is, safe and effective[58], something the scientific literature of the period makes hard to believe. In fact, Parish, in his history of immunization, does not quote Levaditi, Kling and Haber's work. It appears as if there was no real attempt to attribute responsibility for these tragedies, but we do not know exactly when these alarming evaluations were revealed. Leake speaks in vague terms: "*Through those responsible for the production of these vaccines, through several health officers and through others, word has come to the United States Public Health Service of the development, at suggestive intervals following these injections, of cases of paralytic poliomyelitis with high fatality.*"[59]

The unfortunate actors in this drama had various destinies. William H. Park achieved great success with his work on immunisation against typhoid fever, and for promoting measures of hygiene. Most importantly, he had milk pasteurisation implemented in many American cities. According to Paul, it is not impossible that he encouraged his young colleague Brodie to try these hastily-prepared vaccines in man. In 1936, he resigned as director of the Bellevue Hospital Medical College, and from his position at the New York City Department of public Health. He died in 1939, at the age of 75. His one-page biography in the *Dictionary of American Medical Biography* does not mention the episode of his work on anti-poliomyelitis vaccination[60]. Maurice Brodie was probably the principal investigator of this disastrous experiment. Several publications on this vaccine bear his name alone[61], but others are signed by both authors[62]. From one day to the next, Brodie saw himself glorified, only to be disgraced soon afterwards. He was left without work for a time, until he found a mediocre position in Michigan. He died a short time later. Some say he ended his life. Kolmer continued a quite brilliant career. He seems not to have suffered any legal consequences following the serious effects of his ambitious and premature attempt, although five years earlier those responsible for the Lübeck accident (administration of virulent tuberculosis bacilli instead of the Calmette/Guérin attenuated bacilli) had been sentenced to prison terms in Germany. The circumstances of these two dramatic events were different, of course, as was the treatment reserved to their authors.

In truth, poliomyelitis was not as devastating a disease as cowpox or cholera. It made a strong impression on everyone's mind because it was difficult to treat, brought on long and terrible suffering, and left life-long visible sequaella with no hope of a cure, most often in children who suffered the consequences their entire lives. Sometime poliomyelitis broke out in adults. Franklin Delano Roosevelt, the future President of the United States, among others, fell victim to it. At the age of 39, while he was

56. Levaditi, 1936, p. 431.
57. Olitsky, 1936, p. 109.
58. Parish, 1965, p. 276.
59. Leake, 1935, p. 2152.
60. Galishoff, 1984, v. II, p. 578.
61. Brodie, 1934a, p. 594; Brodie, 1934b, p. 300.
62. Brodie, 1935, p. 1089.

vacationing in New Brunswick, he had a severe attack that left him paralysed in both legs. His exemplary attitude, courage and dignity in the face of his handicap earned him great prestige and motivated him to take measures against this terrible scourge. Few countries were as hard hit by polio as the United States. And yet, the epidemic affected a limited number of people in those years: 25,000 cases in 1946, 28,000 in 1948. Of course, these figures are very high, but still relatively modest compared to many other infectious diseases. The disease also had a psychological impact on a nation that had won the war at the price of great sacrifices, and which now believed itself to be out of the way of harm!

Far from the United States, which focused attention on research and trials to develop a poliomyelitis vaccine, *Paris-Match* informed its readers on French and foreign events. On pages 34 and 35 of the May 2, 1953 issue, No 216, it published a long article on a polio vaccination campaign conducted in Casablanca by Pr. Blanc of the *Institut Pasteur* of that city: "*Unquestionably, we witnessed a miracle: Casablanca has avoided a serious poliomyelitis epidemic. But the explanation is still subject to controversy... It seems that the miracle should be attributed to French science. The future will tell if the major experiment of the 1,953 vaccinations in Casablanca was the first victory of man over poliomyelitis, and another extraordinary success in the series of Pasteurian achievements, or merely a mirage on the road to failure.*"[63] Morocco was a country practically free of polio before 1947, the year when two cases occurred; then there were 38 cases in 1950, 53 in 1951, 21 in 1952. When two cases occurred in the same town, over three hundred people were inoculated with Blanc's attenuated virus, provoking "*no reaction of any sort*"[64]. But protection provided by the vaccine could not be evaluated, for there were no more cases in the local population. In February 1953, seven cases of polio observed in Casablanca within a few days provoked a strong reaction. Immediate action was taken: 5,699 children between the ages of 1 and 12 were vaccinated with a vaccine developed in 1947 by repeated passages of the poliovirus to rabbits. Trials on monkeys had established the safety of the vaccine. Moreover, the rabbit-adapted virus stayed in the system of the vaccinated person and protected him for a short time. According to the *Paris-Match* article, this was a sort of immunity by prevention, as in the case of the BCG and tuberculosis, which does not seem very likely. The article describes the first trials in man: "*On June 30, 1948, Prof. Blanc took the most moving decision of his career. He consented to a trial on the first two volunteers. On July 8, analysis showed that they were carriers of an attenuated virus. Since then, they have not presented the least symptom.*"[65] A communication made by Prof. Blanc at the Academy of Medicine on April 23, 1953 described his experiment. The type of virus was not specified, a fact which reduces the value of the work[66]. An important point to mention: it appears certain that the first (truly) attenuated living poliovirus was administered intramuscularly to man on June 30, 1948 by Blanc, before Hilary Koprowski administered his first vaccine using attenuated living virus of type 1 only to the "cotton rat" (*Sigmodon hispidus*), orally, on February 27, 1950[67]. However, Blanc did not proceed to his first oral administration until February 1, 1952[68], following the initial trials of this type conducted by Koprowski.

63. Mezerette, 1953, p. 34.
64. Blanc, 1952, p. 660.
65. Mezerette, 1953, p. 34.
66. Blanc, 1953, p. 230.
67. Blanc, 1952, p. 661.
68. Blanc, 1952, p. 661.

Kolmer had also used an attenuated virus (attenuated or inactivated, it is not clear), but one that was not clearly identified. The *Paris-Match* journalist ends his article with this surprisingly chauvinistic remark: "*Today, Science all over the world has its eyes riveted on Casablanca. In the mad race against the disease of civilisation, Pasteur's France is still ahead.*"[69] The enthusiasm generated by the development of the Salk vaccine and by its French equivalent produced by Lépine (in France), overshadowed their interesting forerunner, the "Blanc vaccine". The virulence attenuation method of the "Blanc virus" and its mode of production were not very different from those of the Sabin, Koprowski or Cox vaccines. But the "Blanc vaccine" contained only one type of poliovirus, making it similar to Koprowski's vaccines, which never contained the three serotypes. The Blanc vaccine seems to have been safe for those who received it.

In 1952, there were 57,740 serious cases of poliomyelitis in the United States. The epidemic was expanding. It is easy to understand the urgency of fighting a disease that was producing an increasing number of severe clinical cases. Its impact on Americans was greatly amplified by the widely publicised measures Franklin Roosevelt was taking against the disease. In 1938, the National Foundation for Infantile Paralysis (NFIP), or National Foundation for short, was created to provide sufficient funds to treat the sick, and to finance the work of all researchers deemed capable of developing a vaccine. A multitude of means was employed, and particularly the "March of dimes", whose objective was to collect dimes. A total of over 260,000 dollars was collected![70] This was a considerable sum, just before the Second World War. In hindsight, it seems that the money went to the right place, but the records are not very clear.

At the end of the Second Word War, at least two types of poliomyelitis virus were known. One of the first projects financed by the National Foundation was to classify numerous strains of this virus. In 1948, three types had been identified. This was a major advance. In 1949, another considerable obstacle was vanquished. John. F. Enders and his team succeeded in culturing, and thus multiplying *in vitro*, polio virus of the three types: type 1 (Brunhilde), type 2 (Lansing) and type 3 (Leon), in cells. Like all viruses, the poliovirus needed living cells to reproduce. The cells used were either those of living animals, in this case monkeys, or cells taken from an organism and cultured *in vitro* in flasks. In the latter case, the most promising cells for producing virus were those taken from monkey kidneys[71]. This was the start of frantic research work intended to obtain an effective poliomyelitis vaccine.

Competition between teams headed by Salk, Sabin, Cox and/or Koprowski and others was fierce. It is clear that all these researchers were seeking the satisfaction of serving humanity, even though they might have had some desire for glory, to varying degrees. No one can blame them for this. On February 27, 1950, Koprowski immunised a human volunteer with no specific antibodies, with his polio vaccine composed of living poliomyelitis virus type II attenuated by intracerebral passage to mice, and then to the Cotton rat. The vaccine was made from a suspension of Cotton rat brain and spinal cord. Nineteen additional vaccinations followed. The vaccinated subjects presented no clinical signs, and responded by showing specific antibody synthesis[72a]. Between

69. Mezerette, 1953, p. 34.
70. Brandt, 1978, p. 257.
71. Robbins *in* Plotkin, 1994, p. 140.
72a. Koprowski, 1952, p. 108.

1950 and 1956, about five hundred children were vaccinated by the Koprowski team. These trials gave rise to all types of commentary: "*Human experiments were already under way. In utmost secrecy the audacious Hilary Koprowski... had fed a live-virus vaccine to institutionalized children.*"[72b], in other words, mentally handicapped children. But it must be said that these children were, in fact, in great danger of being contaminated by the poliovirus. In addition, at the time this type of clinical trial was common practice, and was generally accepted.

In 1953, Salk immunised human beings with poliovirus inactivated by formaldehyde. First, children who had had polio and who were therefore already immunised against the virus, then mentally handicapped children without specific antibodies. A long and painstaking clinical trial of this vaccine was then quickly planned by a Vaccine Advisory Committee (VAT), an offshoot of the private National Foundation. But tensions soon arose between Salk and the VAT. The latter advocated a double blind trial, in which half the participants would receive a placebo (for example, salted water), while the other half would receive a dose of vaccine. Subsequently, the incidence of paralytic poliomyelitis cases in the two groups would be compared. This procedure guaranteed a well-conducted clinical trial. Salk disapproved of this type of assay, considering that each case of polio in the control group would be the responsibility of the experimenters, who had not vaccinated. Accepting this type of trial with a control group was against his personal ethical beliefs, which is understandable.

Finally, Salk's procedure for vaccine inactivation was not always considered effective by other researchers. Salk and others (especially his declared competitor Sabin) engaged in public disagreements in which one could detect serious scientific issues mixed with jealous impulses.

Producing the virus posed a considerable problem: that of passing from semi homemade laboratory methods to semi-industrial methods. The first lots of the Salk vaccine were provided by the Connaught firm of Toronto. Monkey kidney cells suspended in a culture medium were developed in mechanically stirred flasks. Enders, the famous expert on polio virus culture, provides these details: "*Suspended-cell or suspended fragment culture... Recently the suspended-cell culture has been modified to meet the need for the production of large quantities of virus to be used in the preparation of vaccines. Farrell and his associates have shown that representatives of all three antigenic types of poliomyelitis virus can be propagated in bottles containing 500 ml of medium (Mixture N° 199) plus 5 mg of minced kidney tissue. The cultures were made in Povitzky or diphteria-toxin bottles which were placed on a rocking machine at 37° C. The highest titres were obtained between the 2nd and the 7th days after the inoculation of the Mahoney (I) and MEFI (II) strains of virus... This fact is obviously of advantage in the case of materials to be used in the manufacture of vaccines.*"[72c] In practice, Farrell and his associates described roller tube cultures (4-litre bottles containing 500 ml of culture medium and 0.5g of tissue, which were rolled over by means of rollers), or rocked bottle cultures (5-litre bottles containing 500 ml of culture medium and 5g of tissue, rocked by a mechanical to-and-fro movement). An experiment was made using a 20-litre flask containing two litres of culture medium and ten grams of tissue[73]. It is obvious that these North Americans were considerably behind Frenkel and the Dutch scientists working on the foot-and-mouth virus. Connaught carried out his work

72b. Carter, 1966, p. 99; Koprowski, 1960, p. 85.
72c. Enders, 1955, p. 269.
73. Farrell, 1953, p. 273.

between 1952 and 1954[74]. This technique was abandoned when production had to be increased to satisfy the demand. Reactors, large vats made of glass and later of stainless steel, whose capacity could be increased, almost indefinitely, came into use. Frenkel's vats used to culture foot-and-mouth virus probably served as a model. It is difficult to know how to attribute individual credit for the final success achieved in this area, but it is certain that Frenkel had very innovative ideas. In 1951, he was already using 60-litre stainless steel vats[75] while Connaugh worked with 4-litre flasks. Spencer describes monkey kidney cell culture for the preparation of the Salk vaccine in 1955, at the "*Wyeth laboratories situated in Pennsylvania farm country at Marietta, on the Susquehanna River. The production line begins with monkeys which are tested to make sure they are free from disease... To prepare the soil for the 'virus farm', the kidney tissue and nutrient fluid are incubated for six days in five liter bottles...*"[76].

The director of the Mérieux firm, Charles Mérieux, for one, stated that his production of antipolio vaccine was based on the foot-and-mouth virus culture technique developed by Frenkel: "*In 1956, Sabin took me* (Charles Mérieux) *aside and said: 'With your experience with foot-and-mouth disease and with your equipment, you're the one who should produce the vaccine for France'. Of course, I was already thinking the same thing.*"[77] He also said: "*The first vaccine against foot-and-mouth disease was as rustic as Jenner's vaccine; with Fraenkel* (spelled incorrectly), *we went from the glass balloon to the steel vat, from animal production to cellular engineering. This veterinary experience was what allowed me to become a passionate actor in the history of anti-polio vaccination.*"[78] Another developmental path was opened by the Dutchman Anton van Wezel, who created large bacteria fermentors having 300 to 1,000-litres capacity, called "Bilthoven Units", that he adapted to cell culture. The authors of this description, Blume and Geesink, both Dutch, do not mention their countryman Frenkel...[79a]. The question of priority in terms of discoveries would have to be more closely investigated to allow us to draw definite conclusions. None of the American books on the development of polio vaccines, at least those referred to in this chapter, mention Frenkel or van Wezel. They attribute the credit to the Connaught firm which, of course, contributed to this success, at least in terms of culture mediums.

The public and the press, especially the *New York Times*, were enthusiastic. The atmosphere was filled with expectation. On April 25, 1954, the VAT approved the assay, and the decision was immediately ratified by the Public Health Service. But it had been an error to give *carte blanche* to a committee that was both judge and involved party, since it had contributed greatly to finance Salk's work. This work was to some extent (a great extent!) the fruit of the committee's own labour, and there was clearly conflict of interest (*a priori* moral and not financial). The vaccination campaign involved 400,000 American children, half of them enrolled in the immunised group, the other in the unvaccinated control group. Given the impatience of the public, preliminary results were published, in summary, as early as 1955. These results were favourable. The *Boston Daily Globe* published Tuesday, April 12, 1955, bore this heading in large letters, covering the entire title page: "*World hears official report: Polio 90% beaten - Salk vaccine hailed as medical victory - End of dread, crippling disease within*

74. Paul, 1971, p. 418.
75. Frenkel, 1951, p. 187.
76. Spencer, 1955, p. 19.
77. Mérieux, 1988, p. 117.
78. Mérieux, 1996, p. 8.
79a. Blume, 2000, p. 1593.

space of two years now seen a possibility - No fatalities reported among the 460,000 children given the three injections last year - The announcement was made here today with all the buildup and drama of a Hollywood production... Dr. Francis asserted that the vaccine developed by Dr. Jonas E. Salk proved 'incredibly safe' He said that the vaccination was 80 to 90 percent effective against paralytic poliomyelitis, 60 to 70 the disease caused by the most common Brunhilde type of virus, 90 per cent and more effective against the two others strains Leon and Lansing.)"[79b] In a few hours, the Salk vaccine obtained the authorisation to be marketed in the United States. The vaccine was produced in *in vitro* monkey kidney cell cultures, and inactivated with formaldehyde. This, in itself, was not new. Poliovirus culture had been developed by Enders and his colleagues, and inactivation with formaldehyde was a classic procedure. However, Salk could be thanked for making the polio vaccine. The complete results of this clinical trial, deemed excellent, were published in 1957[80]. Some people objected to the manner in which the clinical trial had been conducted, but it would have been surprising to see unanimous agreement in such a debate. What was most severely criticized was no doubt the manner in which government authorities delegated their responsibilities to the National Foundation, doing no more than approving its conclusions[81]. Salk was glorified instantly by a confident American public, proud of its power and aware of its rightful place in this achievement. He and his family were celebrated on the first page of newspapers all over the world. But the major disadvantage of this vaccine was the need to give each person several injections, to ensure good protection. Moreover, the killing of great numbers of monkeys (5,000 per month in the United States alone) was involved in the use of monkey cell cultures to be renewed for each lot of primary monkey culture, with no real possibility of viral control. Five firms were charged with the production of Salk vaccine: Parke Davis and Co; Pitman-Moore; Eli Lilly and Co; Wyeth Inc. and Cutter Laboratories. The criterion applied was to ask these pharmaceutical

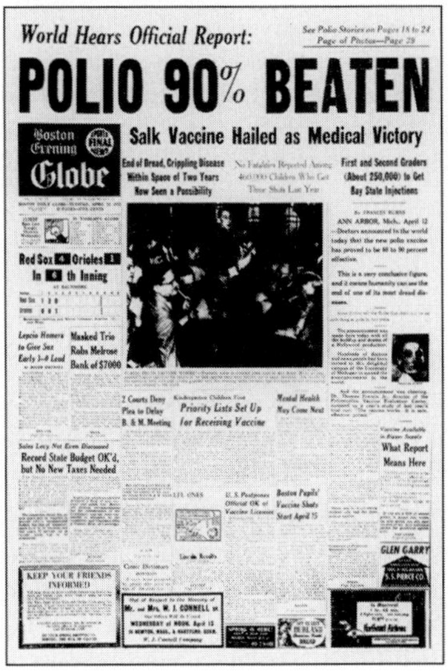
World Hears Official Report:

POLIO 90% BEATEN

Boston Evening Globe

Salk Vaccine Hailed as Medical Victory

End of Dread, Crippling Disease Within Space of Two Years Now Seen a Possibility

First and Second Graders (About 250,000) to Get Bay State Injections

Masked Trio Robs Melrose Bank of $7000

Priority Lists Set Up for Receiving Vaccine

Record State Budget OK'd, but No New Taxes Needed

What Report Means Here

Figure 18. The *Boston Daily Globe* published Tuesday, April 12, 1955, bore this heading in large letters, covering the entire title page: *"World hears official report: Polio 90% beaten - Salk vaccine hailed as medical victory - End of dread crippling disease within space of two years now seen a possibility..."*[79b]. (All rights reserved.)

79b. Boston Daily Globe, April 12, 1955, p. 1.
80. Francis, 1957.
81. Brandt, 1978, p. 257.

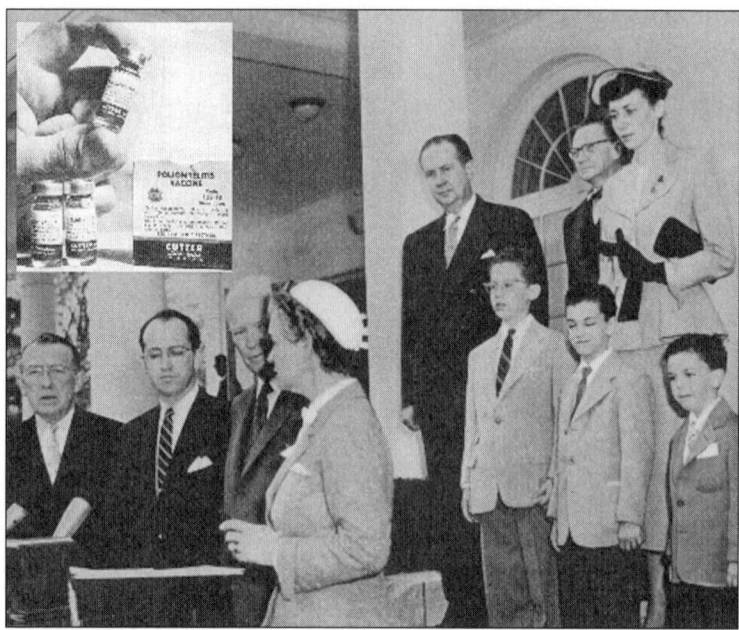

Figure 19. From glory to disaster! The 317th issue of *Paris-Match*, a wide-distribution French weekly, dated April 23-30, 1955, placed doctor Salk "*on the honour roll of humanity*", dedicating six laudatory pages to him. "*On April 22, Salk, before his whole family, is proclaimed 'Benefactor of humanity' by Ike* (Eisenhower)...". The scene shows Ike in the company of Salk and his family. But the 321rst issue of the same magazine, dated May 21-28, 1955 related the "*scandal surrounding the Salk vaccine*". These magazine issues were published three weeks apart. It was a hard fall. The Salk vaccine was not a great discovery. It was conventional for its era, but it had been awaited with great trepidation by millions of people. It won its inventor glory that was well-deserved but exaggerated by the media. Salk's only fault was to express absolute confidence in the safety of his vaccine. His aura had hidden from sight the pitfalls of industrial production of the vaccine, which, we must keep in mind, is as important a stage as all the others. In the insert, vaccine vials from the Cutter Company, containing non activated poliomyelitis virus.

companies to produce eleven consecutive lots of good vaccine, that is, whose virus has been totally inactivated but was still immunogenic, before going on to industrial production.

Salk declared that he considered himself personally responsible for the safety of his vaccine. He was taking a great risk and doing it quite lightly... because inadequately inactivated vaccine lots provoked cases of vaccinal polio, rapidly exposed by Dr. Langmuir of the Communicable Disease Center (CDC) of the Public Health Service. Poliomyelitis caused by the vaccine itself! On April 26, 1955, two weeks after the initial proclamation of the value of the Salk vaccine, five cases of paralytic polio were recorded in children immediately following vaccination. The incriminated vaccine was made by Cutter, in Berkeley, California. Despite rapid recall of the firm's products, 204 cases of paralytic polio occurred (79 among vaccinated children, 105 among members of their families and 20 among those with whom they had close contact); 11 people died[82a]. Due to ill fate, and above all to the inertia of American pharmaceutical products

82a. Paul, 1971, p. 437.

control authorities, tests made on the vaccine lots for the clinical trial conducted by the VAT were stopped at the time of passage to industrial production. These Services did not want to delay the start of the vaccination campaign, wanting it to coincide with the start of the season when the incidence of polio cases was highest. Relying on the VAT, the government had lacked foresight. But the VAT was discharged of responsibility. "*Sen. Wayne Morse, of Oregon, declared that 'The Federal Government inspects meat in the slaughter-houses more carefully than it has inspected the polio vaccine offered by the drug companies to the parents of the nation for inoculating their boys and girls against this dread disease.*"[82b] It is obvious that the Cutter Company was aware of the inactivation problems of some of its polio vaccine lots. It had already recalled nine lots out the twenty-seven it had produced, on its own initiative. Out of the twenty-seven vaccine lots produced by this firm and analysed *a posteriori*, seven contained virus that was not inactivated[83]. And yet, they respected the requirements of that period, which were not very strict[84]. The management of the Cutter firm was guilty of serious negligence at the very least. After this, an additional step was introduced to eliminate virus aggregates not completely inactivated by the means utilised. More stringent quality and safety control measures were required of all manufactures, and later a health surveillance Service was created at the Center for Disease Control (CDC), and then in numerous countries... with a more or less long latency period. This accident threw doubt in people's minds, and discredited the Salk-type inactivated anti-polio vaccine for a long time. The only positive outcome of this tragic event was the considerable reinforcement of federal government controls applying to the products of pharmaceutical companies.

"*Advances in science often meet temporary setbacks, and it is hardly surprising that the Salk polio vaccine ran into trouble. But not often in the history of medicine has a contribution started off with such a dramatic build-up, and then become so suddenly involved in discord and confusion. On April twelfth, at Ann Harbor, Michigan, 500 scientists and 100 reporters assembled for the 'unveiling of Dr. Thomas Francis' report on the vaccine's nationwide field trials of 1954. They heard the vaccine pronounced 'safe, effective and potent' and they hailed it as one of the greatest medical developments of the century. Yet, in less than a month the program had run into incredible difficulties.*"[85] These comments omit specific mention of the deaths and cases of paralysis that were the consequences of this very regrettable episode.

Canada, Denmark, Belgium, Germany and South Africa started production and use of the Salk-type vaccine in 1955. In France, the same year, Lépine developed an inactivated virus vaccine similar to Salk's[86]. But he started with virus strains that were naturally attenuated and less dangerous than Salk's in case of failed inactivation. The Danish did the same thing. The inactivating agents of the Lépine vaccine were formaldehyde and later beta-propiolactone, that also inactivated the SV40 virus "Simian virus 40", subsequently found in lots of Salk and Sabin vaccines.

During the Salk vaccine trials, several other American teams, including those headed by Albert Sabin, Hilary Koprowski and Herald Cox, attempted to develop an

82b. Spencer, 1955, p. 20.

83. Paul, 1971, p. 437.

84. Spencer, 1955, p. 19; Carter, 1966, p. 313; Paul, 1971, p. 434.

85. Spencer, 1955, p. 20.

86. Lépine, 1975, p. 67.

attenuated virus polio vaccine. In 1955, separately, several attenuated virus polio vaccinal strains could be or actually were administered orally to human beings[87]. Potentially dangerous clinical trials started cautiously on populations of a dubious nature, by today's criteria, but which were accepted at the time. These vaccines now had to be tested on a greater number of people. In fact, Americans were all immunised, children with the Salk vaccine and adults by natural immunisation; therefore, assays had to be conducted outside the United States. Sabin, who was of Russian origin and spoke Russian, received an offer from Soviet authorities to try his vaccine in that country. After satisfactory safety trials of the Sabin strain in 1956-1958, three million children were immunised with the Sabin vaccine in May and June of 1959. The results of these tests were excellent[88]. In 1959, 15.2 million Soviet citizens were already vaccinated[89]. Details concerning the side effects of these trials are few[90]; transparency was not always respected in the ex USSR.

The attenuation method for the three strains of Sabin poliovirus was a method similar to that used by Pasteur and his students, and later by followers of the Pasteurian school, and was the method that would be used for future vaccines. Vaccine development was still truly empirical at the time. For instance, the type 1 (Mahoney) vaccine was passed fourteen times in MKTC cells (Cynomolgus monkey kidney cells), then twice in monkey testicular cells, by Salk in 1941. In 1953, this strain was used again by Li and Schaffer, who passed it eleven times in MKTC cells, then several more times in kidney and skin cells. In 1954, Sabin passed this strain five times in MKTC cells, then again in the same cells, this time using the "limit dilution" method, to obtain pure strains that were tested to detect their residual neurovirulence. In 1956, Sabin re-passed one of these strains twice in MKCT cells, and Merck, Sharp & Dohm (the manufacturer), passed them in Rhesus monkey MKTC cells[91].

The clinical results that authorised the marketing of the Sabin vaccine in the United States are not very clear. It is surprising that this vaccine passed the controls of the United States and of many other countries without much difficulty. As early as 1960, the Sabin vaccine was authorised on the America market, on the strength of a report written by Horsmann after a visit to the USSR and to Eastern European countries[92]. A curious way of proceeding! Cox was able to conduct assays in Latin America, and Koprowski conducted trials on the populations of the Belgian Congo (today the Democratic Republic of Congo) and of Rwanda/Burundi. Soon, the Salk vaccine was abandoned... given that it was not being used by the medical profession. With no market and no production, it disappeared from the United States. In 1960, many countries started to produce the Sabin vaccine. A major conference organised in London by the Mérieux firm reviewed the production of this living vaccine. Sabin himself presided over this conference. Problems concerning the monkeys were discussed: their species, their origins, their transport, kidney cell culture constitution, simian virus detection, *in vitro* and *in vivo* safety assays, related controls... everything was discussed in detail[93].

87. Sabin, 1955a, p. 924; Sabin, 1955a & b, pp. 924 & 1050; Sabin, 1955c, p. 297; Koprowski, 1955a, p. 1039; Koprowski, 1955b, p. 335.
88. Smorodintsev, 1961, p. 240.
89. Chumakov, 1961, p. 228.
90. Mérieux, 1988, p. 116.
91. Sutter *in* Plotkin, 1999, p. 364; Sutter *in* Plotkin, 2004, p. 651.
92. Robbins *in* Plotkin, 1999, p. 13.
93. M.R., 1961, p. 141.

On March 15, 1963, Belgium started massive vaccinations with Sabin vaccine, in response to the recommendations of that country's Superior Council of Hygiene.

The Sabin-type oral vaccine had real advantages compared to the Salk-type vaccine. Easily administered by mouth, without syringes and therefore less expensive, better accepted by subjects to be vaccinated and by their parents, giving rapid and long-lasting immunity (usable during epidemics), containing no adjuvants, providing local immunity (that is, at the point of entry of the virus), its virus was excreted by the subject, indirectly "vaccinating" those close to him (without their knowledge): a real marvel! Unfortunately, the Sabin vaccine can cause one case of paralytic polio in 2.4 million doses administered (about one out of 750,000 vaccinated subjects at first administration, according to other sources[94], but this figure seems very pessimistic). The virus returns to its normal virulence (by reverting, that is, by mutating back) and causes poliomyelitis with all its possible disastrous consequences for the subject and/or his family[95]. In fact, only the first administration to a subject without immunity can be dangerous. The booster shots can be composed indifferently of living or inactivated virus. They are harmless in people who already have a minimum of anti-polio immunity, which might not be the case for those in close contact with the vaccinated person. The disadvantage of a living vaccine is its limited stability, requiring a costly transport chain.

Most European countries chose to use living anti-poliomyelitis vaccine. Other countries, like France and the Netherlands, never stopped using the Salk-type inactivated vaccine. In France, the Mérieux Institute manufactured Lépine vaccine and living-virus Sabin vaccine. In 1982, the recommendation in France was to use inactivated virus vaccine for routine immunisations, and attenuated living-virus vaccine in the context of epidemics. Salk-type vaccine preparation was improved by the *Rijksinstituut voor Volksgezondheid* (RIV), and later by the Mérieux Institute. The first did this by using cell-carrying bullets, and obtained a much higher production of virus by volume unit of the culture recipient; the second was able to replace primary (fresh) cell culture of monkey kidney with the continuous cell line monkey kidney production process. This eliminated the need to sacrifice hundreds of animals to produce the vaccine[96]. In time, very serious studies were conducted on the use of the Sabin vaccine, and WHO recommendations are very precise. In countries where polio has already been eradicated, it is preferable, whenever possible, to use the inactivated virus vaccine, to avoid the risk of re-introducing into the natural environment living virus that could revert (very rarely, in fact) to wild virus or recombine with closely related viruses. Since January 2000 (other sources say 1997), the U.S. Advisory Committee for Immunization Practices recommends the vaccination of American children not yet vaccinated with an inactivated virus vaccine. It was only in the year 2000 that this type of vaccine was administered again in France and Belgium, as a first vaccine... One case of vaccinal poliomyelitis was reported in Belgium. A 26-year old mother contracted acute anterior poliomyelitis after her baby received the polio vaccine. This is a case of contact polio of vaccinal origin. The child had been vaccinated with living Sabin virus. This accident provoked severe paralysis in all four limbs, and sequelar paraplegia[97]. Was it necessary to take such a risk in 1989?

94. Greensfelder, 2000, p. 1867.
95. Editorial, 2001, p. 131.
96. Blume, 2000, p. 1593.
97. Derenne, 1989, p. 358.

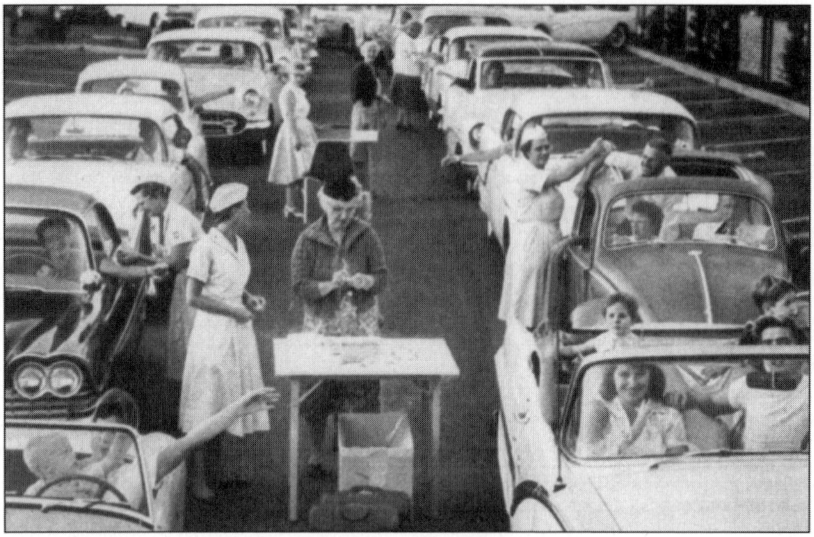

Figure 20. "*Anti-polio auto vaccination in the family car, in Alabama.*" This anti-poliomyelitis vaccination campaign was carried out with Sabin-type attenuated living vaccine. Fear of polio and its sequels contributed greatly to motivating Americans to have themselves vaccinated. The effects were rapid and conclusive. Poliomyelitis disappeared from that country even though no noticeable hygiene improvements can be invoked in such a short period of time. (DR/*Science et Vie*, 549, June 1963.)

The Lépine injectable inactivated-virus vaccine was developed in 1955. In 1957, 4,109 cases of polio were recorded in France. Vaccination became compulsory in 1964. In 1969, 68 cases of poliomyelitis were reported, twenty-six cases in 1978, 2 in 1989 and one imported case (the patient having been contaminated outside France) in 1995. Since 1990, no cases of polio have been contracted in France. But the disease still exists elsewhere in the world. It is possible to contract it in infected countries, and bring it back. Therefore, the populations of countries without polio virus must be protected until the virus is totally eradicated in the whole world.

The history of polio vaccines, made from inactivated virus or conferred attenuated virulence, has not been without its storms. The first major problem arose when Sweet and Hilleman of the Merck Institute for Therapeutic Research discovered a virus contaminating the cell cultures (of Asian monkeys) used to produce the viruses for many lots of vaccine. This virus, "Simian Virus 40" (SV40) can cause tumours in hamsters. It can resist doses of formaldehyde high enough to inactivate poliovirus (Salk vaccine), or can contaminate living vaccine lots (Sabin vaccine) prepared from primary kidney cell cultures of certain monkeys. These vaccines could be dangerous. SV40 was totally eliminated from vaccines in 1963. The Lépine vaccine, produced from cell cultures originating in African monkeys (not contaminated by the SV40 virus), did not encounter this problem. Those who did have this problem were the persons vaccinated with living vaccines contaminated by SV40 virus, between 1955 and 1962. Subsequently, careful surveys showed that the American population inoculated with lots of polio vaccine contaminated by the SV40 virus did not present a detectable rise in cancer incidence. However, the SV40 virus was found in a very few brain tumors,

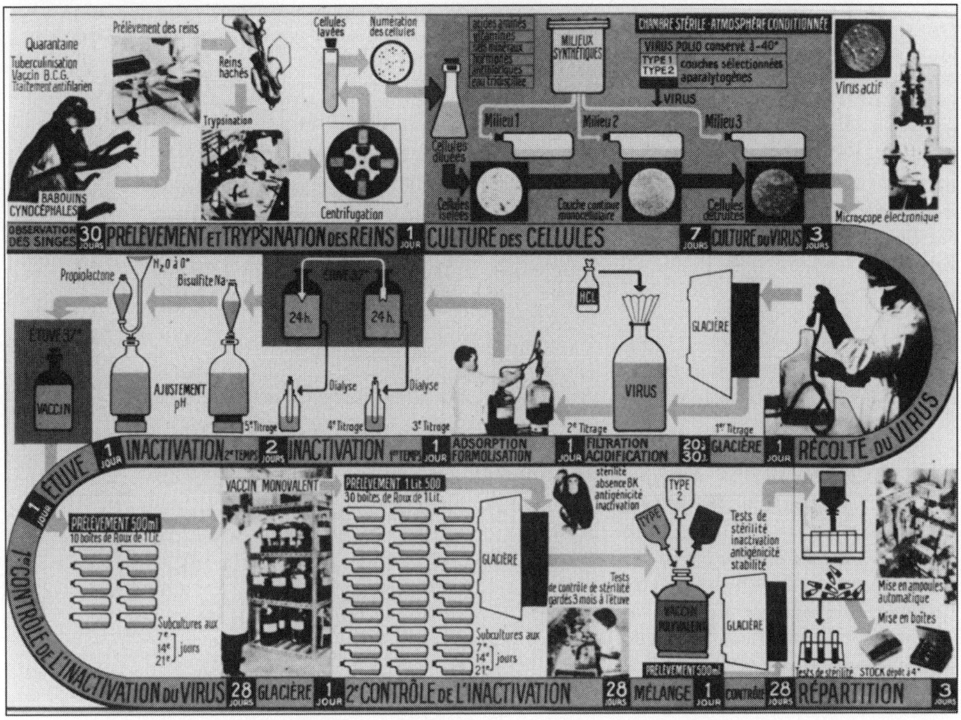

Figure 21. Hachette's *L'Encyclopédie par l'image,* dated 1963, in its "Vaccines and sera" issue, by M. Viette, A. Vallée, Y. Chabert, laboratory heads at the *Institut Pasteur,* shows the stages of anti-poliomyelitis vaccine preparation. The Lépine vaccine was made from strains of poliovirus selected for their non pathogenic effect in humans. The virus was inactivated using formaldehyde and beta-propiolactone. The vaccine was tested twice on cell culture, then for microbial sterility, and finally for immunogenic value. The three types of virus were produced separately, before being mixed and marketed. Production was carried out rigorously but, from today's perspective, the use of Roux bottles seems rather archaic.

osteosarcomas, mesotheliomas and non-Hodgkin lymphomas[98]. What significance should be attributed to these rare positive samples? No statistical study could demonstrate a cause- and -effect relation based on such a low prevalence in a population. What must be weighed in the balance is the possible eradication of poliomyelitis, a serious and relatively common disease, against very rare cases of cancer, very regrettable, of course, if caused by the SV40 virus. Recently, a study presenting serious arguments sheds very strong doubt on the presence of the SV40 genome in human mesotheliomas[99]. When the SV40 was discovered, it was carefully studied and certain portions of its genome were used in very numerous laboratory genetic constructions. During that process, SV40 contamination was found in all types of samples.

The only positive aspect of this troublesome episode was increased control of vaccine production. The first required step was to find less dangerous cells than those of primary cultures. Unfortunately, continuous cell lines were practically all "transformed",

98. Ferber, 2002, p. 1012.
99. Lopez-Rios, 2004, p. 1157.

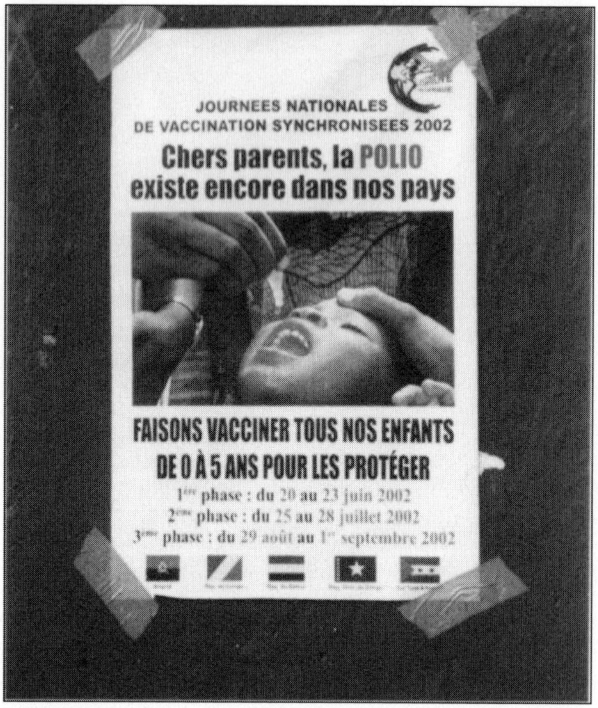

Figure 22. UNICEF and the WHO launched an international poliomyelitis eradication campaign, with very good results (drastic reduction of cases of polio followed by paralysis). But the campaign has not yet achieved the complete elimination of the disease for various reasons. A poster seen in a street of Bukavu, Democratic Republic of Congo, in 2002, reads: "*National days of synchronised vaccination 2002. Dear parents, POLIO still exists in our countries, let us vaccinate all our children between 0 and 5 years, to protect them.*" Three phases were planned: 1rst phase: from the 20th to the 23rd of June 2002; 2nd phase: July 25 to July 28, 2002; 3rd phase: August 29 to September 1, 2002. The countries concerned are Angola, the Republic of Congo, the Republic of Gabon, the Democratic Republic of Congo, and Sao Tomé and Principe. (Author's photograph.)

that is, taken from cancer cells. Between 1960 and 1963, Hayflick of the Wistar Institute of Philadelphia (USA) developed a cell line from human diploid embryonic cells ("WI - 38") that survived about fifty resowings. This gave rise to heated controversy between the NIH Cell Culture Committee of the National Institute of Health of the United States, and Hayflick, and to disagreement with the cell culture committee of the WHO's permanent section of microbiological standardisation. European countries accepted without delay the WI-38 cells (diploid lines of non continuous human fibroblast) for the production of viruses to be used in vaccine manufacturing. The discovery of the presence of SV40 virus in Salk and Sabin vaccines put an end to this dispute. The use, under very strict restrictive conditions, of continuous cell lines was accepted on condition that primary cells (obtained directly from human or animal tissue) be replaced by non contaminated cells[100]. Starting in 1982, the continuous cell line "VERO" Vervet monkey heteroploid, was used in a number of countries.

Another important controversy concerned the assays of a vaccine prepared by Hilary Koprowski for the Lederlee firm, and later at the Wistar Institute. These living vaccine preparations were tested, on a small scale, in their country of origin, and then in Northern Ireland, in Switzerland and in Sweden, where they were not marketed. Dick and his associates in Belfast, in particular, revealed the presence of reversion, that is, the return to virulence of the two Koprowski strains: type I SM and type II TN, excreted in the stool of those vaccinated with these preparations. These two strains, after passages to humans, proved to be capable of inducing paralytic forms of poliomyelitis in

100. Hilleman, 1995, p. 1.

monkeys inoculated with them. These results were published in January 1957[101]. They were strongly contested by Koprowski. Her vaccinations in the Belgian Congo/Rwanda-Burundi, on a very large scale, took place in 1957 and are still subject to controversy.

Several new and very useful vaccines were placed on the market and made it possible to avoid serious diseases and their possible sequelae.

Living vaccines

Living viral vaccines are still used. The first Pasteurian vaccines, against chicken cholera or ruminant anthrax, were "living" vaccines with attenuated virulence. The discovery by Smith and Salmon of "killed" or "inactivated" vaccines was a revelation and a gigantic advance. Chemical vaccines were undeniably less dangerous and were promising for the future. Unfortunately, the immunity they induced was much less solid and long-lasting than that conferred by living vaccines. This is why the development of living vaccines had and still has considerable importance. But their use requires a complete cold chain, a fact that constitutes a major difficulty for their distribution in numerous countries.

At the end of the 1950s, Samuel Katz, John F. Enders and their associates developed the Edmonston strain of the measles virus by cultivating it on human embryonic cells, and on chick cells. Tried on monkeys and then on humans, this strain provided a good measles vaccine, but a variable proportion of vaccinated children had quite severe side effects[102]. A serovaccination composed of this vaccine and of specific antiserum was employed successfully. The strain was further attenuated by Anton Schwartz[103] and Maurice Hilleman[104], and their colleagues. Using the loss of virulence of this strain in monkeys made it possible to obtain an excellent vaccine. Because the measles virus is specific to man, we can hope to eradicate measles in the near future.

The mumps virus was cultivated by R.H. Weller and Enders in 1948, on fragments of chick embryos and in embryonated eggs. The virus was then inactivated with ether or with UV rays. Several thousand persons were vaccinated successfully. Hilleman attenuated the Jeryl Lynn strain of mumps virus cultivated on embryonated eggs, and obtained authorisation for its marketing in 1967. It is the only strain accepted for vaccination in the United States and in Europe, although other promising lines have been developed.

The rubella virus was attenuated by successive passages in culture and, in 1970, several strains were developed. The Wistar-RA 27/3 strain, developed on human fibroblasts by Stanley Plotkin, is used the world over. It was isolated from a contaminated human foetus, and had eight passages on WI-38 cells at 37° C, and additional passages at 30° C. The RA 27/3 vaccinal strain was subjected to a few more passages at low temperature, on the same cells. The rapid attenuation of the virus could be due to the adaptation of the virus to low temperature, and its high immunogenicity could be due to the low number of passages that were necessary[105].

101. Dane, 1957, p. 59; Dick, 1957, p. 65.
102. Katz, 1960, p. 180.
103. Schwarz, 1962, p. 386.
104. Hilleman, 1968, p. 587.
105. Plotkin, 1969, p. 178.

The combination of these three vaccines: measles-mumps-rubella produces immune responses against these three viruses that are equal to those obtained by vaccines administered separately[106], and is used in the whole world.

The chickenpox vaccine (Oka attenuated living strain), developed by Michiaki Takahashi in the 1970s[107], is very effective in healthy subjects. But it can produce serious side effects in immunodeficient subjects[108]. Surveillance of this vaccine since 1995 in the United States confirms that it is very well tolerated: out of about 40 million vaccinated children in that country, five cases of serious side effects were reported. In some countries, it could be appropriate to administer the varicella vaccine routinely to healthy children and, with great caution, to other children[109]. But there is still disagreement concerning universal vaccination in children, given the cost-benefit ratio represented above all by the economics of parental work stoppages, a vaccination protocol requiring two injections, and the uncertainty concerning shingles in the population later. The United States introduced the vaccine in 1995. It is not certain that this vaccine should be recommended for the entire population[110]. In Europe, only Germany opted for this procedure. The rest of Europe limits itself to targeted vaccination.

An example shows the complexity of certain situations, for instance that involving the new rotavirus vaccines. These viruses are the cause of 400,000 to 600,000 yearly deaths in children, due to diarrhoea, in developing countries, and of numerous days of hospitalisation of children in developed countries. Wyeth developed a vaccine that was introduced on the market in August 1998, in the United States and in Finland. This vaccine had 49% to 68% effectiveness in treating infantile diarrhea, and 69% to 91% effectiveness in preventing severe diarrhoea. Shortly after this new vaccine was introduced on the market, medical vigilance networks reported cases of intestinal invagination occurring soon after inoculation with this vaccine, in a percentage of cases superior to about 1 case for 10,000 vaccinations (1 for 2,500, according to another source). The use of this vaccine was suspended by American health control authorities, before being rapidly taken off the market by the manufacturer. About one quarter of children with his serious affection can die of it; this figure represents an unacceptable risk in developed countries for a disease of this seriousness. But the removal of the vaccine from the market had consequences for developing countries, where it could have saved hundreds of thousands of children. In their case, the risk would have been clearly inferior to the benefit. Applying the same criteria in developed (rich) countries and in developing (poor) countries is certainly not ethical. But what company, what organisation would dare to introduce into a developing country a vaccine taken off the market in a rich country[111]? This problem could only possibly be solved by the clear will of international agencies like the WHO or UNICEF. Fortunately, two new vaccines against this gastroenteritis, developed using methods different from those of Wyeth, respectively by Richard Ward and David Berstein of the Cincinatti Children's Hospital (Glaxo Smith Kline Biologicals), and Fred Clark, Paul Offit and Stanley Plotkin in the latter's laboratory at the Philadelphia Children's Hospital (Merck); after

106. Plotkin, 2004, p. 707.
107. Takahashi, 1974, p. 1288.
108. Levin, 2003, p. 954; Levy, 2003, p. 948.
109. Gershon, 2003, p. 945.
110. Bégué, 2002, p. 21.
111. Weijer, 2000, p. 525.

lengthy clinical trials on over 60,000 children[112], authorisation for marketing was obtained in 2006. These vaccines have not yet been made part of routine compulsory vaccinations in France.

Subunit Vaccines

Today, new technologies make it possible to develop vaccines composed only of purified portions of microbial bodies. This is the case for whopping cough vaccine, vaccine against diseases caused by the respiratory syncytial virus, and hepatitis B vaccine.

The first description of whopping cough was probably that made by Guillaume de Baillou when he observed the disease in Paris, in 1578. The disease was listed among causes of mortality in London in 1701. Its pathogenic agent, *Bordetella pertussis*, was discovered by Jules Bordet and Oscar Gengou in 1906. In 1994, the number of whopping cough cases world-wide was estimated at 40 million; the disease had caused 5 million cases of pneumonia, 360,000 deaths and 50,000 serious and permanent nervous-system diseases.

Very quickly, attempts were made to vaccinate against this disease with killed bacteria. "*Whopping cough vaccination, by injection of dead bacteria, has given very encouraging results. In Brussels, the bacilli cultured in Roux bottles are not heated; they are sterilised by dilution in physiologic phenic-acid serum at 0.5 p. 100. The culture medium is agar in which a tenth of its volume of rabbit serum is incorporated. In 1923, Madsen and his associates carried out a very large number of vaccinations in the Faroe Islands; they observed that this method, which does not always prevent the onset of the disease, nevertheless makes it much more benign; mortality is considerably reduced.*"[113] Bordet specifies, later in his book, that the vaccine must be toxin-free, because toxin would produce a local lesion. Other studies have been conducted with vaccines prepared somewhat differently.

The whole-cell anti-pertussis vaccine (that is, containing the whole bacterium) sometimes produced unfortunate adverse effects that were the subject of lengthy discussions[114]. In 1975, in Japan, two children died after being inoculated with this vaccine. The press, and then the population, reacted very strongly and the Japanese Minister of Health suspended the use of the vaccine. Unfortunately, whopping cough cases increased in that country from 206 cases reported in 1971, to 13,105 cases in 1979. A new version of whopping cough vaccine was needed; it was offered by Sato and his associates in 1984. The purification of *Bordetella pertussis* components made it possible to obtain a so-called acellular vaccine, much less reactogenic for vaccinated subjects than the whole-cell vaccine[115]. Similar vaccines are now distributed in many countries, with good results.

Diseases caused by respiratory syncytial virus are highly dreaded. They occur in very young children, provoking respiratory problems: bronchiolitis, bronchopneumonia... The pathogenic agent is a virus. The serious consequences of this disease motivated the search for a means of protecting children. One vaccine candidate was produced from purified virus grown in cell cultures, inactivated by formaldehyde. This vaccine was tested for safety in adult volunteers. Then, it was inoculated intramuscularly to the residents of a children's asylum called Junior Village. During a respiratory syncytial epidemic that

112. Roberts, 2004, p. 890.
113. Bordet, 1939, p. 110.
114. Edwards *in* Plotkin, 2004, p. 492.
115. Sato, 1984, p. 122.

broke out shortly afterwards, the inoculated subjects proved not to be protect at all, and worse still, they were more seriously affected than the unvaccinated children. *A priori*, the circulating anti-virus antibodies against the respiratory syncytial virus were responsible for this paradoxical immunopathologic effect[116]. Of course, these trials were discontinued. What was needed was to induce a different immune response: a cellular response. Several subunit vaccine candidates are under study or at the clinical trial phase.

The hepatitis B vaccine, composed only of the external protein capsule of the virus, is also a subunit vaccine.

"Epidemic jaundice" has a very long history. This disease was first described in medical texts by Hippocrates over 2,000 years ago! It probably included hepatitis B. But it was not until the 1940s that real progress was achieved in understanding this affection. Hepatitis A, also called infectious hepatitis, transmitted by orofecal contamination and having a short, two to six-week incubation period, was distinguished from hepatitis B, transmitted by the inoculation of infected serum, and having a long, six weeks to six months incubation period followed by a disease whose clinical symptoms can vary from serious to benign, or be altogether absent. Other types of viral hepatitis exist and are designated by the letters C,D,E...

The clinical phase of hepatitis B begins with the relatively classic symptoms of all infectious diseases, such as fever, headache, muscle pains, weakness... the virus multiplies in the hepatic cells, which are killed in great numbers. Urine becomes dark and the patient soon becomes jaundiced, remaining in this condition for several days, even several weeks. The patient's state slowly improves, the symptoms disappear and complete recovery follows. Rarely (in less than one percent of cases), fulminant hepatitis develops, due to liver necrosis. In these cases, the disease causes confusion, bleeding, coma and finally death. Sometimes, chronic hepatitis can occur, with very serious consequences: cirrhosis of the liver or even liver cancer. The hepatitis B virus is well known. It is a double-stranded DNA virus, and is enveloppped, meaning that it is composed of several layers containing a great number of antigens. It reproduces in hepatocytes that are killed not by the virus itself but by its host. The latter, through a cytotoxic immune response, kills all infected cells, stopping the propagation of the virus by sacrificing its own infected cells[117].

One of the particular characteristics of hepatitis B is the abundance of viral particles in the blood of the infected person. These particles are easy to detect; this constituted the first method of diagnosis ("Australia antigen" research). But interestingly, these viral particles are produced very quickly. Most of them are incomplete and only consist of the outer envelope of the virus. They do not contain the nucleic acids (DNA) that allow the virus to multiply. These viral particles can be purified in the blood of patients with hepatitis B. They can induce an immune response, as it has been shown first in chimpanzees and later in man by Philippe Maupas, veterinarian, physician and pharmacist from the University of Tours (France)[118].

These purified particles protect against an attack of the normal hepatitis B virus. The first available vaccine against this virus was obtained using this method. This vaccine, called plasma-derived, is still available. However, ensuring its safety requires more testing than is needed for the vaccine obtained by genetic engineering.

116. Kapikian, 1969, p. 405.
117. Denis, 2004, p. 155.
118. Maupas, 1976, p. 1367.

The success of the first vaccine against hepatitis B was followed by a great technological advance. It became possible to purify the nucleic acid coding for the proteins in the hepatitis B virus envelope, and then artificially produce empty envelopes. In order to do so, the small part of the genetic material that codes the viral envelope is introduced in an expression system that, by reproducing, will produce at the same time its own proteins and viral cells. It must be pointed out that proteins of the hepatitis B viral envelope, once produced, cluster together and spontaneously take the form they naturally have, that of small spherical bodies. These empty envelopes are then cleared of the cellular debris of the expression system. The vaccine requires several injections followed by one or several booster shots. Good immunity is achieved in most vaccinated individuals.

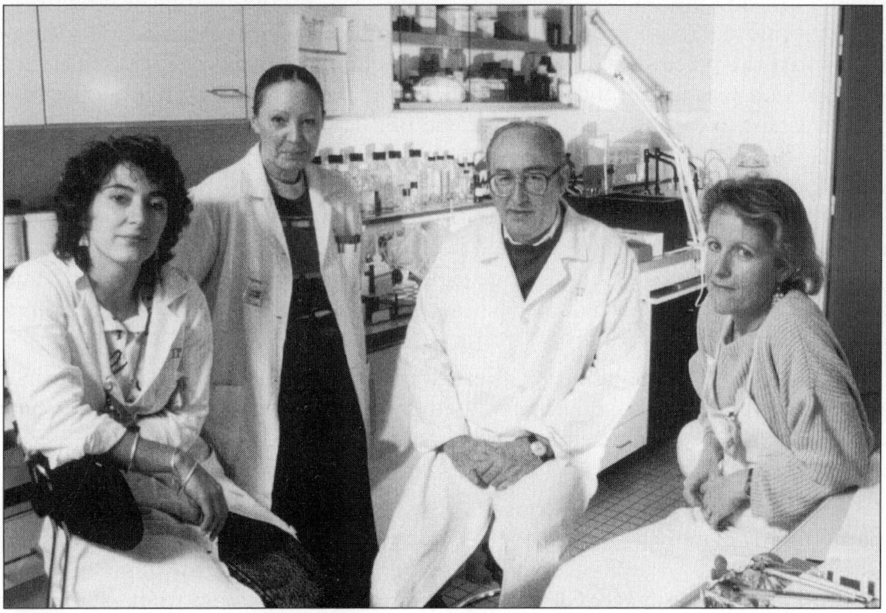

Figure 23. Pierre Tiollais and his team in his *Institut Pasteur* laboratory, at the time of his studies on hepatitis B.

The first recombinant hepatitis B vaccine was prepared by Pierre Tiollais and his colleagues at the *Institut Pasteur*, in 1985, using CHO cells (cells of Chinese hamster ovaries)[119].

Vaccine production by genetic engineering presents many advantages. The first advantage is production unrelated to the material generating the pathogenic agent itself, which eliminates all risk of vaccine-related infection except those due to the system of production: vero-cells, yeast... In this case (for example hepatitis B vaccine), the production system is *in vitro* and is eliminated at the latest at the end of antigen production. The second is certainly the availability of a source of antigens not dependent on patients or on the infectious agents. Biotechnology makes it possible to supply almost unlimited quantities of antigen and thus of vaccine.

119. Tiollais, 1985, p. 1333.

A third advantage of genetic engineering is the possibility of introducing, in the genome of organisms called "vectors" such as living attenuated vaccines (vaccinia, for example), strands of ribonucleic or deoxyribonucleic acid which produce, *in situ*, in the organism to be immunized, the antigen or antigens of another organism (rabies, for instance). The rabies vaccine is the first example of this type of vaccine. The system of production is *in vivo*, in the patient, and must respect all safety standards.

No longer present in Western Europe since the end of the 19th century, rabies originating in Poland reappeared in 1968. Ever since then it has been spreading, and had reached the outskirts of Paris in the 1990s[120].

Vaccinating foxes with a living vaccine administered orally offered a possible solution. Capturing a fox, vaccinating it and releasing it again was tried in Switzerland and in Germany. But only for a time, of course, since it was a monumental task reminiscent of Sisyphus and his rock, and results were negligible. In 1976, Baer and Winkler had demonstrated the possibility of vaccinating foxes orally with living virus. The vaccine was placed in a plastic bag hidden in bait. When the fox bit into it, the bag opened and the vaccine came into contact with the oral mucosa; this immunized the fox for at least a year. Various vaccines were tried by the countries where the problem was present: Germany, Austria, Belgium, France, Luxembourg and Switzerland. One vaccine was a recombinant vaccine developed by the Transgene company in Strasbourg, the Wistar Institute of Philadelphia and the Rhône-Mérieux Group (a division of the present Merial Company)[121]. This is in fact Jenner's vaccine (without the thymidine kinase gene, making it an attenuated-virulence vector) into which a gene (coding the G glycoprotein of the rabies virus) was inserted.

This recombinant vaccine was used after extensive innocuity trials conducted in Belgium, France and Switzerland. Starting in 1988, bait containing the vaccine was dropped over the areas concerned by helicopter. As soon as 1990, rabies regressed thanks to the combined efforts of these countries[122].

The Brussels newspaper *Le Soir* front-page heading on May 22, 2001 read: "Rabies is eradicated" in Belgium[123]. Credit for this can be attributed to a number of people, particularly Pr. Paul-Pierre Pastoret of the Faculty of Veterinary Medicine of the University of Liège, who supervised the implementation of the first trials of the "rabies vaccine" on restricted military grounds.

Numerous vectors, viral or bacterial, have been developed: pox vaccine and other viral vaccines like those using bird viruses, adenovirus, poliomyelitis virus, salmonella, BCG and even the anthrax bacillus... Of course, all these vectors have to be selected and demonstrated to be of low virulence for the species that may be concerned, directly or indirectly, by these vaccinations. This strategy is promising. Several vaccines using second-generation recombinant virus are presently being developed or at the trial stage. A real revolution is in progress. It is very likely that even more effective vaccines with less side effects will be developed against infectious agents. It is to be hoped that they will provide solutions for combatting diseases still difficult to eliminate such as AIDS or the major parasitic diseases like malaria, trypanosomiasis or schistosomiasis...

120. Aubert, 2003, p. 9.
121. Kieny, 1984, p. 163; Wiktor, 1984, p. 7194.
122. Blancou, 1986, p. 373; Brochier, 1991, p. 320; Aubert, 2003, p. 5.
123. Bodeux, 2001, p. 1.

11
Yellow Fever Vaccine

"Most terrifying has been the devastation of yellow fever in its erratic wanderings up and down our coast (USA) *from 1647 until the early part of the present century."*
Paul F. Clark, 1961[1].

The present chapter on yellow fever is relatively detailed, in order to illustrate the interdependence of research on vaccines, and the ethical problems related to their use. Each new development of vaccines is based not only on the characteristics of the disease under study, but also on the state of knowledge available at the time in vaccinology, immunology, microbiology and especially technology... Some references to the work of contemporary researchers who proposed potential new technology of vaccines are given, in order to illustrate this entanglement clearly. The history of vaccinations includes, of course, animal as well as human vaccines. To exclude one or the other would be senseless, since all research, no matter how original, builds on previous research. In sciences, at least in modern sciences, there is always a past reference!

This chapter examines the history of yellow fever vaccination up to the 1960s, that is, to the development of the 17D vaccine and its trials. An excellent review of the present status of the yellow fever vaccine is available in the literature[2].

Yellow fever is "*an acute, specific, infectious, but non-contagious disease, characterized by fever occurring in one, but generally in two, paroxysms; the first of these is of short duration and followed by a brief remission or intermission which is succeeded in turn by secondary fever, accompanied by albuminuria, jaundice, passive haemorrhages from the mucous membranes, and, in severe cases, black vomit*".[3] In time, the aetiology became known. "*Yellow fever is a severe infection which is transmitted from man to man by mosquitoes. The virus is inoculated with the puncture of a mosquito proboscis and spreads in the blood throughout the body. The favourite site for its multiplication is the liver, and the damage produced here is responsible for the jaundice, which gives the name yellow fever to the disease.*"[4]

Yellow fever or Yellow Jack*, Bronze John, Bullam fever, the saffron scourge... is one of the diseases most abundantly described in the literature, because the epidemics were devastating and terrifying. For centuries, this disease, with its unknown origin and means of transmission, for which there was no known treatment and which caused very high morbidity and mortality, remained a constant source of dread for new settlers in endemic areas: Africa, South America and the West Indies. Yellow fever is essentially a tropical disease, which can, in rare circumstances, extend into temperate climates. This disease has caused some disasters that became famous in infectiology; it is still firmly rooted in Africa and parts of America, where monkeys and mosquitoes serve

---

* The yellow quarantine flag on ships.

1. Clark, 1961, p. 46.
2. Monath, 1996, p. 157; Monath, 1996, p. 95; Monath, 2008, p. 959; Monath, 2010, p. 159.
3. Carroll *in* Osler, 1907, p. 336.
4. Burnet, 1959, p. 105.

as a reservoir for it[5a]. Yellow fever is still a serious public health problem, because although it is presently controlled by hygiene and vaccination, it can re-emerge if this health monitoring were to cease.

Many contagious diseases were readily considered infectious even when their pathogenic agent was totally unknown. Smallpox and measles are good examples. They gave rise to the concept of a living, microscopic pathogenic agent that can pass from one organism to another. This concept led to the segregation of patients through isolation, quarantine, etc. However, making this identification was not always easy. For instance, yellow fever was long a subject of confrontation between contagionists and their opponents, the anticontagionists or localists, who attributed "*disease entirely to conditions of the patient or the physical locality of his life or that persons might be attacked because of fear or grief*" [5b]. One of the first localists, perhaps the very first, was a French military surgeon named Devèze (1753-1829), who published a well-documented book[6] attempting to show the non contagious nature of yellow fever. Devèze had spent 15 years in Cap Français (present-day Cap Haïtien), in Haiti and then in Philadelphia during the 1793 yellow fever epidemic which was particularly devastating for the population of that city, causing 4,041 deaths out of a population of 40,000[7]. His observations were accurate. He insisted repeatedly on the spread of the epidemic in dirty, humid neighbourhoods, and on the absence of the disease in the areas on high ground where the hospital was located. His conclusions are in agreement with what we know today about conditions of transmission, facts that were unknown at the time.

Yellow fever was particularly well-known and feared in the United States, where it appeared 35 times between 1702 and 1880, striking almost every year between 1800 and 1879[8]: in Charleston and Philadelphia as early as 1693, then in all the ports of New England up to New Hampshire, and inland as far as Mobile, Memphis, Natchez, St. Francis Ville, Baton Rouge... In 1853, yellow fever caused 7,970 deaths in New Orleans, and 3,093 in 1867, Clark estimates that between 1793 and 1900 there were 500,000 deaths due to yellow fever in the United States[9]. South America was also affected: in Rio, there were 4,160 fatalities in 1850, 1,943 in 1852, and 1,397 in 1886. In Havana, around 1900, the annual death rate fluctuated between 500 and 1,600 deaths.

Africa was the continent most affected by yellow fever epidemics. But Europe was also host to the disease. Some epidemics caused great devastation: the one in Barcelona in 1821 affected 80,000 people and killed about 20,000. In Lisbon, in 1857, over 6,000 people died in a few weeks. Many disease foci were observed: Saint-Nazaire* in 1861 (26 fatalities); Swansea, South Wales in 1865 (17 fatalities), etc.[10]

Sawyer provides a list of yellow fever epidemics between 1905 and 1932. He concludes: "*Yellow fever is firmly entrenched in West Africa and Northern Brazil, and is probably*

---

* It was brought by the ship *L'Anne-Marie* with a cargo of sugar from Havana (Larousse du XIXe siècle, 2e suppl., 1888, p. 1248).

5a. Balfour, 1914, p. 1176.

5b. Newsholme, 1927, p. 80.

6. Devèze, 1820.

7. Osler, 1938, p. 314.

8. Winslow, 1943, p. 352.

9. Clark, 1961, p. 46.

10. Anonymous, 1902b, t. VIII, p. 6418; Manson, 1904, p. 170; Léger, 1928, p. 970; Kazeeff, 1934, p. 421; Joyeuz, 1944, p. 592; Freestone *in* Plotkin, 1994, p. 741.

endemic in the interior of Colombia. Cities long free from yellow fever may yet be revisited by disastrous epidemics if the extensive breeding of stegomyia mosquitoes is permitted."[11]

The greatest catastrophies were often due to the migrations of populations without immunity into high risk areas, before any exact knowledge on the mode of transmission of the disease: armies waging war (the Spanish-American War, although many deaths were also caused by typhoid fever) or displacement of workers during the first Panama Canal project conducted by the French. In 1909, Gorgas wrote: "*Yellow fever has caused more disaster to military expeditions going to these tropics* (American tropics) *than had all the other tropical diseases put together, and it has been equally fatal to non-immune individuals in civilian life.*"[12]

Several countries took a special interest in the yellow fever problem: the United States and Brazil, where epidemics had broken out, as well as Great Britain and France, nations possessing many colonies in Africa. Directly or indirectly, by means of foundations, they organised a number of expeditions, some very well known, others much less, to study yellow fever on location, in infected areas. The history of the fight against yellow fever begins with studies of the transmission of this very likely infectious disease (the existence of viruses was not yet known at the time), that was not, however, clearly contagious.

• **1879.** The United States National Board of Health appointed a **Havana Yellow Fever Commission**, 1880-1882 (often called the **Chaillé Commission**, after its president) composed of Colonel Hardie, Dr. Jean Guiteras and Dr. George M. Sternberg as secretary. The Spanish Governor General of Cuba appointed a local physician, Dr. Carlos Juan Finlay, to cooperate with this commission. Its chief contributions were: i) the exclusion of many of the bacteria that had been claimed to be causative agents of the disease, and ii) stimulation of interest in yellow fever on the part of three influential people: Finlay, Guiteras and Sternberg.

• **1880, February 25.** An U.S. Navy commission is appointed to look into the cause of an outbreak of yellow fever on board the *U.S.S. Plymouth* **(Plymouth Commission)**. The report describes the etiology of the disease as being parasitic: germ, seed, poison of yellow fever are the terms used to designate the causal agent...[13]

Both the pathogenic agent and the mode of transmission of yellow fever were still unknown. The disease was epidemic but not contagious. Toward the end of the 19th century and the beginning of the 20th century, the idea that certain diseases could be transmitted by insects acting as vectors started to emerge[14]. In 1878-1880, Manson identified mosquitoes as responsible for filariasis[15], but given its parasitic origin, this disease could have been an exceptional case[16]. Between 1889 and 1892, Smith and Kilborne showed that ticks transmit bovine Texas fever. It was first example of infectious disease transmission by insects; they published their work in 1893[17]. Manson, Ross, Grassi and Bignami attributed malaria transmission to mosquitoes[18a]. The first

11. Sawyer, 1932, p. 291.
12. Gorgas, 1909, p. 1075.
13. Delaporte, 1991, p. 13.
14. Joyeux, 1937, p. 701.
15. Kelly, 1906, p. 98; Garrison, 1966, p. 716.
16. Delaporte, 1991.
17. Smith, 1893; Nuttall, 1899, p. 71; Winslow, 1943, p. 347.
18a. Manson, 1904, p. 28; Kelly, 1906, p. 100; Winslow, 1943, p. 347.

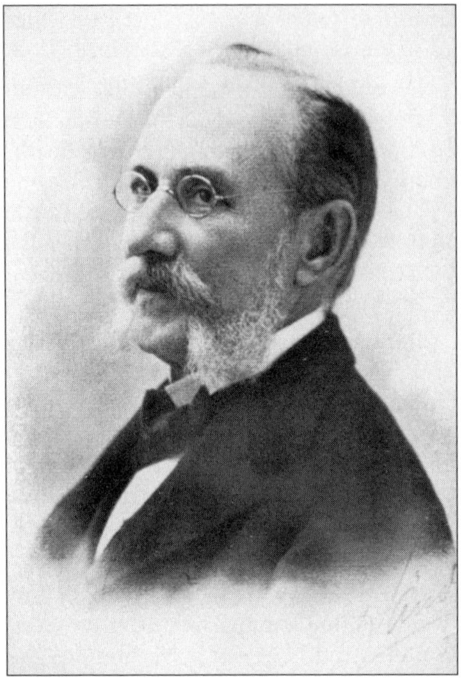

Figure 1. Dr. Carlos J. Finlay who first promulgated the theory of the transmission of yellow fever by the mosquito[18b].

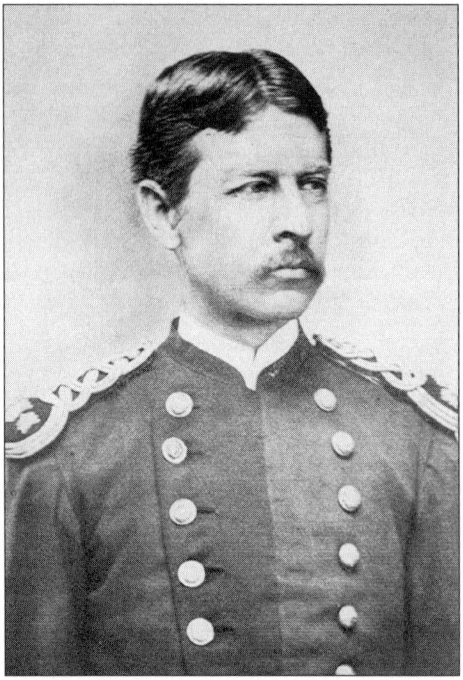

Figure 2. Walter Reed, from a photography taken in 1901[18b].

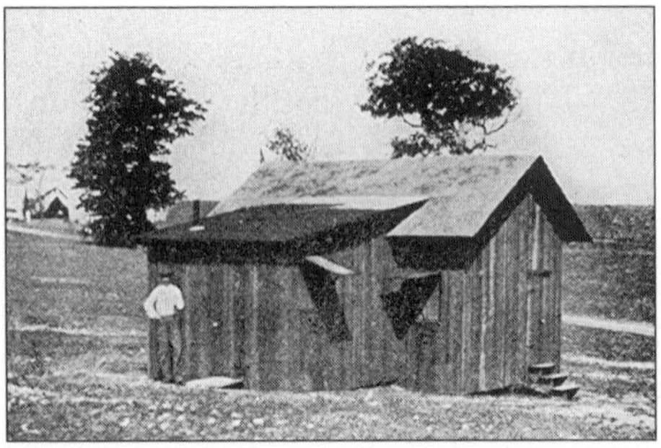

Figure 3. Camp Lazear. Building where the experiments were made which proved that yellow fever is not transmitted by means of infected clothing (fomites). The figure on the left is Dr. Caroll[18b].

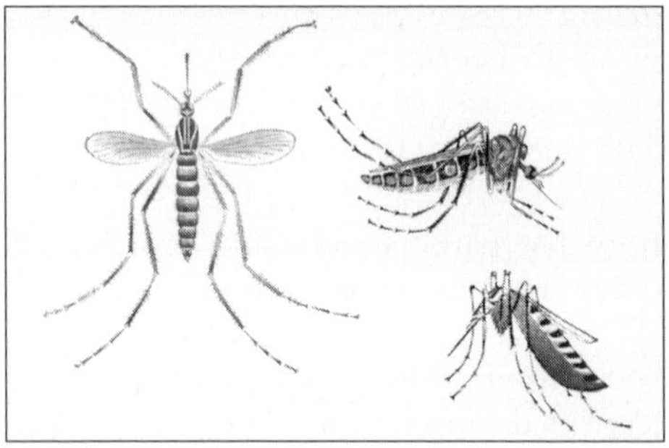

Figure 4. The mosquito *Stegomyia faciata (Aedes aegyptia)*, one of the carriers of yellow fever: left, seen from above; top right, at rest; bottom right, sated[18c].

18b. Kelly, 1906.
18c. Kolle, 1918, t. 2, plate 76.

hypothesis of yellow fever transmission by insects was presented by S.C. Nott of Mobile (Alabama) in 1848[19], to be followed by Daniel Beauperthuis in 1853[20]. Finally, based on contemporary work, the hypothesis that yellow fever is transmitted by mosquitoes was advanced to the scientific world by Dr. Carlos J. Finlay. On August 11, 1881, he correctly stated, in the title of a communication to the Royal Academy of Havana; "*The mosquito hypothetically considered as the agent of transmission of Yellow Fever*"; the same communication was presented on August 14 before the participants to the International Sanitary Conference in Washington[21], and its content was developed in the course of the following years: "*From these considerations, taken in connection with my successful attempts in producing experimental yellow fever by means of the mosquito's sting, it is to be inferred that these insects are the habitual agents of its transmission.*"[22] But Finlay's experiments were not completely convincing. The rate of transmission was relatively low, since Finlay had used mosquitoes a short time after they stung a contaminated person, without letting the virus have the time (about 12 days) to multiply in the mosquito's salivary glands[23].

• **1900.** Sternberg, Surgeon General of the United States Army, appointed a **second Yellow Fever Commission**. The United States occupied Cuba and rightly feared the yellow fever endemic on the island. They sent a mission headed by Walter Reed and including James Caroll, James W. Lazear and Aristides Agramont. A camp named Lazear, after his death of yellow fever, was installed at *Columbia Barracks*. At the time, man was the only species known to be susceptible to yellow fever. Transmission trials were conducted on volunteers, first observed for 15 days, then exposed to the sting of mosquitoes that 6 to 24 days earlier had sucked blood from yellow fever sufferers in the second or third day of their disease. After a 3 to 5 day incubation period, 5 out of 6 subjects presented yellow fever symptoms, while mosquitoes only become virulent after 12 to 18 days[24]. On the other hand, "*the attempts which we have therefore made to infect building N° 1 (infected by fomites) and its seven nonimmune occupants during a period of 63 nights has proven an absolute failure*"[25].

The Reed commission's conclusions (1902) were definite: i) the circulating blood of yellow fever patients is only infectious during the first three days of the disease; ii) the vector mosquitoes are only infectious 12 days after their contaminating sting; iii) the infectious agent crosses Berkefeld filters and is destroyed by exposure to 55° C temperature for 10 minutes; iv) yellow fever is not transmitted by fomites and disinfecting them does not prevent transmission of the disease.

Two missions, one Brazilian (Ribas, Lutz, Barreto, Barros, Rodriguez) and the other French, composed of Emile Marchoux and Paul Simond, two military doctors, and A. Taurelli Salimbeni, under the scientific direction of the Paris *Institut Pasteur*, worked in Rio de Janeiro (November 1901)[26]; they confirmed and completed the results of the Reed commission. An American mission composed of J. Roseneau, H.B. Paerker and Francis and G. Beyer was sent to Vera Cruz (Mexico) to confirm

19. Kelly, 1906, p. 112.
20. Léger, 1928, p. 970; Blanchard, 1934, p. 209.
21. Williams, 1994, p. 170.
22. Finlay, 1886, p. 395.
23. Kelly, 1906, p. 132.
24. Reed *in* Owen, 1911, p. 167.
25. Reed *in* Owen, 1911, p. 166.
26. Marchoux, 1903, p. 665.

the conclusions of a previous commission composed of Mr. Parker, Mr. Beyer and Mr. Pothier, studying the mosquito species that transmit yellow fever[27]. In 1906, Marchoux and Simond, in the course of a second French mission to Rio de Janeiro, completed the previous data, particularly concerning the role of mosquitoes in the transmission of the disease[28]. Hygiene measures were implemented. The fight against mosquitoes produced momentous results. Gorgas was very optimistic: "*It seems to me that yellow fever will entirely disappear within this generation, and that the next generation will look on yellow fever as an extinct disease having only a historic interest. They will look on yellow fever parasites as we do on the three-toed horses - as an animal that existed in the past, without any possibility of reappearing on the earth at any future time.*"[29]

• **1913. The British Colonial Empire, London**, appointed a **Yellow Fever Commission** to gather evidence showing that the disease had long been present and was widely distributed in West Africa[30].

• **1916. The Rockefeller Foundation** appointed a commission headed by Gorgas, which made a survey of yellow fever foci in South America and expressed the opinion that the eradication of yellow fever was feasible. Successful control campaigns had been completed or were in progress in Havana, Vera Cruz, the Isthmus of Panama and Rio de Janeiro[31].

• **1925.** The threat of yellow fever abated for a time: "*As a result of the rapid contraction of the yellow fever areas of the New World during the first 20 years of the period we are discussing (1905 - 1925), a peak of optimism was reached in 1925. It seemed that complete extermination of yellow fever from the Americas and perhaps from the world was practicable and almost in sight.*"[32]

• **1932-1938.** Based on Finlay's work, Reed and his colleagues believed for several years that yellow fever was a house disease due to human-to-human contamination through the agency of the mosquito. By eliminating mosquitoes, including *Aedes (Stegomyia) aegypti*, it was possible to eradicate yellow fever, as had been done in several places such as Havana or the Panama Canal when the project was taken over by the United States. Unfortunately, a yellow fever epidemic broke out in the rural zone and the jungle of the Valle do Chanaan, Espirito Santo, Brazil, in 1932, followed by several others in Colombia, Peru, Bolivia, Paraguay and most of the Brazilian states. A study was undertaken to understand the origin of these epidemics. A report based on the analysis of 24,304 mosquitoes showed that several new species of mosquitoes (*Aedes leucocelaenus* and *Haemagogus capricorni*) were likely to serve as vectors for the yellow fever virus[33a]. This destroyed the hope of eradicating yellow fever by hygiene measures alone (mosquito eradication, isolation of patients), as considered by Soper[33b], and placed major importance on the development of a vaccine suitable, if possible, to large populations[33b]. Unfortunately, in Africa there are also cycles of yellow fever transmission that involve humans and other primates[33c].

27. Marchoux, 1906, p. 16.
28. Marchoux, 1906, p. 16.
29. Gorgas, 1909, p. 1075.
30. Sawyer, 1932a, p. 291.
31. Sawyer, 1932a, p. 291.
32. Sawyer, 1932a, p. 291.
33a. Shannon, 1938, p. 110.
33b. Soper, 1935, p. 2404.
33c. Andrews, 1967, p. 98; Monath *in* Plotkin, 2008, p. 959.

Is Yellow Fever a Microbial or a Viral Disease?

The idea of diseases caused by microscopic beings is ancient, but it was not demonstrated until the second half of the nineteenth century, initially through the first cultures of alcoholic and vinegar ferments achieved by Pasteur, and later thanks to the discovery of several pathogenic bacteria by Koch's and Pasteur's teams, which revolutionized existing concepts. Some of those concerned learned notions of microbiology from competent sources, others were carried away by their enthusiasm and, lacking the appropriate knowledge, undertook risky projects which hindered progress by inundating the literature with questionable or altogether false results.

• **1878.** It appears that Richardson of Philadelphia was the first to use the expression *Bacteria sanguine, febri flavo...*[34].

• **1883.** João Batista de Lacerda, a physiologist from the National Museum of Rio de Janeiro, discovered a vegetable organism, a mushroom called Cogumello, a "polymorphic fungus"[35], *Peronospora luta* as the agent of the yellow fever.

• **1883-1884.** Dr. Domingo Freire, President of the Federal Health Council of Rio de Janeiro, stated that he had found the yellow fever microbe named "*Micrococcus amaril*" or " *Cryptococcus xanthogenicus*"[36].

• **1885.** In Mexico, Dr. Carmona Y. Valle from the Medical School of the University of Mexico confirmed Freire's results[37] and, apparently, suggested a microbial agent, *Peronospora luta*, as that responsible for yellow fever[38].

• **1888.** The Frenchman Gibier presented a slim, refringent, straight or curved bacillus as the agent of the yellow fever[39].

• **1889.** Finlay briefly maintained that the yellow fever microbe is "*Micrococcus tetragenus*".

Sternberg discredited these three potential agents: Freire's was a *Staphylococcus albus*, while the other two were common commensal bacteria.

• **Around 1890**, Cornil pointed out several bacilli found by Billings, resembling those of rabbit septicaemia or chicken cholera, and proposed them as agents of yellow fever[40].

Another false yellow fever agent discovered by Kuczynski and Hohenabel was *Bacillus hepatodystrophicans*[41].

• **1897.** In 1897, Dr. Giuseppe Sanarelli proposed the *Bacillus icteroides* as the agent of yellow fever: "*To-day we can recognise the specific agent of yellow fever; we have it in our hands; we have minutely studied its life, customs, necessities, relations with external agents...*"[42].

34. Léger, 1928, p. 970.
35. De Lacerda, 1883, p. 821.
36. Freire, 1884, p. 804; Manson, 1904, p. 170; Léger, 1928, p. 970.
37. Löwy, 1990, p. 144.
38. Léger, 1928, p. 970.
39. Cornil, 1890, t. II, p. 146; Sternberg, 1892, p. 529; Kelly, 1906, p. 117.
40. Cornil, 1890, t. II, p. 146.
41. Sawyer, 1932a, p. 291.
42. Sanarelli, 1897a, p. 7; Sanarelli, 1897b, p. 433.

Cultures of *Bacillus icteroides* injected to 5 men produced typical cases of yellow fever...[43]. This conclusion was accepted by many researchers. For instance: "*There can be no doubt that Professor Sanarelli's persevering and ingenious researches have given the study of yellow fever an impetus which is sadly needed. They have placed that dreaded scourge more in line with the other specific infective diseases* (by giving it an agent visible under the microscope), *and have opened up the possibility of devising new and hopeful methods of treatment...*"[44]. Sanarelli enjoyed an excellent reputation as a scientist and his data were accepted *a priori* for a long time, before their lack of validity was acknowledged.

- **1888-1889.** "*Bacillus X*" was proposed with many reservations by Surgeon General Sternberg himself[45].
- **1897.** Around the same time, another bacillus was proposed by W. Havelburg, probably a coli bacillus[46].
- **1899.** At the request of Sternberg, Walter Reed and James Carroll compared "*Bacillus X*" with *Bacillus icteroides* and concluded that the first was part of the colon group, while the second was a variety of hog cholera bacillus, with no direct relation to yellow fever[47].

These unfortunate claims, more or less excusable given the research conditions of that period, led researchers down wrong paths and delayed the development of a method of prevention.

The proposal of these different agents also led to disagreements in which certain researchers, such as Sanarelli, distinguished themselves: "*I cannot understand, however, his* (Dr. Sternberg) *obstinate unwillingness to concede that another has succeeded in solving the problem which proved unsolvable to him... I can understand then, that he* (Dr. Sternberg, ironically referred to a few lines earlier as 'illustrious surgeon-general') *would not readily concede success to another when he had himself failed... It would seem only reasonable, then, that Dr. Sternberg, instead of trying to justify his own failure by systematically belittling the results obtained by others... I find it totally inexplicable that Drs Reed and Carroll before attempting to launch such a paradox did not at least look up for a moment some good treatise of bacteriology...*"[48]. Sanarelli's remarks solicited a very lengthy response from Reed and Carroll: "*We pass by, therefore, as unworthy of comment, Sanarelli's insinuation that we could lend ourselves to the support of any controversy between himself and surgeon-general Sternberg; and further, his advice that we should have looked up for a moment some good treatise on bacteriology before attempting to launch such a paradox as that* Bacillus icteroides *should be considered to be a variety of the hog-cholera bacillus.*"[49]

In 1901, Walter Reed and James Carroll learned of the results Loëffler and Frosch obtained in their work on foot-and-mouth disease; they filtered serum of yellow fever patients. They wrote: "*We here desire to express our sincere thanks to William H. Welch, of the John Hopkins University, who, during the past summer, kindly called our attention to the important observations which have been carried out in late years by Loëffler and Frosch relative to the aetiology and prevention of foot and mouth disease in cattle... the specific agent of yellow fever is of such minute size as to pass readily through the pores of a Berkefeld filter.*"[50]

---

43. Manson, 1904, p. 170.
44. Anonymous, 1897, p. 96.
45. Sternberg, 1892, p. 531.
46. Havelburg, 1897a, p. 294; Havelburg, 1897b, p. 525.
47. Reed, 1899a, p. 321; Reed, 1899b, p. 513; Reed, 1900, p. 215.
48. Sanarelli, 1899, p. 193.
49. Reed, 1889a, p. 321.
50. Reed *in* Owen, 1911, p. 149.

Identifying the agent as a virus was very useful, but a major problem still existed at the time: the availability of an animal model, yet to be discovered, to conserve the virus by passage to it, and to be able to study it in the laboratory.

In 1906, Marchoux and Simond showed that it was possible to artificially conserve a strain of yellow fever virus simply by artificial passage to the mosquito, a process requiring the breeding of this Diptera[51], an inexpensive operation, but which had not yet been tried.

• **1909.** Despite the fact that the pathogenic agent had been shown to be filterable, visible agents continued to be designated as the cause of yellow fever, such as the one proposed by Seideling in 1909.

• **1919. Rockefeller Foundation.** The mistaken identification by H. Noguchi, researcher at the Rockefeller Foundation, of a yellow fever agent caused considerable delay in the progress of the search for effective prevention of the disease. He described the treponema *Leptospira icteroides*, which was in fact the agent of leptospirosis (Weil's disease). Noguchi was probably misled by the physicians who had shown him patients not suffering from yellow fever, but from a disease with similar symptoms, since the distinction was sometimes hard to make.

"*Noguchi's views were gradually accepted everywhere.*"[52] Noguchi admitted his error in good faith, and unfortunately died of yellow fever in the course of his subsequent research.

Finally, an Animal Model, even Two!

• **1920. A West African Yellow Fever Commission** of the Rockefeller Foundation was sent in Africa.

• **1925. A Second West African Yellow Fever Commission of the Rockefeller Foundation** was established in Yaba, near Lagos, in Nigeria. Adrian Stokes, coming from London, was one of the physicians assigned to the Commission.

Around 1926-1927, a severe yellow fever epidemic broke out in West Africa[53]. This type of occurrence was devastating in the country or region affected. Laigret describes his arrival to Dakar, where he was sent by the French government to coordinate the fight against the epidemic ravaging the city. He recounts: "*I had just arrived in France* (after a period spent at the *Institut Pasteur* in Saigon, present-day Ho Chi Minh City) *when I was asked to leave for Dakar: I was charged with organising the city's health protection. As soon as I was in Marseille, I understood that the situation in Africa was serious. Maritime trade with the West coast was interrupted. The large trade ships no longer sailed. I embarked on a small-tonnage vessel, whose only other passenger was a Lebanese settler… I was 33 at the time. I was enthusiastic, eager to arrive in Dakar; the ship's captain was much less so, less and less as we approached. He finally declared that he would not enter the harbour and 'dropped' us, the Lebanese and me, one morning at dawn, three miles from the coast, across from Rufisque, onto a vessel that took us to the coast, the two of us and my guinea pig crates*. I found a car to drive us to Dakar. There, I was greeted by an unforgettable sight:*

* Guinea pigs were susceptible to the wrong agent of the yellow fever "discovered" by Noguchi.

51. Marchoux, 1906, p. 16.

52. Léger, 1928, p. 970.

53. Stokes, 1928b, p. 253.

a totally paralysed city, the harbour bereft of ships, merchandise abandoned on the pier, fear in all the faces and utterings of the inhabitants... Helpless, the physicians had stopped offering any treatment, because the population blamed the deaths on the doctor each time the latter had attempted to offer any therapy... I will never forget these nights in Dakar, the city deserted, the streets completely empty, the doors and windows of all the houses shut as soon as the sun set, the prohibition to be outside under pain of an eight-day confinement in a quarantine station for observation... At length, ships were authorised to sail into Dakar in the daytime... one morning a passenger disembarked, came straight to see me and introduced himself: 'Watson Sellards, professor at Harvard University in Boston'... It was the start of a friendship that was to last fifteen years."[54]

• **1928. Rockefeller Foundation.** An essential new element was revealed in 1928 by Adrian Stokes, professor of pathology at Guy's Hospital in London, J.H. Bauer and N.P. Hudson of the **Second West African Yellow Fever Commission** headed by Dr. Henry Beeukes, stationed in Larteh, on the Gold Coast: monkeys were susceptible to contamination by the yellow fever virus. Finally, an animal model had been found. In July 1927, an inoculation of blood from a non lethal case in a man named Asibi (Asibi strain) infected Indian Crown monkeys, and then *Macacus sinicus* monkeys and finally the *Macacus rhesus* monkey, the best experimental yellow fever model, bearing a great resemblance to the clinical picture and the lesions observed in humans[55]. Unfortunately, Stokes died of yellow fever in the course of this research.

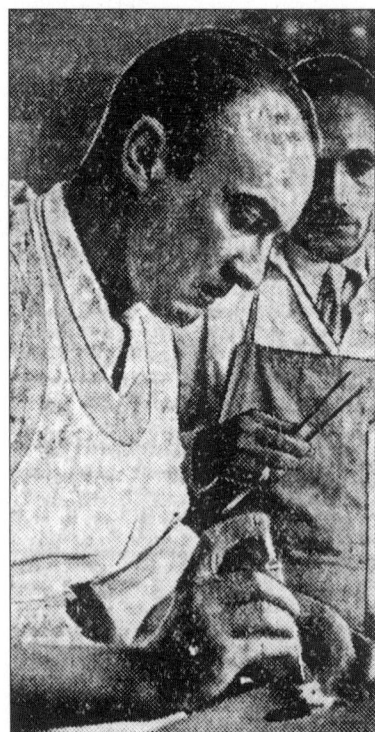

Figure 5. Jean Laigret (1893-1966) inoculating a white mouse intracerebrally. (Reproduced with permission of the "*Académie nationale de Médecine*", Paris.)

54. Laigret, 1953 (1966), p. 2441.
55. Stokes, 1928b, p. 253; Stokes, 1928a, p. 103.

• **1929. *Institut Pasteur* in Dakar (Senegal).** Before falling victim to yellow fever, Stokes had written a note whose content was known by his friend Sellards: rhesus monkeys *(Macacus rhesus)* were susceptible to inoculation by the yellow fever virus. Sellards arrived in Dakar with rhesus monkeys and proceeded, with Laigret, to look for a yellow fever virus strain in a patient with a light form of the disease. The epidemic was fading, Sellards and Laigret were fortunate enough to be called to care for a patient in the very early phase of the disease. This Lebanese man, François Mayali, is at the origin of the "French strain", very graciously designated as such by W. Sellards[56], and which was distributed to all interested researchers[58b]. Sellards took this frozen strain from Dakar to the Wellcome Laboratories in London[58a], where it was conserved by passage to monkeys, performed by Hindle, who then sent it to the *Institut Pasteur* in Paris on May 4, 1928. By using the same process, Dr. Chagas transported virus from the *Institut Pasteur* in Paris to Brazil, where Dr. H. de Beaurepaire Aragão inoculated monkeys at the Oswaldo Cruz Institute.

Transmission of the yellow fever virus to monkeys allowed for at least two new possibilities, one of which was the conservation of the virus in the laboratory. Organs of infected monkeys provided the basic material for developing potential vaccines, and later for vaccine production. This discovery considerably reduced the time needed to obtain results, but it occasioned numerous laboratory infections, and even several deaths. The second new possibility was the transport of the virus over great distances. Transporting the virus made it possible to work in regions without *Aedes aegypti* mosquitoes, and in well-equipped laboratories. This very virulent virus was contagious through contact with contaminated products like the blood or organs of monkeys that had died of the disease.

• **1930. Harvard Medical School, Boston.** The fortunate discovery of a monkey model was followed shortly by another discovery, just as important, made by Max Theiler, a young researcher recruited by A. Sellards, at the Harvard Medical School, who reported in 1930 that white mice are susceptible to be infected by the yellow fever virus (French strain) inoculated intracerebrally, using the same method Pasteur and his team had used with rabies. "*It has been found that if the yellow fever virus is injected into the brain of white mice, a certain number become ill and die. The virus can be propagated in mice indefinitely by the intracerebral injection into normal mice of the brain of an infected mouse**. *Once established in mice the passage virus… In subsequent passages… the virus is highly neurotropic in mice*." Moreover, Theiler noted that "*continuous passage of the virus through mice leads to a gradual loss of virulence for the rhesus monkey*"[59a]. Using successive passages from mouse to mouse, a neurotropic strain was obtained, in contrast with the "natural" strain called viscerotropic. This contribution was crucial for the subsequent development of the yellow fever vaccine.

---

* Max Theiler, at about the 30th mouse passage, contracted the yellow fever, fortunately a light case[58b].

56. Petit, 1929, p. 98; Laigret, 1953 (1966), p. 2441.

57. Mathis, 1928, p. 604 (Mathis was the director of the *Institut Pasteur* of Dakar); Sellards, 1932, p. 229.

58a. Sellards, 1928, p. 713.

58b. Frierson, 2010, p. 77.

59a. Theiler, 1930a, p. 367; Theiler, 1930b, p. 249.

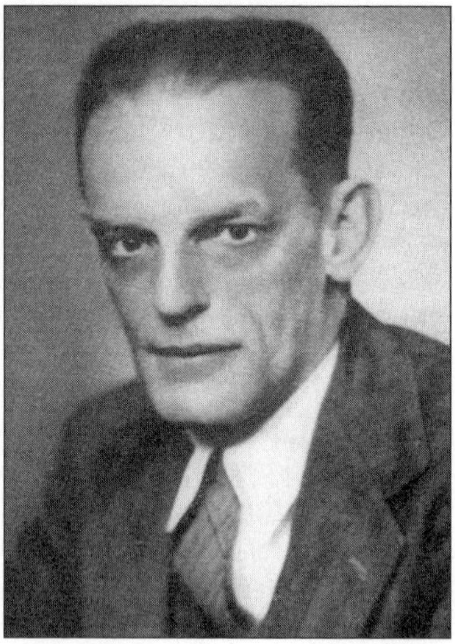

Figure 6. Max Theiler (1899-1972) was awarded a Nobel Prize, in 1951, in Physiology and Medicine for "*his discoveries concerning yellow fever and how to combat it*". Max Theiler can be credited with the transmission of the yellow fever virus to white mice inoculated intracerebrally, with the development of an intraperitoneal protection test in mice and the process of developing the 17D yellow fever vaccine by *in vitro* culture of the virus. Theiler contributed little to inovative techniques, but "*he showed a capacity for a systematized approach and persistence in action. Personal qualities that are essential to good science*"[59b].

• **1931. Rockefeller Foundation, New York.** Development of an intraperitoneal protection test in mice, consisting "*in the inoculation of mice intraperitoneally with yellow fever virus, fixed for mice, together with the serum to be tested, and a simultaneous injection of starch solution into the brain to localize the virus. If the serum lacks protective power the mice die of yellow fever encephalitis*".[60] The introduction of a relatively simple test to detect antiviral yellow fever antibodies proved to be particularly useful for epidemiological surveys on this disease, and for difficult diagnoses differentiating between yellow fever and other diseases like leptospiral jaundice. Finally, the test was used as a yellow fever immunity test for persons worried about their health status, in cases where there was uncertainty about whether or not an attack of yellow fever had occurred, or when the person in question had been vaccinated a long time previously.

Progress in Immunisation

It was a well known fact that reliable immunity existed in people who had had yellow fever: "*Inasmuch as a single attack of yellow fever, however mild, protects, as a rule, from future attacks, there is reason to hope that similar protection would result if a method could be discovered of inducing a mild attack of the disease by inoculation or otherwise.*"[61] In principle, it therefore appeared possible to vaccinate.

There were at least two reasons that incited researchers to develop a method of preventive immunisation against yellow fever. On the one hand, the death of large numbers of people decimated by yellow fever epidemics partly, but never totally, checked by the fight against vector mosquitoes. On the other hand, more pragmatically, the frequent accidental cases of contamination, some among those who volunteered for experimental inoculations at the time when man was the only known susceptible

59b. Norrby, 2007, p. 2779; Feldman, 2000, p. 246.
60. Sawyer, 1931b, p. 533; Theiler, 1933, p. 57.
61. Sternberg, 1892, p. 529.

species, as well as among researchers or medical personnel contaminated accidentally while studying yellow fever, and particularly while inoculating animals. Once it was discovered that it was possible to inoculate the virus to monkeys and later to mice, in only 4 years there were 32 cases of yellow fever infection among laboratory personnel studying the virus, with 5 fatalities among them; Hideyo Noguchi on May 21, 1928 and William A. Young in 1929, both in Accra; Adrian Stokes on September 19, 1927 in Lagos[62]; Paul A. Lewis of the Rockefeller Institute in 1929, and in 1930 entomologists Theodore B. Hayne and Guillet[63]. In addition, A. Maurice Wakeman died of an obscure tropical infection contracted while studying yellow fever in West Africa[64]. Given the long list of those whose devotion cost them their lives, a vaccine was impatiently awaited.

Several immunisation trials were carried out using false pathogenic agents; they were, of course, inconsequential. Following the favourable results obtained with inactivated virus veterinary vaccines, trials were conducted using the same techniques, but were inconclusive. The development of serovaccination, particularly against diphtheria, oriented the research in this direction, producing good protection but involving almost unsolvable problems of antiserum supply and conservation in countries with yellow fever epidemics. The development of a living, attenuated virulence vaccine was a great discovery made essentially by Max Theiler.

Some False Starts

• **1858. Havana, Cuba.** A curious attempt at inoculation with snake venom: "*This discovery originated with Mr. de Humbold. The operation requires venom from an ophidien and is performed on subjects living away from regions where yellow fever is endemic, in order to protect them from this terrible disease. The inoculated subjects develop rather uniform local symptoms; general symptoms are very variable in different individuals, but in a significant number they resemble those of yellow fever* (specifically, slowing of the pulse and a tendency to bleeding from the gums)... *The inoculation has produced the same level of disease seriousness, and thereby of mortality, in non-acclimatised subjects as in acclimatised individuals. Based on statistical data, de Humbold demonstrates that mortality due to the inoculated fever has been lower than that among the non inoculated, at a rate of 3.26 to 15... These results are good... Unfortunately, the commission (governmental, composed of three professors from the University of Havana and the head of the health authority of the Island of Cuba) formally states that the inoculation has produced no worthwhile results.*"[65]

• **1883-1884. Rio de Janeiro.** The Pasteurian era has began with the Germ Theory and the chicken cholera vaccine; Dr. Domingo Freire declares that he has discovered the yellow fever microbe[66]. Very soon, he announces in Paris that 400 people have already received his yellow fever vaccine, with authorisation from the Emperor of Brazil (the one with whom Pasteur had an exchange of correspondence). The vaccinated subjects seemed to be protected from contamination in infected areas. Mr. Rebourgeon, director of the veterinary School in Rio Grande,

62. Pettit, 1928, p. 921; Stokes, 1928b, p. 253; Stokes, 1928a, p. 103.
63. Léger, 1928, p. 970; Laigret, 1953 (1966), p. 2441.
64. Sawyer, 1932a, p. 291.
65. Manzini, 1858, p. 194.
66. Freire, 1884, p. 804.

former student of Pasteur, was a firm advocate of this method. In his presentation before the Rio de Janeiro section of the *Société de biologie*, Domingo Freire claimed to have made 418 inoculations between 1883 and 1884, and 10,881 inoculations in total between 1883 and 1890, all of them free of charge. Apparently, mortality was reduced by a factor of 10 in those who were vaccinated, compared to those who were not. But opinions differed and a commission named by the Brazilian government refused to formulate a judgement on the value of the method[67]. The method was, in fact, an inoculation of *Micrococcus amaril*. According to Freire, its consequences were minimal: "*Intraorbital and supraorbicular pain, slight headache, loss of appetite, rise in temperature, weakness in the limbs.*"[68] Other descriptions are less optimistic, reporting quite severe side effects, including 38 to 39 degree fever, chills, general unwellness, nausea and vomiting. The microorganism was collected after three passages in culture. In 1887, Sternberg, the excellent bacteriologist of the American army, visited Dr. Freire in Rio de Janeiro and saw nothing in his cultures other than the common *Staphylococcus pyogenes albus*, a non or poorly pathogenic bacterium[69]. "*There is no satisfactory evidence that the method of inoculation practised by Dr. Domingo Freire has any prophylactic value.*"[70] Sternberg analyzed Freire's statistics and found them biased in favour of his vaccine. Sternberg refused to attribute any value whatever to Freire's vaccine. This was a hasty experiment, with no controls..., theoretically not very dangerous[71]. But it showed the extent to which in vaccinology scientists with fanciful ideas could become dangerous in the absence of rigorous controls. To Freire's credit, he appears not to have caused his inoculated subjects any serious health problems. The bacterium must have been non pathogenic. In addition, the inoculations were free and performed with the blessing of the Brazilian government[72]. The weak point of this experiment was that the causal role of *Microroccus amaril* in the etiology of yellow fever had never been proven, nor would it ever be subsequently.

• **1885. Mexico.** Sternberg recounts that Dr. Carmona proposed a method of protection against yellow fever: "*It consisted in the subcutaneous injection of material obtained by desiccation of urine of yellow fever patients freely exposed to the air in shallow vessels.*"[73] But results did not live up to expectations: "*In the month of May, of last year (1885), when the yellow fever epidemic was commencing at Vera Cruz, Dr. Carmona, of Mexico, inoculated six prisoners with the dried residue of yellow fever urine. In two of the six, the local symptoms of the inoculation were immediately followed by those of fatal yellow fever, and, a few days later, both died on the same day.*"[74]

67. Freire, 1887a, p. 858; Freire, 1887b, p. 1020; Freire, 1891, p. 579; Lucas-Championnière, 1887, p. 232; Trouessart, 1887, p. 49.
68. Freire, 1884, p. 804.
69. Sternberg, 1895, p. 301.
70. Sternberg, 1892, p. 529.
71. Sternberg, 1895, p. 302.
72. Freire, 1891, p. 579.
73. Sternberg, 1895, p. 301.
74. Finlay, 1886, p. 395.

The First Immunisation Trials (Variolation Rather than Vaccination) with Small Doses of Normal Virus

1881. Havana. Finlay was the first to attempt immunisations, without knowing the agent of the disease, but relying on the accepted idea that a first attack of yellow fever protects from a second attack. Finlay believed that the "low doses" could be used to immunise without making it necessary to take great risks: "*In resolving to experiment upon human subjects, I relied upon the inference that the quantity of virus carried by a single sting must be a minimum dose, capable of producing only the mildest forms of the disease ever observed in nature, and that a number of such bites would be necessary to occasion a dangerous attack.*"[75]. Starting in *June* 1881, and until 1886, Finlay inoculated in succession 24 volunteers, priests who had recently arrived from a region without yellow fever - Spain - with single-sting doses from mosquitoes captured after they had stung a yellow fever patient. Six inoculations (out of the total 24) were followed, within the normal yellow fever incubation period (5 to 22 days), by an attack of fever, the exact counterpart of mild attacks of yellow fever, of which Finlay kept careful notes, and which were proved by subsequent observations to have conferred immunity[76]. However, Finlay remains very cautious about these results, as he clearly states[77]. In 1891 he published a second report, in which he described a group of 33 subjects inoculated using his method, and a control group of 32 subjects. He specifically stated: "*I was fortunate in receiving from two religious communities placed under my medical charge the authorization to practise my inoculations on such members as would be willing to submit to them.*"[78] Finlay confirmed the efficiency of his method, quite original when he started. His approach brings to mind the revolution caused by the Suttons and by others in the field of variolation. Unfortunately, Finlay worked in more or less heavily infested areas, a parameter he could not control. Above all, he was unaware at the time that mosquitoes only become infectious following their contamination after 12 days of incubation. Moreover, yellow fever sufferers only present viremia during the first three days during which they are symptomatic. The value of Finlay's results is difficult to assess; his results are probably inaccurate.

Around 1901. Havana. A Cuban physician, Juan Guiteras, professor of pathology and tropical medicine at the University of Havana, wanted to take up Finlay's immunisation experiments in order to protect new-comers to Cuba. Guiteras was familiar with Reed's work showing that contaminated mosquitoes only become infectious 12 days after the sting that made them infectious. In 1901, Guiteras infected seven volunteers, three of whom died, putting an end to this immunisation attempt. Reed recounts the local consequences of this unfortunate episode: "*on the day of Dr. Carroll's arrival at Havana, August 11, 1901* (a stay in Havana to work on filtration of the agent of yellow fever), *the first patient of the series of seven cases of yellow fever which Dr. Guiteras had produced by bites of infectious mosquitoes, was taken sick. The fatal outcome of three of these cases* (the US nurse, Miss Clara Louise Maass, and two Spanish people, Mr. Carro and Mr. Campa) *produced a somewhat panicky feeling toward experimental yellow fever among the nonimmunes at Havana, which feeling was intensified by the sensational and distorted statements in one of the local Spanish papers. It was, therefore, extremely difficult - in fact, practically impossible - to obtain for inoculation purposes persons who could with reasonable certainty be regarded as nonimmunes.*"[79]

75. Finlay, 1886, p. 395.
76. Finlay, 1886, p. 395.
77. Finlay, 1886, p. 395.
78. Finlay, 1891, p. 264.
79. Reed *in* Owen, 1911, p. 149.

Inactivated Virus Vaccines (Called "Killed Virus" at the Time since their Real Nature Was still Unknown)

In the 1920s, several vaccines against animal diseases caused by a filterable virus were proposed. The techniques developed for these infectious, essentially animal, diseases served as models for other diseases, with variable degrees of success...

1928. Wellcome Bureau in Tropical Medicine. Edward Hindle tried to immunise using the methods described at that time: "*It seems of interest to see whether a protective vaccine could be prepared by using any of the methods employed in the case of other diseases caused by filterable viruses, and in particular those recommended by Todd (1928) for fowl plague, Laidlaw and Dunkin (1928) for dog distemper, and Bedson, Maidland and Burbury (1927) for foot-and-mouth disease.*"[80]* On April 19, 1928, Hindle was the first to vaccinate monkeys against yellow fever. He used a ground spleen and liver mixture from an infected *Macacus rhesus* monkey, emulsified in physiological solution 5 times its volume. A preparation called formalinized vaccine contained formaldehyde in a concentration of 1 per 1,000. A monkey was inoculated and withstood a test inoculation. Another preparation called phenol-inactivated vaccine contained carbolic acid and glycerine. Seven *Macacus rhesus* monkeys were immunised with this vaccine; six withstood the test inoculation[81]. In 1931 Topley and Wilson considered these results very promising[82].

1928. *Institut Pasteur*, Paris. Pettit, Stefanopoulo and Aguesy attempted to use an anavirus (based on Ramon's formula, by adding formol and by aging at controlled temperature; the word "anavirus", used by Pettit and his colleagues, is a reference to "anatoxine", a word used by Ramon [*see chapter* 9]). One monkey was vaccinated with formalinised vaccine, and he withstood a test inoculation. Seven monkeys were vaccinated with a phenol-inactivated vaccine, and six withstood a test inoculation[83]. Pettit, Stefanopoulo and Aguesy point out that Hindle's work preceded their own (June 29, 1928[84]). Hindle warmly thanks A.W. Sellards for providing the yellow fever virus strain he brought from Africa, which was later transfered to the *Institut Pasteur* in Paris.

1929. Wellcome Bureau in Tropical Medicine. Hindle confirms his results: "*The results of my experiments (1928) showed that a phenol-glycerine emulsion of liver and spleen of infected monkeys conferred a very high degree of protection against very large amounts (10,000 to 100,000 minimum lethal doses) of virus. A formalinised suspension also showed the same vaccinating property. These experiments have been extended during the past six months in order to determine the best method of preparing an efficient vaccine for general use, the duration of protection, and some of the factors influencing its potency...*"[85].

1928-1929. Oswaldo Cruz Institute, Rio de Janeiro, Brazil. At the start of 1929, during a yellow fever epidemic, using a slightly modified version of Hindle's formula (that is, inactivated vaccine), Dr. H. de Beaurepaire Aragão vaccinated a very large population, leaving very few written records. According to professor Chagas: "*At first, results were encouraging, but after its* (the vaccine's) *use on a larger scale, it was observed that its action was somewhat irregular...*". In Rio, over 25,000 vaccinations were

---

* See details on these experiments at the end of this chapter.

80. Hindle, 1928, p. 976.
81. Hindle, 1928, p. 976.
82. Topley, 1931, p. 1249.
83. Pettit, 1928, p. 921.
84. Léger, 1928, p. 970.
85. Hindle, 1929, p. 405.

performed during the epidemic... According to Hindle, the fact that only a small number of those vaccinated in Brazil contracted yellow fever shows that the vaccine provided protection[86]. Hindle encouraged these trials: "*Arago* (1928), *working in Brazil with the local strain of yellow fever, confirmed my observations in monkeys and obtained such favourable results that the vaccine was tested in human beings... Between three hundred and four hundred people were vaccinated, including the health officers working in the infected neighbourhoods and people living either in the same houses as, or in the vicinity of, yellow fever cases. While so unwarranted conclusions are drawn, it is noted that none of the vaccinated contracted the disease, although some of them must have been exposed to infection.*"[87] Subsequent comments on these vaccination trials were less favourable, and these "Hindle inactivated vaccines" were eventually forgotten.

1929 and 1930. Laboratories of the International Health Division, Rockefeller Foundation. Sawyer and his colleagues from the Yellow Fever Laboratory at the Rockefeller Foundation (New York) tried various techniques to attenuate yellow fever virus virulence (formaldehyde or tricresol) inoculated them to monkeys and tested with the Asibi virus strain. "*The irregular results convinced us that much further research would be necessary if a safe and dependable vaccine for human beings was to be prepared by the chemical treatment of virulent strains of yellow fever virus.*"[88]

1930. Butantan Institute, Sao Paulo, Brazil. Using Kelser's technique of vaccine inactivation with chloroform, used against rinderpest, J. Lemos Monteiro successfully immunised two *Macacus rhesus* monkeys[89].

1931. Wellcome Bureau of Scientific Research London. In 1929, Findlay (1893-1952) joined Hindle in his laboratory. They immunised several monkeys with two so-called killed vaccines, either by formaldehyde or carbolic acid, although they were not convinced that the method would be effective in the case of yellow fever[90]. In the course of this work, three members of the Wellcome team suffered yellow fever attacks that fortunately were not too serious[91].

1933-1934. Wellcome Bureau of Scientific Research, London. "*Findlay, 1933-34, using virus inactivated by methylene blue and Pointolite lamp after the method of Perdrau and Todd (1933)* found that even at much larger doses 20-30 c.c. no immunity followed in monkeys.*" Findlay and Mackensie tried to immunise monkeys, hedgehogs (an animal species very sensitive to the yellow fever virus) and mice with massive doses of formalinised virus. They concluded that it was impossible to concentrate the virus sufficiently (more or less attenuated virus of the Theiler strain) to obtain a dose equivalent to those that seemed to confer a certain immunity to inoculated mice or to a inoculated hedgehog[92].

Around this period, the yellow fever virus was going to be grown in tissue or cell cultures, a process much easier to control than passages to animals.

---

* See notes at the end of the chapter.

86. Pettit, 1931, p. 522.
87. Hindle, 1929, p. 405.
88. Sawyer, 1932b, p. 945.
89. Monteiro, 1930, p. 695.
90. Findlay, 1931, p. 740.
91. Parish, 1965, p. 262.
92. Findlay, 1936c, p. 205.

1936. Rockefeller Foundation, New York. "*Immunisation against dog distemper (Laidlaw, 1928, p. 209)* (emulsion of 20% virulent infected puppy spleen formalinised at 2.5 per 1,000) *and Rift Valley fever (Mackensie, 1935, p. 65) by the use of inactivated viruses* (using 0.95% formalin) *has revived interest in the application of this method to yellow fever immunization… at the time of these earlier experiments the source of yellow fever virus limited to emulsions of tissues or the blood serum of infected monkeys… More suitable sources of virus have become available in the form of tissue cultures and filtered emulsions of infected mouse brains… Yellow fever virus (Asibi viscerotropic or 'mouse' neurotropic strains) inactived by exposure to ultraviolet light or by formaldehyde did not possess any demonstrable immunizing property.*"[93]

Vaccination attempts using an inactivated vaccine against yellow fever seem to have stopped at this point. It is likely that repeated injections were lacking... and especially a good adjuvant. Finally, the source of virus was infected animal organs, a complex mixture of a small quantity of viral antigens and a large quantity of tissue. The organs used, most often those of monkeys, could provoke very diverse immune reactions in inoculated subjects: in the same species, a reaction limited to alloantigens; in a different species, more or less strong reactions likely to limit the action against the viral antigens...

Serotherapy

Serotherapy was a major therapeutic advance and, for a long time, the only hope of a cure for many patients such as diphtheria sufferers... Unfortunately, the implementation of yellow fever serotherapy was very difficult from a practical standpoint in warm-climate countries with rudimentary medical infrastructures at the beginning of the 20th century.

Fruitless attempts

Around 1900. Sanarelli prepared a hyperimmunized horse serum (14 months of inoculations) and provided interesting statistics that, obviously, were not confirmed because the pathogenic agent was the wrong one[94].

Around 1921. Noguchi prepared a vaccine and a serum using his *Leptospira icteroides*, which unfortunately had no effect during a yellow fever epidemic in 1926-1927 in West Africa[95]. At the request of the French government, around mid August 1927, the *Institut Pasteur* prepared an anti-Leptospira serum based on Noguchi's formula; this serum was sent to Dakar[96]. In their report, Pettit and Stefanopoulo let the reader sense some envy on the part of these two French researchers, given Noguchi's research conditions: he had access to 500 Asian monkeys in his laboratory... in Africa. But by this time Noguchi's pathogenic agent was already questioned[97].

The Right Path

1903. The Marchoux Commission. "*The first attempts in this direction* (passive immunisation) *were made by Marchoux and Simond (1906), who found that the inoculation of*

93. Gordon, 1936, p. 221.
94. Manson, 1904, p. 170.
95. Noguchi, 1921, p. 181; Léger, 1928, p. 970.
96. Pettit, 1928, p. 921.
97. Pettit, 1928, p. 921.

yellow fever serum that had been warmed, or kept at 25° C for eight days, conferred partial immunity against the disease."[98] In fact Marchoux, Salembeni and Simond, with no controls to evaluate the validity of their work, concluded cautiously at the end of their trials: "*Serum from convalescent subjects seems to have therapeutic properties.*"[99]

1927. West African Yellow Fever Commission of the Rockefeller Foundation. In 1927, Stokes used serum from convalescent subjects (one or many?) to protect monkeys from an inoculation of the yellow fever virus[100].

1928-1931. *Institut Pasteur,* Paris. Pettit and Stefanopoulo prepared monkey and horse immunsera against yellow fever, obtaining results similar to Stokes. Monkey serum has greater immunising power than horse serum. About 60 litres of immune serum were sent to French-speaking Africa, to Brazil and to Monrovia. No information about the results obtained with this serum came back. Serovaccinations were also performed successfully on infected monkeys, and 600 flasks (of unspecified volume) of equine immune serum were made available to the authorities (perhaps the 60 litres indicated above)[101]. In 1931, Marchoux, Salimbeni and Simond reported that "*the immunity conferred by the convalescent serum is still considerable after twenty-six days*"[102].

1933. *Institut Pasteur,* Paris. Pettit and Stefanopoulo published a new report on the work they were conducting to produce immune serum against yellow fever in monkeys and horses. Equine sera can reach much higher titre levels than convalescent sera, and can, theoretically, be produced in unlimited quantities[103].

All of these sera were not often used in yellow fever patients, because of the difficulties to overcome practical problems. But they were extensively used in serovaccinations.

Serovaccination: Simultaneous Injection of Living Virus and of Specific Immune Serum

Serovaccination was a stage in the development of vaccinations against various diseases in many countries, and it was used with particular success by William Park to combat diphtheria in New York[104]. Since inactivated yellow fever vaccines were not very effective, if at all, this option had to be attempted. A study conducted by Berry and Kitchen on all cases of laboratory contamination occurring since the introduction of the monkey model in yellow fever showed that out of 32 cases reported in 4 years, 4 fatal cases were due to the "monkey" virus, and one was due to a bite by an infected mosquito. In contrast, the 3 cases unquestionably due to murine virus (Theiler's neurotropic) had been benign[105]. Therefore, this "mouse" virus could be tried in a vaccination or, at least, in a serovaccination. This led Sellards to leave the *Institut Pasteur* in Paris and then, with his colleagues at the *Institut Pasteur* in Tunis, to try to vaccinate against yellow fever with living murine vaccine alone (*see page* 429). This idea is presented in two articles by Sellards, but it does not reflect the actual events[105].

98. Hindle, 1929, p. 405.
99. Marchoux, 1903, p. 665.
100. Anonymous, 1927, p. 615.
101. Pettit, 1928, p. 921; Léger, 1928, p. 970; Pettit, 1931, p. 522.
102. Pettit, 1931, p. 522.
103. Pettit, 1933, p. 67.
104. Park, 1922, p. 1584.
105. Berry, 1931, p. 365; Sellards, 1932a, p. 229; Sellards, 1932b, p. 1609.

1931. Oswaldo Cruz Institute, Rio de Janeiro, Brazil. Dr. H. de Beaurepaire Aragão tried to immunise against yellow fever using an inoculation of human or monkey serum from individuals with immunity to this disease, followed 24 hours later by the inoculation of a lethal dose of virus. Experiments on several monkeys started in 1928 and produced good results[106].

1931. Rockefeller Foundation, New York. The first yellow fever serovaccination trials in humans were conducted by Wilbur A. Sawyer, S.F. Kitchen and W. Lloyd[107], who expressed their concerns clearly: "*The method here presented for vaccination against yellow fever was devised primarily to interrupt the long series of accidental infections of persons making laboratory investigations*."[108] This was not a theoretical problem! These authors relied on data from literature on veterinary vaccinology: "*The practice of injecting virus and immune serum at the same time but in different places has been followed in vaccinating swine against hog cholera and cattle against rinderpest, and in immunizing against other diseases of animals*."[109] Sawyer and his colleagues refer to immunisation obtained in monkeys by injecting a mix of a lethal dose of virus and a specific quantity of serum selected for its neutralising properties. This procedure also set the limits of the possible sphere of application of a method requiring 0.3cc per kilo of body weight of serum from individuals recovering from yellow fever, that is, for an adult, about 20 to 30 cc of human antiserum inoculated under the skin of the abdomen, with the virus mixed in directly (0.2 grams of virulent mouse brain), or given 6 hours later. The virus came from the mouse-adapted French strain fixed in mice between the 105th and the 176th passage. It was given in a 10% suspension of brain matter from a mouse killed by an intracerebral inoculation. All those inoculated gained immunity as solid as that of persons recovering from an attack of yellow fever[110]. Ten persons were vaccinated between May 13 and June 29, 1931[111a]. Sawyer and his colleagues immunised over 20 persons in New York without incident (and 3 more people in Nigeria and in Brazil, with material sent from the United States) starting on May 13, 1931.

1931-1933. Oswaldo Cruz Institute, Rio de Janeiro. H. de Beaurepaire-Aragão vaccinated 5 people using the Sawyer method, slightly modified. Three of these people received an initial injection of 3 cc serum and, six hours later, an inoculation with a mix of 2 cc serum and 0.001 gram of murine brain virus, without any noteworthy accident (*sic*)[112].

1931. Academy of Medicine (Paris). The French government asked the Academy to describe the state of progress in the fight against yellow fever. The report resuming the situation at the time states that vaccination seems to give satisfactory results, but must be improved. As to serotherapy, it seems promising, but is difficult to implement[113].

---

106. Aragão, 1931, p. 1078.
107. Sawyer, 1931a, p. 62.
108. Sawyer, 1932b, p. 945.
109. Sawyer, 1932b, p. 945; Duval, 1929, p. 87.
110. Sawyer, 1932b, p. 945; Pettit, 1933, p. 67; Sawyer, 1934, p. 1072.
111a. Sawyer, 1931a, p. 62. The first subject immunized against the yellow fever, with a combination of antigen/antiserum, was Dr. Bruce Wilson of the International Health Division of the Rockefeller Institute, on leave in Brazil[111b].
111b. Frierson, 2010, p. 77.
112. Aragão, 1931, p. 1078; Aragão, 1933, p. 1471.
113. Pettit, 1931, p. 522.

1931-1934. Wellcome Laboratories, London. After their failed attempts with inactivated virus, Findlay and Hindle turned to serovaccination[114]. They illustrated the success of the method by citing vaccination against rinderspest or hog cholera. At first, starting in November 1932, fifteen people were vaccinated with a subcutaneous injection of 35 to 45 cc of immune serum, followed 4 to 6 hours later by a subcutaneous injection in the arm of 0.5 cc of a 1/10 suspension of the brain of a mouse infected by the yellow fever virus in human serum. The remaining 80 people were immunised intradermally. The protocol used was 1 cc serum intradermally, given in four 0.25 cc injections administered into the four corners of a square with 2.5 cm sides, followed 2 to 4 hours later by a 0.2 to 0.5 cc intradermal injection of a 1/10 brain suspension. This method reduces the cost of immunoserum, is well-tolerated and allows a greater number of immunisations. Findlay applied Sawyer's method to 25, then 50 and finally a total of 200 subjects, on December 31, 1933. By March 31, 1934, 251 persons had already been immunised against yellow fever in London, with good results: "*Immune bodies* (antibodies) *begin to appear in the blood stream 8 to 9 days after immunization; they attain their maximum titre in from 4 to 5 weeks*."[115] From 1933 on, serovaccination was the method recommended by the Ministry of Health in London[116]. Immunity lasted between ten to sixteen months[117].

1931-1936. *Institut Pasteur*, Paris. In September 1931, in France, Sellards introduced the neurotropic yellow fever virus given intracerebrally to white mice. The virus was at its one hundred and twenty-fifth passage. Inoculated intracerebrally, it killed the mice in from five to eight days by producing an ascendant paralysis syndrome[118]. Attempts were made to immunise monkeys with the "Theiler-mouse" virus. Sawyer and his colleagues, who developed serovaccination in May 1933, were hosts to G. J. Stefanopoulo of the *Institut Pasteur* in Paris, who came to their laboratory to learn their technique. The technique was later used at the *Institut Pasteur* in Paris. Pettit and Stefanopoulo prepared an equine immunoserum instead of the human serum, and used it in 10 subjects; 2 others were vaccinated with human serum from recovering patients, with good results[119]. In Prof. Pettit's Unit at the *Institut Pasteur* in Paris, 103 subjects were vaccinated using this technique; this was followed by protection tests in mice. Side effects were limited[120].

1932-1936. Wellcome Bureau of Scientific Research. "*The virus component used from 1932 to the middle of 1936 consisted of a 20 per cent, suspension in normal human serum of mouse brain infected with the neurotropic strain of yellow fever virus...*"[121].

1934. Serovaccination becomes the method of choice. The method used at the Rockefeller foundation (56 vaccinations), at the Wellcome (264 vaccinations), in Brazil (5 vaccinations) and at the *Institut Pasteur* in Paris (12 vaccinations) was Sawyer, Kitchen and Lloyd's serovaccination. "*Given its safety, the protection it confers and its duration (at least two years), the procedure developed by Drs. W.A. Sawyer, S.F. Kitchen and W. Lloyd is presently the one* to be *recommended*." Among those who used this method, there was almost general consensus as to its merit, but this consensus did not go beyond a limited sphere. In addition, a new problem arose: Theiler discovered, in the mice he was

114. Findlay, 1931, p. 740.
115. Findlay, 1933, p. 1009; Findlay, 1934b, p. 43; Findlay, 1934a, p. 437; James, 1934, p. 1048.
116. James, 1933, p. 46.
117. Kazeeff, 1934, p. 421.
118. Advier, 1934, p. 441.
119. Pettit, 1934, p. 1075.
120. Stefanopoulo, 1936, p. 359.
121. Findlay, 1936a, p. 1321.

breeding, a virus capable of causing encephalomyelitis after a 7 to 30-day incubation period, a fact which threw suspicion of serious contamination on yellow fever virus strains passed to mice or produced in mice[122].

1935. *Institut Pasteur*, Paris. A case of meningeal encephalitis arose in Professor Pettit's Unit, after a serovaccination. The woman in question had received 14.5 cm^3 of immune equine serum intramuscularly, followed 4 hours later by a dose of yellow fever neurotropic virus with attenuated virulence (Theiler's murine neurotropic strain). The patient eventually recovered, after a long convalescence[123]. Mollaret and Findlay made a careful study of this case, since the lot to which the inoculated vaccine belonged came from Findlay's London laboratory, which shows the close collaboration that existed between these laboratories. Several hypotheses were formulated; one, an accident due to the equine serum, was eliminated for various reasons. Contamination of the vaccine by a spontaneous murine neurotropic virus was another hypothesis; it was, in fact the one considered most plausible, and the following warning was added: "*We now see the mouse more and more as a dangerous animal.*" Mollaret proposed that to produce viruses for vaccination the guinea pig could replace the mouse in order to avoid a spontaneous murine neurotropic virus, or even better, that a virus could be developed from tissue cultures[124]. Mollaret was probably thinking of the experiments conducted by Mathis, who used the French strain of the yellow fever virus in 155 intracerebral passages to white mice, and in 10 more passages to guinea pigs. "*The yellow fever virus, adapted and fixed to the guinea pig's nervous system, acts like a vaccine when administered by subcutaneous inoculation* (in monkeys)."[125] The *Institut Pasteur* in Paris was thinking of changing experimental animal species, while the Wellcome and the Rockefeller were considering the use of a virus strain passed on tissue culture, a more innovative solution. Moreover, C. Levaditi and H. Plotz, both at the *Institut Pasteur* in Paris, had the know-how needed to carry out such a tissue culture project.

Subsequent serovaccination trials were conducted using modified viral strain techniques, particularly those involving tissue cultures.

1936. Wellcome Bureau of Scientific Research. Start of serovaccination using a strain of neurotropic virus with virulence attenuated through tissue culture. "*From the middle of 1936 onwards an attenuated pantropic strain of virus has been exclusively used. This attenuated strain of ordinary yellow fever virus, first prepared by Lloyd (1936)*[126]*, was to begin with grown in tissue culture flasks containing minced mouse embryo tissues in normal serum Tyrode solution*[127]*. Later minced chick embryo was substituted for the mouse embryo.*"[128]

1937. Wellcome Bureau of Scientific Research. The possibility that a correlation might exist between 2,200 immunisations against yellow fever by serovaccination, and 48 jaundice cases that appeared 2 to 7 months after the inoculation, was considered. "*The symptoms observed have been very similar to those of common infective hepatic jaundice.*"

122. Theiler, 1934a, p. 122; Joyeux, 1937, p. 740.
123. Darré, 1936, p. 169.
124. Mollaret, 1936, p. 176.
125. Mathis, 1934a, p. 505.
126. Lloyd, 1936, p. 481.
127. Findlay, 1936a, p. 1321.
128. Findlay, 1937, p. 297.

Stefanopoulo reported 2 cases of jaundice that appeared between 2 and 3 months after the vaccination of 102 white subjects in Pointe Noire (Gabon), but cases of infective hepatic jaundice were present in that town. No formal conclusion was drawn[129].

Theiler's Neurotropic Mouse-Adapted Virus with Virulence Modified by Various Means

1931. *Institut Pasteur,* Paris. "*Prof. A.W. Sellards, who in the fall of 1931 was working in Prof. A. Pettit's laboratory (Institut Pasteur,* Paris*), wished to be vaccinated with living murine virus alone, and to try the procedure on humans. Dr. E. Roux* (Director of the *Institut Pasteur* in Paris)*, who was consulted regarding this matter, forbade the* Institut Pasteur *to apply this procedure to man, because of its possible dangers.*"[130]

1931. *Institut Pasteur,* Tunis. Laigret continues the account of his recollections (some of which were quoted earlier): "*In 1931 I had just arrived at the* Institut Pasteur *in Tunis, and Sellards wrote me saying that he wanted to continue his studies with me.* [Emile Roux had just forbidden (in the fall of 1931) human trials of the murine vaccine at the *Institut Pasteur* in Paris.] *I spoke about him with* Mr. Nicolle (the director at the time)*. In monkeys inoculated by Sellards with brain from paralysed mice, apparently yellow fever did not appear, and there were reasons to think that they had been rendered immune. If we could reproduce this in humans, we would have the yellow fever vaccine...* Mr. Nicolle *agreed...* (But) *Was there not a risk of introducing yellow fever in the country* (Tunisia)*? Inversely, if trials were conducted in a region where yellow fever was endemic, it would be almost impossible to eliminate the causes of errors due to natural immunisation...* Mr. Nicolle *decided that very cautious trials could be conducted in Tunisia in winter, when there are no mosquitoes... I sent a wire to Sellards telling him to come...* Mr. Nicolle *decided that initially humans would be inoculated with a dilution such that the inoculated quantity would correspond to the millionth parcel of the brain of an infected and paralysed white mouse. Everything went well...*"[131].

Sellards seems to have been the one who proposed that the French neurotropic strain, obtained by repeated passages of the virus to mice intracerebrally, be used. Laigret is at the origin of the use of this strain in large European or African populations.

1932-1934. *Institut Pasteur,* Tunis. Faced with Emile Roux's veto at the *Institut Pasteur* in Paris, Sellards chose a new location and new partners. Laigret recounts: "*Finally, the first human trials conducted cautiously with A.W. Sellards showed that the murine virus* (Theiler's fixed mouse neurotropic strain) *can confer, with no apparent adverse reaction, an immunity easily confirmed by seroprotection tests... but this in no way means that such a virus has become totally incapable of exerting, albeit rarely, a certain action resembling, more or less, its former pathogenic power... I have observed these exceptional reactions on two occasions... Therefore, it is dangerous to inject man with unknown quantities of Theiler's virus. Dilution ratios are not reliable indicators of their virus concentration, which is highly variable from one mouse brain to another... Injecting, at the same time as the virus, an antiserum* (serum from an animal or person cured of yellow fever) *does not reduce the danger in any way...* (an argument against serovaccination, the competing vaccination technique)*. There is only one way to evaluate the activity of brains intended for*

129. Findlay, 1937, p. 297.
130. Pettit, 1934, p. 1075.
131. Laigret, 1953 (1966), p. 2441.

vaccination... and that is to titre their content..." Subsequently, Laigret prepared and used glycerinated or dried vaccines, attempting to reduce the number of injections[132].

1932. *Institut Pasteur,* Tunis. Having tried unsuccessfully a mouse virus killed (inactivated) in formalin[134], in 1932 Sellards and Laigret inoculated augmenting small quantities (1 to 3 injections) of Theiler's murine virus (at the 134th passage to mice) to "*five subjects with chronic nervous disorders for which pyretotherapy* is indicated*". The mouse brains are crushed and made into an emulsion in physiological solution with 10 percent rabbit serum added. This initial solution is passed through a centrifuge for 3 to 4 minutes. The dilution fluid is diluted in turn. A drop of the dilution at 1/10000th regularly kills a mouse inoculated intracranially. When the inoculations are subcutaneous, 1cc of emulsions at 1/10000th or at 1/1000th provokes no reaction; in the same conditions, a dose of 1/100th given to a subject provoked a very slight temperature elevation, and the same inoculation was very well tolerated when given in augmenting doses of 1/10000th to 1/100th, and even 3cc of a 1/10th emulsion. The protective power of serum of inoculated subjects emerges 7 to 34 days after the vaccination. Sellards and Laigret conclude: "*We believe that our results could serve as the basis for vaccination trials carried out in the populations of regions where yellow fever remains a threat.*"[135] Laigret knew (and feared?) the side effects of the Sellards-Laigret, vaccine, and remained very cautious: "*Laigret, seeing febrile reactions in certain subjects inoculated with his vaccine, had prepared a donkey serum in 1932, for the treatment of accidents ensuing from his yellow fever vaccination. For this purpose, a donkey was inoculated with the neurotropic virus in Dakar.*"[136]

1932. *Institut Pasteur,* Tunis. When the first study was complete, Laigret noted that out of 7 new subjects ("*patients eligible for pyretotherapy, in most of whom syphilitic infection of the nervous centres had been established*") inoculated on June 1, 1932 with 1cc dose of mouse brain emulsion at 1/1000, only one presented a slight increase in temperature on June 12; on the 14th day one developed fever and on the 16th day two more had fever with significant general symptoms. The origin of these effects was debated: superinfection, reaction to animal tissue, fluctuation of the virulence of the mouse-adapted strain given intracerebrally. The author concludes that the effects seen in these three subjects indicate that the virulence of the yellow fever mouse-adapted virus is not entirely fixed[137]. However, the subjects never presented viraemia (multiple blood and cerebrospinal fluid tests). Nevertheless, the seriousness of the side effects led Laigret to look for another method of attenuating neurotropic "mouse" virus virulence. To reduce the inoculated doses, the researchers established a mouse-adapted dose: the most infinitesimal quantity capable of infecting a mouse is sufficient to confer immunity to man in 50% of cases[138]. Continuing his studies, Laigret exposed virulent mouse brains to temperatures between 10° C and 20° C for one, two or four days; he then prepared glycerinated suspensions and made dried attenuated preparations (also called dry). This aging process was likened by Laigret himself to that used for rabbit spinal cord by Pasteur[139].

---

* Intermittent increase of body temperature by diathermy, or inoculating with malaria, in syphilis[133].

132. Laigret, 1934b, p. 1078.

133. Sellards, 1932b, p. 1609.

134. Gould's Medical Dictionary, 1941, pp. 513 & 1170.

135. Sellards, 1932b, p. 1609; Sellards, 1932c, p. 2175; Sellards, 1932a, p. 229.

136. Advier, 1934, p. 441.

137. Laigret, 1932, p. 412.

138. Mathis *in* Levaditi, 1938, p. 820.

139. Sellards, 1932a, p. 229; Laigret, 1932, p. 412.

End 1932 - start 1934. *Institut Pasteur,* Tunis. "*Having to return to America to teach, Sellards left us. It had been decided that I would continue the studies in Tunis and that I would send the sera from vaccinated subjects to Sellards, so that he could test them in his Boston laboratory. Thus, we continued to collaborate from a distance... I had succeeded in drying the mouse brains... Thus, I could apply the three-step* (injections) *method... I had vaccinated myself using this method... This work* (the development of the method) *had taken three years... One evening, when Mr. Nicolle came to enquire about my work, he asked me: 'What will you do now?' - 'I have to go to Dakar.' - 'Very well, I will write.' The minister's answers were evasive... At the same time, yellow fever was reappearing in the Ivory Coast, and then in Senegal... Still hesitant, the minister submitted the question of vaccination trials to the President of the Republic* and it is he who authorised my Mission to Dakar where...*"[140].

1933. *Institut Pasteur,* Tunis. Laigret presents the methods of preparation of his glycerinated or dried vaccines. His preparations are titred for their virulence in mice. Neither vaccine kills mice any more, and both provoke the emergence of "protective substances" in laboratory animals; the concept of antibodies had not yet been established; it was to be created in 1937 by Tiselius, who showed that protective serum substances could be found among gamma-globulines. To vaccinate human beings, "*three successive injections are given into the adipous tissue of the abdominal wall, twenty days apart, using three increasingly more virulent vaccines*"[141].

1934. *Institut Pasteur,* Dakar. Much later, Laigret continued to recount these events. He went to the *Institut Pasteur* in Dakar to carry out a mission whose objectives were defined in a decree issued on May 11, 1934[142]. "*... I* (Laigret) *arrived* (in Dakar) *in May 1934. I had brought with me, in refrigerated thermos bottles, enough matter to vaccinate 500 people. I also had what was needed to organise a vaccine production centre at the* Institut Pasteur *in Dakar... I arrived in Dakar one morning at 6 o'clock. In the afternoon, 200 people came to be vaccinated..., and the next day about three hundred more... so we hastened to prepare the vaccine at the* Institut Pasteur. *I left for Kaolack with the new vaccine... a hot and humid region where stegomyias proliferate. There, we had 250 more volunteers. I returned to Dakar to observe febrile reactions. There were very few, all of them benign... After two weeks, it was time for the inoculation of the second, 10-unit vaccine in Dakar. All those who received the first vaccine returned for the second. I spent the following week making lengthy vaccination rounds across Senegal; the last session in Saint-Louis attracted many candidates. A military plane took me back from Saint-Louis to Dakar, where I was anxious to know if there were febrile reactions following the second vaccine. When I landed, I saw only frowning faces. I was told that there were serious reactions, that some people were quite ill... It was almost noon... Losing no time, I left by car to see all those who were ill. Five or six were in bed, but aside from a fever they had no worrisome symptoms. The others were seated at table with their families. They had had a high fever, unpleasant in the stifling heat, but nothing more serious than what they were told to expect... The same unjustified concerns surfaced in Kaolack. Reactions were so numerous and violent that the physician feared that the Lebanese would not come for the second vaccination* (Laigret often refers to the Lebanese, because he gave this conference in Beyrouth in 1953). *They were all there, even bringing new volunteers with them... The many blood samples we took for*

* Probably Albert Lebrun (1871-1950).

140. Laigret, 1953 (1966), p. 2441.

141. Laigret, 1933, p. 198.

142. Sorel, 1936, p. 1325.

serological analysis confirmed progressive immunisation: half the subjects were immunised after the first vaccine, 90% after the second, 99% after the third. We had vaccinated 3,500 people. Only one worried me. A young military pharmacist presented a high fever, sleepiness and stiffness in the neck fifteen days after the second vaccination. It was the first case of meningoencephalitis I was seeing, as a reaction to yellow fever vaccination. Since then, I have seen 10 more cases... all of them resolve after three days... In many places in Senegal, in the same house, in the same family, there were yellow fever cases among the unvaccinated; none of the vaccinated individuals caught the disease. The vaccine was in demand everywhere..."[143]. Laigret was most probably vaccinating adults, and the only case of meningoencephalitis appeared 15 days after the vaccination.

1934. *Institut Pasteur,* Dakar. The Sellards / Laigret (or Laigret / Sellards, and later Laigret vaccination, depending on the authors) was practiced on large populations in West Africa (Senegal, Casamance, Guinea, Ivory Coast, Sudan, Nigeria,[144] using three injections administered 20 days apart, with modified murine virus (Theiler's method) attenuated at 20° C for 4, 2 then 1 day (Laigret's method). Between June 10 and August 15, 1934, 3,196 inoculations were given to white volunteers in West Africa. "*No local reaction was observed. In about one third of cases, after the inoculation of the first vaccine, more rarely after the second, and exceptionally after the third, a febrile reaction is observed. When this reaction occurs, it appears six days after the inoculation that triggers it. It produces a high fever, with headaches, orbital pain and rachialgia, lasting 12 to 30 hours. Individuals who are exhausted by a long stay in the colonies, who are overworked, who present hepatorenal deficiency, have frequently been observed to have this reaction. Women were not subject to it. Overall, 70 percent of the vaccinated received the three inoculations and did not have to interrupt their usual occupations. In two of the vaccinated, we observed: in one, a meningeal syndrome; in the other, myelitis with transient paraplegia. They quickly made a complete recovery. Blood and cerebrospinal fluid from these two patients infected neither macaques nor mice... Neither in Senegal... where mosquitoes abound... there was not the least epidemic spread following vaccinations.*"[145] Obviously, it was feared that the Laigret vaccine might transmit yellow fever to the unvaccinated. That was not the case. This vaccine was well-received and strongly encouraged by the French colonial administrative authorities: "*The government* (of French West Africa) *proposed that a vaccine preparation centre be organised, based on the Tunisian method, at the* Institut Pasteur *in Paris, and that the colonial population have access to 3 vaccination centres: Paris, Marseille and Bordeaux... The essential thing was that the method be the same in the colonies and in France.*"[146] The rest of the article describes the development of the competing method, serovaccination.

1934. Vaccination in French West Africa. About 10,000 people were immunised "*in the course of the past year*" (either the year 1934, or between July 1934 and July 1935), first with the Sellards-Laigret vaccine (phosphate-treated vaccine in 3 injections). The injections were given 20 days apart "*three vaccines composed respectively of murine brain emulsions exposed for 4, 2 and 1 day to normal temperature. All yellow fever vaccinations performed between June 1934 and December 1935... used this technique. During his mission (June-August 1934) doctor Laigret, with the help of a colleague,*

143. Laigret, 1953 (1966), p. 2441.
144. Laigret, 1947, p. 13.
145. Mathis, 1934b, p. 742.
146. Laigret, 1934a, p. 1593.

inoculated 2,164 subjects of both sexes, 792 of whom received two injections and 240 three injections. The procedure was entirely limited to European volunteers and educated natives. When Mr. Laigret left, vaccinations continued to be conducted in the conditions he had established... In total, by December 31, 1935, 28,890 vaccinal injections had been administered, meaning that 5,699 subjects received all three injections, making immunity very likely."[147] Vaccination campaigns against yellow fever were continued by the Director of the *Institut Pasteur* in Dakar, Constant Mathis, and soon over 100,000 people were inoculated[148].

Subsequently, in order to reduce the protocol to two or even one injection, the "virus" was coated with egg yolk and/or olive oil, based on the lipo-vaccine technique developed by Le Moignic and Pinoy[149]. Laigret's new procedure (phosphate-treated vaccine coated with egg yolk, in a single injection) was used after the 3-injection protocol[150]. Trials on 89 subjects divided into three groups, using very high doses of coated virus (30 times the quantity of the highest dose inoculation with the 3-injection method), were conducted without noteworthy difficulty. The most serious side effects were two cases of meningitis and one case of myelitis; they were cured leaving no sequellae. Finally, out of the various protocols that were tried, the one chosen was simple coating with egg yolk of 6,000 minimal murine doses given in one injection[151].

1936. *Institut Pasteur*, Dakar. C. Mathis was clearly biased in favour of the Sellards-Laigret vaccination, although he was perfectly aware of its side effects[152].

1936. *Institut Pasteur*, Paris. Yellow fever vaccinations at this Institute were first performed by Prof. Pettit using serovaccination (1933-1934), then, starting in October 1934, using Laigret's vaccine prepared at the *Institut Pasteur* in Tunis by Laigret himself. Between this date and March 1, 1936, 100 vaccinations were performed. A group of 38 subjects was vaccinated using the 3-injection method with virus attenuated by aging at normal temperature for 4, 2 and 1 day. Not all the vaccinated subjects received all 3 injections 20 days apart. Two serious nervous reactions were observed around the 14th day after the vaccination. A second group of 59 subjects received dry, coated yellow fever vaccine in a single injection, with no serious side effects, and particularly no nervous reactions, at least in the 23 subjects observed. A third small group of 3 individuals presented light side effects. Martin compares his 2 serious side-effect cases with the one reported by Darré and Mollaret, after serovaccination[153].

1936. At Laigret's request, *La Société de Pathologie Exotique* formulated its wishes regarding yellow fever vaccination. "*La Société de Pathologie Exotique expresses the wish that yellow fever vaccination be conducted as it has been in the past, on volunteer subjects; that this vaccination which uses a living neurotropic virus be employed with caution.*"[154] This positive but guarded attitude shows the limits of the acceptability granted the Laigret vaccine, which was only recommended in the face of a threat.

147. Sorel, 1936, p. 1325.
148. Laigret, 1947, p. 13.
149. Le Moignic, 1916, p. 201.
150. Peltier, 1939, p. 657.
151. Nicolle, 1935, p. 312; Nicolle, 1936, p. 28.
152. Mathis, 1936, p. 1042.
153. Martin, 1936, p. 295.
154. Société de Pathologie Exotique, 1936, p. 449.

1936. *Institut Pasteur*, Tunis. Laigret was clearly pleased to announce that 2 subjects vaccinated using the Sellards-Laigret method still showed immunity after 3.5 and 4 years[155b].

1936. Medical Inspector General Sorel, delegate to French West Africa. Nicolle and Laigret's highly optimistic conclusions regarding yellow fever vaccinations, actually very few in number in relation to the entire population, were demolished by Medical Inspector General Sorel: "*Thus, these arguments do not seem to have sufficient weight to constitute proof that the present lull in yellow fever occurrence in French West Africa is due to preventive vaccinations...*"[156a]. He goes on to describe the unsafe nature of Sellards-Laigret vaccinations. Side effects of the vaccine can be classified into two categories: those that appear around the 6th day, and those that appear around the 14th or 15th day. The first are more frequent, ranging from light to serious, and they tend to produce visceral symptoms: fever, headaches, arthralgia, nausea, vomiting, fetid stools, asthenia. The reactions occurring between the 12th and 15th day, not detected when vaccinations initially started (before 1936?), were attributed to concomitant problems such as an attack of malaria or dengue, food poisoning... The vaccinators noted above all the great number of reactions, mostly neurotropic in nature: attack on the 6th day after vaccination, and onset of a 39° C fever on the 15th day, with frontal headache and stiffness of the neck and the spinal column, indicating a meningeal or encephalitic affection, with motor, sensory, psychic or mental, as well as lethargic involvement, sometimes present at the same time. Sorel concluded: "*But we can assert right off with certainty that a clinical study alone is not sufficient proof to convince us that in 12,000 yellow fever vaccinations administered, only four nervous reactions were observed.*"[156b] And he cited 27 detailed clinical observations. Sorel noted the problems but did not identify their cause, which was unknown to him. He submitted two hypotheses: it was either the Sellards-Laigret vaccine or a spontaneous murine virus. He went on to discuss the two types of vaccine used at the time: Findlay's vaccine* (human anti-yellow fever serum and mouse brain) and Pettit's vaccine (animal anti-yellow fever serum and mouse brain), abandoned by Pettit himself because of the infrequent but undeniable risk associated with it. Sorel believed the Sellards-Laigret vaccine to be effective, but stressed that no irrefutable proof of this had been presented. Moreover, he questioned the vaccine's complete lack of danger "*not only in the days immediately following inoculation, but also over the next few months*". He ended by saying: "*Therefore, although we can continue to recommend careful experimental use, with follow-up, of this vaccination to all those placed in real danger of being contaminated by the yellow fever virus, and although we can envisage wide application of the vaccination in areas where the emergence of a few cases of yellow fever leads to fear of an epidemic, we consider it desirable and cautious not to plan at present systematic widespread application of a procedure that is still under study.*"[157] This opinion, expressed by General Sorel, Medical Inspector, in 1936, was, for all intents and purposes, ignored.

1939. *Institut Pasteur*, Dakar. Peltier points out the underlying problem: "*But up until now, due to practical problems for the most part, this vaccine was given almost*

---

* In fact, Sawyer, Kitchen and Lloyd's serovaccination[155a].

155a. Sawyer, 1931a, p. 62.

155b. Laigret, 1936c, p. 172.

156a. Sorel, 1936, p. 1325.

156b. Sorel, 1936, p. 1325.

157. Sorel, 1936, p. 1325.

exclusively to white subjects. Yet the danger of the spread of yellow fever will persist as long as we have not reached the indigenous population, which probably constitutes a major virus reservoir." [158] Therefore, what was needed was to develop a simpler method than the three-injection or even the one-injection method. Having said this, Peltier presented the results of his first trials using a combined yellow fever and smallpox vaccination, administered cutaneously, that is, by scarification. The first trials started in November 1938 and were conducted on monkeys using neurotropic virus administered by scarification on the abdomen, reproducing the experiments conducted by Beeuwkes of the Rockefeller Commission, and described at the Dakar Intercolonial Conference on April 26 or 30, 1928. Results were satisfactory. In January 1939, an experiment on 4 white volunteer adult subjects and two black subjects was successful: the virus was found in the blood of the vaccinated subjects in the ensuing days, and a subsequent seroprotection test was positive for all of them. In May 1939, 741 people had been vaccinated without any adverse effects; 90% were immunised against yellow fever[159].

1939-1940. *Institut Pasteur,* Dakar. The first trials of combined vaccination by scarification in man started in November 1938 and lasted several months; the subjects belonged to black communities where follow-up was easy. 90% of the seroprotection tests were positive; 81% of subjects presented vaccinal pustules and developed no serious side effects. A request for administering the combined vaccine to 100,000 native inhabitants of Senegal was submitted to French West Africa authorities and was accepted. The vaccinations were carried out between May and July 1939. The use of scarification made it possible to vaccinate 800 people an hour and up to 5,000 a day. The yellow fever vaccine was prepared at the Dakar *Institut Pasteur*, and the smallpox vaccine was prepared at the *Institut Pasteur* in Paris or at the Vaccine Institute located on Ballu Street in Paris. 98,873 vaccinations were performed and 2,140 serum samples were taken prior to vaccination. The colonial administration contributed greatly to the success of the vaccination sessions, with the help of the "chiefs of native districts", who had themselves and their families vaccinated first, to set the example. Testing of smallpox as well as of yellow fever vaccinations (1,678 blood samples were tested) confirmed that the Jennerian vaccine combined with the yellow fever vaccine produced the same rate of success as it did when used alone. As for the yellow fever vaccine, 95% of seroprotection tests were positive. The inoculations were very well tolerated, even by infants. There were no signs of neurotropic yellow fever virus transmission by mosquitoes found in the blood of recently vaccinated individuals[160]. In 1940, 400,000 people had already been vaccinated[161].

1941. French West Africa. On December 10, yellow fever vaccination was made compulsory in French West Africa[162]. In Senegal, starting in 1942, the implementation of the quadrennial yellow fever vaccination plan using the Dakar vaccine has led to the absence of reported cases of this disease since 1953, whereas the 12 serious epidemics that had occurred between 1779 and 1942 had claimed numerous lives, and many isolated cases continued to occur over the years. Very soon, serological studies

158. Peltier, 1939, p. 657.
159. Peltier, 1939, p. 657; Husson, 1953, p. 735.
160. Peltier, 1940a, p. 137; Peltier, 1940b, p. 146.
161. Husson, 1953, p. 735.
162. Husson, 1953, p. 735.

conducted by the *Institut Pasteur* in Dakar revealed an immunisation rate of 74%, even 55% in some regions and 39% in children under 10 years.

1944. *Institut Pasteur,* Dakar. 11 million inhabitants had received the Dakar yellow fever vaccine. Tests on 2,490 subjects showed that immunity was acquired by 95% of those vaccinated[163].

1945. *Institut Pasteur,* Dakar. The United Nations Relief and Rehabilitation Administration (UNRRA) entrusted an international commission with the task of comparing the Dakar vaccine to the 17D vaccine (*see later its origin*). Three groups of 200 military men, who had arrived directly from France, were vaccinated. The Dakar vaccine came out ahead in immunisation tests (*see immunisation or protection tests, page 418*), with 98.94% positive results in a group of 200 subjects who had received combined Dakar and smallpox vaccine, 97.3% in the group that received the Dakar vaccine alone, and 64.29% in the 17D group. The Dakar vaccine was certainly a very high-immunogenicity vaccine, but its side effects were poorly tolerated by adults and were intolerable in children, especially very young children. The 17D strain used in this trial was still in its early years of use. The results of this rudimentary comparison were primarily intended to evaluate the immunogenicity of the Dakar vaccine, rather than test the 17D strain. Based on the Commission's report, the UNRRA Standing Committee on Health approved the yellow fever vaccine produced by the Dakar *Institut Pasteur* for international certificates; on September 11, 1946, the World Health Organization followed suite[164].

1947. *Institut Pasteur,* Dakar. The colonial administration was very happy with the results: "*The absence of yellow fever in the French territories of West Africa is now almost entirely the result of mass vaccinations of both the European and native population. Since 1941, about 15 million vaccinations were performed - a figure which corresponds almost to the total populations under census in those territories. Vaccination against yellow fever, however, had been practiced in the French territories of Western Africa since 1934, the vehicle being the neurotropic virus of the mouse, first by the procedure of Sellards-Laigret (vaccine phosphate in three injections) and later by the Laigret process (vaccine phosphate mixed with egg yolk)... to replace subcutaneous inoculation... with inoculation by the simple application of virus to cutaneous scarifications. The combined vaccinations were performed first on the Macacus rhesus and then in man... and subsequently, attention was gradually directed to subjects of both sexes and all ages, including more than 50 children from six months to one year old... The results of the last experiment were published in March, 1939. Even under those optimum conditions, it has been confirmed beyond any doubt that: 1. It is almost impossible for the neurotropic virus to develop or even to maintain itself in the Stegomyia. 2. When, by any chance, the neurotropic virus is so maintained the Stegomyia is unable to transmit it by biting, even to the most sensitive of animals - the Macacus rhesus- and much less to man... A vaccination campaign comprising 100,000 inhabitants of Senegal was authorized and undertaken during the months of May, June and July, 1939... The vaccines were very well tolerated. The neighbouring population was very carefully observed, and no manifestation of yellow fever, not even the slightest, has been noticed despite the prevalent breeding of the Stegomyia... The results of the vaccination against smallpox were controlled 8 days after the performance. The tests for*

163. Husson, 1953, p. 735.
164. Husson, 1953, p. 735.

sero-protection... Among 1,630 sera thus tested, 1,559 were found positive, or 95.6 per cent..."[165].

1947. *Institut Pasteur,* Tunis. Laigret continues to have faith in "his vaccine": "*After twelve years, we can confirm that the vaccine does not produce reactions of a serious nature. There is often high fever, but not immediately following the inoculation. When it occurs, it is only on the sixth or seventh day. The febrile episode is no more severe than an ordinary malaria attack; it lasts a few hours, rarely a whole day. No complications have been observed. The frequency of a febrile episode occurring on the sixth or seventh day is about 25 to 30 percent in humans. The ratio is smaller in women and children.*

A meningeal reaction constitutes a more serious incident, but it is rare, and even more rare today than at the start of our vaccinations. I have personally seen 13 cases. Overall, its frequency is certainly under one case in 10,000 vaccinated individuals. It appears around the fifteenth or the eighteenth day after vaccination, in the form of high fever, delirium, generally moderate stiffness of the neck, convulsions in children. Lumbar puncture extracts a fluid rich in lymphocytes. Thus, the incident replicates a lymphocytic meningeal syndrome. Recovery is spontaneous, occurring without fail within three or four days."[166]

1951. *Institut Pasteur,* Dakar. In 1951, production of Dakar vaccine included: 100 lots prepared, 88,100 phials produced for 9 million vaccinations, 37 lots of vaccine titred. In addition, 638 neutralisation tests were conducted, 633 of which were conclusive[167].

1953. *Institut Pasteur,* Dakar. Forty-two million subjects were vaccinated or revaccinated, about 110,000 of them of European origin; immunisation rates were very good. Side effects were not serious; they appeared early (5th or 6th day) or late (12th to 15th day), were meningoencephalitic in nature, and disappeared within 5 to 6 days. Vaccination was not recommended for children under 2 years, and children under 10 years in areas where viral diseases (mumps, measles, encephalitis...) were known to exist. The 17D vaccine (*see below*) was to be used in cases where the Dakar vaccine was contraindicated[168]. The method of production of the Dakar vaccine was described in detail by Husson and Koerber in 1953. The breeding of albino mice provided 15,000 animals aged 2.5 months, yearly. A system reducing the number of passages of the mouse-adapted virus to 3 in 5 years, that is, an elementary but incomplete seed lot system, was used. Brains from a passage were vacuum-dried at - 20° C, placed in vacuum sealed tubes and stored at - 20° C. Three times a week, a lot of 90 mice were inoculated with virus from a phial. The brains of mice paralysed the fourth and fifth day after inoculation were extracted and then dried and crushed in a sterile chamber, before being placed in 100-dose vials in a glove box. The vials were stored at + 4° C, and had a validity period of 2 months. Numerous sterility tests were performed throughout the production process. Several titrations were conducted during production or during vial storage (in temperate to extreme weather conditions). The vials could be transported (10 days maximum) at normal temperatures. The vaccine was reconstituted in a gum Arabic phosphate solution[169].

---

165. Peltier, 1947, p. 1026.
166. Laigret, 1947, p. 13.
167. Husson, 1953, p. 735.
168. Husson, 1953, p. 735.
169. Husson, 1953, p. 735.

This vaccine could be considered the prototype of a very efficient, economical, useful, home-made type vaccine. Its major disadvantage was the appearance of numerous serious side effects, about which Sorel had warned the concerned authorities as early as 1936.

1952. Board of Health Laboratory, Canal Zone. At the end of November 1948, a yellow fever epidemic broke out in the Atlantic region of Panama and in Costa Rica. The vaccination campaign that ensued used both the 17D vaccine and the vaccine from the *Institut Pasteur* in Dakar. The article provides no other details, and mentions no special problems related to the Dakar vaccine[170].

1953. Virus Research Institute, Lagos. "*In 1951-1952 an epidemic of yellow fever occurred in Southern Nigeria and neurotropic yellow fever vaccine was used as a method of control. This was the first occasion on which this type of vaccine had been employed on a large scale in Nigeria. The number and severity of reactions was high, so that the use of this vaccine has been discontinued. Therefore, although observations on some aspects are inadequate, it has not been possible to accumulate much data on others and they may be considered inadequate for critical scientific assessment. Nevertheless, they are all presented here as an indication of what can happen after the use of this vaccine... Cases of reaction following vaccination came from the African population in a limited area in Southern Nigeria, where a vaccination campaign was in progress to effect the control of epidemic of yellow fever. Most of the cases, however, came from areas which were not touched by or affected only to a very small degree by the epidemic... The observations on the incidence are reliable since they were made in a town where the people are hospital minded and where the registration of deaths is enforced. Neurotropic reactions were characterized by encephalitis with a high mortality rate. Five subjects were brought for autopsy within one hour of death... The histological picture is similar to that produced by other viruses which cause encephalitis in man... The low content of virus in the brain is consistent with findings in other viral encephalitis...*"[171]. These autopsies were the first to show cerebral tissue lesions. They made it possible to isolate certain yellow fever viruses in these tissues; previous research had only examined spinal fluid. Finally, the Dakar vaccine was associated with vaccinia, which could itself cause encephalitis. However, despite the fact that vaccinations were performed in the city, there is no specific data concerning the exact number of persons vaccinated, nor the number of side effects, except the febrile episodes seen in 1,238 people, and the initials of the 5 individuals who died. Strangely, this very useful article serving as a warning is lacking some essential information...

MacNamara's article also reports: "*An incidence in children of three to four per thousand vaccinations is recorded, and a case fatality of about 40 per cent. Adults, however, also were affected, but at a much lower rate; the oldest recorded age of a patient being 31 years.*"[172] But he gives no other details.

About 56 million doses were inoculated up to 1953 using the Dakar vaccine: the equivalent of two doses per inhabitant of French West Africa, on average. Thanks to this vaccine, in 1952 yellow fever was almost entirely eliminated in French West Africa, but not in Ghana or Nigeria, its neighbouring countries[173].

170. Elton, 1952, p. 170.
171. MacNamara, 1953, p. 199.
172. MacNamara, 1953, p. 199.
173. Monath *in* Plotkin, 2004, p. 1095.

The Neurotropic Strain (Dakar) Stopped Being Used as a Vaccine

1965-1966. The Francophone Medical Society of Black Africa (*Société médicale d'Afrique noire de langue française*) dedicated a session to a yellow fever epidemic that occurred in the Diourbel region in Senegal between October and December 1965. The alert was given in November, when a case of yellow fever, diagnosed with certainty, occurred after 12 years of freedom from the disease. The region affected by the epidemic included about 140,000 inhabitants, 38% of whom were children between 0 and 10 years. The region was infected with swarming *Aedes (Stegomyia) aegypti*. There had been no yellow fever epidemic in Senegal since the 1927 epidemic that produced 190 cases and caused 135 fatalities. Since then, there had been sporadic incidents of isolated or clustered cases responsible for some fatalities; these incidents reached their peak in 1937, when there were 37 cases and 30 deaths. Starting in 1939, the development of the Dakar vaccine by scarification, and its compulsory use within quadrennial programs of compulsory vaccination, achieved the gradual elimination of yellow fever from Senegal. The last cases reported were: 1 in 1942, 3 in 1943, and 2 in 1953. However, in 1960, when the danger of an epidemic seemed to have been eliminated, this achievement was marred by the number of fatal encephalitis cases following vaccination, particularly in those who were vaccinated for the first time, mostly young children. In 1960, it was decided that children under 10 years would be excluded from vaccination campaigns. Serological surveys conducted starting in 1962 showed significant fluctuations in the protection rates observed in populations, depending on age and place of residence; the surveys also showed that, alarmingly, the virus of sylvatic origin continued to circulate in certain areas of Senegal. Surveys on yellow fever-related mortality were hard to conduct because of the diversity of the symptoms: from benign fever to typical hepatonephritis, because of concomitant hepatitis epidemics, as well as language problems. The first cases appeared in October 1965, and the alert was given on November 12, after the autopsy of a young girl. The start of the epidemic apparently killed about 140 people, 90% of them children under 10 years, before prophylactic measures (vaccinations and the fight against mosquitoes) were taken. Vaccinations were performed initially in the primary epidemic area, in large cities and in the port and airport of Dakar. The Dakar vaccine was used for subjects over 10 years.

In two months, 4 tons of DDT were sprayed and the hunt for mosquito nests and for their larvae was highly effective. Very quickly, 1,989,000 vaccinations were performed, 1,869,000 with the Dakar vaccine and, in children, 120,700 with the Rockefeller 17D vaccine, whose national and international availability was limited. Health control checkpoints were set up on communication routes: roads and railways, with stringent control of passenger anti-yellow fever certificates, and turning back of non immunized persons.

The 1965-1966 yellow fever epidemic made between 2,000 and 20,000 victims, depending on the reports consulted, with a 10 to 15% mortality rate, that is, between 200 and 3,000 deaths - a range illustrating the limitations of this type of survey in terms of reliability. This epidemic was probably due to a virus of sylvatic origin, as well as to the stopping of vaccinations in the population under 10 years. It might also be the case that routine vaccination was perturbed by the establishment of Senegal's independence in 1960.

A decision was made to produce 17D vaccine, and vaccination of children with this virus was considered in 1963.

In November 1965, when the epidemic alert was given, 400,000 children had to be vaccinated urgently with the 130,000-dose available stock of 17D vaccine. In the area where the epidemic originated, the minimum age for compulsory vaccination was reduced to 2 years, and to 5 years for children in Dakar and in Cap-Vert, when it was not possible to vaccinate them using 17D vaccine. The *Institut Pasteur*, with the assistance of the USAID (United States Agency for International Development) and all the public health services in Senegal, started the vaccinations. The children were summoned by radio messages to come together at specified gathering points, and mobile teams vaccinated in remote centres that were too far from designated gathering points or cities. Vaccinations with the Dakar vaccine were performed in the usual conditions, especially in permanent centres in Dakar. Taking into account the percentage of error to be expected in a vaccination campaign of this scope, 90% of the population was vaccinated[174]. The attempt to define the rate of immunity against yellow fever in a certain Dakar population led to the conclusion that 90% of tested subjects had accepted to be vaccinated and had acquired immunity[175].

On the other hand, this victory over the emerging epidemic was accompanied by a great number of encephalitic events following vaccination with the Dakar strain vaccine. This was a foreseeable risk, since Laigret and others had drawn attention to it from the beginning of the development of the neurotropic strain Sellards-Laigret produced at the *Institut Pasteur* in Tunis and then at the *Institut Pasteur* in Dakar. When he reported on the 20,000 vaccinations performed in 1948, Peltier had considered this a negligeable problem, given the seriousness of the yellow fever threat for the population. The 1952 mass vaccination campaign in Nigeria[176] attracted attention to this risk previously considered minor, and led to the decision to stop vaccinating children under 10 years, who were the most frequent victims of these events.

The 1965 campaign conducted in Senegal resulted in immunisation with the Dakar vaccine starting at the age of 2, instead of 10 years. Between November 17 and December 7, 1965, 498,887 vaccinations by scarification were performed in the Cap-Vert region. In 1966, the report of the Board of public health of the Republic of Senegal recommends, in its conclusions: "*All the population, including the children, should be vaccinated. The Rockefeller 17D vaccine can be used in mass campaigns.*" This required a suitable structure, complex and expensive, with a cold chain for vaccine storage and with injection material[177]. Later, when a certain quantity of 17D vaccine became available, 67,326 children in the Dakar region were vaccinated subcutaneously.

Dakar hospitals treated 248 patients with encephalitis after yellow fever vaccination, and registered a mortality rate slightly below 10% (23 deaths). Rey and his associates add: "*But if the mass campaign had taken place in the usual context, we would have had to add about thirty almost fatal cases (very serious cases where death was only avoided through assiduous hospital care). The mortality rate would have risen to 22%. To these negative consequences of vaccination, we must add the fact that the*

174. Ba, 1966, p. 550.
175. Vézard, 1966, p. 557.
176. MacNamara, 1953, p. 199.
177. Wone, 1966, p. 500.

neurological prognosis of the survivors is still unclear: some of them still present anomalies after four months." Most of these patients were of African origin, and a minority were Lebanese or "Portuguese" of mixed race. No adverse effects were seen in "European" children, almost all of whom had already received the 17D vaccine at a prior date. The patients were between 1 and 20 years old, with the predominant majority ranging between 2 and 11 years. Despite the unexpected arrival of very many sick children, quite exact data were gathered concerning them[178]. The various vaccine lots and vaccination centres were excluded because no important parameters emerged in the collected data.

The 498,887 vaccinations with Dakar vaccine performed in the Cap-Vert region resulted in 231 cases of encephalitis, that is, 46 cases out of 100,000 vaccinated subjects. For first vaccinations, Rey and his associates report the risk in children between 3 and 11 years inoculated with Dakar vaccine to be 1 case in 720 vaccinated subjects, that is, about 1 to 2 cases out of 1,000. MacNamara found that in a similar age range (below 10 years) there were 3 to 4 adverse events in 1,000 vaccinated subjects. The results of Rey (1 to 2 cases out of 1,000 subjects), those of MacNamara (3 to 4 serious adverse events for 1,000 subjects) and those of Sankalé (1 out of 500 to 1,000) are not very different when compared to the results of surveys presently conducted in European countries and in North America[179].

The average incubation period was 12.5 days, ranging between 1 to 30 days. In addition to Dakar, a survey was conducted in Diourbel (25,000 inhabitants), where 35,000 vaccinations with Dakar vaccine and 10,000 with 17D vaccine were performed in children, 15,000 of them below 10 years old (5,000 with Dakar vaccine, 10,000 with 17D), and in Thiès (60,000 inhabitants) were 130,000 vaccinations were performed, including in 15,000 children between 4 and 10 years, using Dakar vaccine, and 1,500 children under 4 using 17D vaccine. Early reactions occurring on the 5th and 6th day were seen in 17% of those vaccinated with Dakar vaccine, and in 11% of those vaccinated with 17D vaccine. Two fatalities from early-onset encephalitis occurred following vaccination with 17D vaccine, one of them being an anaphylactic type reaction. Reactions occurring later (12th to 15th day) were cases of meningoencephalitis (19 cases) in children under 10 years old vaccinated for the first time with Dakar vaccine. "*Even if only half the cases were identified, the frequency ratio of meningoencephalitis cases due to the Dakar vaccine can be evaluated at about 1 out of 30,000 vaccinated subjects in all age groups, and at 1 out of 500 or 1,000 vaccinated children under 10 years.*"[180a]

In 1966, Bres and Robin presented a list of benign, serious and even lethal meningoencephalitic reactions, to which we can add those that occurred during the 1965 Dakar vaccination campaign (Table I).

178. Bert, 1966, p. 591; Bres, 1966, p. 610; Collomb, 1966a, p. 575; Collomb, 1966b, p. 587; Lemercier, 1966, p. 601.
179. Bres, 1966, p. 610; MacNamara, 1953, p. 199; Sankalé, 1966, p. 617.
180a. Sankalé, 1966, p. 617; Payet, 1966, p. 597.

Table I. Meningoencephalitic reactions (benign, serious or lethal) that occured during vaccination campaigns (Bres & Robin)[180b & c].

Site	Year	Cases	Number of deaths	Vaccinations	Remarks on the vaccinated
Brazzaville	1944	102	18	102,000	60% under 10 years
Dakar	1950	20	2	?	Children (ages not specified)
Costa Rica	1951	13	3	?	Under 13 years
Hunduras	1952	2	?	1,200	?
Nigeria	1952	83	32	142,000	Under 10 years in the case of 29 deaths
Congo-Léopoldville	1958	98	9	116,000	Children (under 10 years?)
Cameroun	1959	76	9	57,000	Under 10 years
Dakar	1965	234	23 (in hospital environment)	498,887	Children between 2 and 11 years (in 90% of cases)

When looking at these 1965 data, it must be kept in mind that 27 years had passed since 1939, when the vaccine was first used, that 158,000,000 doses had been produced since that time, and that, according to Bres and Robin, at least two thirds of these doses had been used. Mass vaccinations in Ghana (1951-1952) with 922,000 doses of vaccine provided by the Dakar *Institut Pasteur*, and in Ethiopia (1960-1962), where 1,250,000 persons over 10 years were vaccinated, must be included in these data. Numerous hypotheses were advanced to explain these wide fluctuations: insufficient dosages, different neurotoxicities of the yellow fever virus vaccine depending on the number of passage in mice (125th passage in 1931, 132nd passage in 1932, 256th to 258th in 1947, different strains of yellow fever virus, simultaneous action of a pathogenic agent...[181].

The *Institut Pasteur* in Dakar stopped producing Dakar vaccine in 1982.

Murine Vaccine with Virulence Modified in Tissue Culture

1932. The yellow fever virus, adapted to mice by the intracerebral technique, and the least pathogenic for man, had become neurotropic; this constituted a major obstacle to its use for vaccinations, be it using the serovaccination technique (Sawyer) or Laigret's "super-attenuated" (?) pure virus method. Adverse postvaccinal events in children under 10 years vaccinated for the first time could not be ignored; they rarely occurred in adults. Serovaccination with Theiler's neurotropic viral strain and with human or animal immunosera (from recovering subjects) seemed to cause few postvaccinal adverse events, but the possibility of such occurrences could not be excluded.

In 1907, the development of cell and tissue cultures outside living organisms became well established thanks to Harrison[182], Carrel and many others. Soon, the idea of

180b. Bres, 1966, p. 610.
180c. Sankalé, 1966, p. 617; Payet, 1966, p. 597.
181. Bres, 1966, p. 610; Rey, 1966, p. 560; Sankalé, 1966, p. 617.
182. Nicholas, 1961, p. 130.

cultivating "viruses" in *in vitro* systems, and of attempting to modify them, emerged. The need to reduce the virulence and the neurotropic character of the Theiler murine strain was at the origin of this type of approach.

Theiler's laboratory based its work on Rivers and Ward's studies on cowpox virus culture in medium composed of minced chick embryo tissue (1g) suspended in Tyrode's solution (40-50 ml). These authors summarized their work as follows: "*Indeed, the virus* (cowpox) *that has been cultivated for 2 years in the manner described induced little or no reaction in rabbits. Material from these cultures, however, gave rise to typical vaccinal pustules in man. This observation appears to us to be of importance and among other things seems to indicate that a virus of a desired character for human use can be produced by culture methods. In view of the findings presented at this time, it is believed that the change in the reactivity of the virus for the rabbit was not due entirely - and perhaps not at all - to a gradual diminution in the amount of virus in successive sets of cultures, but to some alteration in the character of the virus itself.*"[183] Rivers and Ward were considering the possibility of diminished virulence, an idea not yet elucidated at the time, although it was not new: the cowpox virus was considered the causal agent of smallpox, transformed by passage to bovines. But these authors were not considering the option of modifying virus tropism.

1932-1933, Rockefeller Foundation, New York. In 1932, Eugen Haagen and Max Theiler grew a neurotropic strain (produced by means of repeated passages in mouse brain) of the yellow fever virus. At first, they obtained a successful culture by using the hanging drop technique, but they did not produce a continuous series. The latter was eventually obtained using rabbit kidney, or rabbit or guinea pig testicle cells, in Tyrode solution with monkey serum in Carrel flask[184].

Finally, they were able to grow the virus in a mixture of normal (*monkey*) serum and Tyrode solution in which were suspended small fragments of fresh tissue of minced chicken embryos 8 to 10 days old in Carrel flask.[185] Haagen and Theiler specified: "*The infectivity tests were always done in mice. All mice inoculated intracerebrally with the 22nd subculture showed typical symptoms of encephalitis with paralysis.*"[186] When grown in chick embryo cells, the neurotropic virus remained neurotropic.

1934-1936. Rockefeller Foundation, New York. Lloyd and collaborators repeated Haagen and Theiler's studies, starting with a natural yellow fever strain, instead of a neurotropic strain. But he arrived at the same result, that is, no clear change in virus tropism[187].

1935-1936. Wellcome Laboratories, London. Findlay and Clarke[188] showed that repeated passages of the neurotropic strain in monkey liver (of species susceptible to the virus) produce the reversal of the virus to a pantropic strain: "*It is thus obvious that the pathogenicity of the yellow fever virus may vary within wide limits in accordance with the particular environment in which the virus lives, neurotropism being accentuated by growth in brain tissue, pantropism by growth in the liver.*"[189] "*In a further*

183. Rivers, 1931, p. 453; Rivers, 1933, p. 635.
184. Plotz *in* Levaditi, 1938, p. 1134.
185. Haagen, 1932, p. 435.
186. Haagen, 1932, p. 435.
187. Lloyd, 1936, p. 481.
188. Findlay, 1935, p. 579.
189. Findlay, 1936, p. 213.

experimental trial of the truth of this concept, Findlay (1935) has passaged both the neurotropic and viscerotropic (pantropic) yellow fever viruses through a (in vivo) *transplantable mouse carcinoma. In this environment of young, actively growing, relatively undifferentiated cells of mouse, Findlay has already gained some evidence that the pantropic virus is losing its viscerotropic activity.*"[190] In fact, in 1936 Findlay published a very detailed list of examples of virulence or tropism modification in a large number of viruses causing human or animal diseases[191]. This very careful bibliographical work indicated that it could perhaps be possible to obtain a vaccinating yellow fever virus strain with no risk of serious neurotropic side effects, which represented the most serious postvaccinal adverse events.

The Origin of the 17D Strain

1935. Rockefeller Foundation, New York. According to Lloyd, "*for a more detailed study, the virus chosen, initially pantropic, grown in flasks in a medium consisting of minced murine embryonic tissue, gradually lost its pathogenic viscerotropic power. This strain was passaged over 130 times in the same medium over a period of 21 months.*"[192]

This yellow fever viral strain was used to immunise 20 people, by means of the serovaccination method developed by Sawyer and his associates[193]. The subjects received between 23,000 and 170,000 minimal lethal doses (MLD) for mice, with human immunoserum ranging between 0.5 and 0.6 cm^3 per kilo of body weight. Side effects following vaccination were quite benign or absent, despite a large number of MLDs. Protective antibody titres grew rapidly for two weeks, but decreased very rapidly as well[194].

This indicated that affinity in the yellow fever virus could be modified using suitable techniques, the simplest of which was cultivated in a selected culture medium. This procedure was carried out by Lloyd, Theiler and Ricci in 1936[195].

1936. Rockefeller Foundation, New York. Lloyd, Theiler and Ricci grew the "Asibi pantropic", "French neurotropic" (305 mouse brain passages) and "French neurotropic" (105 mouse brain passage) yellow fever virus strains in several selected culture media (minced tissue of mouse embryo, chicken embryo and adult mouse testis), suspended in Tyrode solution with serum in 25 or 50 cc. Erlenmeyer flasks, according to Carrel, Rivers and Ward[196]. "*Pantropic yellow fever virus has been cultivated for more than 130 subcultures in media consisting of serum-Tyrode solution and minced tissue of mouse embryo, chicken embryo or adult mouse testis... Neurotropic yellow fever virus of both relatively early and late mouse passage has been cultivated for more than 120 subcultures in a medium of serum-Tyrode solution and containing minced chicken embryo tissue... The cultivated strains of pantropic yellow fever virus have exhibited consistently in* Macacus rhesus *a progressive loss of the power to provoke yellow fever following inoculation... The antigenic power for immune man of the neurotropic virus of mouse brain origin and the cultivated pantropic virus of mouse embryonic tissue origin is approximately the same... The results of the immunization of 26 persons with pantropic yellow fever virus cultivated in mouse embryonic tissue, in the presence of an existing passive immunity produced by the concomitant injection of a titrated*

190. Lloyd, 1936, p. 481.
191. Findlay, 1936b, p. 213.
192. Lloyd, 1935, p. 2365.
193. Sawyer, 1931a, p. 62.
194. Lloyd, 1935, p. 2365.
195. Lloyd, 1936, p. 481.
196. Carrel, 1927, p. 848; Rivers, 1931, p. 453; Rivers, 1933, p. 635.

quantity of human immune serum are recorded. The sera of thirteen individuals in this group which were titrated for protective antibodies during the period from 14 to 28 days following inoculation showed titres ranging from 8 to + 256."[197] Lloyd, Theiler and Ricci grew various yellow fever virus strains, without modifying their immunising effect, but the viruses... "*exhibited consistently a progressive loss of power to provoke yellow fever following inoculation*" in *Macacus rhesus*[198].

1936. Rockefeller Foundation. Sawyer's serovaccination is still used; the strain chosen, cultivated on *in vitro* living cells, has lost much of its viscerotropic virulence without acquiring the high degree of neurotropism resulting from repeated passages in mouse brain. Because human antiserum was difficult to obtain and the dose required was 40cc for a medium-weight subject, it was replaced by hyperimmune monkey serum[199].

1936-1937. Rockefeller Foundation. Theiler and Smith continued the Lloyd, Theiler and Ricci experiments. In June 1937, the strain cultivated in mouse embryonic tissue medium was resown more than 240 times over a period of 3 years. It was designated as 17E[200]. After 18 cultures, a subline was introduced into a medium containing minced whole chick embryo, and maintained through 58 subcultures; the medium was then modified and the brain and spinal cord were removed from the embryo before mincing. The virus remained in the medium throughout, for over 160 subcultures. This strain was named 17D[201]. Theiler and Smith continued these experiments and wrote: "*Experimental evidence is presented to show that prolonged cultivation of yellow fever virus in vitro results in a change in its pathogenicity, and that this change varies with the type of tissues used for cultivation... Three different types of tissues were used... They included whole mouse embryo, chick embryo from which the head and spinal cord had been removed, and testicular tissues of mice and guinea pigs...*"[202]. The changes in the pathogenicity of the virus cultivated in medium containing tissues of chick embryo from which the head and spinal cord had been removed were very pronounced. The neurotropic virulence of the virus was lost to a large extent, between the 89th and the 114th passages... Its neurotropism was also much diminished between the 114th and the 176th passages...[203].

1936 or 1937. Rockefeller Foundation. Three animal species, very susceptible to the yellow fever virus, were tested: mouse, monkey and hedgehog. So, monkeys inoculated by peripheral routes did not develop encephalitis; those inoculated intracerebrally developed histopathological changes, but only 5-19% succumbed to encephalitis. The animals developed antibodies and were resistant to the test inoculation with Asibi virus. These studies showed that virus grown for more than 200 subcultures in chick embryo from which the head and spinal cord had been removed would be harmless for man. Four persons immunised against yellow fever were inoculated with doses of between 44,000 and 330,000 MLDs of 17D virus. Subsequently, 8 non-immunised subjects were vaccinated with doses between 50,000 and 3,000,000 MLD. Reactions were minimal and sera taken 2 to 4 weeks after inoculation showed the presence of yellow fever antibodies[204].

---

197. Lloyd, 1936, p. 481.
198. Lloyd, 1936, p, 481.
199. Theiler, 1936, p. 2354.
200. Theiler, 1937a, p. 767.
201. Theiler, 1937a, p. 767.
202. Theiler, 1937b, p. 787.
203. Theiler, 1937a, p. 767.
204. Theiler, 1937b, p. 787; Smith, 1937a, p. 801.

1936. Wellcome Laboratories, London. Starting in November 1932, Findlay and his associates vaccinated 951 persons against yellow fever, using serovaccination: 736 in London and the rest in Africa. The living virus used was the neurotropic strain in the first few years, and later the pantropic virus attenuated over several years in tissue culture. The 17D strain was introduced in Great Britain in 1936; Colonial Service employees were vaccinated with this strain. A few cases of jaundice were observed. The initial doses of antiserum were of human origin; subsequently, they were of equine origin, according to Pettit and Stefanopoulo. Mouse embryos in the culture were replaced with chick embryos, as a precaution against the lymphocytic choriomeningitis virus that can be present in healthy-looking mice. The virus used was harvested after a single passage in mice, performed cerebrally[205].

1936. *Institut Pasteur*, Paris. Lépine drew attention to the problem of a murine virus (several strains of lymphocytic choriomeningitis virus had already been identified), and maintained that these viruses are frequent and deserve the attention of those who perform yellow fever vaccinations[206].

1937. Rockefeller Foundation. A second article written by Theiler and Smith describes immune reaction in monkeys, and the protection they acquire against the very virulent yellow fever virus after inoculation with the 17D viral strain. Results were very satisfactory and side effects were minimal[207]. A third article by these authors analyses the contrasting effects of previous cultures and shows that: "*There is evidence to indicate that a prolonged cultivation of the virus in mouse embryo brain medium increases its neutrotropic properties*."[208]

Soon afterwards, Smith, Penna and Paoliello presented the results of over 59,000 vaccinations with the 17D strain without immune serum, 95% of which conferred immunity. Antibodies appeared between the 7th and the 21rst day after inoculation. Side effects were limited to headaches and slight fever. The virus was detected in the blood on the 5th, 6th or 7th day after vaccination[209].

Large-Scale Production of the 17D Yellow Fever Vaccine

To facilitate large-scale production, Theiler was able to transfer the 17D strain from chick tissue culture to the developing egg itself, using Goodpasture's technique.

1937. Rockefeller Foundation, New York. In 1937, various viruses were grown on embryonated eggs, and the technique had been mastered. Wild yellow fever virus strains, as well as strains adapted to *in vitro* tissue culture, had all been easily cultivated in embryonated eggs[210]. The vaccine was prepared by grinding up chick embryos infected with the living attenuated 17D strain, and drying the culture from the frozen state. The vaccine was reconstituted in sterile normal saline, and a single dose, usually 0.5ml, was injected subcutaneously[211].

205. Findlay, 1936a, p. 1321; Lloyd, 1936, p. 481.
206. Lépine, 1936, p. 236.
207. Theiler, 1937b, p. 787.
208. Smith, 1937, p. 801.
209. Smith, 1938, p. 437.
210. Elmendorf, 1937, p. 171.
211. Gell, 1962, p. 756.

By 1939, over 1 million people had received the 17D vaccine without severe complications[212]. In 1940, the 17D vaccinal strain had already been used to immunise 40 million people. It was undoubtedly one of the most widely-used vaccines in the world[213].

During the Second World War, the 17D vaccinal strain was used to immunise the allied troops stationed in West Africa. Unfortunately, between March and September 1942, among the 2.5 million vaccinated American soldiers, there were 28,600 cases of jaundice and 62 deaths. A small quantity of so-called normal serum was used to dilute the vaccine; several lots of this serum were contaminated by a hepatitis virus[214]. Burnet's figures are quite different: "*The first widespread recognition of the condition* (serum hepatitis or homologous serum jaundice) *came in the early months of 1942 when about 80,000 American servicemen developed jaundice for no apparent reason. Investigation showed that the factor common to all units in which cases of jaundice developed was that they had been inoculated with certain batches of yellow fever vaccine.*"[215]

This was confirmed by Clark: "*This vaccine* (17D), *too* (just like the Dakar strain), *has its serious difficulties with 20,585 cases of jaundice, some of them fatal, occurring among about 2.5 million American troops vaccinated. Subsequent studies showed that these reactions were not due to the mutant yellow fever virus, but to the fact that some lots of the supposedly normal human serum used as a diluent in the preparation of the vaccine contained contaminating serum hepatitis virus. Since the omission of this human serum, the serum jaundice has not followed the use of the acqueous base of 17D vaccine.*"[216]

The 17D vaccine encountered difficulties, like all other vaccines. In time, "substrains" of the 17D strain emerged; one of them was not providing proper immunisation, another produced cases of encephalitis, causing the death of one child[217]. In 1942, in a group of 35,073 vaccinated subjects, 273 suffered abnormally severe reactions to yellow fever vaccine inoculations, and 199 of them showed evidence of neurological involvement. This reaction pattern was very different from the one that emerged in previous field studies. The increased pathogenicity was attributed to a series of 20 passages in tissue culture, and three to five passages in chick embryo of the original 17D substrain, during which a reversion to virulence had occurred[218]. Avian leukosis virus contaminants were discovered in vaccine lots and eliminated by various methods.

Panthier (1956) reported 7 cases of nervous reactions, detected in a population of over 100,000 vaccinated subjects; only infants less than one year old presented these reactions. Three of these cases could have been due to a variation in a substrain, similar to that described by Fox (1942). The author recommended that, with the exception of special epidemiological emergencies, yellow fever vaccination should not be given to children under one year[219].

A few cases of encephalitis in infants following vaccination with 17D yellow fever virus were reported by Smith in 1954, one case was described by Haas (1954) and another by Scott (1954); Parish reported a case in 1954 as well. "*The incidence of the*

212. Monath, 1999, p. 815.
213. Parish, 1965, p. 262.
214. Parish, 1965, p. 262.
215. Burnet, 1959, p. 172.
216. Clark, 1961, p. 64.
217. Parish, 1965, p. 269.
218. Fox, 1942, p. 117.
219. Panthier, 1956, p. 477.

complications is not known. In Glasgow over the period January 1, 1950 to December 31, 1954, 17,040 persons of all ages were vaccinated with 17D yellow fever virus with no more than an occasional report of malaise or sickness. Of this 17,040, however, only 103 were children of 3 months or younger and only 174 were under the age of 7 months. If it is a complication of young infants the incidence may be underestimated if it is taken in relation to the total numbers of persons vaccinated irrespective of age."[220]

As early as 1951, the WHO expert committee on yellow fever vaccine recommended that the seed lot system with primary and secondary seeds be used for vaccine production. In 1969, the WHO International Health Regulations demanded the use of the 17D vaccine for the issuing of vaccination certificates. In 1975, the WHO stipulated that 17D vaccine strains be identified and controlled.

Aside from these cases, only two cases of encephalitis were reported in the medical literature (1960 and 1966) in the United States, following the use of the 17D vaccine prepared using the seed lot system and distributed in many tens of millions of doses[221].

1953-1954. *Institut Pasteur,* Paris. Panthier described the material developed to prepare the yellow fever vaccine, strain 17D, that was obviously widely used[222].

Discussion and Controversy Surrounding the Various Yellow Fever Vaccine Protocols. The Neurotropic Strain Vaccine Ceased to Be Used. A Consensus Regarding the 17D Vaccine...

For several years, methods of vaccination that included the Rockefeller Foundation's serovaccination, that of the Pasteur Institutes in Tunis and Dakar, as well as Theiler's 17D strain, were in competition. The arguments defending a particular method were sometimes scientifically grounded, and sometimes more emotional than rational... But the discussion became centred around the Sellards-Laigret-Peltier Dakar method as soon as the procedure was developed in 1932...

1934. Wellcome Laboratories. Findlay published an assessment of the technique developed by Laigret and used on rhesus monkeys; the author concluded: "*Experiments are recorded on the immunization of rhesus monkeys against yellow fever by Laigret's method, which involves attenuation of the virus by exposure for varying periods at 20° C. The development of immunity appears to be correlated with the circulation of living neurotropic virus in the peripheral blood stream. One of the monkeys developed encephalitis after an injection of supposedly attenuated virus. In view of the danger attendant on the circulation of active neurotropic virus in the blood stream this method is not recommended for human immunization.*"[223] Findlay's conclusions were probably correct but they had to be compared to Laigret's.

1934. *Institut Pasteur,* Dakar. Laigret responded to his critics in these terms:

"*Aside from the method we applied in West Africa, there is only one other... This method is serovaccination. It uses the yellow fever murine virus, following an immune serum injection. It involves neither attenuation nor titration. It is a blind procedure. The reactions it produces are complex. Some are due to the virus; they resemble those seen after inoculation with the virus alone. In addition, some reactions are due to the serum: fever, rashes, etc. Repeat inoculations become impossible because of the anaphylactic effects: this explains why the*

220. Thomson, 1955, p. 182.
221. Freestone, 1994, p. 481.
222. Panthier, 1956, p. 616.
223. Findlay, 1934c, p. 983.

immunity obtained is of shorter duration: antibodies disappear from the blood after the sixth month following serovaccination. Moreover, the serovaccination principle has been disqualified for a long time."[224] He also commented: "*The practice of injecting, at the same time as the virus, an antiserum* (human or animal serum from a subject cured of yellow fever) *in no way diminishes the danger...*"[225].

1934. Dakar Faculty of Medicine. Blanchard, the director of this Faculty, described clearly the tendencies existing in medical schools.

The first, encountered in Tunis and represented by Sellards and Laigret initially, and later by Laigret alone, advocated and defended the use of the vaccine from virus with attenuated virulence but high neurotropism, administered in small titrated quantities, often called Dakar vaccine or strain, comparing it to Sawyer and Kitchen's serovaccination; the latter is, in fact, the one chosen by the Pasteur Institute in Paris (vaccination method used by Pettit and Stefanopoulo) to immunise "colonial" subjects leaving for West Africa. According to Blanchard, this method was not effective enough[226]. Clearly even within "France", there were two schools of thought (two Pasteur Institutes: in Paris and in Dakar) which were politely but firmly opposed.

1935. International Health Division, Rockefeller Foundation. "*It was considered an essential factor that a certain time after the vaccination the virus not be detected in the peripheral circulation. This safety criterion was adopted after numerous experiments on rhesus monkeys... After subcutaneous injection of the yellow fever neurotropic virus, a small percentage of rhesus monkeys develop encephalitis and die. In our laboratory, we have observed that when we inject extremely low doses of virus, encephalitis has a greater chance of developing... We prevent encephalitis by injecting, at the same time as the virus, suitable quantities of immunoserum... this discussion on the safety of vaccination methods started in response to Laigret's announcement that he vaccinated a large number of people against yellow fever by using a living neurotropic virus alone. There were no fatalities, contrary to what we might have expected based on our experiments on monkeys, and there were few very strong reactions due to central nervous system involvement... based on these experiments, as well as those conducted by Findlay, we can see that Laigret's method, with its three forms of preparation, leads to various degrees of virus inactivation, rather than to the attenuation of the virus... There are many indications that the hematocephalic barrier of young animals is more permeable to certain agents than that of adults... the ideal yellow fever vaccine has not yet been developed. Laigret has shown very clearly that the yellow fever neurotropic virus can be used, at least in adults, with only a slight risk of producing effects on the central nervous system. His method could probably be simplified... At present, the method using the neurotropic virus and immunoserum at the same time appears to be the method of choice...*"[227]. Theiler and collaborators were to continue looking for a third method, with reason...

1935. Wellcome Laboratories. "*In view of the danger attendant on the circulation of active neurotropic virus in the blood stream this method* (Laigret-Sellards) *is not recommended for human immunization.*"[228]

1936. Wellcome Laboratories. Later, Findlay concluded an article by making the following recommendation: "*At present, it is not advisable that the pantropic virus cultivated*

224. Laigret, 1934a, p. 1593.
225. Laigret, 1934b, p. 1078.
226. Blanchard, 1934, p. 223.
227. Theiler, 1934b, p. 347; Theiler, 1935, p. 1342.
228. Findlay, 1934c, p. 983.

in tissue should be used alone, since we have experimental proof that the attenuated virus can be easily reactivated."[229a]

1936. Wellcome Laboratories. "*Simplification in yellow fever immunization has been accomplished by the procedure of Sellards and Laigret*[229b]*, later modified by Laigret*[229c] *in which active but allegedly attenuated virus was used without serum. The safety of this procedure has been questioned by Theiler and Whitman*[229d] *and its efficiency by Findlay*[229e]*.*"[230]

1936. *Institut Pasteur*, Brazzaville. Febrile reactions with jaundice were relatively frequent in equatorial Africa. Saleun and Ceccaldi raised the question of whether there might exist a viral disease that provokes in man clinical symptoms and organic lesions similar to spirochetosis and yellow fever[231]. Viral hepatitis was not very well known at that time, and this complicated the fight against yellow fever.

1936. *Institut Pasteur*, Tunis. Laigret defended his vaccine. He reminded his readers of the difficulties inherent to the development of any vaccine, especially a "living vaccine": "*The accidents associated with the smallpox inoculation no longer count in the face of the benefits of Jennerian vaccination.*

The undeniable risk of what was called laboratory rabies does not diminish the value of the Pasteurian preventive treatment for those have been bitten. G. Blanc in Morocco and our own team in Tunisia and Algeria performed thousands of vaccinations against exanthematic typhus with living virus whose safety is not absolute; this did not prevent us from showing that such vaccinations are useful. Girard's living plague vaccine deserves the same favourable conclusion. At present, at least 12,000 people have been vaccinated against yellow fever; out of these 12,000 individuals, 4 have had nervous reactions, with no ensuing fatalities. Adverse events following yellow fever vaccination can in no way be compared for an instant to the dangers of yellow fever… It has been claimed that injecting a protective serum beforehand would prevent such incidents… Mr. Darré and Mr. Mollaret have just reported on a case of meningoencephalitis during yellow fever serovaccination… serovaccination has not kept its promise. Using serum as an adjunct to the vaccine only adds the disadvantages of a needless serotherapy to those of the living virus… Yellow fever is disappearing in Africa. This is the only thing to consider."[232]

Following the publication of a report[233] by General Sorel, French Medical Inspector, evaluating 3-stage Sellards-Laigret vaccinations between June 1934 and December 1935, whose conclusions were rather reserved, Laigret responded by saying that the four or five postvaccinal meningeal reactions known to have occurred in a total of 20,000 vaccinations were cured leaving no sequellae[234].

Laigret continued to argue for risk/benefit evaluation on the scale of entire populations, and not on an individual scale. Mollaret (*Institut Pasteur*, Paris) responded to this by saying that "*the low percentage of yellow fever vaccination accidents presently observed is not to be considered negligeable*", and by recommending additional studies to improve the

229a. Findlay, 1936a, p. 1321; Lloyd, 1936, p. 481.
229b. Sellards, 1932b, p. 1609.
229c. Laigret, 1934b, p. 1078.
229d. Theiler, 1935, p. 1342.
229e. Findlay, 1934c, p. 983.
230. Gordon, 1936, p. 221.
231. Saleun, 1936, p. 661.
232. Laigret, 1936a, p. 230.
233. Sorel, 1936, p. 1325.
234. Laigret, 1936b, p. 823.

safety of the Laigret vaccine; he added: "*Personally, I remain convinced of the need to continue vaccinating against smallpox as well as yellow fever.*"[235] Moreover, Lépine (*Institut Pasteur*, Paris) insisted on the benefits of the Laigret vaccine: "*The principle of vaccination cannot be called into question even if its benefits are obtained at the cost of a few incidents or accidents seen with any vaccination method, but especially with vaccines containing living viruses.*"[236] But he stressed the problems associated with this vaccination.

1938. *Institut Pasteur*, Dakar. Mathis responded more objectively to the arguments against the Dakar vaccine: "*These various vaccines have been criticised for their potential to transmit yellow fever to unvaccinated individuals without any proof of the validity of this hypothesis. These vaccines have also been criticised for producing serious side effects, including postvaccinal nervous reactions that Mathis considers normal signs of experimental yellow fever.*"[237]

It is tempting, of course, to compare MacNamara's article to earlier publications by Peltier or Laigret. "*Our first trials in man, which began in November 1938 and were carried out over the next months in hundreds of black subjects belonging to communities with easy access for follow-up (Dakar Marine, schools in Dakar and Rufisque), produced 90 percent positive results for seroprotection; 81 percent of subjects were carriers of vaccinal pustules. No serious general reaction was observed.*"[238]

In 1940, 98,873 combined vaccinations (yellow fever and smallpox) were performed by scarification in French West Africa. "*On certain days we vaccinated over 5,000 people, including subjects of both sexes and of all ages, from infants to the elderly... Inoculations were very well tolerated, even by infants.*" Peltier's second publication gives precise details concerning vaccination sites and the number of subjects vaccinated[239]. "*The facility and safety of the new method* (yellow fever vaccination) *having thus been established and in view of the numerous dangers confronting the troops stationed in French West Africa, the public authorities decided in the latter part of 1941 to make the vaccination against yellow fever by the method of the* Institut Pasteur *of Dakar compulsory for all the military and civilian populations of those regions... On January 1, 1946, the total of simple or mixed vaccinations against yellow fever reached the figure 14,330,735 for a total population of about 16 million inhabitants... French Africa is beginning to reap the fruits of the effort... thus there were 17 confirmed cases in 1941, 10 in 1942, 12 in 1943, 2 in 1944, one doubtful case in 1945, and none at all during the first semester of 1946. Among these cases of yellow fever, 6 were in individuals who were supposed to have been vaccinated by the Dakar method. It is probable that almost all of these cases have to do with persons hostile to the vaccinations who deliberately wiped off the vaccines immediately after the scarification...*"[240].

In 1953, Laigret wrote: "*It was the first time* (in 1934) *I saw a case of meningoencephalitis due to yellow fever vaccination. Since then, I have seen 10 other cases...*"[241].

If we pursue an approximate but reasonable train of thought, considering that at least 20 million people of African and European origin were vaccinated with the vaccine produced by the *Institut Pasteur* in Dakar, and that 10 percent were children (under 10 years), which is, *a priori*, a minimal percentage, MacNamara's figures would translate

235. Mollaret, 1936b, p. 234.
236. Lépine, 1936, p. 236.
237. Mathis *in* Levaditi, 1938, p. 820.
238. Peltier, 1940a, p. 137.
239. Peltier, 1940b, p. 146.
240. Peltier, 1947, p. 1026.
241. Laigret, 1953 (1966), p. 2441.

into 6,000 and 8,000 cases of postvaccinal encephalitis and between 2,400 and 3,200 fatalities, which could not fail to be known by those responsible for vaccination campaigns and would be difficult to hide from health authorities and from the national and international press. The first encephalitis symptoms would have appeared 10 to 13 days after vaccination, and fatalities would have occurred between 11 and 23 days later. These approximate figures raise questions about the numbers reported on the one hand by Laigret and Peltier, and on the other hand by MacNamara and Stones. Perhaps a different inoculation technique or a mutant virus are factors to consider, but the latter would only have appeared when MacNamara performed his vaccinations... or the facts reported by both Laigret and/or MacNamara could be incorrect...

On the other hand, the yellow fever vaccine produced by the *Institut Pasteur* in Dakar caused many and serious adverse reactions, and was dangerous for children, especially very young children. The arrival of a safer vaccine, the 17D strain, made it possible to stop using this dangerous vaccination in children under 10 years starting in 1960.

A more temperate perspective was expressed by Clark in 1961: "*The Dakar neurotropic mouse-adapted strain, studied extensively by Peltier and associates, has been employed in over 20 million vaccinations in French African colonies from 1939 to 1948 with resulting successful antibody formation and reduction in incidence of the disease. Unfortunately a number of severe reactions have developed following use, some of them fatal. A safer vaccine is the 17D relatively avirulent, mutant virus developed by Max Theiler of the Rockefeller Foundation. This vaccine was tested severely during World War II when thousands of troops, British and others, were vaccinated and subsequently exposed to possible infection, with exceedingly few cases of the disease developing; also in South America in the general population and among yellow fever workers where the incidence was formerly high, they now work with safety. This vaccine, too, has had its serious difficulties with 20,585 cases of jaundice, some of them fatal, occurring among about 2.5 million American troops vaccinated. Subsequent studies showed that these reactions were not due to the mutant yellow fever virus, but to the fact that some lots of supposedly normal human serum used as a diluent in the preparation of the vaccine contained contaminating serum hepatitis virus.*"[242]

The Rockefeller 17D vaccine has been repeatedly improved since the 1950s. Accounts of this work described by Monath are available in the literature[243].

Conclusion

"*Manifestly there is no royal road in establishing control of any disease.*"
Clark, 1961[244].

Yellow fever is a good illustration of the difficulties encountered in the study of a serious disease with poorly known characteristics, epidemic or endemic, whose pathogenic agent is not clearly identified and whose reservoir is uncertain, for which a vaccine is difficult to develop because the pathogenic agent involved is highly virulent, with no animal model initially, then the monkey - difficult to handle, and finally the mouse, and recourse to tissue cultures...

242. Clark, 1961, p. 64.
243. Monath *in* Plotkin, 2008, p. 959.
244. Clark, 1961, p. 64.

Man's fight against yellow fever was chaotic, long, painful, fraught with difficulties... To whom should the yellow fever vaccine be attributed? To Finlay for the hypothesis of transmission by mosquitoes, to Reed for identifying a viral origin, to Stokes for the "monkey" model, to Theiler for the "mouse" model? The first vaccinations were performed by Sawyer, Kitchen and Lloyd; mass vaccinations were conducted by Sellards and Laigret. Haagen, Lloyd, Smith and Theiler are responsible for tissue cultures and Smith for clinical trials... so many people...

It is difficult to take a definite stand in favour of one of the two schools: Sellard-Laigret (pure virus, more or less modified) and Sawyer (serovaccination), at least in the context of the time when they were being used. By contrast, it is clear that Theiler's work considerably improved yellow fever immunisation methods, achieving good immunity combined with greatly reduced, albeit not absent, adverse effects, except for the very young child.

Vaccinology has not often attracted the attention of the Nobel Foundation and of those who constitute the successive committees selecting Nobel Prize winners. Many are eligible, few are selected. A Nobel Prize was awarded to Max Theiler, inventor of a yellow fever vaccine, who undoubtedly deserved it; but was he the only one to deserve it? The necessarily restrictive nature of this prize is antitethical to any historical perspective. It involves excessive oversimplification well-suited to the mass media that use it as an eye-catching headline...

For a long time, excellent relations existed between the teams working on yellow fever: loans of strains, recognition of priority... Then this climate deteriorated, due to the responsibility associated with the use of different vaccination techniques... although in the 1930s, 40s and 50s it was accepted that the end justifies the means, within certain limits and in some circumstances...

Should we aim for the application of the "precaution principle", so dear to politicians, that would banish all "bad" technological risk, accepting only what is natural, ecological and ideally without any risk at all? Such a prospect seems very distant. The fight against yellow fever is an example that raises all these questions.

The danger of postvaccinal reactions associated with the Dakar vaccine administered by scarification was probably underestimated for several years after the introduction of this vaccine in 1939, and then overlooked[245] in the face of the danger of yellow fever itself. MacNamara's article, following that of Sorel, revealed the danger of the Dakar vaccine[246], but the questionable quality of the data collected, as MacNamara himself acknowledges, probably delayed awareness of the problem on the part of various health authorities that produced or used the vaccine. The 17D Rockefeller vaccine, on the other hand, was above all suspicion... at least when it was first used. But can prevention ever be free of any risk?

In 1995, in Peru, there were 440 cases of yellow fever, and 169 fatalities, before the contagion could be stopped. Similar epidemics break out almost every year in different countries. Yellow fever is a re-emerging disease in Africa and South America. The 17D vaccine is still very beneficial for persons being exposed to the virus[247]. Yellow fever remained a fearsome disease for a long time. It was eventually brought under control through the fight against mosquitoes and the use of vaccinations.

245. Peltier, 1947, p. 1026.
246. Sorel, 1936, p. 1325; MacNamara, 1953, p. 199.
247. Kirkpatrick, 2003, p. 369.

Notes on the Vaccination Techniques Used as a Model by Researchers Working on the Development of a Yellow Fever vaccine

• **Note 1:** "*Todd* (1928) *for fowl plague, Laidlaw and Dunkin (1928) for dog distemper, and Bedson, Midland and Burbury (1927) for foot-and-mouth disease.*"

1927. Bedson, Maitland and Burbury used a formalinized antigen at only 1 per 12,000, adjusted to a pH of 7.6 and stored 48 hours at 26° C or 28° C[248].

1928. National Institute for Medical Research, Hampstead, London. Attempts to immunise fowls against fowl plague with heated formalinized virulent materials (blood, spleen, etc.) were unsuccessful. Solid immunity against the disease can reliably be produced in fowls by the injection of three doses, at a one-week interval, of a phenol (or tricresol) glycerine vaccine prepared from the liver of birds killed by the disease[249].

1928. National Institute for Medical Research, Farm Laboratories, Mill Hill. Laidlaw and Dunkin explored the possibilities of vaccinating against dog distemper. The best formula consists of injecting a 10 percent organ (liver, spleen, mesenteric ganglion) suspension in saline solution, from a dog killed by the disease, inactivated with sufficient formalin to produce 1 in 10,000 formaldehyde. A dog treated with dead vaccine alone shows resistance to the distemper virus, but not complete immunity. A vaccinated dog that subsequently receives living virus becomes immune[250].

• **Note 2:** "*Findlay* (1933-1934), *using virus inactivated by methylene blue and a Pointolite lamp after the method of Perdrau and Todd* (1933...)"[251].

1933. National Institute for Medical Research, Hampstead, London. Perdrau and Todd successfully immunised ferrets and dogs against dog distemper by photodynamic inactivation of an extract of infected ferret spleen using methylene blue[252].

• **Note 3: 1929, College of Medicine, Tulane University, Ma.** "*The dessicated virus-serum* (from hog cholera) *can be utilized in conjunction with immune serum dessicated or fresh to produce an active immunity in the hog. The virus-powder is first thoroughly dissolved in the fresh immune serum or in the dissolved dessicated immune serum in the proportion of one part virus to 2 parts serum. This admixture of virus and immune sera in no way prevents the production of an active immunization of the host following its subcutaneous injection...*"[253].

248. Bedson, 1927, p. 5; Maitland, 1927, p. 93; Verge *in* Levaditi, 1943, p. 265.
249. Todd, 1928, p. 101.
250. Laidlaw, 1928, p. 209.
251. Findlay, 1936c, p. 205.
252. Perdrau, 1933, p. 78
253. Duval, 1929, p. 87.

Conclusion

The history of vaccinations has been the subject of very few works, with the exception of relatively short texts at the beginning of general books on vaccinations, like *Vaccines*[1] or *Veterinary Vaccinology*[2]. H.J. Parish's book *A History of Immunization*[3] deals only with human vaccines, examining them one by one, which is interesting but does not provide a general overview of vaccine development. Edited by Stanley A. Plotkin and Bernardino Fantini, "*Vaccinia, Vaccination, Vaccinology: Jenner, Pasteur and their successors*" is an excellent book that brings together, in particular, the recollections of several major actors in the history of vaccinology[4]. Veterinary vaccines have not been of much interest except for the historic vaccines: chicken cholera, ruminant anthrax, swine erysipelas, developed by Pasteur himself. The book "*History of the surveillance and control of transmissible animal diseases*", written by Jean Blancou[5], fills this gap, but does not deal with human vaccines.

The present work attempts to provide a coherent view of the history of vaccinations, both human and veterinary, based, as much as possible, on reliable sources; unfortunately, this book does not discuss all vaccines... There are much too many: against bacteria, against viruses, against parasites and now against numerous molecules...

As early as December 1903, in his presidential address to the Society of American Bacteriologists, Theobald Smith, considered one of the greatest American bacteriologists, said: "*At this point, I cannot abstain from referring to the major influence exerted by the study of infectious diseases in inferior animals on bacteriology... As long as a stupid distinction between human and animal pathology will be maintained, a distinction rooted in past ignorance, progress will be slow.*"[6] New infectious diseases in humans often originate in animal diseases: spongiform encephalopathy, SARS (Severe Acute Respiratory Syndrome), avian or swine flu - examples abound. Animal diseases played an essential role in the history of vaccinations. Finally, because of less strict ethical requirements applied to animal studies, veterinary vaccines have contributed greatly to the development of vaccinology, as well as animal... and human health, even though the efforts dedicated to them were modest compared to those made to develop human vaccines. Even today, "*One World, one Medicine*" is a slogan rather than a reflection of reality.

The history of vaccinations... is not any easier to explore than the history of other sciences. Vaccinations have brought about profound changes in the evolution of human societies. *A priori*, it might seem easy to recount their history. But this is not always the case. The description of discoveries and their origins will always be a delicate task. No discovery came from nowhere, at least not in biology or medicine. But how do we distinguish precursors from inventors, and inventors from imitators?

---

1. Plotkin, 1994, 1999, 2004, 2008.
2. Pastoret, 1997.
3. Parish, 1965.
4. Plotkin, 1996.
5. Blancou, 2003.
6. Smith, 1903 (1981), p. 233.

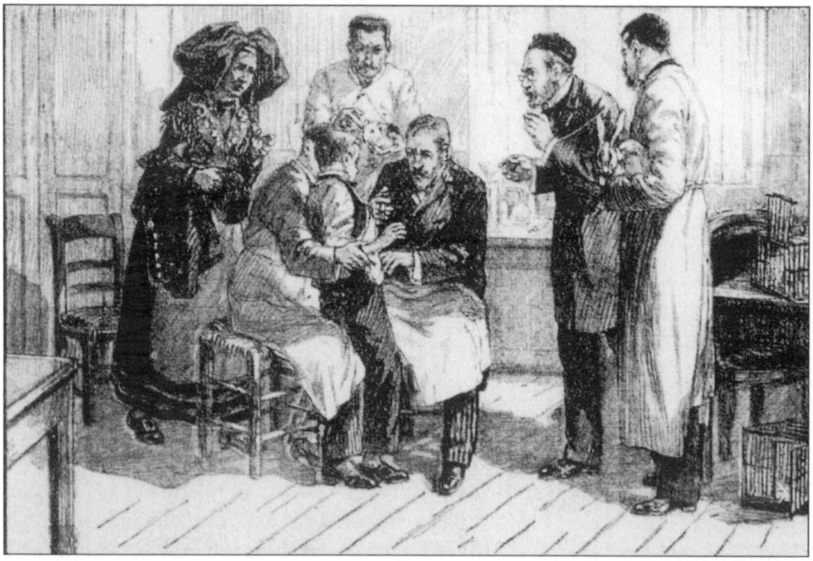

Figure 1. "*Pasteur* (second from the right), *assisted by Dr. Grancher, inoculates the famous virus for the first to the little Alsacian boy Meister, who had contracted rabies.*" (Drawing by Lecoultre.) The article that follows in *Le Pèlerin* bears the heading: "*But the greatest, the most brilliant of Pasteur's scientific discoveries is without any doubt that of the rabies vaccine. But is it effective in all cases? Experiments conducted on bitten dogs bring confirmation. Will this still hold true the day when he will attempt the same experiment, the same treatment, in man?*" The article and the illustration both reflect the veneration of which Pasteur was the object in France and in many other countries. Little Meister and his mother, wearing Alsacial traditional garb, seem particularly out of place in this decor; the assistants, one holding a rabbit, the other a guinea pig, are just as incongruous... (*Le Pèlerin*, issue 2333, November 5, 1922.) Pasteur, Koch and Lister were the founders of three fundamental fields of medicine: vaccinology, microbiology and asepsis (Metchnikoff, 1939).

At first, a vaccine is an idea. Then it must become a substance. Is the birth of a vaccine the initial brilliant idea, the first risky implementation, the small-scale application (Pilot production) or industrial production? Is it the first administration to man or to a specific animal species? Is it effectiveness against a specific disease? ...

What value should be attributed to an original source: a scientific article; the laboratory notes of a scientist; reported data from a conference, not bearing the signature of its author; comments made during a private conversation, showing the priority of a concept or of results... It is difficult to decide...

In addition, in vaccinology as in other scientific domains, there are disputes and claims concerning most discoveries: cowpox/vaccine: Jenner, Jesty, Pearson...; chicken cholera: Pasteur, Roux...; ruminant anthrax: Pasteur, Roux, Toussaint...; rabies: Pasteur, Roux, Galtier...; cholera: Ferran, Gamaleïa, Haffkine...; typhoid fever: Pfeiffer/Kolle, Wright... anatoxine/toxoid: Ramon, Glenny...; poliomyelitis: Salk, Koprowski, Sabin...

The truth is sometimes difficult to discern, because we rarely have access to laboratory notes like Pasteur's. When one reads the notes of an author, such as those of Pasteur, certain things are clearly apparent. Pasteur wrote the notes to reread them later. But the evolution of his ideas is more difficult to follow. The examples cited in this book are a very small portion of the whole body of notes. The choice was obviously personal.

Historically, the arrival of Lady Montagu-type inoculation (variolation) was considered a major medical event, despite the undeniable disadvantages that hindered the dissemination of the smallpox to a great extent. How was acceptable risk at a given time determined? The established limit evolved considerably over time. This factor was evaluated from the start of variolation use, on the one hand by comparison with other risks, as well as by the reasons for taking the risk. Surprising comparisons were sometimes made: "*It is impossible to build four or five-storey houses, & even taller churches, without great risk for many various artisans; & that is not all: the church must have a bell tower reaching to the sky & inviting thunder, this tower must bear a cross topped with a rooster; there is certainly more risk in setting this rooster in place than in being inoculated, & this rooster offers no protection from anything. If inoculation was to be banished, many common occupations would reasonably have to follow suit: divers, miners, roofers... seamen, tree pruners, firefighters, pyrotechnicians, builders, &c. &c., where & how can & should they be stopped?*"[7]

This question of risk/benefit remains unanswered, since the answer would depend on many factors, including treatment possibilities! Kenneth Calman, who was then head of the Health Department of the United Kingdom, proposed a classification of the risk into six levels: "high", over 1%; "moderate"; "low"; "very low"; "minimal"; "negligible"; as well as a certain number of qualifications like "avoidable/unavoidable", "justifiable/unjustifiable", "acceptable/unacceptable", including untested medications, last-resort medications, etc.[8] This was an excellent idea, but as Calman himself says, it had to be illustrated by examples. Calman's own example, American foot-ball, would not be suitable in francophone countries, although it might be understood in the Province of Quebec, in Canada. It would be useful to classify health risks by probabilities associated with daily occurrences such as taking the lift, bicycling, being struck by lighting,

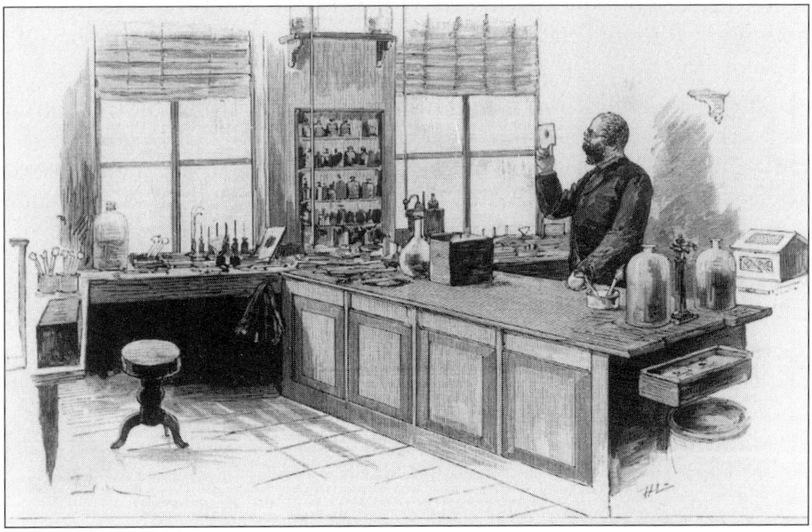

Figure 2. "*Dr. Koch in his laboratory. (Drawing by Mr. Marold, based on the sketch of our Berlin correspondent.)*" (*L'Illustration*, issue 2490, November 15, 1890.) Koch and his students discovered a great number of human and animal pathogenic agents. They played a crucial role in the foundation of microbiology.

7. Médecin, 1768, p. 10.
8. Anonymous, 1996, p. 371.

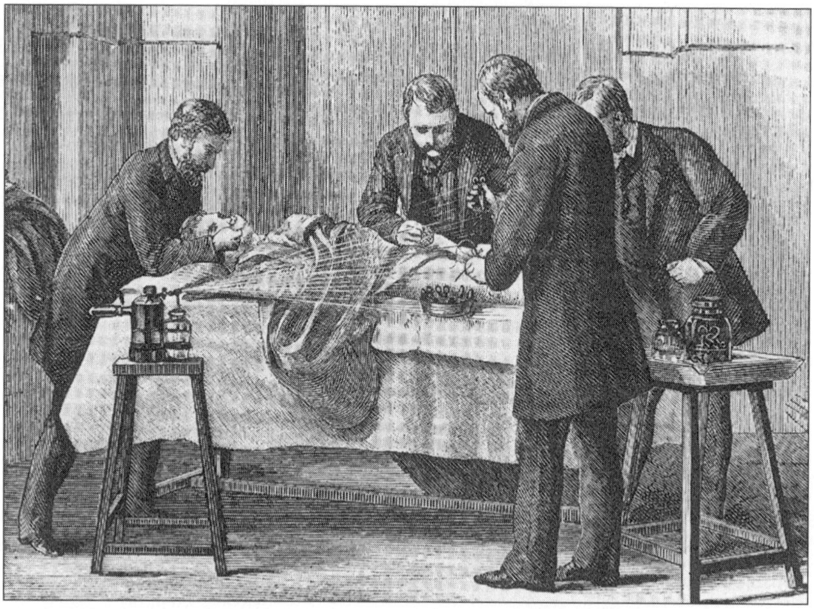

Figure 3. "*The first cases which he* (Joseph Lister) *treated using antiseptic principles were compound fractures of the legs, in 1865.*" (Reference Handbook of the Medical Sciences, 1885, t. 1, page 259.) Surgery was transformed by Lister's discovery.

winning the national lottery... In most if not all cases, the figures would have no meaning for the person to be vaccinated. Distances of a million or a billion light-years mean nothing to the uninitiated. A vaccination risk of 1 out of 1 million doses has some vague reality, but 1 out of 10 million, or less, no longer has any.

Information that is easy to understand would be very welcome. Statisticians are cautious; they write statements such as: "*Although a risk above that incurred by the general population has not been demonstrated in a cohort vaccinated with a given vaccine, a low correlation cannot be excluded...*" Of course, this is interpreted as an unacknowledged risk. For such risks to be meaningful, they would have to be accompanied by precise figures, and compared to other risks familiar to the public. This requires considerable work. For example, hepatitis B vaccines, in France particularly, have been the object of close surveillance, leading to this conclusion: "*Faced with the impossibility of excluding all cause-and-effect relations, several pharmaco-epidemiological studies have been conducted. Their sometimes contradictory findings do not allow the exclusion of a low risk.*"[9] This study reveals no case of demyelination disease in children under 2 years, the age recommended for this vaccine. It is extremely disappointing to have the study conclusions indicate that a low risk cannot be excluded, a statement that suggests nothing concrete to the reader, but discourages him from receiving the vaccine at any age.

Variolation was an impressive discovery, but its disadvantages were considerable. Jennerian vaccination, completely unexpected, was also a major step forward, the great naturalist Cuvier pointed out: "*Thus, even if the discovery of vaccine were medicine's only discovery in our era, it would be sufficient to permanently inscribe our times in the history*

9. Imbs, 2003, p. 1489.

of sciences, and to immortalise Jenner's name by conferring him a place of honour among the major benefactors of humanity."[10]

Even more impressive was the impact of the almost simultaneous discovery of pathogenic microbes and Pasteurian vaccines. These novelties aroused much enthusiasm. The discovery of bacterial animalcules (and filterable viruses) and of the means of combating them by antisepsis and asepsis on the one hand, and by vaccines and sera on the other, constituted a veritable revolution. We had come a long way: just before the validation of germ theory and the application of its consequences, Dr. Chenu's statistics on the treatment of the Crimean War wounded speak clearly. Between 1854 and 1856, out of 1,681 individuals who underwent femur resection, 92% did not survive; out of 1,321 wounded who underwent tibia resection, 71% died, most often of gangrene or of septicemia[11]. These percentages are enormous! But the discovery of surgical antisepsis and antitetanic serum radically changed the prognosis of many surgical procedures, especially in times of war. Progress was rapid, but stopped... before reaching a peak of 100%. Today, we still have a small but significant number of nosocomial infections. In hospitals, respect of the rules of hygiene would save more lives than gene theory which is, nevertheless, a major element in the development of certain future therapies.

Some infectious diseases could be eradicated because man is their sole reservoir; smallpox and measles are examples in point. Other diseases could be eradicated because we have effective vaccines against them. Unfortunately, their use is not always seriously implemented. Infectious foci subsist in certain countries, while other countries have eliminated the disease: congenital rubella, diphtheria, whopping cough, *Haemophilus influenza* B meningitis, hepatitis B... In France, there have not been any cases of diphtheria, and practically no cases of measles or whopping cough for many years. It would be possible to eliminate the measles, mumps and rubella by vaccinating (with MMR) over 95% of the child population under the age of 2. The United States and Finland used this method to successfully eradicate measles. In France, some work remains to be done, because the vaccination rate is only 86%, with large areas where the coverage is less than 80%...

Since its beginnings with Lady Montagu, Jenner and Pasteur, vaccinology has made immense progress in a short time. It has saved innumerable human lives (as well as animal lives). Cross-reaction vaccines (vaccinia and smallpox...), attenuated living vaccines (chicken cholera, ruminant anthrax, BCG...), killed bacteria vaccines (cholera, typhoid, plague...), anatoxines/toxoids, subunit vaccines (component(s) of pathogenic agents)... all these vaccines belong to the Jennerian and Pasteurian tradition. Their technology is largely based on this tradition. Their development was hindered by limited knowledge available in genetics, immunology, bacteriology, virology and parasitology... Finally, production methods were still rudimentary. For a long time, vaccines were prepared on a small-scale, locally, in less than safe conditions... because their transport without maintenance of a cold chain, at room temperature and at the speeds possible at the time was difficult, if not impossible. Markets were limited. Thus, when Wright's typhoid fever vaccine was adopted by the British armed forces, one part was produced in England and transported to India, and another part was made "on the way" in Calcutta and Agra[12]. A booklet was published in view of standardising vaccinal

10. Cuvier, 1810, p. 349.
11. Quoted by Metchnikoff, 1939, p. 9.
12. Wright, 1900, p. 122.

preparations to be administered to the troops[13]. Each province, each regiment... made its own vaccines. Of course, in these conditions, batches of vaccine were not uniform, despite the precautions that were taken. Quality control was rudimentary or inexistent.

Vaccinology continued to improve, often as a result of accidents. The price of progress continued to be high! But the criteria of vaccine production quality, safety, reliability and effectiveness were raised under the pressure of stricter controls. At the same time, the price of vaccine development, production, distribution and administration increased proportionally. Gradually, manufacturing of vaccines progressed from small-scale production to production by State agencies or by private companies under the supervision of specialised government agencies.

Vaccines have changed the world. They have been partly responsible for world population growth. They have reduced the suffering of populations, but have not been able to stop it completely. The benefits of vaccination programs in poor countries would have to be reinforced by a more equitable world economy, to which the rich countries would have to make greater contributions.

Vaccinology in the widest sense of the word is about three centuries old and is founded essentially on the principles of microbiology and immunology. These two sciences, born about a hundred years ago, have known exponential development in recent years, thanks to molecular biology. Unfortunately, vaccinology does not advance at the same pace, because transposing theory into practice is difficult. Prevention, particularly of infectious diseases, has always depended on hygiene and on vaccinations. The expense is high, but this kind of investment is profitable. In many cities, at least in developed countries, hygiene campaigns date back to about 1850-1900. Hygiene conditions have improved, but the work must be continued and the protection offered the population must be reinforced by a free vaccination program provided not on a compulsory basis but through persuasion and even benefits (insurance, payment) granted by the society that reaps part of the benefits of the program.

Man is constantly expanding his territory on the planet, to the detriment of other species; he disturbs ecological balances, thereby creating new infectious diseases of animal origin, that affect the human species. Vaccinology faces great challenges in setting limits to this presently uncontrolled tendency.

A society's maturity is reflected more clearly in disease prevention than in the treatments it can offer its citizens when needed, when it is already late, and at times too late...

13. Lamb, 1906.

Overview of the Protagonists of this Story

ARLOING Saturnin (1846-1911). French veterinarian, doctor of medicine, doctor es natural sciences. Professor at the Veterinary School in Toulouse, then in Lyon. He became director of the Veterinary School in Lyon, and professor of experimental medicine at the Lyon Faculty of Medicine. His scientific areas of interest included human and bovine anthrax, gas gangrene, puerperal fever and surgical instrument sterilisation, as well as the fight against animal viruses, among others[1].

AUZIAS-TURENNE Joseph-Alexandre. French physician born in Pertuis (Vaucluse) in 1819, died in Paris in 1870. In 1842, he defended his thesis in medicine. In 1861, he founded a dispensary at 356 Saint-Jacques Street, where he treated venereal disease patients free of charge. He discovered "syphilisation" (from his personal perspective on the technique)[2]. His writings were published after his death, in 1878, by his friends, under the title "*La Syphilisation*". Apparently, Loir brought Pasteur this work, sent by Mr. d'Andecy, secretary general of the "*Crédit foncier*" (an old French bank), a friend of his father's, and one of the executors of Auzias-Turenne's will[3]. According to Loir, the book became Pasteur's favourite, and provided Pasteur with many ideas. This might be so, but it is not certain. Auzias-Turenne had published many articles in well-known scientific journals of that period, and particularly in the *Comptes-Rendus de l'Académie des Sciences* (Paris). Auzias-Turenne bequeathed his skeleton to the University of Christiania (Norway), which asked to take possession of it[4], a fact denied by his friends[5]. Today, his remains are buried in the Montparnasse Cemetery in Paris.

BEHRING Emil Adolf von (1854-1917). German military physician and bacteriologist. He completed his medical studies at the Medical School of Health in Berlin. In 1889, he left the army and entered the Berlin Institute for Hygiene, headed by Robert Koch. In 1890, he discovered antitoxins and the principle of serotherapy, with Kitasato. He was awarded the 1901 Nobel Prize in physiology and medicine for this work. Behring also focused his research on tuberculosis and tetanus.

BIGGS Herman M. (Trumansburg, N.Y., 1859 - New York, 1923). This American physician was an important figure in the development of public hygiene and the prevention of infectious diseases, especially tuberculosis. He was the first director of the Carnegie Laboratory of the Bellevue Hospital Medical College, where he was a professor. He headed a very useful mission in France to promote the fight against tuberculosis, in 1917, at the end of the First World War.

BOECK Carl Wilhelm (1908-1875). Professor of surgical medicine, and of skin and syphilitic diseases in Christiana, Norway[6].

BORDET Jules Jean Baptiste Vincent (1870-1961). Belgian physician and microbiologist. Noted for his discoveries in the field of immunity: complement-fixation reaction, and aviary diphtheria microbe. He discovered *Bordetella bronchoseptica* (the whooping cough microbe) and gave his name to the genus Bordetella. He founded the *Institut Pasteur* in Brabant (Belgium), and was awarded the Nobel Prize in 1919.

BOULEY Henri-Marie. Born in Paris on May 17, 1814. Having obtained his veterinary diploma in 1836, he began to practice his profession with his father, before joining the teaching staff of the Alfort School. In January 1866, he was named Inspector General of the French veterinary Schools[7].

1. Courmont, 1911, p. 261.
2. Larousse du XIXe siècle, 1878, 1rst Suppl.
3. Auzias-Turenne, 1878, last page; Loir, 1938, p. 102.
4. Hahn *in* Berthelot, 1885-1892, t. 4, p. 835.
5. Auzias-Turenne, 1878, p. XXII.
6. Dupont, 1999, p. 87.
7. Neumann, 1896.

His remarkable natural distinction was coupled with competence, erudition, oratorical talent, wit and joviality. Converted rather late to Pasteurian principles, he became an enthusiastic and fanatical disciple of Pasteur's discoveries[8], while keeping a benevolent and protective, if sometimes blind, eye on the work of his young colleagues. But he was very fond of controversy, even to the point of excess. He was Commander of the *Légion d'Honneur*, member of the Academy of Medicine (1855) and of the Academy of Sciences (1868). In 1884, he succeeded Claude Bernard at the Museum of Natural History, where he held the Chair of Comparative Pathology. "*This same year, Mr. Bouley was elected President of the Academy of Sciences for 1885. It was the first time that such a distinction was conferred on a veterinarian... He presided at the Academy of Sciences for the last time during the famous session where Mr. Pasteur presented the results of his rabies research.* He had arranged to be brought to the Institute on the threshold of death..."[9]. He succumbed to a cardiac illness on November 20, 1885.

BOURREL Jean-Aimé (1822-1892). Former military veterinarian, he opened a practice in Paris and specialised in the treatment of domestic carnivores with rabies or suspected of having rabies.

BOYLSTON Zabdiel (1679-1766). Boston physician and inoculist, invited for a stay in London (1724-1726) by Sir Hans Sloan, to bring the benefit of his experience in inoculation. Elected member of the Royal Society. "*At the urging of the Rev. Cotton Mather and with the support of most of the town's ministers and many of the colony's well-to-do, but with strong opposition from much of the general public, the Boston selectmen, and most of the city's doctors, led by William Douglass, the town's best educated and most distinguished physician, conducted the first large-scale inoculation in the Western world during the Boston epidemic of 1721.*"[10]

BROUARDEL Paul-Camille-Hippolyte (1837-1906). Obtained his medical diploma in 1865 and the "*agrégation*" in 1869; became professor of forensic medicine in 1879, and then dean of the Faculty of Medicine of Paris.

BURNET Franck Mac Farlane (1899-1985). Australian virologist and immunologist. Author of numerous publications and theories: the distinction between "self" and "non-self" (1949) and clonal selection theory (1957), for which he was awarded the Nobel Prize in 1960.

CALMETTE Léon-Charles-Albert (Nice, 1863 - Paris, 1933). At 20, he entered the Health Service of the French Navy and served in China, Gabon... In 1890 he was transferred to the Health Service of the colonies and as a result, was enrolled in a training program at the *Institut Pasteur* in Paris. Very quickly, he was sent to set up the *Institut Pasteur* in Saigon (Hô-Chi-Minh-City), which he directed until 1893. At that period, he started his work on serpent venom. In 1895, he founded the *Institut Pasteur* of Lille, inaugurated in December 1899. In Lille, he studied the biological treatment of wastewater, antivenom sera, tuberculosis... In 1910, with Edmond Sergent, he founded the *Institut Pasteur* of Algiers... with Guérin, he developed the BCG, a tuberculosis vaccine.

CAMPER Pieter (1722-1789). Dutch physician, anatomist and naturalist. His work encompassed very diverse subjects, from the observation of air in the bones of birds to inoculation against bovine pleuropneumonia[11].

CARRO Jean de (1770-1857). Physician from Geneva, living in Vienna and later in Carlsbad, where he died. He was an active participant in the distribution of the Jennerian vaccine.

CHAMBERLAND Charles-Edouard (Chilly-le-Vignoble 1851 - Paris 1908). He graduated from the *Ecole Normale Supérieure* in 1874, was a professor at the Nîmes lyceum in 1874-1875, before entering Pasteur's laboratory as an assistant in 1875 (or 1876 or even 1877, depending on the source). He became one of Pasteur's loyal disciples. He participated in most of the master's laboratory work, but does not seem to have initiated these projects, because biology and medicine were not his main interests. However, his creative imagination found free expression in his physics projects. His physics thesis established the fundamental rules of sterilisation in bacteriology[12]. Pasteur put him in charge of vaccine production in his laboratory. His "claim to fame" was the filter that bears his name. The

8. Anonyme, 1884a, p. 120.
9. Decaisne, 1885, p. 790.
10. Kaufman, 1984, vol. 1, p. 87.
11. Thomas, 1893, p. 541.
12. Chamberland, 1879.

term "Chamberland filter" was followed by the term "Pasteurian system"... Chamberland was an intelligent and cordial man. Pasteur Vallery-Radot described him as follows: "*A dreamer, a dilettante by nature seeing life with the eyes of a philosopher, through the smoke of his inevitable pipe, he liked being disturbed in his laboratory; we would go there to exchange ideas, and come away with a valuable, new perspective*."[13a] Charles Chamberland is buried in the Chilly-le-Vignoble cemetery, where his imposing bust presides over his tomb.

CHANTEMESSE André (1851-1919). One of Pasteur's first disciples. He made an outstanding contribution to the development of typhoid fever vaccine. Member of the Academy of Medicine (Paris).

CHAUVEAU Jean-Baptiste-Auguste (1827-1917). Student at the Alfort Veterinary School, then professor and later director of the Lyon Veterinary School, in 1875. Under his authority, the School was shaken by lively student revolts. Given his exceptional qualities, he was promoted doctor *honoris causa* by the Lyon Faculty of Medicine, which named him professor of experimental and comparative medicine. In 1886, he succeeded Bouley as professor of comparative pathology at the Museum of Natural History (Paris). Chauveau was a great physiologist, who worked closely with Etienne Marey, from Beaune. They were the first scientists to record heart contraction movements in horses, using cardiac probes. Chauveau admired and supported Pasteur's work, but he was not a flatterer. He defended the work of his student Toussaint more or less against Pasteur. Member of the Academy of Medicine (1891) and of the Academy of Sciences (1886), Chauveau was a remarkable and very worthy scientist.

COLIN Gabriel (1826-1896). Professor at the Alfort Veterinary School. Author of an excellent Treatise of comparative physiology of domestic animals (*Traité de physiologie comparée des animaux domestiques*), whose success justified three editions. He was awarded the Breant Prize in 1880 for "his work on septicemia and anthrax"[13b]. He took an adversarial position on nearly all new ideas and new techniques. He fought relentlessly against Claude Bernard's work, as well as that of Chauveau, Pasteur and others... Colin was an interesting figure, but his renown is due solely to his quarrels with Pasteur!

DAVAINE Casimir-Joseph. French physician (1812-1882). Although his medical practice was his principal occupation, he also wrote a considerable number of scientific works of excellent quality. Member of the Academy of Medicine in 1868.

DEZOTEUX François (1724-1803). French physician, zealous promoter of inoculation[14].

DIDAY Paul. Born in Bourg (Ain), in 1812. Physician who became head surgeon of the Antiquaille Hospice, before opening a private practice in Lyon.

DUCLAUX Emile (Aurillac, 1840 - Paris, 1904). A graduate of the "*Ecole Normale Supérieure*", holding a teaching title in physics sciences, he entered Pasteur's laboratory as an assistant. Doctor es sciences in 1865. He was named professor of chemistry at the Tours lyceum, then in Clermont-Ferrand (where he met Roux, whom he appreciated greatly). He made many trips to Alais (Alès), and to Pont-Gisquet, to work with his master, Pasteur, who was studying the diseases of silkworms. After the French defeat in 1870, Pasteur took refuge in Clermont-Ferrand, at Duclaux's home. It is there that they undertook their studies on beer, at the Kühn Brewery in Chamalières. In 1873, thanks to Pasteur's support, Duclaux was named professor of physics at the University of Lyon. In 1875, he married; the couple had three children. At the birth of the third child, the mother died of puerperal fever, and the child survived only briefly. In 1878, he was attributed the meteorology chair of the Agronomic Institute (Paris). He gave biological chemistry lectures at the Sorbonne, and later at the *Institut Pasteur*... He met Roux by chance, when the latter was an impoverished medical student, and hired him as an assistant. At Pasteur's request, Roux entered the *Ecole Normale Supérieure* laboratory, which needed an inoculator and... medical expertise[15].

Duclaux was a wise, kind, modest and hard-working man. According to his second wife, he received a letter from an elected official, vice-president of the French senate, Scheurer-Kestner, asking for his

13a. Pasteur Vallery-Radot, 1950, p. 500.

13b. Gosselin, 1881a, p. 598.

14. Thomas, 1893, p. 817.

15. Cressac, 1950, p. 58.

opinion on the Dreyfus affair. Duclaux, who was not very interested in politics, replied like a scientist: "*What I think is that if those of us who attempt to solve scientific problems would conduct our enquiry in the manner that seems to have been applied in this affair, it would be only by chance that we would arrive at the truth.*" Duclaux considered the accusation unfounded. Given the prevailing attitudes of the times, this very reasonable stance provoked virulent reactions in the anti-Dreyfus press, which caused Duclaux to define his position more clearly. Thus, he unintentionally became a Dreyfusian militant, and soon afterwards vice-president of the League for the defence of human and citizen's rights (*Ligue des droits de l'homme*). Pursued by the government for having organised a gathering of over twenty persons, he was indicted and condemned to a suspended fine of 16 francs. Three years later, he received the Commander's ribbon of the *Légion d'Honneur*. What demon possessed Duclaux, a well-established member of good society, living comfortably, to go from one public assembly to another? "*I often ask myself how, given my easy-going and not particularly daring temperament, I let myself be persuaded to become a militant.*" A few years later, after having defended the memory of James Darmesteter, a Dreyfus partisan, the latter's widow came to see him to thank him in person. She was to become Duclaux's wife in 1901 (1902?). In the years that followed, Duclaux's health deteriorated, and he passed away in 1904. In Aurillac, at his request, his coffin went directly from the train station to the cemetery, with no ceremony at the church or the City hall, to everyone's discontent. No incense, no speeches or military honours, no decorations, no flags! [16] Political factions of the right as well as the left were extremely offended. Really, this man remained asocial even in death...

His deferential friendship for his master, Pasteur, remained true despite highs and lows. In a letter dated March 23, 1893, Duclaux sent Pasteur his "resignation" from the position of assistant director of the *Institut Pasteur*: "*The misunderstanding that arose tonight between us, although neither of us wished it, renders delicate the position of assistant director of the* Institut Pasteur, *to which you have assigned me. It would not be suitable for an assistant director to appear to be in disagreement with his Director, especially when the latter's name is Mr. Pasteur, and the Board would not judge it appropriate for me to keep my position. It would look as if I was desperately holding on, when in fact, as you know, I did not solicit or even desire this position. Therefore, allow me to submit my resignation* (sic)." Duclaux proposed that he remains a Unit head, but nothing else [17]. Skies were sometimes cloudy on Dutot Street! But the letter does not mention the reason for the disagreement, which unfortunately remains unknown. In any case, things soon went back to normal...

DUCLAUX Mary, born Agnès-Mary-France Robinson (1865?-1947). Englishwoman of Anglican faith, she was very cultured and beautiful. Well-read, intelligent, a poet, she wrote a French literary column in the austere *Times* newspaper. In 1901 (or 1902) she married Emile Duclaux, who left her a widow for the second time two or three years later. Thanks to her intimate ties with two Pasteur successors who headed the *Institut Pasteur*, her testimonial regarding this institution is very valuable. In her book *La Vie d'Emile Duclaux*, she drew some accurate portraits of the protagonists of the Institute.

EHRLICH Paul (1854-1915). German physician. Highly intelligent, recognized for his decisive contribution to the development of haematology, immunology and chemotherapy. Nobel Prize in 1908.

FERRAN Y CLUA Jaime (Jaume in Catalan). Spanish physician and bacteriologist, born in Cordoba de Ebro (near Tarragone) in 1852, where his father practiced medicine; he died in Barcelona in 1929. He completed his medical studies in Barcelona and received his degree in 1873. He started a private practice in Pla de Parradès, before moving to Tortosa, where he was afflicted with boredom. Apparently, he was very disheartened by the mediocrity of medical knowledge in his era. He found the practice of medicine tedious. He became friend with José J. Landerer, an astronomer who introduced him to photography. At about the same time, he met Innocent Pauli, with whom he practiced the art of photography. Landerer published articles in *Les Comptes rendus de l'Académie des Sciences* of Paris. Ferran had occasion to read this publication, and discovered Pasteur's work, which solicited his enthusiasm. Some excellent authors like Zinsser [18], Plotkin [19] and Parish [20] cite him as a student

16. Vermenouze, 1992, p. 111; Heyman, 1992, p. 203.
17. NAF 18103, item 76.
18. Zinsser, 1918, p. 487.
19. Plotkin, 2004, p. 4.
20. Parish, 1965, p. 80.

of Pasteur, but this is inaccurate. What he was, in fact, was a declared disciple. He focused all his interest on the new bacteriology. It was at this period that he started his work on the cholera bacillus, and conducted his anti-cholera vaccination campaigns. Once the epidemic was over, he returned to Tortosa. In 1886, he was named director of the *Laboratori Microbiologic Municipal de Barcelona*, recently created to implement the Pasteurian anti-rabies treatment. "*Starting with the idea that the fixed virus is a rabies virus perfectly adapted to the rabbit, Ferran has decided some time ago to use fresh cord to immunise man.*"[21] After experiments on dogs, Ferran went on to humans, and called his method "supraintensivo", while Pasteur's was simply intensive, in the most serious cases. He introduced Pasteurian anthrax vaccination in Spain. During his career, he claimed to have developed (?) vaccines against cholera, typhoid fever, diphtheria, plague, tuberculosis, tetanus, typhus and rabies; and to have discovered the anti-diphtheria serum six years before Behring. Convinced of bacterial pleomorphism, he described cholera bacillus cycles[22], as well as a tuberculosis bacillus different than that of Koch[23]. These discoveries were never confirmed by other authors[24].

Jaime Ferran was an unconditional admirer of Pasteur's work, and he found it hard to understand that Pasteur did not show the same enthusiasm in defending his (Ferran's) projects. On September 23 or 25, or in October (the date is difficult to read) 1888, he wrote to Pasteur: "*Never ceasing for an instant to have the greatest admiration and respect for you, beyond the fact that my success is due to M. Pasteur who, by his writings, has inspired and guided my work, I deem it just that the name of the illustrious scientist of whom France is proud with good reason, be associated with the glory of this discovery* (the discovery of the rabies microbe, evidently, an error). *It can sometimes happen in a battle that a certain soldier takes a fortress, but the victory rightly belongs to the general who led the troops to glory.*"[25] In this sense, in a note entitled "*Note on the rabies microbe, its isolation, its pathogenic effects*", sent to the Academy of Sciences (Paris) on December 1, 1888, his concluding remarks were: "*If, as we are convinced, our research on the rabies microbe enters the field of science as a useful and important discovery which will provide other experimenters with the occasion of making new conquests, we declare clearly and formally that a large part of the glory that could come to us rightly belongs to Mr. Pasteur, to whom modern science owes so much and whose work served as a guide to our modest efforts.*"[26] Pasteur apparently responded with some scepticism. On January 4, 1889, Ferran answered him by saying that a commission named by the Royal Academy of Medicine of Barcelona was mandated to study his work on rabies[27]. Of course, the rabies virus is not a bacterium. This was as false as the "glory" given to Pasteur. But Ferran's letter is quite interesting. He describes his method of work, obtaining samples, bacillus culture, pathogenic effects, and he even includes three good quality microphotographs. He specifies that when it is inoculated under the skin, his "rabies bacillus" does not multiply and "*This is why the chemical rabies vaccine, so impatiently awaited, is perhaps the only one to be used in all institutes...*"[28]. Of course, Pasteur could not have been very pleased.

Rabid wolf bites were very dangerous, and it was difficult to prevent the onset of the disease. Ferran attributed this to leucocytes (white blood cells) that become infected at the virus injection points, and carry the virus to nerve centres. What was needed, he felt, was to avoid the migration of leucocytes away from the sites of fresh virus injection. On the advice of Dr. Bertran y Rubio, he added a small quantity of mercury albuminate to his vaccine, mixing it with a mercury chloride solution at 1 per 2,000. Injection of this vaccine provoked a light inflammatory reaction *in situ*, which attracted the leucocytes rather than pushing them away[29]. It is unlikely that this hypothesis was valid, but Ferran's idea is interesting and shows his inventive spirit.

21. Marie, 1909, p. 290.
22. Trouessart, 1886, p. 193.
23. Ferran, 1912, p. 106.
24. Bornside, 1982, p. 399.
25. NAF 18103, item 263.
26. NAF 18103, items 187 to 195.
27. NAF 18103, item 265.
28. NAF 18094, items 187 to 195.
29. Anonyme, 1924, p. 883.

In 1899, a plague epidemic broke out in Porto. Ferran was sent there to study it, with Drs. Vinas and Grau. The report was published under the title *La Peste bubonica*. His work was important but contested, even in Catalan country.

In 1905, at the age of 52 or 53, Ferran was divested of his position as Director of the Barcelona Microbiology Laboratory... for unspecified reasons. He retired from professional life and travelled in Europe and America. He died in Barcelona in 1929. His native village, Corbera de Ebro, erected an attractive monument in his honour.

FINDLAY G.M. of the Wellcome Bureau of Scientific Research, London. He conducted studies on viral diseases and particularly on yellow fever.

FINLAY Carlos J. (1833-1915). Cuban physician, son of a Scottish father and a French mother; educated in Germany, France and the United States. President of the Superior Board of Health of Cuba. He made a major contribution to the elimination of yellow fever in many regions by identifying the mosquito (certain species) as the (possible) vector of this disease.

FRENKEL Herman (1891-1962). Dutch veterinarian, Director of the State Veterinary Research Institute in Amsterdam. He made a remarkable contribution to the production of virus.

GALTIER Pierre-Victor (1846-1908). Professor at the Lyon Veterinary School, specialising in infectious diseases, health surveillance and jurisprudence. He was Pasteur's precursor in the field of rabies. His findings were very useful to Pasteur, who borrowed much data from him without providing the reference. "*Galtier received official recognition late: the Bréant Prize (Academy of Sciences - 1887), the Barbier Prize (Academy of Medicine - 1887), election to the Academy of Medicine (1901).*"[30] He was appointed officer of public instruction in 1906. According to Théodoridès[31], "*a few years later, a testimonial of esteem from abroad came as a reward. In October 1907, he received an invitation from the Institut Carolinska in Stockholm, asking him to send them all of his publications on rabies, in view of their submission for the 1908 Nobel Prize in physiology and medicine. Unfortunately, Galtier was already ill and died in Mulatière, near Lyon, on April 24, 1908, at the age of 62, and could not receive this consecration of his work.*" This nomination of Victor Galtier for the Nobel Prize is often mentioned by various excellent authors, either as a possibility or as a quasi-certainty[32]. When consulted on the subject, the Nobel Foundation stated that Galtier was never nominated for the 1908 Nobel Prize[33]. The nomination process was probably interrupted by Galtier's death. But things have to be placed in perspective. In 1908, the two chosen winners were Ehrlich and Metchnikoff. The work of these two founding fathers of immunology and Galtier's admittedly good work bear no comparison. This is regrettable but true. Galtier's name does not appear in many Larousse dictionaries[34]. A zealous (but incompetent) employee of Larousse Publishing discovered the scientist recently, and entered his name. The description reads: "... *he developed the first ruminant vaccine against this disease* (the rabies)"[35], which is not true. Galtier demonstrated that sheep (and a little later cattle), and therefore very likely animals predisposed to contracting rabies, could acquire a state of immunity against this disease, if they are given intravenous "variolation" using virulent rabid dog saliva. This is not negligible, but it is not rabies "vaccination" in the sense that word had at the time, or in the sense in which it is used today.

Prof. Goret resumed the situation most accurately: "*Mrs. Weckerlin - Galtier, biographer of her father, respectfully provides us with the epilogue of this brief homage: 'Pierre-Victor Galtier's candidacy remained a simple proposal, but such an honourable proposal that it represented the only reward his noble nature could have desired'.*"[36]

Rosset ended one of his articles by saying: "*Pierre Victor Galtier is indeed a precursor of the anti-rabies vaccination and he deserves our recognition.*"[37] This is true, just and fair.

30. Rosset, 1985, p. 41.
31. Théodoridès, 1986, p. 198.
32. Goret, 1965, p. 362; Théodoridès, 1972, p. 167; Debré, 1994, p. 448; Darmon, 1995, p. 326; Robin, 2002, p. 235.
33. Jörnvall, 2000.
34. Larousse, 1897-1904; 1928-1930.
35. Larousse, 1960-4; 1987-89.
36. Goret, 1969, p. 75.
37. Rosset, 1985, p. 48.

GATTI Angelo (1730-1798). Italian physician, professor of medicine at the University of Pisa. He learned the variolation technique in Constantinople, where the method employed was much simpler and safer than the European technique. While travelling, he stopped in Paris and quickly became a fashionable variolator.

GLENNY Alexander Thomas (1885-1965). He built his entire career working for the Wellcome Research Laboratories. "*Much of the Glenny's work was concerned with immunization against diphtheria, which only 25-30 years was a dreaded disease… It is no exaggeration to say that his work on primary and secondary responses, together with the introduction of alum-precipitated toxoid, was a major factor in the success of the immunization campaign launched by the Ministery of health during the late war… Glenny whole life was concentrated on his work*, which *he loved almost fanatically*."[38] He was elected fellow of the Royal Society in 1944 and was awarded the Addingham gold medal and the Jenner medal of the Royal Society of medicine in 1953.

GRANCHER Jacques-Joseph (1843-1907). Son of a tailor from Felleton, a town in the Creuse (France). He obtained his doctorate in medicine by defending a thesis on "*L'Unicité de la tuberculose*" ("*The Unicity of tuberculosis*"). He received his "*agrégation*" in 1875. He worked as hospital physician, and then as professor at the pediatric diseases clinic of the Faculty of Medicine (Paris), in 1885. He acquired a considerable private clientele thanks to his exceptional knowledge of tuberculosis. A wealthy Cuban woman came to consult him in Paris. Grancher fell in love with the lady's only daughter, Rosa, and married her in 1879. The couple had a private villa built at 36 Beaujon Street (Paris), and gave sumptuous receptions there. But malicious gossip whispered that the atmosphere was stiff and the guests bored. Grancher was not one to tolerate laissez-aller attitudes.

Grancher was introduced to Pasteur at the Copenhagen conference in 1884. He studied Pasteur's new ideas and became his disciple. Pasteur found a place for him in an annex of his laboratory. According to Loir[39], Pasteur had no particular liking for him, considering him an epicurean, since he brought an armchair (imagine!) into the laboratory! Loir, Pasteur's nephew, recounts: "*Grancher has sent beautiful armchairs to this laboratory, and particularly a rocking chair… I told Pasteur about it and he came to see it. He could not understand that someone could think of having comfortable seats in a laboratory…*"[40]. Moreover, he smoked cigars that bore his name, because his wife had tobacco plantations in Cuba[41]. How could Pasteur take such a fanciful figure seriously? Nevertheless, Pasteur was extremely happy to call on him to inoculate his rabies vaccine to young Meister and to the first candidates for the anti-rabies treatment. Grancher's help proved to be crucial. He had the courage to believe in the master and to inoculate the Pasteur vaccine to others and even to himself. "*It was less well-known what passion and conviction he needed to take the medical responsibility for all the inoculations he performed personally during the first ten months of anti-rabies vaccinations…*"[42]. Pasteur was very grateful to him. At the time when very violent disputes with Peter were going on, René Vallery-Radot kept repeating to Grancher what his father-in-law was saying: "*What pains me more than I can say… is to have spoiled the very happy life of Mr. Grancher* (until Meister's arrival). *Mrs. Grancher will end up seeing me as a peace-disturber in the life of her dear husband.*"[43] They became friends, but did not always agree, as the Brown-Séquard treatment by injection of testicular extract illustrates. Speaking of this treatment, Grancher writes to Pasteur: "*But… I do not share your optimistic view concerning testicular juice inoculations… I am quite annoyed* (sic) *to be of such a radically opposed opinion to yours, and perhaps you will soon convert me…*"[44]. It's elegantly said, but clear.

Grancher played an important role in the development of the *Institut Pasteur*. He became secretary, vice-president and then president of its Board of Directors, until his death. His last contribution was the creation of the project for the prevention of tuberculosis in children, the Grancher project[45]. The project consisted of protecting children between 3 and 10 years old from almost certain contagion

38. Anonymous, 1965, p. 798; Oakley, 1966, p. 1130.
39. Loir, 1938, p. 27.
40. Loir, 1938, p. 27.
41. Loir, 1938, p. 71.
42. Achard, 1923, p. 533.
43. NAF 18110, item 101.
44. NAF 18103, f.P. 83.
45. Brouardel, 1934, p. 127.

in families with tuberculosis by removing them from their homes and placing them in a healthy rural environment. Grancher died at the age of 64, after a long illness that distressed Pasteur[46]. He became a member of the Academy of Medicine in 1892. His bust is an attractive addition to the main staircase of this Academy.

GUÉRIN Camille (1872-1961). French veterinarian and microbiologist. Assistant, laboratory head, and later Unit director at the *Institut Pasteur* in Lille. He left that city reluctantly in 1928, to take up the same position at the *Institut Pasteur* in Paris. He worked for the most part in collaboration with Calmette. Their greatest success was the development of the BCG or Bacillus Calmette-Guérin (at first, "biliated Calmette-Guérin"). Guérin was Calmette's disciple, and later his associate and his successor.

HAFFKINE Waldemar-Mordecai (1860-1930). Doctor ès sciences, he was faced with an anti-semitism that kept laboratory doors closed to him in his native country. He emigrated to Switzerland, then joined his master and fellow countryman Metchnikof at the *Institut Pasteur* in Paris. He succeeded Yersin as tutor for the course in technical microbial science. In 1892, he developed an anti-cholera vaccine. The viceroy of India invited him to vaccinate the population. Between 1893 and 1896, he went from city to city, vaccinating against cholera. A plague epidemic was raging; Yersin had discovered its bacillus and brought it to the *Institut Pasteur*. Haffkine used the plague vaccine developed by Calmette, Borrel and himself, perhaps somewhat modified or improved. In 1897, when he published the results of his Indian plague vaccination campaign, he identified himself as being from the *Institut Pasteur* (Paris), but called his vaccine plague prophylactic fluid (because the word "vaccine" was still reserved for cowpox in Great Britain).[47] In 1902, a massive vaccination campaign was tarnished by nineteen deaths from tetanus. Haffkine was demoted for serious misconduct, and cleared five years later! In 1909, he received the title of winner of the Bréant prize and received a sum (arrears) of 4,000 francs (about 12,800 euros) for his work on cholera and bubonic plague vaccinations. Roux, rapporteur for the Bréant prize Commission of the Academy of Sciences (Paris), was full of praise for Haffkine's work on the anti-plague vaccine[48]. In 1915, retired and tired of problems such as the use of beef broth in the preparation of his vaccine (the cow is a sacred animal in India), and a certain hostility on the part of the English colonial population, he returned to France, where he spent most of the last fifteen years of his life essentially involved in Zionist projects[49]. He died in Lausanne, in a rented room. Waldemar Haffkine was made Companion of the Indian Empire by Queen Victoria, and was hailed by Lord Joseph Lister as a "savior of humanity"[50].

HINDLE Edward (1886-1973). Beit Memorial Research Fellow in Tropical Medicine; the fellowship was granted by the Wellcome Bureau of Scientific Research.

HUSSON Henri-Marie (1772-1853). In 1799, he obtained his doctorate in medicine at the "*nouvelle Ecole de santé*" in Paris. He was appointed associate librarian. In 1800, when the vaccine was imported into France, he was named Secretary of the committee responsible for assessing and spreading the benefits of this wonderful discovery. When the committee was placed under the authority of the Minister of the Interior, Husson was maintained in his post of Secretary of the Central Vaccine Committee by Count Chaptal, and later by his successors. In 1806, Husson was named physician of Hôtel-Dieu Hospital, and in 1809 was appointed physician of the imperial lyceum. After he successfully vaccinated the imperial prince, he was made Knight of the Order of Reunion Island (1811). He also received the titles of Knight of the *Légion d'Honneur* (1814) and of member of the Royal Academy of Medicine.

INSTITUT PASTEUR. It was founded on March 1, 1886, at the incitement of the Academy of Sciences (Paris) and thanks to an international collection campaign that raised 2,586,680 francs (about 8,285,000 euros). The Institute was legally established by a decree issued on June 4, 1887. Pasteur's fervent wish was that his institute be independent of government supervision (and

46. Gautier, 1908, p. 451.
47. Haffkine, 1897, p. 1461.
48. Roux, 1909, p. 1258.
49. Mollaret, 1993, p. 344.
50. Lutzer, 1987, p. 366.

subsequently from the influence of politicians). But, from the start, the Institute's work was subsidised by financial aid from the Ministry of Public Instruction and the Ministry of Agriculture. These funds were intended to reward, at least partly, the *Institut Pasteur* for its contribution to the well-being of the nation and of humanity.

The patients (bitten individuals) were seen in Pasteur's laboratory, which was originally located on Ulm Street. Injections were administered in the master's office at the *Ecole Normale Supérieure**. These premises quickly became too small. Pasteur used donations to build an annex on Vauquelin Street in the disused Rollin College. That is where the *Institut Pasteur* was born: "*The State Council* (Conseil d'Etat) *officially recognized the* Institut Pasteur *as a public utility establishment... The* Institut Pasteur *was housed on Vauquelin Street, not far from the Ecole normale, where* M. *Pasteur's laboratory is located, and where the method destined to become so beneficial was created. There was no inauguration ceremony. We simply settled into the new building* (a temporary wood building) *to continue the work that had been started.*"[51] It is more than likely that Pasteur had no wish whatever to consider this hut his future *Institut*, with good reason.

The search for a suitable site was difficult. At the end of the March 5, 1886 meeting of the municipal council of the city of Paris, the Strauss council submitted a proposition paying homage to Pasteur and opening negociations in view of creating a vaccinal institution against rabies. But the battle was not yet won. The vote was positive despite opposition from Cattiaux, Officer of health ("*officier de santé*") and municipal councillor of the 19th arrondissement, and from a Dr. Navarre. A plot of land and a building of the old Rollin College were to be placed at Mr. Pasteur's disposal, with a hundred-year lease. But opposition to Pasteur grew over time. The proposed site was reduced from 5,000 to 2,500 square metres, and the lease was reduced from one hundred to thirty years. The committee looked elsewhere and chose to locate on Dutot Street, for the benefit of the future *Institut*, which would otherwise have been dependent on the whims of an assembly. Before all else, Pasteur wanted his freedom and the freedom of his institute.

One and a half million francs of the funds collected by the international campaign were used to buy the land, to construct the first buildings and to furnish and equip them. As soon as it was completed, the Institute led to the construction of other establishments in the area around it. One of these was "*a small canteen somewhat ambitiously named Hotel of the* Institut Pasteur; *a few wine merchant shops are also already serving the same type of clientele*"[51]. They might have been helpful for boosting the courage of those who were about to enter the rabies Unit! The Institute located on Dutot Street** was inaugurated on November 14, 1888 under the name "*Institut Pasteur*" or the "Anti-rabies Institute" of Paris. The ceremony took place in the old library, displaying busts of the most generous donors. Over a thousand people gathered in the library (or wherever they could). Ladies were not invited[52] (*sic*), and those among them who were donors were only present as statues! Among the distinguished (masculine) guests, some names are still familiar: Carnot, Jules Ferry, Léon Say, Berthelot, Chauveau, Ricord, Poubelle, Vallery-Radot... Speeches were made by Bertrand, perpetual secretary of the Academy of Sciences, Grancher and Mr. Christophle, governor of the "*Crédit foncier*". Mr. Pasteur answered with a speech of his own, read by his son, in which he thanked the donors and his associates. He glorified science in the service of humanity[53]. Pasteur was much complimented in the press of his era. "*This establishment, unique in the world, is not only a temple of science, but also a sanctuary of charity and devotion.*"[54]

JENNER Edward (1749-1822). A truly great man, with undeniable qualities and a few faults. He was a good observer, dilettante and generous. His greatest achievement was to demonstrate that cowpox, a cow disease communicable to man but producing only relatively light symptoms, offered protection from subsequent attacks of variola. This was the start of vaccinology. Edward Jenner was an exceptional and likable man[55].

* This office can still be visited upon request.

** A section of Dutot Street was to be called Dr. Roux Street after the death of the latter.

51. Figuier, 1888b, p. 547.
52. Anonyme, 1888b, p. 742.
53. Anonyme, 1888b, p. 742; Sagnet *in* Berthelot, 1885-1892, t. 26, p. 72.
54. Tissandier, 1888, p. 402.
55. Bazin, 1997, 2000; Fisher, 1991.

1749: May 17 (May 6 in our present Gregorian Calendar), birth of Edward Jenner.

1754: Death of Edward Jenner's parents. The Royal College of Physicians of Great Britain gives a favourable opinion on inoculation (variolation) to prevent smallpox.

1757: Edward Jenner is a pupil at Wotton-under-edge Grammar School and is inoculated.

1758: Edward Jenner is a pupil at Cirencester Grammar School.

1761: Apprenticeship of Edward Jenner to M.J. Ludlow, a surgeon in Chipping Sodbury.

1770: Edward Jenner resides with John Hunter, in St. Georges'Hospital, London.

1772: Return of Edward Jenner to Berkeley. Start of a country surgeon's practice. He meets Edward Gardner, who becomes his great friend and confidant.

1774: Benjamin Jesty vaccinates his wife and two children.

1775: Edward Jenner studies hibernating hedgehogs.

1778: Edward Jenner studies the blocking of coronary arteries in angina of the chest.

1783: Edward Jenner takes part in the launching of a hydrogen balloon.

1785: Edward Jenner buys Chantry Cottage, his house at Berkeley, for £600.

1787: Edward Jenner studies the habits of cuckoos.

1788: March 6. Edward Jenner marries Catherine Kingscote. Foundation of the Gloucestershire Medical Society.

1789: Eward Jenner is elected as a Fellow of the Royal Society. Birth of Edward and Catherine Jenner's first child, named Edward (1789-1810).

1792: Edward Jenner, Diploma in Medicine at the University of St Andrews, Scotland.

1794: Birth of Edward and Catherine Jenner's second child, named Catherine (1794-1833).

1795: Edward Jenner narrowly escapes death following an attack of typhoid. First move to Cheltenham.

1796:
- May 14, first inoculation (vaccination) of a child, James Phipps, by Edward Jenner.
- July 1, variolation of James Phipps by Edward Jenner. Total success of the first ever vaccination. Phipps is immunised and protected against smallpox.

1798: Edward Jenner pursues his studies of cowpox and vaccine. His first book, *An Inquiry into the Causes and Effects of the Variole Vaccinae*, summarising his work, is published. First inoculation of vaccine lymph in London by Henry Cline.

1799: Publication of Jenner's "*Further Observations*", his second book.

1800:
- Spread of Jennerian vaccination to most European countries.
- July, first vaccination in the United States, in Boston.
- Waterhouse's History, the first book on vaccination in America.
- Woodville invited to vaccinate in France after investigation by the French Medical Committee.
- December, public testimonial of twenty-two British physicians supporting vaccination in England.

1801:
- The Mediterranean fleet of the Royal navy is vaccinated.
- Thomas Jefferson, President of the United States, has his family vaccinated.

1802:
- May 14, first vaccination in Bombay, India
- June 2, first government donation to Edward Jenner of the sum of £10,000.

1803:
- February 17, formation of the Royal Jennerian Society for the Extermination of the Smallpox, in London.
- November 30, departure of the Spanish expedition carrying vaccine to South America, then to the Far East.
- Vaccination made compulsory in Sweden.

1806: Second parliamentary enquiry into vaccination and donation of £20,000 to Edward Jenner.

1808: Formation of the National Vaccine Establishment.

1809: Massachusetts passes bill financing free vaccination in the state.

1813: December 15, Edward Jenner, Honourary Doctor of Medicine at the University of Oxford.

1815: - September 13, death of Catherine Jenner, wife of Edward Jenner.
- Final departure from Cheltenham.

1820: Edward Jenner has his first heart attack.

1823: January 26, death of Edward Jenner.

Jenner was often severely criticised and even fiercely attacked, but he did receive many small signs of recognition. The first came in 1801, which is astonishing given the date of the publication of his results which was at the end of 1798. According to Baron, the very first letter, dated February 20th, came from forty-four marine officers of Plymouth dockyard; another, dated May 29th, was sent by the physicians of Novara, in Italy. Yet another, on August 4th, came from the *Institut de France* (signed by Cuvier) and finally, on September 14th 1801, he was awarded a diploma and became a Member of the Royal Society of Sciences of Göttingen. This last distinction would seem the most interesting for it came from abroad and represented a genuine official honour. The others either originated in England or were simple tokens of people's gratitude[56].

The Society of Medicine of Bordeaux, in a report on the vaccine presented to the Citizen Councillor of State, prefect of the department of the Gironde, firmly recommended substituting vaccination for variolation and finished by stating: "*It awarded to Dr. Jenner the title of non-resident Associate, as a mark of high esteem and of recognition in consideration of the great benefits he has rendered to humanity.*" This report is dated 25 Fructidor of the year 9 of the Republic, *i.e.* September 12, 1801[57], two days prior to his election as member of the Royal Society of Sciences of Göttingen. *A priori*, these two distinctions accorded by learned societies less than three years after his first vaccine publication appeared, were to be the very first attributed to Jenner. It is somewhat strange that Jenner perhaps never knew of his membership in the Bordeaux Society, for it was not mentioned by Baron, his first biographer, who inherited his personal papers. However, because the letter bore a date of the French revolutionary calendar and had to transit through a neutral country, it is possible that neither Jenner, nor Baron was able to convert the date to the Gregorian calendar, or even that Jenner never received the letter. Nevertheless, the fact that a citizen of an enemy country was taking a position in French scientific society (the peace of Amiens had not yet been concluded) was quite surprising and showed that Jenner's discovery surpassed even rivalry between warring nations. The first honorary degree from America was a "Diploma of Fellow of the American Society of Art and Science in Massachusetts, signed John Adams, President"[58].

JUPILLE Jean-Baptiste (1872-1923). He was the second person to receive Pasteur's rabies vaccine. He earned the Montyon Prize for devotion and virtue (awarded by the *Académie française* on November 19, 1885) by combating a dog that was (probably) rabid, and was threatening his young companions. A courageous young man. Married and the father of two children, he was employed first at *Institut Pasteur* in Garches, then at the anti-rabies laboratory on Dutot Street, and finally in Dr. Roux's service. Duclaux named him concierge of the *Institut Pasteur* in 1897. In 1918 he retired to his little villa in Joinville-le-Pont, on the outskirts of Paris, where he lived until his demise[59].

KITASATO Shibasaburo (1852-1931). Japanese physician, excellent bacteriologist trained in German-style bacteriology in Japan and later in Germany, under Robert Koch. He worked on the tetanus bacillus; with Behring, he discovered the principle of serotherapy. Back in Japan, he founded an infectious disease Institute. He was made Baron, and held a ministerial position.

KOCH Robert, German physician (1843-1910). Although he worked in private practice, he pursued an interest in biology, and particularly in the agent of anthrax. Very quickly, he achieved great recognition. He was one of the main founders of infectious germ theory. In 1882, he discovered the tuberculosis bacillus and received an endowment of 100,000 marks from the German Empire. On

---

56. Baron, 1838.
57. Grassi, 1801.
58. Baron, 1838, t. 2, p. 450.
59. Anonyme, 1898, p. 226; Horiot, 1995.

the subject of anti-anthrax vaccination, Koch attacked Pasteur's work very violently. One of his articles was translated into French in *La Revue Scientifique*, which also published Pasteur's reply. Koch's article uses the form of address "Mr. *Pasteur*" over sixty times, but states that everything this Mr. Pasteur says is mistaken. "Mr. *Pasteur is very far from... does not say if... does not examine..., is content to..., the weak points of his method..., his faulty method..., having made the same mistake again...,* Mr. *Pasteur's methods have to be recognized as inexact..., lets himself be influenced by prejudices...,* Mr. *Pasteur is not a physician* (sic)..., Mr. *Pasteur believes he has discovered the etiology of anthrax...,* Mr. *Pasteur's pretentions...*"[60]. These quotes are only part of Koch's objections. His text is insulting to Pasteur and difficult to accept coming from a very great scientist. Pasteur's answer was polite and sometimes ironic: "*German chickens are perhaps more complacent than French chickens... Isn't it pleasant, in fact, that you can so lightly accuse me of not knowing how to obtain pure cultures!...*"[61]. The inability of Pasteur's team to obtain pure bacterial or yeast cultures was often reported by early and modern writers. But all of Pasteur's work in microbiology proves the contrary.

In 1883, while on a scientific mission in Egypt and India, Koch discovered the cholera bacillus or coma bacillus. At Thuillier's funeral, he was one of the pallbearers. In 1885, Koch was appointed professor at the Faculty of Medicine and director of the new Hygiene Institute at the University of Berlin. In 1892 he achieved great fame when he announced that he had discovered a specific agent that could cure patients of tuberculosis. The secrecy surrounding his work[62] and his product, and even more so the disappointing results he obtained, gave rise to resounding controversy[63]. Koch's insistence on the absence of a relation between human and bovine tuberculosis was a major error[64]. However, Robert Koch was and remains an exceptional figure of the early bacteriological era. In 1905, he received a well-deserved Nobel Prize.

KOLLE Wilhem (1868-1935). German physician, Koch's assistant at the Institute for infectious diseases in Berlin. Professor of hygiene and bacteriology at the University and director of the Bern Institute for the study of infectious diseases. In 1906, he succeeded Ehrlich as director of the Institute for Experimental Therapy in Frankfurt.

KOPROWSKI Hilary (1915-). American physician born in Warsaw, Poland. At the end of the Second World War, after a short stay in Brazil, he immigrated definitively to the United States. He became director of the Wistar Institute in Philadelphia in 1957 and occupied this position until 1991. He played a crucial role in the development of the oral poliomyelitis vaccine and of rabies vaccine. Hilary Koprowski is also an accomplished musician.

LA CONDAMINE Charles-Marie de (1701-1774). Military man, then assistant chemist at the Academy of Sciences (Paris). He took part in the 10-year expedition sent to the Equator to measure part of the Earth's meridian*. Very curious by nature, La Condamine had himself be given 25 cane strokes on the soles of his feet, after ostensibly stealing a trinket at the market of Constantinople (present day: Istanbul), to see if this punishment was really painful. During Damiens'torture before the latter was quartered for having attempted to assassinate a French king, La Condamine paid the executioner to make him one of his assistants... On the other hand, he exerted considerable effort to promote smallpox inoculation, and he was able to have considerable influence thanks to his remarkable personality.

LAIGRET Jean (1893-1966). Physician of the French colonial troops and microbiologist. In 1914, when he was still a medical student, he was recruited as auxiliary army physician; he was decorated with the Cross of War (*Croix de guerre*) for bravery. He was sent to Dakar in 1927 as chief of Hygiene Services, when a yellow fever epidemic broke out[65]. Laigret's character was sometimes difficult, as documented by a letter written by the Governor General of French West Africa to the Minister of the colonies: "*In addition, not content to grossly insult his immediate superior, Mr Laigret took the liberty*

---

* First basis of the meter unit.

60. Koch, 1883a, p. 65; Koch, 1883b.

61. Pasteur, 1883, p. 74.

62. Metchnikoff, 1939, p. 106.

63. Vapereau, 1893.

64. Vermey, 1902, p. 182.

65. Laigret, 1953 (1966), p. 2441.

of criticising in a caustic and inopportune manner the actions of the Dakar District Governor, and mine, even bringing into question the Deputy of Senegal. Such a recalcitrant attitude, which sets an unfortunate example for the entire health corps, must be reprimanded even more severely given that nothing justifies it... I am therefore asking you to insist that the Minister of War remove Doctor-Captain Laigret from the advancement roster..." The governor was obviously upset... but the letter does not specify the cause of Laigret's discontent. He collaborated with Watson Sellards, who joined him in Dakar. In 1931, he was assigned to the *Institut Pasteur* in Tunis, under the supervision of Charles Nicolle. Between 1932 and 1934, he and Sellards developed a yellow fever vaccine, that Laigret modified several times subsequently. Before his death, Jean Laigret was made Officer of the *Légion d'Honneur* and colonel in the Reserves[66].

LANDSTEINER Karl (1868-1943). In 1900 he discovered the major ABO blood types that made it possible to perform blood transfusion from one person to another. In 1930 he received the Nobel Prize in medicine for this work.

LÉPINE Pierre (1901-1989). French physician, professor and head of the virology department at the *Institut Pasteur* in 1940. Starting in 1950, he studied poliomyelitis viruses and, in 1957, a few weeks after Salk, presented an inactivated vaccine.

LISTER Joseph (1827-1912). He started his career as a surgeon at the Glasgow Hospital. The ravages of purulent wounds, of gangrene, of erysipelas were terrible in hospitals. Lister made a decisive discovery when he read Pasteur's writings about the origin of putrefactions being found in the germs present in the environment.

A means had to be found to kill bacteria without harming tissue. One of his colleagues suggested the use of diluted carbolic acid to kill germs. This was the start of antisepsis in surgery, a veritable revolution in the field[67]. Lister was a major contributor to the triumph of germ theory and its application to surgery.

LITTRÉ Emile (1801-1881). French physician (without a thesis, because he never bothered to write one), a truly learned man, translator of Hippocrates, author of a very famous dictionary of the French language, co-editor of the Capuron-Nysten-Littré dictionary of medicine; he was involved with this dictionary from the 10th edition (1855) to the 14th edition (1878). His name was maintained on subsequent editions.

LOIR Adrien (1862-1942). He was Mrs. Pasteur's nephew, and was to be the "hands" of Pasteur between 1882 and 1888, as well as being, for a number of years, his envoy all over the world. He studied medicine while working in Pasteur's laboratory. His first mission, in 1885, was in Saint-Petersbourg, where he created a rabies treatment centre which would become the Experimental Medicine Institute. Loir went to Australia in 1888 to deliver this continent from the scourge of devouring rabbits. The mission was a failure. Before leaving Australia, Loir made a successful demonstration of anthrax vaccine (in Australia, anthrax was called Cumberland disease). Loir's presentation was very commendable. The Australians, convinced by Loir's experiments of the value of Pasteurian vaccines, called Pasteur to the rescue to fight the anthrax that was decimating their livestock. In 1890, Loir returned to Australia. He settled on Rodd Island, facing Sydney, and succeeded in producing anti-anthrax vaccine and bovine pleuropneumonia agent for variolation using the Willems method (Loir refering to Willems as Dutch was an error, since Willems was Belgian). Loir described this work in detail in several articles, and then again in his memoires[68]. When he was passing through Paris in 1892, he defended his thesis[69]. Interesting details about Loir's mission in Australia can be found in an article by Chaussivert[70], as well as on Internet.

On September 7, 1893, a beylical decree created a Regency wine-making laboratory in Tunisia to improve local wine production, which was suffering from the climate. Duclaux assigned Loir to this project. He quickly set up a rabies treatment Unit, a vaccine-production centre and a laboratory for chemical and bacteriological researches. A beylical decree, issued on April 11, 1894, officially created

66. Jean Laigret file, Académie nationale de Médecine (Paris).
67. Fisher, 1977.
68. Loir, 1892, pp. 85 & 134; Loir, 1938, p. 113.
69. Regelsperger, 1908, p. 15.
70. Chaussivert *in* Morange, 1991, p. 242.

an anti-rabies institute; Loir was appointed its director. It was the first such institute in North Africa[71]. On February 14, 1900, the establishment was named *Institut Pasteur* and given civil entity status. Loir was officially designated its director.

A little over a year later, the newspaper *L'Eclair* of May 29, 1901 published this distressing news item: "*A telegram from Tunis informs us that yesterday morning at nine thirty, in front of the laboratory of the Regency Institute, Mr. Panet, a technician, fired four shots with a handgun at Mr. Loir, who was just arriving. All the shots reached their target. The murderer was immediately arrested. The first enquiries revealed that this employee suffered from delusions of persecution. A few days earlier he had resigned from his job with much ado and had told certain people that he was being followed by a Jew, and that this life had to stop. But no one had believed that he could go so far as to attempt to kill a universally respected physician. Dr. Loir is Pasteur's nephew; he was general commissioner of the Tunisian Exposition. He is married and the father of two children. He was taken to hospital and the bullets were extracted. No vital organs were struck; it is expected that doctor Loir will survive.*"[72] What a surprising turn of events! Fortunately for him and his family, Loir recovered. He left Tunisia in 1902.

Loir, who spoke English since his stay in Australia, was to take his knowledge and his experience to the inhabitants of South Africa and Rhodesia. In 1902, at the request of Lord Grey and Dr. Jameson, he founded a *Institut Pasteur* in Boulouwayo, to fight a rabies epidemic. In 1903 he was named professor at the Colonial School of Agriculture (France). In 1906, he was given the General Biology and Pathology Chair at the Faculty of Medicine in Montreal (Canada). Back in France, Loir carried out several more missions abroad[73]. He was Director of the Hygiene Office in Le Havre from 1908 until his death.

Loir wrote an enjoyable and interesting account of his work with Pasteur, entitled *A l'ombre de Pasteur* ("*In Pasteur's Shadow*"). He wrote it when he was about 76, fifty years after he left Pasteur's laboratory. The memories are very distant... He seems to better remember small incidents than historical events. Portions of his text have often been taken literally by commentators of Pasteur's work. In fact, the reader has reason to be sceptical - and sometimes even very skeptical - about the contents of this book written so long after the events it describes. Loir himself comments: "*I never thought, during the long period when I worked closely with him* (Pasteur), *to take notes other than the ones he dictated to me, and which he kept.*"[74] Loir was not in possession of these notes when he wrote his book. In his memoire, the incidents are probably true, but can the same be said about the historical facts? It is clear that most of them are not such accurate reflection of reality. Taking them literally to elaborate major arguments is a very questionable practice. Are Loir's memoires deliberately misleading? Not necessarily.

MATHER Cotton (1662 or 1663 - 1728 or 1729). Protestant clergyman who studied medicine at Harvard College. Married three times, in 1686, 1703 and 1715, father of 15 children. "*Having learned of its successful use in the Middle east in the transactions of the Royal Society of London, and from an African slave he owned*", he convinced Zabiel Boylston to use inoculation (variolation) during the serious smallpox epidemic raging in Boston in 1721[75].

MÉRIEUX Charles (1907-2001). French virologist and entrepreneur from Lyon. He devised an efficient technique for mass production of vaccines against diseases such as polio, meningitis, diphtheria, tetanus, foot-and-mouth disease, etc.

During World War II, he expanded operations at his father's microbiological laboratory in order to distribute blood plasma to members of the French Resistance, and a serum for malnutritioned children. In 1947 he founded the French Institute of Foot-and-Mouth Disease (IFFA) with Herman Frenkel's help (see chapter 10), later renamed the Mérieux Institute.

Mérieux collaborated on vaccine projects with Dr. Hilary Koprowski, American virologist, with whom he developed a safer and more efficient human rabies vaccine. In the early 1980s he started a training organisation, Bioforce Development, to prepare professionals for public health emergencies, especially in third-world countries.

71. Anonyme, 1894, p. 87.
72. Anonyme, 1901, p. 386.
73. Loir, 1907, p. 1393; Regelsperger, 1908, p. 15; Loir, 1930, p. 551.
74. Loir, 1938, p. 5.
75. Kaufman, 1984, vol. II, p. 503.

METCHNIKOFF or METCHNIKOV Elie or Ilia (1845-1916). In 1882, he discovered the phenomenon of phagocytosis in starfish larvae. He created a theory of cellular immunity, based on this phenomenon, but his theory was not easily accepted. He was an unconventional man, whose ideas were sometimes preposterous. For instance, he maintained that "*according to some facts I was able to gather, it seems that men of genius are rarely the first-born in their families; the latter are usually weaker than their younger siblings; mortality and criminality are higher among first-borns, while their younger siblings more often turn out to be geniuses*"[76]. Needless to say, he was the fifth child in his family. But some of his other views were closer to the truth. For instance, he was a staunch advocate of a doctrine which held that the intestinal flora was responsible for reducing longevity in human beings. "*Convinced of the harmful nature of our intestinal flora, over 18 years ago I started an experiment on myself, in order to combat its damaging effect: I abstain from all raw food and, moreover, I have introduced into my diet lactic microbes capable of preventing intestinal putrefaction.*"[77] In one of his last writings, he went on to say: "*Rational microbiotics is a science of the future; but for the moment I will have to be content with a normal life at the age of 70.*"[78] Had he been asked why he was growing old, he would have answered that it was because he did not start his diet early enough! A man ahead of his time... at least on the subject of lactobacilli, which have now become a flourishing business, but not as new as advertisers would have us believe. A likeable figure and a great scientist. He was one of the fathers of immunology, and won a well-deserved Nobel Prize.

NICOLLE Charles (1866-1936). Metchnikoff's student, in 1903 he was chosen for the position of Director of the *Institut Pasteur* in Tunis. He kept this position for over thirty years. His first contribution was the discovery of exanthemic typhus prevention. This disease was endemic in many poor countries, and took the form of a deadly epidemic in the armed forces. He received the Nobel Prize in 1928. He also discovered the important phenomenon of occult (non apparent) diseases.

NOCARD Edmont-Isidore-Etienne (1850-1903). At the age of 26, according to Roux, he was "*... a tall and robust young man, natural and easy-going, whose appearance mirrored his character. He looked honest, intelligent and kind, had a charming smile and a rather sensuous mouth*"[79]. Professor of surgical pathology (1878) at the Alfort Veterinary school, and later of public health and contagious diseases (1887), he was Director of the School between 1887 and 1891, to the great vexation of Gabriel Colin, whose deep-seated hostility toward Pasteur and his ideas was well-known. Roux continues: "*For over twenty years the lives of Edmond Nocard and mine were practically inseparable.*"[80] Nocard turned out to be a brilliant student of Pasteur's. But as Director of the Alfort School, he never really won the confidence of the students, who were sometimes turbulent. He became a Unit head at the *Institut Pasteur*, without leaving Alfort. He proved that human tuberculosis is communicable to birds, and that bird tuberculosis is communicable to mammals of different species; that the virulence of the same tuberculosis bacillus varies depending on the host animal species; that human and bovine tuberculoses have the same pathogenic identity. He identified the contagious bovine pleuropneumonia agent known for a long time as PPLO for pleuropneumonia-like-organism. He used tuberculin as a means of early diagnosis of bovine tuberculosis. With Bang, he proposed to diagnose glanders by using a mallein test. Nocard participated in the development of applied serotherapy, in particular the prevention of tetanus. He identified numerous bacteria, and those of the Nocardia family bear his name. A beautiful monument in his honour is located in the park of the Alfort School[81].

NOGUCHI Hideyo (1876-1928). Of Japan, member of the Rockefeller Institute (1914). Highly reputed researcher who, unfortunately for him, discovered the wrong rabies micro-organisms (1913) and of yellow fever (1918-1924). He died of yellow fever while trying to verify his previous studies[82].

ODIER Louis (1748-1817). Very respected physician from Geneva. He studied medicine in Geneva and Edinburg. He was an enthusiastic promoter of Jennerian vaccination, in Switzerland and in France.

---

76. Metchnikoff, 1939, p. 70.
77. Metchnikoff, 1939, p. 156.
78. Metchnikoff, 1939, p. 158.
79. Roux, 1906, p. 487.
80. Roux, 1906, p. 487.
81. Pilet, 2003, p. 1397.
82. Garrison, 1966, p. 588.

PARK William Hallock (1863-1939). Physician and Public health microbiologist; he studied in New York and in Vienna. He played a particularly important role in the fight against diphtheria, by creating a coherent and active immunisation program against this disease among pupils of New York schools, using toxin-antitoxin (serovaccination). The William Hallock Park Memorial Library was named after him[83].

PASTEUR Louis (Dole, 1822-Garches, 1895). Pasteur was born in a family of craftsmen or farmers, modest and honourable[84]. He was born in Dole, but his family soon moved to Marmoz, and then to Arbois, when Louis Pasteur was 5 years old. He remained attached to the family home in Arbois, which he converted and cared for lovingly. He studied at the Arbois College, then at the Besançon lyceum. He eventually entered the *Ecole Normale Supérieure*[85] where, very quickly, he starts to do laboratory work, for which he has a passion. His work is remarked by distinguished masters, who were to help his career considerably. He goes on to obtain one diploma after another: *agrégation* in physical sciences (1846), and doctoral theses in physics and then in chemistry (1848). He is named professor of physics at the Dijon lyceum, where he cannot continue his laboratory work. Therefore, he leaves this position to become a supply teacher at the faculty of sciences of Strasbourg, where he can hope to continue his experimental work. He married one of the daughters of the University Rector, Marie Laurent. The couple had five children: Jeanne (1850-1859), Jean-Baptiste (1851-1908), Cécile (1853-1866), Marie-Louise (1858-1934) and Camille (1863-1865), three of whom dead in their childhood years. But Pasteur still lacked the working conditions he felt he needed. In 1854, at the age of 32, he accepted the positions of chemistry professor and dean of the Faculty of Sciences of Lille.

1853: Pasteur is made Knight of the Order of the *Légion d'Honneur*.

1856: First studies on fermentation alcohol (beet production).

1857: Study on lactic fermentation, followed by attribution of the functions of scientific studies administrator and director at the *Ecole Normale Supérieure*. Pasteur moves to Paris to fulfil the requirement for candidature to the Academy of Sciences.

1858: Study on tartaric acid fermentation.

1861: Discovery of anaerobiotic life (without oxygen), studies on acetic fermentation.

1862: Pasteur (age 40) is elected to the Academy of Sciences (mineralogy section). Emile Duclaux enters his laboratory.

1863: Pasteur is made Officer of the Order of the *Légion d'Honneur*. Start of the creation of a team of researchers to work with him.

1865: Start of work on pasteurisation; start of work on silkworm diseases.

1867: Lister developed antiseptic surgery, based on Pasteur's work.

1868: Pasteur is made Commander of the Order of the *Légion d'Honneur*.
Pasteur (age 46) has his first hemiplegia attack.

1871: Research on beer.

1872: Retirement from teaching position at the Sorbonne, for personal health reasons.

1873: Pasteur (age 51) is elected to the Academy of Medicine.

1874: First annuity granted to Pasteur: 12,000 francs a year.

1875 (1876 or 1877): Charles Chamberland becomes a laboratory assistant for Pasteur.

1876-1877: Study on septic vibrion and anthrax.

1878: Pasteur's status is raised to Grand Officer of the Order of the *Légion d'Honneur*. Emile Roux enters Pasteur's laboratory.

1880: Elected member of the Central Society of Veterinary Medicine; chicken cholera virus-vaccine development; start of work on rabies.

---

83. Kaufman, 1984, t. II, p. 578.

84. Moreau, 2000.

85. Moreau, 2003.

1881: Pouilly-le-Fort experiment; Pasteur (age 59), member of the *Académie française*.

1882: Adrien Loir enters the *Ecole Normale Supérieure* laboratory.

1883: Second annuity granted to Pasteur.

1885: Vaccination of Joseph Meister against rabies, then vaccination of Jean-Baptiste Jupille.

1886: Alexandre Yersin enters Roux's laboratory.

1888: Inauguration of the *Institut Pasteur*, on Dutot Street.

1891: Foundation of the *Institut Pasteur* in Saigon.

1892: Ceremony in honour of Pasteur at the Sorbonne.

1894: Last stay in Arbois.

1895: Pasteur (age 73) leaves his Paris Institute in June, to go to Villeneuve-l'Etang (*Institut Pasteur* in Garches), where he died on September 28; on October 5, a national funeral was held.

His scientific publications and his speeches constitute his official image, the image he was careful to preserve. In the eyes of the world, he wanted to be a man of science only. But his correspondence is more eloquent. He also dictated the account of a good portion of his life, in the book written by his son-in-law, René Vallery-Radot: Mr. *Pasteur, histoire d'un savant par un ignorant*. He dedicated most of his summer holidays in 1883 to this account of his life. "*Of course René is demanding, but his work is advancing... one more month and his book will be finished.*"[86] "*I have to converse with him from morning to night, and to go over forty years of my life. It's quite tiring, but he is so pleased...*"[87]. "*... René is quite well, I tell you, and even very well, because he is happy to have finished his book, but not as happy as I am. What a vacation I've had! I did not even take an hour for my own studies. I am more tired than when I arrived. But this book had to be written: now it is. Thanks God!*"[88]

This book is an official version of Pasteur's life, with the human side of the story totally absent. René-Vallery-Radot wrote this biography of his father-in-law and his work according to the latter's wishes. The second book, *La Vie de Pasteur*, by the same author, describes Pasteur and his works as the son-in-law wanted to see them. Pasteur was no longer there to contradict him, but who knows if he would have done so? Both books are interesting, but to be considered with some reservation, since the author has a clear favourable bias. The master's laboratory notebooks, his notes and letters to friends sometimes reveal his reasoning. Some of his remarks are surprising. All of these documents were given to the French National Library (*Bibliothèque nationale*) archives by Louis Pasteur Vallery-Radot[89] in 1964, to be made available to the public. We have the right, and even the duty, to study them, sometimes with the feeling of committing an indiscretion, because these notes were not written to be seen by the public, except a few pages, written in careful handwriting and intended (?) to be shown. There are also many texts from his friends and family, from admirers and opponents. They must be taken in context.

Pasteur was awarded many prizes. In 1856, the Royal Society of London awarded Mr. Pasteur the Rumford Medal for his research relative to the polarization of light... In 1869, he was elected one of the fifty foreign members of the Royal Society of London[90].

PETER Michel (1824-1893). Michel Peter married Céline Belin, Adrien Loir senior's niece. Therefore, Michel Peter was the latter's nephew by marriage. Adrien Loir senior had married Amélie Laurent, whose sister Marie Laurent married Louis Pasteur. Adrien Loir senior was Louis Pasteur's brother-in-law. Louis Pasteur and Michel Peter, of the same age, were doubly related. But these rather remote family ties did not encourage the friendship that might have developed between the two men. The families knew each-other but did not often come together[91]. Adrien Loir senior had a son, named Adrien Loir as well, who was later to be Pasteur's "hands" for several years, and who would write his memories under the title *A l'ombre de Pasteur*.

86. Pasteur, Cor., t. 3, p. 372.
87. Pasteur, Cor., t. 3, p. 383.
88. Pasteur, Cor., t. 3, p. 401.
89. Pasteur Vallery-Radot, 1964, p. IX.
90. Americanized, 1892, vol. X, p. 6729.
91. Loir, 1938, p. 31.

Michel Peter was an accomplished man. Born in Paris of poor parents, he started out as apprentice in the Lahure printing shop, after his primary school studies. He started his professional career as a simple printer. Self-taught, in four years he was able to complete the Baccalaureate ès sciences program and obtain his diploma. While he worked as shop manager in the same printing shop, he started to study medicine. Doctor of medicine at 35, he was remarked by Trousseau. He ended his career as holder of a chair at the Faculty of Medicine, head of clinical departments in several hospitals successively, member of the Academy of Medicine, Commander of the *Légion d'Honneur*. He was known for being an agreeable man. He had remarkable oratorical skills. Unfortunately, he considered that applying laboratory experiments to pathology was heresy. Only clinical practice counted.

Michel Peter developed the theory of "spontaneous generation of morbidity", which he opposed to the germ theory. In a speech given before the Academy of Medicine, he said, addressing himself to Pasteur: "*I mean to say that your virus* (anthrax virus) *is prepared and manipulated by you, Monsieur, and by your co-workers. I agree that while you are here, it will be prepared well. But when you will no longer be here? What will become of your attenuated virus when it will be left in the hands of the possible malpractice of careless and irresponsible technicians, and above all, what will become of those inoculated?... I have said, and I repeat, that all this research on microbes are not worth the time spent on them or the fuss made about them, and that after all the work nothing would be changed in medicine, there would only be a few extra microbes... Research and experiments that prove that we are not only surrounded by inoffensive bacteria, but also filled with equally inoffensive bacteria; that these bacteria only become morbid within us and by our intermediary... However, I must say in conclusion that this matter concerns neither* M. *Pasteur nor myself, but medicine, which is threatened by the invasion of incompetent, and rash persons given to dreaming. This is why I have intervened, and it is why I will intervene again and again.*"[92] Michel Peter remained very constant in his opposition to Pasteur, to the point of being obsessively painstaking and ridiculous. But when he died, the obituary notices were very respectful, because he was an excellent physician.

PFEIFFER Richard Friedrich Johannes (1858-1926). German bacteriologist and hygienist, pupil of Koch. He worked in many areas of bacteriology and immunology. In 1896, he developed a vaccine against typhoid fever.

PINEL Philippe (1745-1826). French physician. Appointed to the Bicêtre Infirmery, then to the Salpêtrière Hospital; member of the Institute and professor of internal pathology at the Faculty of Medicine in Paris. He has become famous for freeing the asylum patients in his charge from their chains, and treating them like other patients. He took an early interest in Jennerian vaccination. Member of the Academy of Medicine.

PLOTKIN Stanley (1932-). American physician. While working at the Wistar Institute in Philadelphia, he developed many vaccines; notably, in the 1960s, the rubella vaccine RA27/3 strain, now used wordwide. He also developed experimental vaccines against cytomegalovirus, polio and varicella. He collaborated with Wistar scientists Hilary Koprowski and Tadeusz Wiktor on an anti-rabies vaccine; and with H. Fred Clark on a vaccine against rotavirus.

Stanley Plotkin is the author of the multi-edition standard textbook "Vaccines", and has written over 600 articles. His awards include the Sabin Foundation Medal (2002), the title of Knight of the *Légion d'Honneur* (1998), the Distinguished Physician Award of the Pediatric Infectious Disease Society (1993), Associate member of the French Academy of Medicine (2009). He is currently an advisor at the pharmaceutical firm Sanofi Pasteur.

RAMON Léon-Gaston (Bellechaume, 1886 - Garches, 1963). After completing his studies at the Alfort Veterinary School, he spent a year in the chemistry-pharmacy laboratory of that school. It was there that he learned that a thimbleful of formalin in a litre of milk was enough to prevent milk from turning, without changing its taste or consistency. According to Prof. Clément Bressou, this was the origin of Ramon's tendency to use formalin like a magic potion in numerous circumstances[76]. Ramon entered the contagious diseases laboratory directed by Henri-Vallé, successor of Edmond Nocard. He quickly developed a passion for research. On Vallé's recommendation, he entered the Garches *Institut Pasteur* to produce antidiphtheric and anti-tetanus sera. During the First World War, from the Veterinary School of Toulouse where the Garches annex had taken refuge, he delivered

92. Peter, 1883, p. 560.

six million doses of anti-tetanus serum... This demanding and repetitive task allowed him to observe and discover phenomena that would win him world renown. In 1917, he married Marthe Monon, grandniece of Emile Roux. In two years, his name became well-known thanks to crucial discoveries: the flocculation reaction in 1922, human anatoxine vaccines, the adjuvant substances of immunity, the associated vaccines in 1923, 1924 and 1926. He was named director of the *Institut Pasteur* in Garches in 1926. Upon Emile Roux's death, he became assistant director of the *Institut Pasteur*, and then its director in 1940, a responsibility he renounced at the end of the same year for health reasons. He left the directorship of the Garches annex, and the *Institut Pasteur*, in 1944... In May 1949, he was elected unanimously by forty nations Director General of the International office of Epizootics (OIE), nowadays "World Organisation for Animal Health", a position he held until his retirement in 1959. He was given the Grand Cross of the *Légion d'Honneur*, and received the gold medal of the National Centre for Scientific Research (CNRS). He spent his retirement years in Garches. He is buried in Bellechaume[93], his native village.

REED Walter (1852-1902). American doctor born in Gloucester County, Virginia. He was a graduate of the medical department of the University of Virginia, assistant surgeon in the United States Army (1875). He completed specialized studies in bacteriology and pathology at the John Hopkins Hospital. During the Spanish-American war, he was president of the Board of medical officers charged with investigating and reporting on the prevalence of typhoid fever in the Army. His greatest achievement in the field of science was his contribution to the cause, spread and prevention of yellow fever[94].

RICORD Philippe (1800-1889). French physician, chief surgeon at the Midi Hospital (for venereal diseases), specialist of venereal diseases.

ROSSIGNOL Hippolyte (1837-1919). French veterinarian, he was a skilled practitioner and a talented writer. He became known through his active participation in the Pouilly-le-Fort experiment, which took place on his farm. Initially he did not believe in bacteriology, but he was converted by Pasteur: "*I was an unbeliever myself, but in the face of obvious proof I had only one thing left to do: admit my error, and I did.*"[95]

ROUX Pierre-Paul-Emile (1853-1933). He started his medical studies in Clermont-Ferrand. It was there that he met Duclaux, professor of physics; he became his volunteer assistant. Roux left for Paris to complete his studies; there, financial difficulties drove him to choose medical studies in the military branch, at Val-de-Grâce (Paris). According to Mary Cressac, Roux's niece, Roux was not suited for the discipline characterising that milieu. By deliberately antagonising military authorities, he had himself expulsed at the start of 1877[96]. Roux took various jobs to earn a living. These difficult years ended in 1878 when Roux accidentally met Duclaux, who had just been named professor of meteorology at the Agronomic Institute. Duclaux remembered him very well and hired him as a volunteer assistant. Roux was now closer to the "Pasteur clan". And he had a modest but steady income. Some time later, Duclaux recommended Roux to Pasteur as "*animal inoculator*", a task that physicists and chemists who had graduated from the *Ecole Normale Supérieure* on Ulm Street were unable to perform, having never learned such procedures. Roux entered the Pasteurian universe in 1878, probably in November. His work became indessociable from Pasteur's, in the domain of infectious diseases. His role was essential. In fact, some descriptions of him are surprising. Legroux wrote: "*Emile Roux's character was fundamentally opposed to Pasteur's, he was neither orderly nor very eager in his work, but he had a lively and clear intelligence, adapting very quickly; he was educated and skilled; he was quick to anger, perhaps the only trait he shared with his master?*"[97] What are we to believe?

Roux's great achievement was clinical serotherapy of diphtheria, which earned him international glory. He studied many subjects. He worked successfully on tuberculosis, on "*soluble chemical products*" (toxins), syphilis... In 1892, he was promoted to the rank of Commander of the *Légion d'Honneur*. He received numerous prizes.

93. Bressou, 1970.
94. Owen, 1911, p. 32.
95. Rossignol, 1881b, p. 290.
96. Cressac, 1950, p. 55.
97. Legroux, 1942, p. 39.

At the same time, Roux was a sensitive and sentimental man. He fell in love with a young English woman named Mary, in 1880 or 1881. Having been recommended by Mary Robinson, she was studying French and chemistry in Duclaux's laboratory. Roux found himself praising "*the unequalled complexion of English girls when they are pretty*". In 1884 and 1885, he made several trips to visit the young girl's parents in the suburbs of London. Mary died shortly afterwards of "galloping" tuberculosis. Roux had already had a first pulmonary attack, with fever and blood expectoration. He was tended with great solicitude by Olga Metchnikoff. A deep friendship developed between Roux and this woman with "*dazzling shoulders*" (still in Roux's own words, revealing him to be an admirer of beauty even at death's door)[98].

Roux's tuberculosis remains a troubling episode. Certain data seem to prove that he inoculated himself with tuberculosis in 1883, to study the evolution of the disease. Thus, he might have contaminated Mary with his own experimental tuberculosis, and might have been unwittingly responsible for her death. This could explain his determination to defeat infectious diseases, his work, his fear of germs, his behaviour toward others and particularly women, as well as toward society in general. It might also be partly responsible for his asceticism. According to his family, he recovered relatively quickly from his disease, and was not contagious. But for most of his life he expectorated blood and pus, a symptom attributed to chronic bronchitis. Legroux states that Veillon, Borrel and himself could not identify the Koch bacillus in his sputum, despite repeated exams over many years. Roux, a responsible man, was careful not to kiss children, and used only his own tableware[99].

His niece tells us that he was very fond of the company of the women he visited regularly. She adds: "*Emile Roux, sentimental by nature, brought up by his mother, by Marie Lecoux, and by his sister Marie, understood women and loved them. He had unending indulgence for their excentricities.*"[100] The same grandniece also recounts that he had several other sentimental relationships that seemed solid, lasting and profound. This aspect of Roux's personality clearly humanises the impression conveyed by classical portraits of him, whether they be ink drawings or oil paintings.

His two main interests were science and politics. He was a staunch republican, a Dreyfus partisan and a great admirer of Clemenceau. Born into a family of practicing Catholics, he was a non-believer, but respected the Church and its members. He chose nuns for tending his hospital, and was careful to provide them with all the comfort they needed. He sent them to vacation on a property of the *Institut Pasteur*. He was opposed to the separation of the Church and the State.

Emile Roux was an exceptional man. His attitudes to Ferran and Haffkine were in conflict with Pasteur's. He seems to have had a natural sense of justice. The *Institut(s) Pasteur* provided his living and was (were) his passion. He succeeded Pasteur at the Academy of Medicine in 1896, and was elected Member of the Academy of Sciences in 1899. He was president of the Public Hygiene Board, as well as of numerous commissions of the Ministry of Public Health or of Municipality of Paris[101]. He died on November 3, 1933 and was honoured with a national funeral[102]. His contributions to France, and especially medicine, are inestimable. His tomb is located in the alley of trees of the *Institut Pasteur* gardens, among those who formed his community.

SABIN Albert Bruce (1906-1993). American bacteriologist and physician of Russian origin. After World War II, he was professor at the University of Charleston in Cincinnati, and at the Weizmann Institute. In 1961, his attenuated poliomyelitis vaccine became the world standard in the fight against this disease.

SALK Jonas Edward (1914-1995). American physician. He obtained his doctorate from the University of New York in 1939. He worked with Thomas Francis on immunisation against influenza. In 1947 he became the head of the virus laboratory at the University of Pittsburg, and started his research on poliomyelitis; in 1953, he published his first findings concerning human immunisation. In 1954, his inactivated injectable polio vaccine became widely used for a time and was brought back into use in the past few years.

98. Cressac, 1950, p. 77.
99. Cressac, 1950, p. 154.
100. Cressac, 1950, p. 187.
101. Dujarric de la Rivière, p. 345.
102. Mollaret *in* Dumesnil, 1947, p. 212; Cressac, 1950.

SALMON Daniel-Elmer (1850-1914). He obtained his degree in veterinary medicine from the University of Cornell in 1872. Head of the Bureau of Animal Industry, he conducted several surveys on animal diseases and their influence on public health. With Theobald Smith, he demonstrated that inanimate substances could confer immunity. He discovered the Salmonella bacteria, which bear his name.

SCHICK Bela (1877-1967). Hungarian pediatrician at the University of Vienna. In the United States, he developed a very useful intradermoreaction test for detecting immunity to diphtheria.

SELLARDS Andrew Watson (1884-1942). American physician, microbiologist, a member of the Department of Tropical Medicine of the Harvard Medical School.

SMITH Theobald (1859-1934). The son of German emigrants, graduate of Cornell University (PhD) and of Albany Medical School (MD), he was attracted to microbiology and immunology. He is often considered one of the greatest American bacteriologist and expert in comparative pathology. Ehrlich and Koch's writings, in German (his native tongue), orient him toward research. On December 1, 1883, he was hired as an assistant at the veterinary division of the U.S. Department of Agriculture in Washington, D.C., under Daniel E. Salmon. With the latter, he demonstrated the possibility of conferring immunity using an inanimate substance. He discovered the role of ticks in the transmission of bovine Texas fever; this was the first demonstration of transmission of a pathogenic agent by a vector arthropod. Smith worked at several American Universities: Columbia (George Washington University), Harvard medical School and the Rockefeller Institute.

SPERINO Casimiro. Italian physician. Author of scientific books and articles on syphilis and public health surveillance, which include *De la prostitution dans la ville de Turin* and *La Syphilisation*. Member of the medico-surgical Academy of Torino. Physician at the Torino "Syphilicome" starting in 1837.

STOKES Adrian (1887-1927). Professor of Pathology at Guy's Hospital, London[103]. "*I came into still closer contact with him* (A. Stokes). *He appealed to me as one of the most reliable, original, energic, and lovable of the officers engaged in bacteriological research at the front...*"[104].

TAKAHASHI Michiaki. Director of the Foundation for Microbial Diseases of Osaka University. Inventor of the varicella vaccine, a vaccine isolated from the vesicles of a 3-year old Japanese boy with a typical case of chickenpox. The vaccine, named Oka after the boy, was extensively used in Japan, Kora, USA, France, Thailand and elsewhere.

TERRILLON Octave (1844-1895). He obtained his "*agrégation*" from the Faculty of Medicine of Paris. For two years, he treated the wounds of patients coming to receive Pasteur's anti-rabies treatment.

THEILER Max (1899-1972). South African of Swiss origin, then American physician*. He worked at the Department of Tropical Medicine, Harvard Medical School, in Cambridge, Mass., and later at the Rockefeller Foundation in New York. He created the "Mouse Protection Test" for yellow fever as a diagnostic tool in epidemiology. In 1927, he and his colleagues demonstrated that the yellow fever agent is a filtration virus. He developed the "strain 17D" vaccine against yellow fever. In 1951, he won the Nobel Prize in medicine and physiology "*for his discoveries concerning yellow fever and how to combat it*".

TIOLLAIS Pierre Jean René Noël (1934-). French physician, molecular biologist and oncologist. Professor of biochemistry at the Faculty of Medicine, University of Paris VII, as well as at the *Institut Pasteur* in Paris, where he was director of a Research Unit.

Starting in 1978, he sudied the hepatitis B virus. He and his team cloned the *E. coli* viral genome and determined its sequence. They were the first to describe the genetic organization of the HBV. In1980 they obtained CHO cell lines transfected by the cloned viral DNA, producing the surface antigen of the virus in particle form, which led to the production of the first hepatitis B vaccine obtained by genetic engineering, a real revolution in vaccinology.

---

* Max Theiler was the fourth son of Sir Arnold Theiler, veterinary bacteriologist who headed the South African services to farmers. He discovered the virus responsible for African horse sickness, a deadly disease, and the aetiological agent of the Theileriosis (*Theileria parva*).

103. Parish, 1965, p. 265.

104. Cummins, 1927, p. 956.

Pierre Tiollais is a member of several Academies. Since 1999, he has been honorary professor of the Shanghai Institute of Biochemistry, Chinese Academy of Sciences.

THUILLIER Louis (1858-1883). Graduated from the *Ecole Normale Supérieure* in 1877, he immediately entered Pasteur's laboratory as "*préparateur agrégé*". He took part in anti-anthrax experiments in France, Germany and Hungary. He gained distinction for his studies on swine erysipelas, having discovered the causal agent of the disease. With Pasteur, he developed a relatively effective vaccine against this disease. In 1883, he consented to be part of the Pasteurian studies mission to Egypt, where cholera was raging, with Roux, Straus and Nocard. He died of cholera on Wednesday, September 19, 1883. His correspondence with Pasteur, during his travels in German-speaking countries, is interesting and instructive[105].

TOUSSAINT Jean-Joseph-Henry (1847-1890). He graduated from the School of Veterinary Medicine of Lyon in 1869, and started his career as anatomy instructor, remaining Chauveau's assistant. In 1876, he became professor of anatomy, physiology and elementary zoology at the Veterinary School of Toulouse. Doctor es natural sciences (1877) and doctor of medicine (1878). In 1879, he became professor of physiology at the Medical School of Toulouse, in addition to his other teaching functions. He conducted laboratory work with great passion, and published articles on many varied subjects: the prehistoric horse of Solutré, veterinary surgery, physiology, infectious diseases, etc. In 1880, he sent a note concerning immunisation of animals against anthrax to the Academy of Sciences. In 1880, his first vaccinations of sheep against anthrax brought him flattering renown. Foreign member of the Royal Academy of Agriculture of Torino, member of the order of Academic Palms, envoy of the French Ministry to the Cambridge Conference, honorary associate of the Royal College of Veterinary Surgeons of London, foreign member of the Royal Society of Medical Sciences of Brussels, Knight of the *Légion d'Honneur* in 1882. He received many prizes from the Academy of Sciences and the Academy of Medicine, as well as the gold medal of the Central Society of Veterinary Medicine. Despite support from many colleagues, including the unconditional support of Bouley and Chauveau, two renowned scientists, he was unable to withstand competition with Pasteur and his team. Dr. Caubert, director of the Medical School of Toulouse, commented: "*In 1882, under the weight of the great ideas it carried, his brain gave way*". The health problems to which he was subject starting in 1885 forced him to give up teaching in 1887. He died on August 4, 1890 in Toulouse[106]. His death was sad: "*At the age of 34, disease, attacking the brain of this passionate researcher, brutally interrupted a career sufficiently rich to make it seem as if it was that of a man with the future before him. Then, slowly, secretly, nature went on to destroy this brain that it had so superbly organised; darkness descended on this source of light; at first, waves of love for truths yet to discover persisted; finally, darkness came, all light went out and only the body survived by several years this mind, powerful and original, which, without disdaining the work of others, was more inclined to follow the train of its own thoughts.*"[107]

Inventor of the first anthrax vaccine, his name is respected, but a little forgotten. His memory is overshadowed by that of Pasteur. But Toussaint provoked this destiny by confusing rapid execution with precipitation. His work on the identity of the chicken cholera bacteria and of acute experimental septicemia was discredited. His discovery of the microbe of sheeppox was unfortunate[108]. There are several examples of the fact that Toussaint, probably overwhelmed with work, published too quickly. Arloing comments: "*Toussaint believed that he had observed the abundant presence of tuberculosis virus in vaccinal lymph taken from a tubercular cow. Factors of error probably slipped into Toussaint's experiments, because all attempts made since then to confirm his hypotheses have been negative.*"[109] It is unfortunate that this exceptional and intelligent scientist ended his career in some confusion, perhaps partly due to his health problems. He was a complex but very worthy man.

TRONCHIN Théodore (1709-1781). Born in Geneva, where he started his studies before pursuing them in London and Leyden, where he was a pupil of Boerhaave. He obtained his medical degree at the age of 21, and settled in Amsterdam. He remained in that city for 25 years, before returning

105. Anonyme, 1883a, p. 322; Thuillier, 1968.
106. Neumann, 1896; Wrotnowska, 1975.
107. Charrin, 1890, p. 654.
108. Toussaint, 1881b, p. 362.
109. Arloing, 1891, p. 154.

to Geneva, where he became consultant to royalty and famous figures like Voltaire. He was an ardent advocate of inoculation and it is said that he performed over 20,000. In 1762, he was named physician of the Duke of Orleans and was housed at the "*Palais royal*" in Paris until his death[110].

VALENTIN Louis (1758-1825). Student surgeon in the *Roy-Infanterie* regiment. He was sent to Saint Domingo as physician in chief of the French armies. He lived in *Cap Français* (now *Cap Haïtien*) for 7 years, before going to the United States, where he worked in various hospitals. In 1799 he retired to Nancy and travelled in Italy and in England[111].

VALLERY-RADOT Marie-René (1853-1933). Pasteur's son-in-law, eulogist of his work. Pasteur was impressed with him as soon as they met, and spoke warmly of him: "*It will be my way of praying to God and offering him a thousand thanks for having made our path cross that of this dear and worthy young man who will one day be (and who already is in the eyes of those who can see clearly) a man of distinction in French literature.*" And again "*submitted* (a letter) *to my dear master in literature R.V.R.* (René Vallery-Radot)..."[112]. The latter was certainly a handsome man. His writing style had literary merit. Most of his books, rather conventional, have been forgotten... *Le Journal d'un volontaire d'un an* cannot be said to have more than anecdotal interest[113]. In 1879, he married Marie-Louise, Pasteur's youngest daughter. Secretary of Minister Freycinet in 1879, he received the *Légion d'Honneur* in 1880. His letters, in the possession of the "*Bibliothèque nationale de France*", are undeniably commonplace. He writes to his mother-in-law that she is the best in the world, signs the letter René Vallery-Radot and adds Jean Baptiste n° 2[114], that is, a second son of the Pasteur couple. He decided on his own to make his father-in-law's work known, and profited from this decision.

His first biography, Mr. *Pasteur, histoire d'un savant par un ignorant*, was dictated (probably not word for word, but in terms of content) and reread by Pasteur himself, as he points out in his correspondence. The book can serve as a reference concerning Pasteur's ideas up to 1884, when this work was published. Pasteur himself said of it, in a letter to Chautemps, written on July 31, 1886: "*Everything in it is accurate and written in a charming style*"[115]. However, as the book review in the March 15, 1884 issue of *La Revue Scientifique* pointed out at the time, the book is of no interest on a human level. But what were the human aspects of Pasteur, at least in terms of how he wished to be remembered? Vallery-Radot intended only to popularize Pasteur's scientific ideas and glorify his father-in-law, and indirectly, his family. The book contains no interesting details about the master's life, his students or his laboratory. It leaves the reader with a sense of incompletion.

Vallery-Radot's monumental work is *La Vie de Pasteur*, reprinted at the least thirty times by Flammarion and then Hachette, between 1900 and 1962... The book is written to glorify the master and is full of passages of doubtful accuracy. The author skilfully builds the legend of his father-in-law, systematically showing him in a favourable light vis-à-vis his opponents or competitors. Pasteur no doubt owes a large part of his glory and popularity to his son-in-law. Vallery-Radot was a skilful flatterer who indirectly served the scientific reputation of France, because his book on Pasteur's life was translated in many languages and widely distributed. He was obviously a biased writer, but a good writer, since a poorly-written 692-page book on such a dry subject would not have been so successful. The author can mainly be reproached with his systematic silence concerning the intellectual life, particularly in biology, of Pasteur's contemporaries, other than to criticize them. When the book came out, it received flattering reviews. Lucas-Championnière expressed unreserved praise: "*The personal history of great men is a valuable lesson for us all. Pasteur's life contains incomparable examples and Mr. Vallery-Radot's book inspires liking for Pasteur the man in the hearts of those who have long had limitless admiration for the scientist... The reader follows, like the captivating plot of a novel, the life of this simple and good man with patriotic sentiments, with exquisite tenderness for his family, depicted so brilliantly and faithfully... Thus, when one finishes reading this pleasurable book, one can't help thinking, as I said earlier, that to his other joys, Pasteur was able to add this incomparable happiness of having found a true biographer.*"[116]

110. Tronchin, 1906.
111. Dupont, 1999, p. 558.
112. Pasteur, Cor., t. 3, pp. 105 & 125.
113. Vallery-Radot, 1874.
114. NAF 18110, item 85.
115. Pasteur, Cor., t. 4, p. 78.
116. Lucas-Championniera, 1901, p. 401.

William Osler, one of the most respected physicians in the Anglo-Saxon world, prefaced the American translation of *La Vie de Pasteur*: "... *But after having read for the third or fourth time* La Vie de Pasteur, *I am of the opinion, recently expressed by an anonymous author of a marvellous homage in the* Spectator, *'that he was the most perfect man ever to have entered the realm of Science'*."[117] Obviously, the classification of men of science in their realm is a difficult task. René Vallery-Radot can be congratulated for having sung the praises of his father-in-law, even if at times they were rather far removed from reality.

VAN ERMENGEN Emile-Pierre-Marie (1851-1932). He obtained his doctorate in medicine in 1875, from the Catholic University of Louvain. He studied in Paris (Claude Bernard and Ranvier's laboratories), and then in London, Edinburg, Vienna and Berlin (Koch's laboratory). Back in Brussels, he opened a private practice and availed himself of a bacteriology laboratory. In 1885, he was sent to Spain to study Ferran's anti-cholera vaccination method. In 1888 he became a professor of bacteriology at the University of Gand, where he worked and taught until 1919, when he was elected perpetual secretary of the Royal Academy of Medicine of Belgium. He published numerous studies on bacteriology. He is the author of *Bacillus botulicum*. Van Ermengem was a very cultured man; he spoke six languages[118].

VIALA Eugène. Pasteur's trusted laboratory technician.

WATERHOUSE Benjamin (1754-1846). He studied medicine in Newport, in Edinburg and in London. After he completed his medical studies, he spent a year studying the laws of nations in Leyden. He was one of the first three professors at the Harvard Medical Institution. He came from the Quaker community of Rhode Island and was a partisan of Jefferson, that is, an anti-federalist. He completed his medical studies during the American War of independence. He "*seems to have had an unfortunate feeling of superiority, due to his long training in Europe, and he adopted a pedantic manner which brought upon him only ridicule and enmity*"[119]. Forced to leave his teaching position at Harvard, he occupied several positions in the Marines successively. He played an important role in the introduction of Jennerian vaccination in New England, taught natural history and medicine, and preached against the excessive use of alcohol and tobacco[120].

WILLEMS Louis (1822-1907). Belgian physician, graduate of the University of Louvain, he played an outstanding role in the fight against bovine pleuropneumonia.

WOODVILLE William (1752-1805). British Doctor of medicine (1775). In 1792, he became director at the smallpox hospital, in London. The base of Jenner's statue in Boulogne-sur-Mer bears an inscription that reminds the French that it was Woodville who personally brought them the vaccine and the technique for using it.

MONTAGU (Lady Mary Wortley-Montagu) (1689-1762). Known for the letters she wrote on a long trip to Constantinople, across Europe and touching on Asia and Africa. A French translation of her letters, with very interesting commentary, was published by Moulin and Chuvin[121].

WRIGHT Sir Almroth Edward (1861-1947). He started his university studies at Trinity College in Dublin by completing a four-year modern languages program (1878-1882), which made him fluent in French, German and Spanish. He obtained a doctorate in medicine in 1883. He went to Germany to continue his education; there, he focused on the study of coagulation. Eventually, he was appointed to the Chair of pathology of the Army Medical School on Netley. Being a civilian, he immediately found himself in conflict with his superior David Bruce, who had discovered *Brucella melitensis* while stationed in Malta.

Despite their overt opposition, Wright and Bruce co-authored several publications. Wright was very inventive. He designed a micro-method for the study of blood, by using glass tubes with capillary ends. Wright was stationed in various places, including Malta and South Africa. In 1881, Pasteur conducted his famous experiment in Pouilly-le-Fort; Wright worked on brucella. He immediately

117. Osler, undated, p. I.
118. Bulloch, 1938, p. 364.
119. Viets, 1930.
120. Bazin, 2000, p. 98.
121. Montagu (Moulin & Chuvin), 1991.

conceived the project of immunisation against this disease. He first tried to inoculate a killed brucella preparation to monkeys. Apparently satisfied with the results, he tested the preparation on himself and... developed a very serious case of brucella which lasted several months. At the start of 1893, Haffkine seeked help from Wright, who was back in London, to conduct trials of his method of anti-cholera immunisation with killed bacilli in India, then under British administration. Haffkine obtained Wright's support. At the same time, Wright decided to take typhoid fever as his subject, as he himself puts it in his writings. In 1902, Wright (about 41 years old) decided to leave his functions in the military administration and apply for the positions of pathologist and bacteriologist at St. Mary's Hospital Medical School in London. In 1906, Wright was knighted, elected member of the Royal Society and named director of the Department of Therapeutic Inoculation. The department started to sell vaccines, directly or through the English branch of the Parke Davis firm. At that time, Wright became interested in autovaccines. Autovaccines and the opsonic index were the subjects to which Wright dedicated the last part of his career. He is remembered as a great British bacteriologist and immunologist[122].

YERSIN Alexandre (1863-1943). French physician of Swiss origin. He studied in Lausane, then in Paris. After he cut himself during the autopsy of a man who died of rabies, he had to submit to anti-rabies treatment at the *Institut Pasteur*, where he subsequently became Emile Roux's assistant. For several years he travelled as a physician on the ships of the "*Messageries maritimes*" and discovered the Far-East. In 1892, when Calmette appointed him to the Colonial corps, he had to acquire French nationality. During a mission in Hong-Kong, he identified the plague bacillus. Having discovered Nha Trang Bay, he founded a *Institut Pasteur*, where he studied human and animal diseases, particularly rinderpest. Yersin also studied the daily habits of the local inhabitants. He introduced the rubber tree and the quinine tree to Vietnam[123]. His memory is still honoured in Vietnam.

122. Grainger, 1958, p. 179.
123. Mollaret, 1993.

Glossary
or Evolution of Some Medical Concepts over Time

Abbreviations: Am.: American (sometimes only printed in the USA); Br.: British; Fr. French; Dict.: Dictionary; Med. Dict.: Medical Dictionary.

APHTISATION. Procedure through which the foot-and-mouth virus was artificially transmitted from a diseased animal to another susceptible animal[1].

BACTERIDIUM. "*Type of bacterium in the shape of short sticks that are immobile at all stages of their existence.*" (Fr. Littré Dict., 1898)[2] Pasteur used the world "*bactéridie*" coined by Davaine, to designate the anthrax bacillus.

"*Bactéridie*" was translated as "*bacteridium*" by Billings. (Am. Billings Med. Dict., 1890)[3].

BACTERIUM. "*General term used to designate inferior, microscopic organisms responsible for causing infectious diseases in man and animals.*" (Fr. Littré Dict., 1898)[2].

"*Any microorganism having form of short rod or cylinder*" (Am. Billings Med. Dict., 1890)[3].

CONTAGION. It is important to distinguish the period before and/or after germ theory and its acceptance. According to Diderot and d'Alembert, in the "*Encyclopédie*" ou "*Dictionnaire raisonné des sciences, des arts et des métiers*" (1751-1772): "*Contagion, quality of a disease by which it can pass from the affected subject to a healthy subject, & produce in the latter a disease of the same kind. Contagious diseases are transmitted either by immediate contact, or by contact with clothing, furniture or other infected objects, or even by means of the air that can carry over quite considerable distances certain miasmas or morbific germs. These miasmas are more or less light, more or less mobile, depending on the type of contagious disease to which they belong: those of scabies, for instance, hardly spread beyond the surface of the affected area; those of rabies, that can only be transmitted by immediate application of the saliva of the rabid animal to the wounded area...*" The essential nature of the phenomenon was still unknown at that time.

"*Contagion. More generally, that subtle matter which proceeds from a diseased person or body, and communicates the disease to another person, as in cases of small-pox, measles, &c., diseases which are communicated without contact. This contagion proceeds from the breath of the diseased, from the perspiration or other excretions.*" (Am. Webster Dict., 1854)[4].

Contagion, "*The communication of a disease by contact, direct or indirect; that excessively subtle matter which proceeds from a diseased person or body, and communicates the disease to another person.*" (Br. Annandale Dict., 1899)[5].

Germ theory, a fundamental contribution to medicine, is the fruit of the labours of several contributors: Davaine, Koch, Lister and, of course, Pasteur. It is the scientific basis of the term "contagion" in its modern sense.

---

1. Blancou, 2003, p. 60.
2. Littré, 1898, p. 131.
3. Billings Medical Dictionary, 1890, part 1, p. 141.
4. Webster Dictionary, 1854, p. 257.
5. Annandale Dictionary, 1899, p. 150.

The idea of contagion or of microbial transmission of disease has long been linked with philosophical considerations: "*A tacit or overt feeling made people fear the release of the sick in case ideas of transmissibility should be kindled in the masses.*" (Desnos *in* Fr. Jaccoud Med. Dict., 1867)[6].

CONTAGIONIST. "*One who believes that cholera, plague, and yellow fever are spread by contagion.*" (Am. Billings Med. Dict., 1890)[7].

ENDEMIC. Persistence of a disease in a population or in a region, in a constant or periodic manner. At times, an endemic can become an epidemic. However, the word "*endemic*" can take different meaning, such as: "*Diseases which are peculiar to localities or situations, such as ague* (intermittent fever) *to Lincolnshire, goître to Switzerland, and plica polonica* (curious condition of hair...) *to Poland.*" (Br. Haydn Med. Dict., 1874)[8].

HETEROGENESIS. "*Didactic term, Production of living beings from organic or inorganic substances, without seeds or ovules, also called spontaneous generation.*" (Fr. Littré Dict., 1873)[9].

HYDROPHOBIA. Original name used for rabies until about 1830. This word was still used by Pasteur: "*On December 10, 1880, I was invited by Doctor Lannelongue, surgeon at the Sainte-Eugénie Hospital, to visit a poor child five years old suffering from hydrophobia...*"[10]. He was speaking of rabies.

IMMUNITY. In the legal sense, the word immunity has long been used to designate persons or residents of a locality benefiting from a derogation to the law. The idea of immunity in the medical sense seems to have emerged later, with variolation or vaccination. The phenomenon of non recurrence of certain more or less contagious diseases had been known for a long time, but had not been closely studied, although it had been given practical applications (variolation, clavelisation...).

In its 1803 report, the (French) Central Vaccine Committee spoke of immunity: "*In this action so peaceful and inoffensive* (that of vaccine inoculated to man), *it* (the committee) *nevertheless recognized a great power; that of modifying animal economy and of destroying in us this universal and constant disposition that renders us susceptible to be affected by the contagion of smallpox.*"[11] The idea of immunity induced by man is suggested, even if the word is not used, and the phenomenon not explained.

The world immunity emerged late, but before Pastorian vaccines. Zundel, in his revision of the Hurtrel-d'Arboval dictionary, defined immunity in these terms: "*Conditions due to which some individuals escape falling prey to an ambient contagion... Immunity can be created by preventive inoculations, as can be seen with sheeppox and pleuropneumonia.*" (Fr. Hurtrel d'Arboval Med. Dict., 1875)[12].

Interestingly, at about the same time, the term immunity in medicine was sometimes used in a sense close to the legal sense: "*It is also said, in a general sense, of certain exemptions, of certain advantages: We do not know to what factors to attribute the immunity of which this district benefits during the cholera.*" (Acad. fr. Dict., 1878)[13]. Or "*Preservation from a disease: Certain areas enjoy remarkable immunity during the most deadly epidemics.*" (Fr. Larive Med. Dict., 1889)[14].

IMMUNITY (Theories of...) There existed a theory of evacuation of the smallpox germ that most people carried from birth (see chapter 1), and a theory of fermentations likening smallpox to a process such as fermentation in bread or wine... According to Silverstein, Rhazes (850-923) was the first to give a tentative explanation of non recurrence of an infectious disease (smallpox)[15]. But no solidly founded scientific basis was provided. More elaborate theories arrived... after Pasteurian vaccines.

Nutritive matter exhaustion theory. On February 9, 1880, before the Academy of Sciences, Pasteur described the results obtained with inoculations of chicken cholera bacillus with attenuated virulence. Pasteur invokes the following theory to explain the results: "*... The muscle that was infected became,*

6. Desnos, 1867, t. 7, p. 332.
7. Billings Medical Dictionary, 1890, part 1, p. 141.
8. Haydn Medical Dictionary, 1874, p. 167.
9. Littré, 1873, t. 2, p. 2016.
10. Pasteur, O.C., t. VI, p. 559.
11. Comité, 1803, p. 417.
12. Hurtrel d'Arboval, 1875, t. 2, p. 266.
13. Académie française (Dictionnaire de l'), 1878, t. 2, p. 9.
14. Larive, 1889, t. 2, p. 20.
15. Silverstein, 1989, p. 7.

after its healing and repair, in some way incapable of cultivating the microbe, as if the microbe, through the previous culture, had eliminated in the muscle some principle that life does not bring back and whose absence prevents the development of the tiny organism. In my opinion, this explanation, to which the most concrete facts lead us at this time, will likely become general, applicable to all virulent diseases."[16] This idea was not new. It had already been put forth several times, before Pasteur did so, by Auzias-Turenne: "*Viruses attack the whole system and often end up exhausting it, by exhausting themselves; they destroy it or leave it, when they no longer find nourishment.*" And elsewhere: "*But a fertile ground can be exhausted and become inadequate after prolonged culture of the same virus.*" And again: "*Thus, viruses exhaust certain terrains; afterwards they cannot return there and thrive before a certain period of time, often very long.*"[17] McLaughlin attributed the same theory to Klebs[18]. Pasteur gradually lost faith in this theory.

Theory of impregnation of Chauveau (1880)[19], of the added substance[20], of counterpoison[21], of retention[22] or of harmful substances secreted by the bacilli themselves, which remain in the tissues and prevent their own development. This theory, first proposed by Chauveau for natural immunity on June 28, 1880, opposed the exhaustion theory based on the fact that Algerian sheep, naturally resistant to low doses of anthrax bacteria, were killed by a massive dose of these bacteria. Chauveau deduced from this that a substance prevented bacteria from growing in the system of resistant animals. However, a larger dose of infecting agent can overcome this immunity. Chauveau then extended his theory to acquired immunity. His definition was relatively clear: "*This resistance could be the result of the impregnation of different organic milieus by soluble poison or by any other residual dissolved matter, coming from the first microbial evolution.*"[23] Inhibiting substances were, in principle, produced by the bacteria themselves. Chauveau spoke of "*harmful substances, ptomaines or other soluble matters...*"[24], without being more specific.

Theory of vaccinating matter. On January 29, 1885, Pasteur wrote: "*I tend to think that the apparent rabies virus must be accompanied by a matter that, by impregnating the nervous system would render it unsuitable for the culture of apparent microbe. This would explain vaccinal immunity. If this is so, the theory might very well be general.*"[25] Pasteur tried unsuccessfully to test this idea. In his "*letter on rabies*" written on December 27, 1886, he wrote: "*Lastly, let us not lose sight of the very original and so productive theory of Mr. Metchnikoff. Is vaccinal substance, if it exists, contained in dead microbes?*"[26] It was an excellent hypothesis, but not in keeping with reality.The new Pasteurian theory was close to that of impregnation.

Theory of acclimatization. Proposed around 1890 by Ferran, Chauveau, Charrin[27] and others, this theory defines: "... *infection as an intoxication by one poison or another, attributing the refractory state to an inborn indifference to microbial toxins in the case of natural immunity, and to a kind of acclimatization, of mithridation, in the case of acquired immunity.*"[28]

Theory of susceptible cells. Introduced by Wolff around 1890, this curious theory supposes that cells are susceptible, to varying degrees, of being attacked by pathogenic agents or by their secretion or decomposition products. A first attack destroys precisely the cells susceptible to attack, leaving the others intact. At the time of a subsequent attack, the pathogenic agent finds no target. If vaccination with a low virulence virus is performed, the pathogenic agent destroys the most susceptible cells, and a second vaccine will destroy all predisposed cells remaining after the first attack. Loss of immunity is presumed to be correlated with the return of susceptible cells[29].

---

16. Pasteur, O.C., t. VI, p. 301.
17. Auzias-Turenne, 1865 (1878), pp. 709 & following.
18. McLaughlin, 1892, p. 158.
19. Galtier, 1897, p. 185.
20. Achalme, 1894, p. 163.
21. Larousse, 1888, p. 1421.
22. Anonyme, 1892c, p. 445.
23. Chauveau, 1888, p. 66.
24. Chauveau, 1888, p. 67.
25. NAF 18019, f.P. 9.
26. Pasteur, O.C., t. VI, p. 645.
27. Arloing, 1891, p. 263.
28. Achalme, 1894, p. 177.
29. Anonyme, 1892c, p. 445.

Theory of immunisation by dead or chemical substances. Presented by Toussaint on July 12, 1880, presented again by Ferran and Pauli to the Academy of Sciences (Paris) at the January 18, 1886 session, but each time with debatable proof. Confirmed by Salmon and Smith in September 1887; they apparently published identical findings as early as 1884. At that time, this theory included no physiological mechanism.

Theory of phagocytes, forerunner of cell theory. This is the main theory based on the "*vitalist idea*". It was Metchnikoff who developed this cell theory, that he himself considered still imperfect[30].

Theory (humoral) of immunity. According to Parish, Nuttall and Flügge were the first to formulate the humoral theory of immunity[31]. Unfortunately, this author gives no bibliographic references. The humoral theory of immunity emerged, in fact, from the major studies of Behring and Kitasato, and from the discovery of the bactericide power of blood or serums, by several scientists, Fodor, Flügge, Nuttall and Buchner among them.

Rapidly, cell theory and humoral theory were confronted, analysed, debated and opposed to one-another, until finally they were integrated into a more and more coherent whole by involving natural immunity and inducible immunity.

INFECTION. "*In medicine, the terms infection and contagion are used as synonymous in a great majority of cases... Infection is used in two acceptations; first, as denoting the effluvium or infectious matter exhaled from a person of one diseased, in which sense it is synonymous with contagion; and secondly, as signifying the act of communication of such morbid effluvium by which diseases are transferred.*" (Am.Webster Dict., 1854)[32].

INFECTIOUS DISEASE. Salmon (1896): "*An infectious disease can be defined as any disease due to the introduction in the system of tiny organisms of vegetable or animal nature, having the ability to multiply infinitely and to produce particular poisons that are the principal factors responsible for pathological changes.*"[33]

INOCULATION. " *Inoculate, the act of inoculating.*" and "*Inoculate, to propagate by insertion.*" (Am. Perry Dict., 1777)[34].

"*Procedure through which smallpox, vaccinia or any other virus was artificially transmitted*" (Fr. Capuron Med. Dict., 1806)[35].

"*The practice of transplanting the small-pox.*" (Am. Walker Dict., 1828)[36].

INSERTION. "*The act of placing any thing in or among other matter, the thing inserted.*" (Am. Walker Dict., 1828)[37].

MEDIATE (contact). "*Which only has any relation to, or contact with something through another element between them. As opposed to immediate.*" (Acad. fr. Dict., 1835)[38].

MIASMA. "*Among physicians, denotes the contagious effluvia of pestilential diseases, whereby they are communicated to people at a distance.*" (Encl. Britannica, 1771)[39].

"*Miasma. Miasmata have lately claimed the attention of pathologists, as there are the causes of some of the most fatal fevers to which mankind are subject... Each infectious disease has its own, diffused round the person which is attacked, and liable to convey the disease at different distances, according to the nature of the complaint, or to the predisposition of the object exposed to it.*" (Am. Parr Med. Dict, 1819)[40].

MICROBE. Word invented by the surgeon Sédillot[41]. Portions of a letter written by Littré to M. Sédillot in answer to the latter's request that Littré offer an opinion about this term are reproduced

30. Metschnikoff, 1887, p. 321.
31. Parish, 1965, p. 6.
32. Webster Dictionary, 1854, p. 601.
33. Salmon, 1896, p. 371.
34. Perry Dictionary, 1777, p. 229.
35. Capuron, 1806, p. 183.
36. Walker Dictionary, 1828, p. 1238.
37. Walker Dictionary, 1828, p. 210.
38. Académie française (Dictionnaire de l'), 1835, t. 2, p. 183.
39. Encyclopaedia Britannica, 1771, vol. III, p. 205.
40. Parr Medical Dictionary, 1819, vol. 1, p. 987.
41. Sédillot, 1878, p. 634.

in Pasteur's laboratory notebook 7, copied in Pasteur's own hand[42]: "*I would give preference to microbe*" (letter written by E. Littré on February 26, 1878).

PLEUROPNEUMONIA, exudative; also called epizootic peripneumonia[43a].

SEROSITY. The quality possessed by serous fluids. (Am. Dorland Med. Dict., 1994)[43b].

VACCINA. See Vaccinia (Am. Dorland Med. Dict., 1942)[44]; (Am. Dorland Med. Dict., 1994)[45].

VACCINE. "*Pertaining to cows; derived from cows.*" (Am.Webster Dict., 1849)[46].

"*1. Pertaining to the cow. 2. Vaccinal. 3. Lymph, scab, or any substance containing the virus of cowpox.*" (Am. Dorland Med. Dict., 1942)[47].

"*Substance which, when inoculated to an individual, confers immunity against a parasitic disease, just as vaccinia confers immunity against smallpox. The vaccine is either a concrete agent (microbe), or a soluble product. When used alone, this term maintains its original meaning, that is, it designates the agent of vaccinia transmission.*" (Fr. Garnier Med. Dict., 1920)[48].

"*A suspension of attenuated or killed microorganisms (bacteria, viruses, or rickettsiae), or of antigenic proteins derived from them, administred for the prevention, amelioration, or treatment of infectious diseases.*" (Am. Dorland Med. Dict., 1994)[49].

(SMALLPOX) VACCINE. "*A live vaccinia virus vaccine of calf lymph or chick embryo origin used for immunization against smallpox.*" (Am. Dorland Med. Dict., 1994)[50].

VACCINIA. "*Cow-pox...*" (Am. Gould Med. Dict., 1941)[51].

"*Cowpox; a disease of cattle regarded as a form of smallpox.*" (Am. Dorland Med. Dict., 1942)[52].

"*The cutaneous and sometimes systemic reactions associated with vaccination with smallpox vaccine.*" (Am. Dorland Med. Dict.)[53].

VACCINATE. At first, this term was not used at all, even for cowpox vaccination. In December 1799, Henry Jenner, Jenner's nephew, wrote: "*I would inoculate with pleasure, free of charge, the* (disease called) *vaccinia.*"[54] A few years later, and for at least half a century, the use of this term was to be limited to the use of cowpox/vaccine against smallpox. "*For the moment, I will confine myself to putting forth these ideas on the general significance of vaccinia, in the hope that they might serve one day to generalise the method, since it is not impossible, in fact, that all infectious diseases, the plague, typhus, typhoid fever, cholera, dysentery, measles, scarlet fever and even rabies will one day have, like the typhus of horned animals, their own vaccines: the promise is there in theory; let us hope that experience will confirm it!*"[55] But the hope of having vaccines against all infectious diseases already existed.

VACCINATION. This term was used in the limited sense of inoculation against smallpox for a long time. In 1849, Diday was probably the first to use this word for the inoculation of a substance intended to immunise against a disease other than smallpox. Later, the term was widely used in the context of syphilization by different authors. "*But I suppose that sooner or later medicine will discover a means of prevention, a cholera vaccine (I am not inventing the word, I read it somewhere)...*"[56]. In what

42. NAF 18013, p. 14.
43a. Larousse du XIXe siècle, 1874, t. 12, p. 1178.
43b. Dorland's Medical Dictionary, 1942, p. 1512.
44. Dorland's Medical Dictionary, 1942, p. 1582.
45. Dorland's Medical Dictionary, 1994, p. 1787.
46. Webster Dictionary, 1849, p. 1101.
47. Dorland's Medical Dictionary, 1942, p. 1582.
48. Garnier, 1920, p. 615.
49. Dorland's Medical Dictionary, 1994, p. 1787.
50. Dorland's Medical Dictionary, 1994, p. 1788.
51. Gould's Medical Dictionary, 1941, p. 1441.
52. Dorland's Medical Dictionary, 1942, p. 1583.
53. Dorland's Medical Dictionary, 1994, p. 1789.
54. Jenner, 1800c (1998), p. 19.
55. Guérin, 1863, p. 834.
56. Monteils, 1874, p. 278.

sense is the word vaccine used here, in 1874? It is probably a reference to the advocates of syphilization and their use of the word vaccination; in any case, it certainly does not refer to Pasteur's work, which was published a few years later. What is certain is that Pasteur was the one who gave the word "vaccination" its current meaning.

However, in English, the word retained its initial meaning for a long time[57]: "*The act, art, or practice of vaccinating, or of inoculating persons with the cow-pox or kine-pox.*" (Am. Webster Dict., 1883)[58].

"*The introduction of vaccine into the body for the purpose of inducing immunity. Coined originally to apply to the insertion of smallpox vaccine, the term has come to mean any immunizing procedure in which vaccine is injected.*" (Am. Dorland Med. Dict., 1994)[59].

VACCINATOR. "*Vaccinist, one who inoculates for the cow-pox.*" (Am. Dunglison Med. Dict., 1854)[60].

VARIOLA. "*It* (small-pox) *is called, technically, variola.*" (Am. Webster Dict., 1854)[61].

VARIOLATE. "*1, Having small pustules like those of variola. 2, To inoculate with smallpox.*" (Am. Gould Med. Dict., 1941)[62].

VARIOLATED. "Having or having had smallpox." (Am. Gould Med. Dict., 1941)[63].

VARIOLATION. Inoculation of variola, performed for preventive purposes. This word entered the medical vocabulary late; in 1908 it was found in the Littré and Gilbert medical dictionary. Just as the word "vaccination" has come to designate any vaccine, the word "variolation" can be used for any inoculation of a wild pathogenic germ, for preventive purposes.

"*Variolation, Inoculation (small-pox).*" (Am. Dunglison Med. Dict., 1866)[64].

VARIOLIC. Suffering from smallpox. "*The same as variolous.*" (Am. Webster Dict., 1883)[65].

VARIOLOID. "*A name recently given to a particular variety of the small-pox.*" (Am. Webster Dict., 1854)[66].

VARIOLOVACCINE. " *A vaccine lymph or crust obtained from a heifer which has been inoculated with smallpox virus.*" (Am. Gould Med. Dict., 1941)[67].

VARIOLOUS. "*Pertaining to or designating the small-pox; having pits or sunken impressions like those of the small-pox.*" (Am. Webster Dict., 1854)[68].

"*Variolous. Relating, belonging to variola.*" (Am. Dunglison Med. Dict., 1866)[69].

VIRULENCE. In Pasteur's era, Bouchard (1889) wrote: "*But what is virulence?... It is the outcome of various characteristics... The infectious disease is not directly a function of the microbe... The microbe can have the function of secreting a toxic chemical substance which, when absorbed by man or animal, makes them sick... Infectious agents can cause harm simply by a mechanical action. They can obstruct the capillaries of certain organs by their abundance... To survive, they need to have matter to consume. Thus, a vital competition is established between the cells of the parasites and the cells of the infected organism, which have to abide these new guests at their table.*"[70]

"*Virulence: The relative infectiousness of a micro-organism, or its ability to overcome the defences of the host.*" (Am. Dorland Med. Dict., 1944)[71].

57. Bazin, 1997, p. 156.
58. Webster Dictionary, 1883, p. 1458.
59. Dorland's Medical Dictionary, 1994, p. 1787.
60. Dunglison's Dictionary of Medical Science, 1854, p. 892.
61. Webster Dictionary, 1854, p. 1044.
62. Gould's Medical Dictionary, 1941, p. 1447.
63. Gould's Medical Dictionary, 1941, p. 1447.
64. Dunglison's Medical Dictionary, 1866, p. 1010.
65. Webster Dictionary, 1883, p. 1463.
66. Webster Dictionary, 1854, p. 1226.
67. Gould's Medical Dictionary, 1941, p. 1447.
68. Webster Dictionary, 1854, p. 1226.
69. Dunglison's Medical Dictionary, 1866, p. 1011.
70. Bouchard, 1889, p. 58.
71. Dorland's Medical Dictionary, 1944, p. 1608.

VIRULENCE ATTENUATION (artificial). This notion does not seem to have been considered in relation to variolation. The preferred practice was to choose a virus from benign smallpox. It was, in fact, "*healthy smallpox*" as opposed to "*serious smallpox*". And yet the notion of attenuation of the virulence of a germ was suggested from the start of studies on cowpox. The French Central Vaccine Committee, in its 1803 report, rejected this idea: "*It was thought that an even more considerable effect would be produced* (smallpox)*; specifically, the modification, the alteration of this virus by vital power, and its transformation into a new and distinct leaven, entirely new* (vaccinia)*. No observation, no hint, no comparison makes it possible to draw this conclusion. Nothing proves that the virus was denatured in this manner.*"[72]

In Pasteur's era, no satisfactory theory could explain virulence variations. However, a distinction was made between virulence and immunogenic properties: "*As for the use, for preventive inoculations, of the conservation of vaccinal property in previously pathogenic microbes, whose virulence has been not only more or less attenuated, but completely extinguished or, more precisely, rendered unable to manifest itself, we can reasonably suppose that any pathogenic microbe that has become non infectious, in the common sense of the word, can conserve the ability to create conditions of immunity.*"[73] Thus, it was no longer necessary to have the symptoms of a disease in order to induce immunity. Molecular biology was to provide explanations for this a hundred years later.

VIRUS. "*Latin word retained in French, meaning venom or poison. The word 'virus' is used to designate a malignant, pernicious quality, contrary to nature: this is the case for the smallpox virus, the scurvy and scrofula viruses, the rabies virus, etc.*"[74]

In 1809, Chabert, professor at the *Ecole vétérinaire impériale d'Alfort*, wrote: "*What is the nature, what is the character of the hydrophobic virus? Will we see it, and through the eyes of what doctors, as a phosphoric or electric venom for which saliva is the vehicle... This venom is a sulfurous and incandescent volatile alkaline... these explanations are incomprehensible* (already in 1809!)*... Spontaneous rabies is produced by the convulsive spasms and erethism that accompany great passions... The danger to which a breast-fed child is exposed when he takes the nipple of his wet-nurse, incontinent after she was seized with a movement of terror or anger.*"[75]

Over time, the properties attributed to a virus became more finely defined: "*We must specify the meaning of this word virus. We give this name to the product of a morbid secretion which, when inoculated, can reproduce in another individual a disease similar to that which produced it; to do this, it needs a more or less lengthy incubation period. It differs from venom in that the latter is the product of a natural secretion in a healthy animal, that it is not reproduced by the disease it causes; and finally that it needs no incubation to produce its effects, its action being instantaneous.*"[76]

"*Virus. Active or contagious matter of an ulcer, pustule, &c; poison*" (Am. Webster Dict., 1849)[77].

Thanks to the work of Delafond, Davaine, Pollender and Koch, *Bacillus anthracis* became better known. Pasteur wrote: "*Our first study examined the disease known as anthrax... This disease... is produced by microbes, by small microscopic organisms which develop in superior beings in whom they produce disorders which bring about disease and death. These microbes constitute the virus...*"[78]. In 1884, Pasteur was still using the word "virus" in the sense of "pathogenic agent". "*Active principle of contagion... today we associate this term with morbid principles that have the ability to develop in a healthy subject the same pathology in which they were generated... their most ordinary state is liquid; sometimes they are found in a gaseous state, and at times also in solid state; ... Science can still only emit hypotheses on the nature of virulent principles... According to these theoreticians, the tissues or humors that become virulent do not differ substantially from others; the only difference is an intimate molecular modification that physical and microscopic means are unable to reveal.*" (Fr. Larousse Dict., 1876)[79].

72. Comité, 1803, p. 414.
73. Boillot, 1889, p. 30.
74. Buchan, 1802, t. 5, p. 607.
75. Chabert, 1809, p. 257.
76. de Saint-Martin, 1823, p. 147.
77. Webster Dictionary, 1849, p. 1114.
78. Pasteur, O.C., t. VII, p. 368.
79. Larousse du XIXᵉ siècle, 1876, t. 15.

Larousse, a very cultured positivist, abandoned this position some time later: "… *There is therefore a veritable classification of viruses, based on natural history, which places them definitively in the category of living beings*." (Fr. Larousse Dict., 1888)[80]. A major step forward in the knowledge of viruses between 1876 and 1888…

In time, and with the discovery of microbes, the meaning of the word changed: "*Virus: name given, before the discovery of pathogenic microbes, to the substance that contains the agent of contagion and is capable of transmitting the disease. Today, this term is still used to refer to contagious diseases whose micro-organism has not been isolated.*" (Fr. Garnier Med. Dict., 1920)[81].

"*One of a group of minute infectious agents… characterized by a lack of independent metabolism and the ability to replicate only within living host cells…*" (Am. Dorland Med. Dict., 1994)[82].

ZYMOTIC DISEASE. "*Zymotic: An epithet proposed for any epidemic, endemic, or contagious affection. Zymosis is used to signify such an affection.*" "*Zymosis, Fermentation.*" (Am. Dunglison Med. Dict., 1854)[83].

"*The term Zymotic has recently been applied by Dr. Farr to epidemic, endemic, infectious, and contagious diseases, and has comprised smallpox, measles… Viewing the Greek term to mean a leaven by which the organic nervous system… may be infected or contamined… the term well designates an extensive class of diseases, although its application implies a hypothesis…*" (Am. Copland Med. Dict., 1859)[84].

"Zimotic Disease: *Epidemic, endemic, contagious, or sporadic diseases, supposed to be produced by some morbific principle acting on the system like a ferment.*" (Br. Annandale Dict., 1899)[85a].

"*Zymotic diseases, causing to ferment. The term is suggestive of a fermentation in the blood, occasioned by the introduction into the system of a specific or peculiar virus. The term is used synonymously with 'acute specific disease'*" (Br. Hoblyn's Med. Dict., 1899)[85b].

note=varnote+1. The meaning of the expression, which is still in use, changed over time.

"*Zymotic diseases, an infectious disease*" (Am. Gould Med. Dict., 1941)[86].

"Zimotic Disease: *caused by or pertaining to zymosis. Zymosis: 1 Fermentation. 2 The development of any zymotic disease; the propagation and development of an infectious disease, known by the growth of bacteria and their products. 3 Any infectious or contagious disease.*" (Am. Dorland Dict., 1942)[87].

In the 28th edition, the word "Zymotic" has been eliminated. What remains is: "*Zym(o) a combining form denoting relationship to an enzyme, or to fermentation*" (Am. Dorland's Med. Dict., 1994)[88], which disappears in the 29th edition (Am. Dorland Med. Dict., 2000)[89].

---

80. Larousse du XIXe siècle, 1888, Suppl. 2, p. 1991.
81. Garnier, 1920, p. 624.
82. Dorland's Medical Dictionary, 1994, p. 1826.
83. Dunglison Medical Dictionary, 1854, p. 927.
84. Copland Medical Dictionary, 1859, vol. IX, p. 1563.
85a. Annandale Dictionary, 1899, p. 784.
85b. Hoblyn's Dictionary of Medical Terms, 1899, p. 838.
86. Gould's Medical Dictionary, 1941, p. 1489.
87. Dorland's Medical Dictionary, 1942, p. 1640.
88. Dorland's Medical Dictionary, 1994, p. 1859.
89. Dorland's Medical Dictionary, 2000, p. 1596.

Bibliography

There exist an immense number of documents related to the history of infectious diseases and vaccination. Whenever possible, the sources used in this book are original, although it is difficult to ensure flawless authenticity. In 1833, Bousquet was already remarking: "*The history of vaccine is altered almost everywhere, because the authors copy each-other without bothering to go back to the original source!*"[1] Copy and paste is not such a modern practice!

Pasteur's work, particularly on vaccines, is described based on his publications, his correspondence, texts written by his associates, and above all his laboratory notebooks. Numerous quotations or references (over 200) are given; they can be checked at the Bibiothèque Nationale de France, where the original documents can be consulted.

The author analysed a number of books and articles more or less antithetical to Pasteur, the man: Cadeddu, Decourt, Geison and others... The study of these texts is largely absent from this work, since they concern primarily the person of Pasteur, rather than the development of vaccines. These texts are not directly related to the main subject of this work... They will be the subject of a separate project. The data constituting the foundation of this *Vaccination: a History* have been collected by the author. Of course, new revelations could modify certain points in this book. **The author would be very interested in receiving new data, that he has not found, or even diverging opinions on his text, as long as they are documented.**

The abbreviations employed have been reduced to a minimum: BN or BNF: (French) *Bibliothèque nationale*; NAF for "*nouvelle acquisition française*"; f.P. for folio written by Pasteur; thus (NAF xxxxx f.P. x) means (BNF, NAF number xxxxx, for example 18019, f.P.x); BANM: *Bibliothèque de l'Académie nationale de Médecine* (Paris); Arch. Acad. Sc.: *Archives de l'Académie des Sciences* (Paris); O.C.: "*Œuvres complètes*"; Cor.: Correspondence; t.: tome; v.: volume. The many references relating to the Pasteur Fund of the *Bibliothèque nationale* and the complete works or the correspondence of Louis Pasteur are given directly in the text, to avoid additions to the bibliography. For the convenience of the interested reader, the codes of certain uncommon works of the *Bibliothèque de l'Académie nationale de Médecine* (Paris) have been added to the ordinary references. Of course, this library offers many other works of interest. Complete references are given. In his biography of Littré, Hamburger wrote: "*Littré had asked that the complete reference of the chosen quote be given as well: it was not enough to sign it Racine, it was also necessary to know if it was taken from 'Bérénice' or from 'Les Plaideurs'. Hachette found these specifications excessive and useless, to say nothing of the fact that they tended to multiply errors; but Littré maintained his position.*"[2] Of course, the present work is not comparable to the works of this famous lexicographer, but history always demands the same precision. The page numbers given are those of the quotations used, or the first page of an article when the entire text is pertinent to the reference. No page number is given when the entire work is used as a reference. Small case letters have sometimes been added to year references, in case of possible confusion between several references: 2000a and 2000b for instance. Finally, two publication dates are sometimes given, the original and, in parentheses, the edition used by this author: (*de la Condamine, 1763 [1764], p.* 9), text read in 1763 and printed in 1764. Similarly, additional indications are given when they can shed light on the occurrence of certain events. Approximate conversions of francs (of different values depending on the years) into euros were made using the *Quid* 2004 conversion table. Francs used before 1900 were converted using the 1900 values, giving a very approximate result, of course.

1. Bousquet, 1833, p. 4.
2. Hamburger, 1988, p. 152.

A.B., Nouvelles expériences de vaccination des singes contre la tuberculose, La Revue scientifique (revue rose), 1925, 63e année, page 563.

ABBOTT Samuel W., A reference handbook of the medical sciences, William Wood and company, New-York, 1889, volume VII, pages 509-559.

ABILDGAARD et WIBORG, Extrait d'une lettre écrite de Copenhagen à M. Huzard, le 9 juillet 1791, Sur l'inoculation de la petite vérole, Instructions et observations sur les maladies des animaux domestiques, par MM. Chabert, Flandrin et Huzard, tome V, 3e édition, Paris, Madame Huzard (née Vallat La Chapelle), 1813, pages 349-351.

ACADEMIE FRANÇAISE, Dictionnaire de..., Librairie de Firmin-Didot et Cie, Paris, édition de 1835 (6e édition) en 2 tomes ; Librairie de Firmin-Didot et Cie, Paris, 1878 (7e édition) en 2 tomes.

ACHALME P. Dr, Immunité dans les maladies infectieuses, Rueff et Cie éditeurs, Paris, 1894, 254 pages.

ACHARD Ch., Joseph Grancher. Eloge prononcé à l'Académie de médecine dans la séance annuelle du 11 décembre 1923, Bulletin de l'Académie nationale de médecine, 1923, 87e année, tome XC, pages 533-546.

ACHARD Ch., Les maladies typhoïdes, Masson et Cie, Paris, 1929, 305 pages.

ADAMS Joseph, An inquiry into the laws of different epidemic diseases..., printed for J. Johnson, London, 1809, 159 pages.

ADDRESS FOR THE ROYAL JENNERIAN SOCIETY, printed and sold by W. Phillips, London, 1803, 70 pages.

ADVIER médecin commandant, Etude expérimentale de la fièvre jaune, Annales de médecine et de pharmacie coloniales, 1934, tome 32, pages 441-472.

AMERICANIZED ENCYCLOPAEDIA BRITANNICA, Belford-Clarke Co. Publishers, Chicago, 1892, in X volumes.

ANDRAL, VELPEAU, JOBERT de LAMBALLE, Cl. BERNARD, CLOQUET, SERRES rapporteur, Prix Bréant rapport sur le concours de l'année 1865, Comptes rendus des séances de l'Académie des sciences, 1866, tome LXII, numéro 10, pages 538-545.

ANDREWES C.H., Yellow Jack, in the The natural history of viruses, Weidenfeld and Nicolson, London, 1967, pages 98-106.

ANNANDALE Charles, A concise dictionary of the English language, New and enlarged edition, Blackie & Son limited, London, 1899, 848 pages.

ANONYME, De la conduite à tenir, au sujet de l'Inoculation, à M***, lettre datée du 20 septembre 1754, Journal de Médecine, chirurgie et pharmacie, numéro de mai 1755, 2e edition, 1783, tome II, pages 314-317.

ANONYME, L'inoculation de la petite vérole déférée à l'église et aux magistrats, *name of printer or publisher not given*, 1756, 213 pages.

ANONYME, An inquiry into the causes and effects of the Variolae vaccinae, & c... par Edouard Jenner, Londres 75 pages, 1798, Bibliothèque britannique ou Recueil, Sciences et arts, Genève, 1798, tome 9, pages 258-284 et 367-399 *(footnotes are signed (O) for Odier)*.

ANONYME, Instruction sur la vaccine, Comité médical de l'inoculation de la vaccine établi à Paris, réunion du 19 pluviôse an IX (18 février 1801), 7 pages [BANM, Vaccine généralité 1, dossier 2].

ANONYME, Note du comité sur les eaux aux jambes, Bulletin sur la vaccine, du Comité central sur la vaccine, numéro 19 de mai 1812, pages 14-15.

ANONYME, Dictionnaire des sciences médicales, composé des meilleurs articles puisés dans tous les dictionnaires et traités spéciaux qui ont paru jusqu'à ce jour, chez J. Dewaet, Bruxelles, 1828-1830, 13 volumes.

ANONYME, Vaccine en Angleterre, Nouveau journal des connaissances utiles, 1853, tome I, numéro 3, page 64.

ANONYME, Pleuropneumonie épizootique. – Inoculation, repris du Journal agricole de Verviers, Annales de médecine vétérinaire, 1854, pages 586-587.

ANONYME, De l'unicité du virus chancreux démontrée par la syphilisation, Gazettes des hôpitaux, 37e année, numéro 6 du samedi 16 janvier 1864, page 22.

ANONYME, Chronique scientifique, La revue scientifique, 2e série, numéro 41 du 10 avril 1875, pages 979-980.

ANONYME, M. Louis Thuillier, Le Journal illustré, 20e année, numéro 41 du 7 octobre 1883a, pages 322 et 325.

ANONYME, Causerie bibliographique, La revue scientifique, 1883b, tome XXXI de la collection, 3e série, tome V, pages 724-725.

ANONYME, Causerie bibliographique, Revue scientifique (revue rose), 1884a, tome XXXIV de la collection, 3e série, tome VIII, pages 120-121.

ANONYME, Château de Villeneuve-l'étang, Le Monde illustré, numéro 1446 du 13 décembre 1884b, pages 372 et 374.

ANONYME, sans titre, Le Figaro, numéro 139 du 18 mai 1884c, page 1.

ANONYME, Revue-Chronique. Lettre et rapport de la commission désignée pour vérifier les expériences de M. Pasteur sur la rage, La Science pour tous, numéro 33 du 16 août 1884d, pages 258-259.

ANONYME, La rage à l'occasion de la découverte récente de M. Pasteur, L'Illustré pour tous, choix de bonnes lectures, numéro 397 du 20 décembre 1885a, pages 251-254.

ANONYME, Dernier épisode des inoculations du docteur Ferran. Gangrène des bras. Neuf amputations, L'union médicale, 1885b, 3e série, tome 40, pages 553-554.

ANONYME, Le choléra en Espagne, Le Monde illustré, numéro 1475 du 4 juillet 1885c, pages 473 et 478.

ANONYME, Les salaires à Paris, Revue scientifique (revue rose), 1885d, 22e année, page 671.

ANONYME, Le docteur Ferran, Le Journal illustré, 22e année, numéro 31 du 2 août 1885e, pages 253-254.

ANONYME, La méthode Pasteur et les savants anglais, La Nature, numéro 736 du 9 juillet 1887, page 94.

ANONYME, Sciences médicales, Le vaccin du choléra, La Science illustrée, 1888a, tome 2, 2e semestre, pages 230-231.

ANONYME, Inauguration de l'Institut Pasteur, L'Univers illustré, numéro 1757 du 24 novembre 1888b, pages 737, 740 et 742-743.

ANONYME, Le diagnostic de la rage des animaux après la mort, Journal des praticiens, 1889, tome III, page 64.

ANONYME, Le docteur Koch et la tuberculose, Le Petit Parisien, supplément littéraire illustré, 1890a, 2e année, numéro 94, pages 7-8.

ANONYME, Le docteur Koch, Le Journal illustré, 27e année, numéro 48 du 30 novembre 1890b, pages 378-380.

ANONYME, M. Stanthope, le journaliste américain qui s'est fait inoculer le virus anticholérique, Le Journal illustré, 29e année, numéro 40, 2 octobre 1892a, pages 313 et 315.

ANONYME, Découvertes et inventions nouvelles, M. Stanhope, Le Magasin pittoresque, supplément au numéro 20, 1892b, page 43.

ANONYME, Une nouvelle théorie de l'immunité, Revue scientifique (revue rose), 1892c, tome XLIX, page 445.

ANONYME, Inauguration au Pharo d'un institut anti-rabique, L'Univers illustré, numéro 2023 du 30 décembre 1893, pages 789 et 794.

ANONYME, L'Institut antirabique à Tunis, La Nature, numéro 1101 du 7 juillet 1894, page 87.

ANONYME, Les vaccinations antirabiques à Saigon, Revue scientifique (revue rose), 1895a, 32e année, 4e série, tome III, numéro 10, pages 316-318.

ANONYME, Statistiques de l'Institut Pasteur de Chicago, Revue scientifique (revue rose), 1895b, 32e année, 4e série, tome III, numéro 15, page 478.

ANONYME, La découverte de la vaccine, Revue scientifique (revue rose), 1895c, 4e série, tome IV, page 346.

ANONYME, La vaccination obligatoire au Japon, Revue scientifique, tome IX, numéro 17 du 23 Avril 1898a, page 536.

ANONYME, Le premier inoculé de Pasteur, La Chronique médicale, 5e année, numéro 1 du 1er janvier 1898b, pages 226-227.

ANONYME, Attentat contre un médecin, La chronique médicale, reprenant un article de l'Eclair du 29 mai 1901, 8e année, page 386.

ANONYME, Le professeur Virchov dans son cabinet, La Vie illustrée, numéro 204 du 12 septembre 1902a, page 385.

ANONYME, Nouvelles scientifiques et faits divers, les inoculations préventives contre la fièvre typhoïde dans l'armée anglaise en 1889, La Science illustrée, 1902b, tome XXIX, 1er semestre, numéro 731, page 15.

ANONYME, Léopold II et la vaccine, nouvelle reprise de Gil Blas, La Chronique médicale, 10e année, numéro 4 du 15 février 1903, page 110.

ANONYME, La défense contre la fièvre aphteuse, Le Pèlerin, numéro 1809 du 3 septembre 1911, pages 29-30.

ANONYME, M. Hideyo Noguchi, Le Miroir, numéro du 28 septembre 1913, page 3.

ANONYME, Ferran y Clua (Jaime), Enciclopedia Espana Universal Illustrada, Calpe, en 80 tomes, 1924, tome 23, pages 883-886.

ANONYMOUS, Of the (Middelsex) County' Hospital for the Small Pox, The Gentleman's Magazine, London, June 1747, volume XVII, pages 270-271.

ANONYMOUS, M. Louis Pasteur..., Life, May 29th 1884, page 296.

ANONYMOUS, Notes and News, Protective inoculation for anthrax, The veterinary journal and Annals of comparative pathology, September 1887a, page 227.

ANONYMOUS, Notes and News, Inoculation for contagious pleuro-pneumonia in goats, The veterinary journal and Annals of comparative pathology, September 1887b, page 227.

ANONYMOUS, The bacillus of yellow fever, The British Medical Journal, 1897, July 10, page 96.

ANONYMOUS, Protective inoculation against plague and cholera, The British medical journal, July 1, 1899 issue, pages 35-36.

ANONYMOUS, Vaccination, Americanizer Encyclopedia Britanica, Belford-Clarke Co. Publishers, Chicago, 1902a, volume VIII, pages 6119-6121.

ANONYMOUS, Yellow fever, Americanizer Encyclopedia Britanica, Belford-Clarke Co. Publishers, Chicago, 1902b, volume VIII, pages 6418-6419.

ANONYMOUS, Report of the german commission on antityphoid inoculation, The Lancet, May 27 1905, pages 1453-1454.

ANONYMOUS, The history of inoculation and vaccination for the prevention and treatment of disease, Lecture memoranda, Australasian medical congress, 1914, Aukland N.Z., Burroughs Wellcome & Co., London, 304 pages.

ANONYMOUS, Adrian Stokes, The British Medical Journal, October, 1, 1927, page 615-618.

ANONYMOUS, Alexander Thomas Glenny, The Lancet, October 16, 1965, page 798.

ANONYMOUS, UK medical chief suggests "safe" does not mean "no risk", Nature, volume 383, issue 6599, October 3,1996, page 371.

APERT Dr, Vaccins et Sérums, Ernest Flammarion Editeur, Paris, 1922, 282 pages.

ARAGAO, H. de BEAUREPAIRE, Vaccination par le sérum et le virus dans la fièvre jaune, Comptes rendus de la Société de biologie, 1931, tome 108, pages 1078-1080.

ARAGAO, H. de BEAUREPAIRE, Emploi de virus vivant dans la vaccination contre la fièvre jaune, Comptes rendus de la Société de biologie, 1933, tome 112, pages 1471-1473.

ARLOING, CORNEVIN et THOMAS O., Recherches expérimentales sur l'inoculation du Charbon symptomatique et sur la possibilité de conférer l'immunité par l'injection intra-veineuse, Journal de médecine vétérinaire et de zootechnie, 1880a, tome XXXI de la collection, pages 561-569.

ARLOING, CORNEVIN et THOMAS, Sur l'inoculabilité du charbon symptomatique et les caractères qui le différencient du sang de rate, Comptes rendus des séances de l'Académie des sciences, 1880b, tome XC, pages 1302-1305.

ARLOING Dr S., Les virus, Félix Alcan éditeur, Paris, 1891, 380 pages.

ASHWORTH-UNDERWOOD E., Edward Jenner, Benjamin Waterhouse and the introduction of vaccination into the United States, Nature, 1949, volume 163, pages 823-828.

AUBER Charles-Edouard, Découverte nouvelle d'un procédé simple et facile pour conserver pendant plusieurs années le fluide vaccin intact, l'avoir toujours disponible, et l'exporter dans les pays les plus éloignés, sous la ligne, aux tropiques et aux pôles... suivie d'une dissertation sur les succès de la vaccine dans les cas de Fièvre quarte, Chez Moreau, à Paris, An XIII-1805, 92 pages.

AUBERT A., Discours préliminaire d'un rapport sur le cowpox ou petite vérole des vaches... par W. Woodville et traduit par A. Aubert, chez l'auteur, à Paris, an VIII (1799), 66 pages.

AUBERT A., Notice historique sur la vaccine, extrait du journal de médecine, vendémiaire an IX, in Recueil de mémoires, d'observations et d'expériences sur l'inoculation de la vaccine, chez Magimel, à Paris, an IX (1801a), 57 pages.

AUBERT A., Rapport sur la vaccine, ou Réponse aux Questions rédigées par les Commissaires de l'Ecole de Médecine de Paris, sur la pratique et les résultats de cette nouvelle Inoculation en Angleterre et dans les Hospices de Londres, où on l'a adoptée, chez Richard, Caille et Ravier libraires, à Paris, an IX (1801b), 72 pages.

AUBERT Michel, Du diagnostic de la rage vulpine à son élimination, bilan de l'activité du Laboratoire d'études sur la rage et la pathologie des animaux sauvages de Nancy en matière de rage, Bulletin de l'Académie vétérinaire de France, 2003, tome 156, pages 5-14.

AUZIAS-TURENNE M., Sur la communication de la syphilis à des quadrumanes, des carnassiers et des rongeurs, Comptes rendus des séances de l'Académie des sciences, 1844, tome XIX, page 916.

AUZIAS-TURENNE M., Note sur l'inoculation de la syphilis aux animaux, Comptes rendus des séances de l'Académie des sciences, 1850, tome XXXI, pages 719-720.

AUZIAS-TURENNE M., Cours de syphilisation, 7 leçons données du 31 novembre 1851 au 11 janvier 1852, à l'Ecole pratique de la Faculté de médecine de Paris, Gazette médicale de Toulouse, 1852, 2e volume, pages 33-45, 105-126, 221-237, 325-341 et 389-406, 3e volume, pages 105-116 et 277-290.

AUZIAS-TURENNE, cité par Malgaigne, in RICORD, BEGIN, MALGAIGNE, VELPEAU, DEPAUL, GIBERT, LAGNEAU, LARREY, MICHEL LEVY, GERDY, ROUX, avec les communications de MM. AUZIAS-TURENNE et C. SPERINO, La syphilisation et de la contagion des accidents secondaires de la syphilis, chez J.-B. Baillière, Paris, 1853, page 35.

AUZIAS-TURENNE, Lettre à Monsieur le rédacteur en chef de l'Union médicale datée du 22 août 1851, in Lettres sur la syphilis adressées à M. le rédacteur en chef de l'Union médicale par M. Ricord, aux bureaux de l'Union médicale, Paris, 1856, 2e édition, pages 362-371.

AUZIAS-TURENNE, La syphilisation, publication de l'œuvre du docteur Auzias-Turenne faite par les soins de ses amis, Librairie Germer Baillière et Cie, Paris, 1878, 907 pages.

AUZIAS-TURENNE, citations reprises des comptes rendus du Congrès médical international, séance du 23 août 1867, in Syphilisation par J. Rollet in Dechambre, 1884, 3e série, tome 14, pages 678-691.

AVERY Oswald T. & GOEBEL Walther F., Chemo-immunological studies on conjugated carbohydrate-proteins. V. The immunological specificity of an antigen prepared by combining the capsular polysaccharide of type III *Pneumococcus* with foreign protein, Journal of experimental medicine, 1931, volume 54, pages 437-447.

BA H., CHAMBON L., CAUSSE G., LY C., SECK M. et DIAGNE Mar, La vaccination, la campagne de vaccination, conditions et résultats, Bulletin de la société médicale d'Afrique noire de langue française, 1966, volume XI, pages 550-554.

BALFOUR Andrew, The wild monkey as a reservoir for the virus of yellow fever, The Lancet, 1914, volume 183, pages 1176-1178.

BALIBAR Françoise et PREVOST Marie-Laure, Pasteur, cahiers d'un savant, CNRS éditions et Zulma éditions, Paris, 1995, 246 pages.

BALLHORN M. et STROMEYER M., Traité de l'inoculation vaccine avec l'exposé et les résultats des observations faites sur cet objet, chez Guillaume Rein, à Leipsic, 1801, 152 pages.

BALWIN Edward R., Tuberculosis : history and etiology, in Modern Medicine its theory and practice, edited by William Osler and Thomas McCrae, volume III, Lea Brothers & co., Philadelphia and New-York, 1907, 960 pages.

BALZER F. et DUBREUILH W., Variole, in Nouveau dictionnaire de médecine et de chirurgie pratiques, tome 38, Librairie J.-B. Baillière et Fils, Paris, 1885, pages 306-405.

BARON John, The life of Edward Jenner, M.D., LL. D. F.R.S., physician extraordinary to his majesty *Geo.* IV, foreign associate of the national institute of France, &c. &c. &c. Henry Colbrun, Publisher, London, 1838, 2 volumes.

BARREY C.A., Recherches sur les moyens de détruire la petite vérole ou mémoire sur la vaccine, de l'imprimerie de Chalandre, à Besançon, an IX (1800), 22 pages [BANM, 1800, n° 33 634 (4)].

BARRIER G., Compte rendu des travaux du VIIIe Congrès international de médecine vétérinaire, Recueil de médecine vétérinaire publié à l'Ecole d'Alfort, 1905, tome LXXXII, pages 619-667.

BASSET Professeur J., Essai sur l'immunité, Vigot frères, Paris, 1936, 86 pages.

BAXBY Derrick, Edward Jenner's Unpublished Cowpox Inquiry and the Royal Society: Everard Home's Report to Sir Joseph Banks, Medical History, 1999, volume 43, pages 108-110.

BAYLE A. L. J. et GIBERT C. M., Dictionnaire de médecine usuelle et domestique, Louis Vives, 3e édition, Paris, 1870, 2 tomes.

Bazin Hervé et Rousseau Jean, Immunoglobulines in Allergologie, édité par Jacques Charpin et Daniel Vervloet, Flammarion Médecine Sciences, 3e édition, Paris, 1992, pages 17-32.

BAZIN Hervé Pr. Ce bon docteur Jenner, l'homme qui vainquit la variole, Editions Josette Lyon, Paris, 1997, 182 pages.

BAZIN Hervé, The eradication of the smallpox, Academic Press, London, 2000, 246 pages.

BAZIN Hervé, Saint Hubert, guérisseur de la rage de l'homme et des animaux, Bulletin de la société française d'histoire de la médecine et des sciences vétérinaires, 2007, tome 7, pages 104-126.

BAZIN Hervé, L'Histoire des vaccinations, John Libbey Eurotext, Montrouge, 2008, 471 pages.

BAZIN Hervé, Louis Pasteur, Editions Alan Sutton, Saint-Cyr-sur-Loire, 2009, 128 + XVI pages.

BEAUVAL L., Les traitements du choléra, La Science illustrée, 1893, tome 11, pages 25-27.

BEDSON S.P., MAITLAND H.B. and BURBURY Y.M., Further observations on foot-and-mouth disease ? Section A Experimental studies of immunity in guinea-pigs to foot-and-mouth disease. Journal of comparative Pathology and Therapy, 1927, volume 40, pages 5-28.

BEGUE Pierre, Vaccination en France, rationnel et évolution du calendrier vaccinal La vaccination, Annales de l'Institut Pasteur/Actualités, 2002, pages 21-36.

BEHRING von Emil und KITASATO Shibasaburo, Ueber das Zustandekommen der Diphtherie-Immunität und der Tetanus-Immunität bei Thieren, Deutsche Medizinische Wochenschrift, 1890a, volume 16, pages 1113-1114.

BEHRING von Emil und KITASATO Shibasaburo, Untersuchungen über das Zustandekommen der Diphteria-Immunität bei Thieren, Deutsche Medizinische Wochenschrift, 1890b, volume 16, pages 1145-1148.

BELHOMME L. et MARTIN Aimé, Traité pratique et élémentaire de pathologie syphilitique et vénérienne, A. Coccoz, Paris, 1864, 690 pages.

BERRY G.P. and KITCHEN S.F., Yellow fever accidentally contracted in the laboratory A sudy of seven cases, The American journal of tropical medicine, 1931, volume XI, pages 365-434.

BERT J. et COLLOMB H., L'électroencephalogramme dans l'encéphalite vaccinale (vaccination antiamarile), Bulletin de la société médicale d'Afrique noire de langue française, 1966, volume XI, pages 591-596.

BERTHELOT Marcelin, sous la direction de... La grande encyclopédie, inventaire raisonné des sciences, des lettres et des arts, secrétaire général: André Berthelot, Société anonyme de la grande encyclopédie, Paris, 1885-1892, 31 volumes.

BERTHELOT A., Nouvelles données sur la vaccination préventive des enfants nouveau-nés contre la tuberculose par le B.C.G., La Revue scientifique (revue rose), 1927, 65e année, pages 404-405.

BIGGER Joseph W., Man against microbes, The English University Press ltd, London, 1939, 304 pages.

BILLINGS John S., The national medical dictionary, Lea brothers & Co., Philadelphia, 1890, 2 volumes.

BIZIMANA N., Epidemiology, surveillance and control of the principal affectious animal diseases in Africa, Revue Scientifique et technique, Office International des Epizooties, 1994, volume 13, pages 397-416.

BLACK's medical dictionary, by John D. Combrie, A. & C. Black limited, London, 1914 reprinted 1916, 858 pages.

BLACK's veterinary dictionary, by William C. Miller and Geoffrey P. West, Adam and Charles Black, London, 1967, 8e edition, 1015 pages.

BLAKE John B., Public Health in the Town of Boston 1630-1822, Harvard University Press, Cambridge, 1959, 278 pages.

BLANC Georges et MARTIN Louis-André, Innocuité pour l'homme du virus poliomyélitique fixé au lapin. Hypothèses sur le pouvoir protecteur d'un tel virus, Bulletin de l'Académie nationale de médecine, 1952, 3e série, tome 136, pages 655-663.

BLANC Georges et MARTIN Louis-André, Premiers essais de prophylaxie de la poliomyélite par un virus vivant fixé au lapin. Innocuité de la méthode, Bulletin de l'Académie nationale de médecine, 1953, 3e série, tome 137, pages 230-234.

BLANCHARD Maurice, Précis d'épidémiologie. Médecine préventive et hygiène coloniale, Vigot frères, Paris, 1934, 415 pages.

BLANCOU J., KIENY M.-P., LATHE R., LECOCQ J.-P., PASTORET P.-P. SOULEBOT J.-P., DESMETTRE P., Oral vaccination of the fox against rabies using a recombinant vaccinia virus, Nature, 986, volume 322, pages 373-375.

BLANCOU J., Early methods for the surveillance and control of rabies in animals, Revue scientifique et technique de l'Office International des Epizootie, 1994, volume 13, pages 361-372.

BLANCOU Jean, Histoire de la surveillance et du contrôle des maladies animales transmissibles, Office international des épizooties, Paris, 2000, 366 pages, translated in english, History of the surveillance and control of transmissible animal diseases, Office international des épizooties, Paris, 2003, 362 pages.

BLONDEAU et D'OLIER, Association française pour l'avancement des sciences, session de 1880, Reims, section des sciences médicales, Le progrès médical, 1880, tome VIII, pages 712-718.

BLOOMFIELD Arthur L., A bibliography of internal medicine, Communicable diseases, The University of Chicago Press, Chicago, 1958, 560 pages.

BLOT rapporteur, Rapport présenté à M. le Ministre de l'agriculture et du commerce par l'Académie de médecine sur les vaccinations pratiquées en France... pendant l'année 1872, Imprimerie nationale, Paris, 1875, 217 pages... pendant l'année 1874, Imprimerie nationale, Paris, 1876, 179 pages.

BLUME Stuart and GEESINK Ingrid, A brief history of poliomyelitis vaccines, Science, 2000, volume 288, pages 1593-1594.

BOCHEFONTAINE M., Effets produits chez l'homme et les animaux par l'ingestion stomacale et l'injection hypodermique de cultures des microbes du liquide diarrhéique du choléra, Comptes rendus des séances de l'Académie des sciences, 1885, tome C, pages 1148-1151.

BODEUX Phlippe, La rage est éradiquée, Le Soir, numéro 118 du mardi 22 mai 2001, pages 1 et 18.

BOECK W., Manière d'appliquer la syphilisation dans les hôpitaux de Christiania, Gazette des hôpitaux, 34e année, numéro 19 du 14 février 1861a, pages 78-79.

BOECK W., Note sur la syphilisation, Gazette des hôpitaux, 34e année, numéro 83 du mardi 16 juillet 1861b, pages 330-331.

BOECK Professor, On syphilisation printed from Lancet, Sept. 9 and Oct. 14, 1865, pp. 284, 425, The retrospect of practical medicine and surgery, edited by W. Braithwaite and James Braithwaite, Uniform American edition, New-York, published by W. A. Townsend, January 1866, volume LII, pages 212-220.

BOECK, *text reproduced by Alfred Fournier* in Inoculation in Nouveau dictionnaire de médecine et de chirurgie pratiques, 1874, tome 19, pages 97-138.

BOILLOT A., Action des microbes sur les êtres vivants (Académie des sciences, séance du 20 mai 1889), La Science illustrée, 1889, tome 4, page 31.

BOIVIN André et DELAUNAY Albert, L'organisme en lutte contre les microbes, Gallimard, 3e édition, 1947, 425 pages.

BONJEAN Jh., Monographie de la rage à l'usage de toute personne sachant lire, Imprimerie Châtelain, Chambéry, 1878, 238 pages.

BORDET Jules, Traité de l'immunité dans les maladies infectieuses, Masson et Cie éditeurs, Paris, 1920, 1re édition, 720 pages; 1939, 2e édition, 879 pages.

BORDET Monsieur le professeur (Jules), Les forces spirituelles: Roux et Calmette, *conference held in Brussels on February 23, 1934*, Conferancia – Journal des annales de l'Université, 28e année, numéro XIV du 1 juillet 1934, pages 69-84; *offprint included in the* "Travaux de l'Institut Pasteur du Brabant, 1927-1940".

BORDET Paul, Immunologie, Flammarion Médecine-Sciences, Paris, 1972, 1175 pages.

BORNSIDE George H., Jaime Ferran and preventive inoculation against cholera, Bulletin of the History of Medicine, 1981, volume 55, pages 516-532.

BORNSIDE George H., Waldemar Haffkine's Cholera Vaccines and the Ferran-Haffkine Priority Dispute, Journal of the History of Medicine and Applied Sciences, 1982, volume XXXVII, pages 399-422.

BORREL A., Etudes sur la clavelée, Sérothérapie et séroclavelisation, Annales de l'Institut Pasteur, 1903, tome 17, pages 732-762.

BOSTON DAILY GLOBE, Tuesday, April 12, 1955, volume CLXVII, number 102, 52 pages.

BOUCHARD Ch., Thérapeutique des Maladies infectieuses Antiseptie, *General pathology Course given at the Faculty of Medicine in Paris in 1887-1888, reproduced and published by Dr. P. Le Gendre*, Librairie F. Savy, Paris, 1889, 382 pages.

BOUCHUT M., Discussion de la communication de M. le Dr H. Toussaint intitulée "Vaccinations charbonneuses", Association française pour l'avancement des sciences, 9e session, Reims, séance du 19 août 1880, Au secrétariat de l'association, Paris, page 1025.

BOULEY H. et REYNAL, continué par André SANSON, L. TRASBOT et Ed. NOCARD, Nouveau dictionnaire pratique de médecine, de chirurgie et d'hygiène vétérinaires, Labé éditeur puis Asselin et Houzeau libraires, 1856-1894, 22 volumes plus un supplément d'André Sanson et L. Trasbot, 1897.

BOULEY H., La rage, moyens d'en éviter les dangers et de prévenir sa propagation, *conference given at one of the scientific evenings at the Sorbonne*, Asselin et Cie, Paris, 1870, 88 pages and La rage, Revue des cours scientifiques, 1870, 7e année, pages 337-350 et 360-368.

BOULEY M., Observations à l'occasion du procès-verbal, Bulletin de l'Académie nationale de médecine, 44e année, 2e série, tome IX, séance du 27 juillet 1880a, pages 753-754.

BOULEY M., Communications : I Inoculations préventives du charbon, Bulletin de l'Académie nationale de médecine, séance du 21 septembre 1880b, 44e année, 2e série, tome IX, pages 942-954.

BOULEY M., Observations à l'occasion du procès-verbal, I Procédé de vaccination contre le charbon, Bulletin de l'Académie nationale de médecine, séance du 3 août 1880c, 44e année, 2e série, tome IX, pages 791-796.

BOULEY M., Observations à la suite de la note précédente de M. Pasteur, Comptes rendus des séances de l'Académie des sciences, 1880d, tome XCI, pages 457-459.

BOULEY M., Observations à l'occasion du procès verbal de la séance du 1er mars 1881, Bulletin de l'Académie nationale de médecine, séance du 8 mars 1881a, 45e année, 2e série, tome X, 1re partie, pages 300-325 *including a note written by Toussaint in response to Mr. Colin: "De l'immunité pour le charbon ", a note written by Pasteur and interruptions by Mr. Colin.*

BOULEY M., Observations à l'occasion du procès verbal de la séance du 14 juin 1881, Bulletin de l'Académie nationale de médecine, séance du 21 juin 1881b, 45e année, 2e année, tome X, pages 803-836.

BOULEY M., Dépôt sur le bureau de l'Académie, Bulletin de l'Académie nationale de médecine, séance du 28 juin 1881c, 45e année, 2e série, tome X, 1re partie, page 847.

BOULEY M., Observations à l'occasion du procès-verbal, Bulletin de l'Académie nationale de médecine, séance du 28 juin 1881d, 45e année, 2e année, tome X, pages 854-855.

BOULEY H., Observations à la suite de deux communications de M. Pasteur, Comptes rendus des séances de l'Académie des sciences, 1881e, tome XCII, page 668.

BOULEY A., Le progrès en médecine par l'expérimentation 1880-1881, Asselin et Cie, Paris, 1882a, 672 pages.

BOULEY M., Prix Barbier, in Rapport général sur les prix, Bulletin de l'Académie nationale de médecine, 46e année, 2e série, tome XI, séance du 1e août 1882b, pages 861-863 et 886.

BOULEY, rapporteur, PASTEUR, Paul BERT, VULPIAN, GOSSELIN, Commissaires du prix Vaillant, De l'inoculation comme moyen prophylactique des maladies contagieuses des animaux domestiques, Comptes rendus des séances de l'Académie des sciences, 1883, tome XCVI, pages 914-916.

BOULEY A., La nature vivante de la contagion. L'inoculation préventive de la rage, la Revue scientifique (revue rose), 1884, tome XXXIV de la collection, 3e série, tome VIII, pages 353-366.

BOUQUET Henri, Vaccination, Larousse mensuel, numéro 63 de mai 1912, page 420.

BOURGUIGNON H., Appel à des expériences, dans le but d'établir le traitement préservatif de la fièvre typhoïde et des maladies infectieuses inrécidivables, par inoculation de leurs produits morbides, Comptes rendus des séances de l'Académie des sciences, 1855, tome XLI, pages 544-545.

BOURIAT M., Instruction sur la clavelisation, Bulletin de la société d'encouragement pour l'industrie nationale, 10e année, de l'imprimerie de Madame Huzard, Paris, juillet 1811, pages 173-178; Extrait du Bulletin de la Société d'Encouragement pour l'industrie nationale, numéro LXXXV, de l'imprimerie de Mad. Huzard, à Paris, janvier 1812, 15 pages. [BANM, no 39 612 D (4)].

BOURNAND Fr., Un bienfaiteur de l'humanité, Pasteur, sa vie, son œuvre, Tolra éditeur, Paris, 1896, 350 pages.

BOUSQUET J.-B., Traité de la vaccine et des éruptions varioleuses ou varioliformes, ouvrage rédigé sur la demande du gouvernement, chez J.-B. Baillière, Paris, 1833, 367 pages.

BOUSQUET secrétaire, Rapport présenté à M. le ministre de l'agriculture et du commerce par l'Académie royale de médecine sur les vaccinations pratiquées en France pendant l'année 1854, Imprimerie nationale, Paris, 1857, 101 pages.

BOUSQUET M., Rapport présenté à son excellence M. le ministre de l'Agriculture, du commerce et des travaux publics par l'Académie impériale de médecine sur les vaccinations pratiquées en France pendant l'année 1856, Imprimerie impériale, Paris, 1858, 71 pages.

BOUSQUET M., Sur la transmission de la syphilis par la vaccine, Bulletin de l'Académie impériale de médecine, 1865, tome XXX, pages 486-499.

BOUTRY Maurice, La variole à la cour de Marie-Thérèse d'Autriche, La chronique médicale, 10e année, numéro 10 du 15 mai 1903, pages 305-318.

BOYLSTON A.W., Clinical investigation of Smallpox in 1767, The New England Journal of Medicine, 2002, volume 346, pages 1326-1328.

BRANDT Allan M., Poliomyelitis, Politics, Publicity, and Duplicity: Ethical Aspects in the Development of the Salk Vaccine, International Journal of Health Services, 1978, volume 8, pages 257-270.

BRES P. et ROBIN Y., Méningo-encéphalites après vaccination antiamarile avec le vaccin par scarification de Dakar, Etude virologique (résultats préliminaires) et considérations étiopathologiques, Bulletin de la société médicale d'Afrique noire de langue française, 1966, volume XI, pages 610-616.

BRESSOU Clément, La vie exemplaire de Gaston Ramon, in Hommage à Gaston Ramon, Institut Pasteur de Paris, 1970, 21 pages.

BRETONNEAU, Memoirs on Diphteria, selected by Robert Hunter Semple, The new Sydentam Society, London, 1859, page 229.

BRINES Robert, Two hundred years on: Jenner and the discovery of vaccination, Immunology Today, 1996, volume 17, issue 5, pages 203-204.

BROCHIER B., KIENY M.-P., COSTY F., BAUDUIN B., LECOCQ J.-P., LANGUET B., CHAPPUIS G., DESMETTRE P., AFIADEMOMYO K., LIBOIS R., PASTORET P.-P., Large scale eradication of rabies using recombinant vaccinia-rabies vaccine, Nature, 1991, volume 354, pages 520-522.

BROCHIN, Grippe, in Dictionnaire encyclopédique des sciences médicales, G. Masson & P. Asselin et Cie, Paris, 4e série, tome 10, pages 709-749.

BROCQ-ROUSSEU M., Notice nécrologique de M. Piot Bey (1857-1935), Bulletin de l'Académie nationale de médecine, 99e année, tome 113, 3e série, numéro 6, séance du 12 février 1935, pages 213-214.

BRODIE Maurice, Active immunization in monkeys against poliomyelitis with germicidally inactivated virus, Science, 1934a, volume 79, pages 594-595.

BRODIE Maurice, Active immunization of children against poliomyelitis with formalin inactivated virus suspension, Proceedings of the society of experimental and biological medicine, 1934b, volume 32, pages 300-302.

BRODIE Maurice and PARK William H., Active immunization against Poliomyelitis, Journal of the American Medical Association, 1935, volume 105, pages 1089-1093.

BROUARDEL P., Rapport sur les essais de vaccinations cholériques entrepris en Espagne par le Dr Ferran, présenté au ministre du commerce par MM. P. Brouardel, Charrin et Albarran, Bulletin de l'Académie nationale de médecine, séance du 7 juillet 1885, 2e série, tome XIV, pages 902-933.

BROUARDEL M., sans titre, Bulletin de l'Académie nationale de médecine, 1887, 51e année, 2e série, tome XVII, pages 43-49.

BROUARDEL G. et ARNAUD J., L'organisation antituberculeuse française, Masson & Cie, 1934, 260 pages.

BRYCE James, Pratical observations on the inoculation of Cowpox, printed for William Creech, T.N. Longman and O. Rees, T. Cadell jun. and W. Davies, Edinburgh, 1802, 236 pages.

BUCHAN William, Domestic Medicine or a Treatise on the Prevention and Cure of Diseases by Regimen and Simple Medicines Adapted to the Climate and Diseases of America by Isaac Cathrall, printed by Richard Folwell, Philadelphia, 1799, 512 pages.

BUCHAN G., Médecine domestique ou traité complet des moyens de se conserver en santé, et de guérir les maladies par le régime et les remèdes simples, 5e édition, (traduit de l'anglais par J.D. Duplanil), à Paris, chez Moutardier, an X-(1802), 5 tomes.

BULLOCH William, The history of bacteriology, Oxford University Press, Oxford, 1938, unabridged reprint by Dover publications Inc., New-York, 422 pages.

BURKE Richard W., The Equine Diseases of India, printed at the Star Press, Jubbulpore, 1887, 63 pages.

BURNET Etienne Dr., La lutte contre les microbes, Librairie Armand Colin, Paris, 1908, 318 pages.

BURNET F.M., Influenza virus on the developing egg: I Changes associated with the development of an egg-passage strain of virus, British journal of experimental pathology, 1936, volume XVII, pages 282-293.

BURNET Sir Macfarlane, Natural history of infectious disease, At the University Press, Cambridge, 1959, 2nd edition, 356 pages.

BURRALL F.A., Asiatic cholera, William Wood & Co., New-York, 1866, 155 pages.

BYNUM W.F., The scientist as anti-hero, Nature, 1995, volume 375, pages 25-26.

CADEDDU Antonio, Pasteur et le choléra des poules: révision critique d'un récit historique. Historical Philosophical Life Science, 1985, volume 7, pages 87-104.

CADILHAC Paul-Emile, Le cinquantenaire de l'Institut Pasteur, L'Illustration, numéro 5012 du 25 mars 1939, pages 363-369.

CAFFE, DALLY, GALLARD, MARCHAL (De Calvi), LANOIX, TARDIEU, REVILLOUT, etc., Discussion sur la variole et la vaccine, 1870, Conférence médicale de Paris, Adrien Delahaye, Paris, 1872, 191 pages.

CAFFEM AGA, Pièce concernant l'inoculation & la manière dont elle est pratiquée dans les royaumes de Tripoli, Tunis & Alger, in Recueil de pièces concernant l'inoculation de la petite vérole, & propre à en prouver la sécurité & l'utilité, chez Desaint & Saillant, à Paris, 1756, pages 138-139.

CALMETTE A., L'infection bacillaire et la tuberculose chez l'homme et (chez) les animaux, Masson et Cie éditeurs, Paris, 1920 (1re édition), 619 pages; 1922 (2e édition), 644 pages; 1936 (4e édition, revue et complétée par A. Bocquet et L. Nègre), 1024 pages.

CALMETTE A., Vaccination préventive de la tuberculose de l'homme et des animaux par le BCG. Rapports et documents, Masson et cie, Paris, 1932, 366 pages.

CAMPER M., Mémoire sur l'épizootie de la Hollande, Histoire de la société royale de médecine, Mémoire de médecine et de physique médicale, année 1779, pages 321-323.

CAMUS L., La vaccine à l'Académie de médecine (de 1820-1920), Centenaire de l'Académie de médecine, Masson, Paris, 1921, pages 239-278.

CANTWELL M., Tableau de la petite vérole, chez Jean-Thomas Hérissant, à Paris, 1758, 234 pages.

CAPELLE secrétaire de correspondance, Rapport sur la vaccine présenté au citoyen Conseiller d'état, Préfet du département de la Gironde au nom de la Société de médecine, chez Pinard, à Bordeaux, an IX (1801), 42 pages [BANM, no 33 634 (13)].

CAPSTICK P.B., GARLAND A.J., CHAPMAN W.G., MASTERS R.C., Production of Foot-and-Mouth Disease Virus Antigen from BHK21 clone 13 cells grown and infected in Deep Suspension Cultures, Nature, 1965, volume 205, pages 1135-1136.

CAPURON Joseph, Nouveau dictionnaire de médecine, de chirurgie, de physique, de chimie et d'histoire naturelle, Imprimerie De Moronval, à Paris, 1806, 483 pages.

CARPANETTO Dino, Il preguidizio sconfitto La vaccinazione in Piemonte nell'eta francese 1800-1814, Societa di studi Buniviani, Pinerolo, 2004, 235 pages.

CARREL A. et RIVERS T.M., Comptes rendus de la société de biologie, 1927, volume XCVI, pages 848-850.

CARTAZ A. Dr, Le choléra en Espagne, les vaccinations du Dr Ferran, La Nature, numéro 630 du 27 juin 1885, pages 58-59.

CARTAZ A. DR, La rage, traitement prophylactique de M. Pasteur, La Nature, numéro 666 du 6 mars 1886, pages 211-214.

CARTAZ A., Le traitement de la diphtérie, travaux de monsieur Roux, La Nature, numéro 1113 du 29 septembre 1894, pages 282-283.

CARTER Richard, Breakthrough – The saga of Jonas Salk, Trident Press, New-York, 1966, 435 pages.

CATALOGUE raisonné de divers Ecrits qui ont paru concernant l'Inoculation de la petite Vérole, in Recueil de pièces concernant l'Inoculation de la petite Vérole, & propres à en prouver la sécurité & l'utilité, chez Dessaint & Saillant, à Paris, 1756, pages 271-319.

CHABERT, FLANDRIN et HUZARD MM., Instructions et observations sur les maladies des animaux domestiques... Librairie vétérinaire de Madame Huzard, Paris, 1809, 4e édition, tome 1, 480 pages.

CHAMBERLAND Ch., Recherches sur l'origine et le développement des organismes microscopiques, thèse présentée à la Faculté des sciences de Paris pour le grade de docteur es sciences physiques, soutenue le 5 avril 1879, Gauthier-Villards, Paris, 1879, 94 pages.

CHAMBERLAND Ch., Rôle des êtres microscopiques dans la production des maladies, La revue scientifique, 1882, tome XXIX de la collection, 3e série, tome III, pages 450-460.

CHAMBERLAND Ch., Le charbon et la vaccination charbonneuse d'après les travaux récents de M. Pasteur, Bernard Tignol, Paris, 1883a, 316 pages.

CHAMBERLAND Ch. et ROUX E., Sur l'atténuation de la virulence de la bactéridie charbonneuse, sous l'influence des substances antiseptiques, Comptes rendus des séances de l'Académie des sciences, 1883b, tome XCVI, pages 1088-1091.

CHAMBERLAND et ROUX MM., Sur l'atténuation de la bactéridie charbonneuse et de ses germes sous l'influence des substances antiseptiques, Comptes rendus des séances de l'Académie des sciences, 1883c, tome XCVI, pages 1410-1412.

CHAMBERLAND Ch., Annales de l'Institut Pasteur, cité dans La revue scientifique, (revue rose) 1894, 31e année, 1e semestre, page 571.

CHABOSEAU NAPIAS Louise, L'Institut Pasteur de Tokyo, Revue générale des sciences, 1909, volume 20, pages 692-693.

CHAPTAL, Lettre du Ministre aux préfets – Prospectus, Société pour l'extinction de la Petite-Vérole en France, par la propagation de la vaccine – Arrêté du Ministre de l'Intérieur, portant formation d'une Société centrale de Vaccine – Règlement adopté par le ministre de l'intérieur, pour le comité de la Société centrale de vaccine, in Ministère de l'intérieur, Société pour l'extinction de la petite vérole en France par la propagation de la vaccine, Paris, le 14 germinal an 12 (2 avril 1804).

CHARPENTIER P.-C, Les microbes, Vuibert et Nony Editeurs, Paris, 1909, 355 pages.

CHARRIN Dr., Notice nécrologique, H.Toussaint, Revue générale des sciences pures et appliquées, 1890, tome 1, pages 654-656.

CHAUVEAU, VIENNOIS, MEYNET P., Vaccine et variole, nouvelle étude expérimentale sur la question de l'identité de ces deux affections, Recueil de médecine vétérinaire, 1865, 5e séries, volume II, pages 417-448 and 513-559.

CHAUVEAU A., Etude expérimentale des conditions qui permettent de rendre usuel l'emploi de la méthode de M. Toussaint pour atténuer le virus charbonneux et vacciner les espèces animales sujettes au sang de rate, Journal de médecine vétérinaire et de zootechnie, 1882, tome XXXIII de la collection, pages 337-343.

CHAUVEAU A., De l'atténuation directe et rapide des cultures virulentes par l'action de la chaleur, Comptes rendus des séances de l'Académie des sciences, 1883a, tome XCVI, pages 553-557.

CHAUVEAU A., De la faculté prolifique des agents virulents atténués par la chaleur, et de la transmission par génération de l'influence atténuante d'un premier chauffage, Comptes rendus des séances de l'Académie des sciences, 1883b, tome XCVI, pages 612-616.

CHAUVEAU A., De l'inoculation préventive avec les cultures charbonneuses atténuées par la méthode du chauffage rapide, Comptes rendus des séances de l'Académie des sciences, 1883c, tome XCVII, pages 1242-1245.

CHAUVEAU A., De la préparation en grandes masses des cultures atténués par le chauffage rapide pour l'inoculation préventive du sang de rate, Comptes rendus des séances de l'Académie des sciences, 1884a, tome XCVIII, pages 73-77.

CHAUVEAU A., Du chauffage des grandes cultures de bacilles du sans de rate, Comptes rendus des séances de l'Académie des sciences, 1884b, tome XCVIII, pages 126-130.

CHAUVEAU A., L'inoculation préventive du choléra, La revue scientifique (revue rose), 1885, 22e année, 3e série, numéro 12, pages 353-360.

CHAUVEAU M.A., Sur le mécanisme de l'immunité, Annales de l'Institut Pasteur, 1888, tome 2, pages 66-74.

CHAUVEAU M.A., Remarques sur la note de M. Ferran (note de la séance du 15 octobre 1892), Comptes rendus de la Société de biologie, 1892, volume 44, pages 773-774.

CHRONIQUE, Le traitement de la rage aux Etats-Unis, La Nature, numéro 687 du 31 juillet 1886, page 142.

CHRONIQUE, Les Instituts Pasteur en Russie, La Nature, numéro 1236 du 6 février 1897, pages 158-159.

CHUMAKOV M.P., VOROSHILOVA M.K., DROZDOV S.G., DZAGUROV S.G., LASHKEVICH V.A., MIRONOVA L.L., RALPH N.M., SOKOLOVA I.S., DOBROVA I.N., ASHMARINA E.E., SHIRMAN G.A., FLEER G.P., ZHEVANDROVA V.I., KOROLEVA G.A., TOLSKAYA E.A., YANKEVICH O.D.(Moscow), VASILYEVA K.A., KUSLAP T.R. (Tallinn), PODSEDLOVSKY T.S., USPENSKY Y.S. (Vilnius), BOIKO V.M. (Tashkent) and SINYAK K.M. (Lvov), On the course of mass immunization of the population in the Soviet Union with the live poliomyélite virus vaccine from Albert B. Sabin's strains, in Poliomyelitis, papers and discussions presented at the fifth international poliomyelitis conference, Copenhagen, Denmark, July 26-28, 1960, compiled and edited for the International poliomyelitis congress, J. P. Lippincott company, Philadelphia and Montreal, 1961, pages 228-239.

CITRON Julius Dr., Immunity – Methods of diagnosis and therapy and their practical application, translated from the German and edited by A. L. Garbat, P. Blakiston's son & Co., Philadelphia, 1912, 209 pages.

CLARK Paul F., Pioneer microbiologists of America, The University of Wiscontin Press, Madison, 1961, 369 pages.

CLAUDE Daniel, La fièvre aphteuse, La Nature, 1952, numéro 3208, pages 87-88.

CLEMENT Abel, Vaccinothérapie de quelques lésions pyogènes du cheval et du mulet, Thèse pour le doctorat vétérinaire (Diplôme d'état) soutenue devant la Faculté de médecine de Paris en 1927, Imprimerie J. Bonnet, Toulouse, 1927, 59 pages.

CLERC Alexis, Hygiène et médecine des deux sexes, Sciences mises à la portée de tous, Editeur?, vers 1900, tome 1, 809 pages.

COCHU, Observations sommaires lues le 21 novembre 1763 dans l'assemblée des commissaires, nommés par la Faculté de Médecine de Paris, au sujet de l'inoculation de la petite vérole, chez F.A. Quillau, à Paris, 1765, 19 pages.

COLIN M. (d'Alfort), Sur un prétendu moyen de conférer l'immunité contre le charbon, Séance du 1er mars 1881, Bulletin de l'Académie nationale de médecine, 1881, tome X, pages 279-284.

COLOMBIER M., Instruction sur la rage, puis Notes sur le traitement méthodique de la rage, Journal de Médecine, chirurgie, pharmacie, &c, 1785, tome LXV, pages 185-239.

COLON François, Essai sur l'inoculation de la vaccine ou moyen de se préserver pour toujours et sans danger de la petite vérole, chez l'auteur, rue du Faubourg Poissonnière, n° 2, à Paris, de l'imprimerie de Testu, an IX (1800), 36 pages [BANM, n° 33 634 (3)].

COLLOMB H., REY M., DUMAS M. et BERNE C., Syndromes neuro-psychiques au cours des encéphalites postvaccinales (vaccination antiamarile), Bulletin de la société médicale d'Afrique noire de langue française, 1966a, volume XI, pages 575-586.

COLLOMB H., DUMAS M. et GIORDANO C., Encéphalites postvaccinales (vaccination antiamarile) Etude neuro-radiologiques, Bulletin de la société médicale d'Afrique noire de langue française, 1966b, volume XI, pages 587-590.

COMITE CENTRAL DE VACCINE, Rapport du... établi à Paris par la Société des souscripteurs pour l'examen de cette découverte, chez Mme Ve Richard, Paris, 1803, 460 pages.

COMITE MEDICAL pour l'inoculation de la vaccine, Expériences faites à Paris, in Recueil de mémoires, d'observations et d'expériences sur l'inoculation de la vaccine, chez Magimel, à Paris, an IX (1800), pages 35-41.

COMITE MEDICAL pour l'inoculation de la vaccine, Rapport fait au Préfet du Département de la Seine par le Comité Médical de la Société des souscripteurs, pour l'inoculation de la vaccine, *printing location not indicated*, 1801, 14 pages [BANM, n° 39 612(4)].

COMMISSION nommée par MM. les Préfets de la Seine et de police, Rapport sur la marche et les effets du Choléra-Morbus dans Paris et les communes rurales du département de la Seine, année 1832, Imprimerie royale, 1834, 205 pages plus tableaux et pièces annexes.

COMMISSION DE L'ACADEMIE ROYALE DE MEDECINE, J.B.E.H., SIMONDS, GAUDY, Van DOMMELEN, HUFNAGEL, COMMISSION DE PAVIE, ANONYME, Annales de médecine vétérinaire, 1854, pages 33-56, 293-321, 421-422, 429-435, 443-445, 508-513 et 597-613.

COMMITTEE The (from the National Vaccine Establishment) A bill [as amended by the Committee] to prevent the spreading of the infection of the Small Pox, ordered to be printed 3d June 1808, 2 pages.

CONKLIN W.J., Cow-pox, A reference handbook of the medical sciences edited by Albert H. Buck, William Wood & Company, New-York, 1886, volume II, page 318.

CONSEIL SUPERIEUR D'HYGIENE PUBLIQUE DE FRANCE, Travaux, Recueil des actes officiels et documents intéressant l'hygiène publique, 1908, tome 37 (année 1907), pages 696-698.

CONTE A., Police sanitaire des animaux, Librairie J.-B. Baillière et fils, Paris, 1895 (1re édition), 515 pages & 1906 (2e édition), 532 pages.

COPEMAN S. Monckton, Vaccination: its natural history and pathology, being the Milroy lecture for 1898 delivered before the Royal College of Physicians of London, Macmillan and Co., London, 1899, 257 pages.

COPLAND James, Small-pox, A Dictionary of Pratical Medicine, edited by Charles A. Lee, volume VIII, Harper and Brothers Publishers, New-York, 1856, pages 883-922.

COPLAND James, Vaccination, A Dictionary of Pratical Medicine, edited by Charles A. Lee, volume IX, Harper and Brothers Publishers, New-York, 1859, pages 1415-1428.

COPLAND James, Syphilis, A Dictionary of Pratical Medicine, edited by Charles A. Lee, Harper and Brothers Publishers, New-York, 1859, volume IX, pages 1459-1495.

COPLAND James, Zymotic diseases, A Dictionary of Pratical Medicine, edited by Charles A. Lee, Harper and Brothers Publishers, New-York, 1859, volume IX, page 1563.

CORNIL A.-V., et BABES V., Les bactéries et leur rôle dans l'étiologie, l'anatomie et l'histologie pathologiques des maladies infectieuses, Félix Alcan, éditeur, Paris, 3e édition, 1890, 3 tomes.

COTHENIUS M., Sur les préservatifs les plus sûrs de la petite vérole, Collection académique, composée des mémoires, actes ou journaux des plus célèbres Académies & Sociétés littéraires... à Paris, chez Panckoucke, 1774, tome 12 de la partie étrangère et tome 3 des mémoires abrégés de l'Académie Royale de Prusse, pages VII-IX et 156-171.

COURMONT J., Nécrologie, S. Arloing, Revue des sciences pures et appliquées, 1911, tome 22, page 261-262.

COURMONT J. et PANISSET L., Précis de microbiologie des maladies infectieuses des animaux, Octave Doin et fils éditeurs, Paris, 1914, 1054 pages.

COULOMB secrétaire général, Lettre du Ministre de l'intérieur aux Préfets de départements, Journal du galvanisme, de vaccine, etc., an XI (1803), tome 1, pages 183-189.

COUNCILMAN William T., Smallpox, Modern medicine its theory and practice in original contributions by american and foreign authors, edited by William Osler and Thomas McCrae, Lea Brothers & co., Philadelphia and New-York, 1907, volume II, pages 250-300.

CREIGHTON Charles, Jenner and vaccination: A strange chapter of medical history, Swan Sonnenschein & Co., London, 1889, 360 pages.

CREIGHTON Charles, A history of epidemics in Britain, volume 2: from the extinction of plague to the present time, at the university press, Cambridge, 1894, 883 pages.

CRESSAC Mary, Le docteur Roux, mon oncle, L'arche, Paris, 1950, 243 pages.

CROOKSHANK Edgar M., History and pathology of vaccination, volume I: A critical inquiry & volume II: Selected essays, H.K. Lewis, London, 1889, 2 volumes.

CROSS John, A history of the variolous epidemic which occured in Norwich in the year 1819, and destroyed 530 individuals; with an estimate of the protection afforded by vaccination, and a view of past and present opinions upon chicken-pox and modified small-pox, printed for Burgess and Hill, London, 1820, 296 pages.

CROUIGNEAU J. Dr, Rapport sur les vaccinations pratiquées dans la Côte d'Or de 1801 à 1861 présenté à M. le Préfet, manuscrit de 267 pages [BANM, Vaccine 32, dossier 3].

CRUZEL J. Traité pratique des maladies de l'espèce bovine, 1e édition, P. Asselin, Paris, 1869, 919 pages, 3e édition par F. Peuch, Asselin et Houzeau, Paris, 1892, 752 pages.

C.T., Les paysans russes chez M. Pasteur, l'Illustration, numéro 2248 du 27 mars 1886, page 212.

CULLERIER et RATIER, Prophylaxie de la syphilis, Encyclopédie des sciences médicales, Répertoire général de ces sciences, au XIXe siècle, Société encyclographique des sciences médicales, Bruxelles, 1843, tome 26, pages 64-65.

CUMMINS S. Lyle, Correspondence, The British Medical Journal, 1927, November 19, page 956.

CUNY Hilaire, Louis Pasteur The man and his theory, Fawcett Publications Inc., New-York, 1966, 192 pages.

CUVIER M., Rapport historique sur les progrès des sciences naturelles depuis 1789, et sur leur état actuel, présenté à Sa Majesté l'Empereur et Roi en son Conseil d'Etat, le 6 février 1808, de l'imprimerie impériale, Paris, 1810, 394 pages.

D'ALEMBERT, Extrait du mémoire de M. d'Alembert, de l'Académie françoise, &c. lu à l'Académie royale des sciences, le jour de la rentrée sur l'application du calcul des probabilités à l'inoculation de la petite vérole, Journal de Médecine, de Chirurgie et de Pharmacie, 1761, tome XIV, pages 73-82.

DALMAS A., Choléra, in Dictionnaire de médecine ou répertoire général des sciences médicales, Béchet jeunes, Paris, 2e édition, 1834, volume 7, pages 451-543.

DANE D.S., DICK G.W.A., CONNOLLY J.H., FISHER O.D., McKEOWN Florence, BRIGGS Moya, NELSON Robert and WILSON Dermot, Vaccination against poliomyelitis with live virus vaccines 1.A trial of TN type II vaccine, British Medical Journal, 1957, volume 1, pages 59-65.

D'AQUAPENDENTE Hierosme Fabrice, fameux médecin, chirurgien, & professeur anatomique en la célèbre Université de Padouë, Œuvres chirurgicales divisées en deux parties dont la premiere contient le Pentateuque chirurgical, l'autre toutes les opérations manuelles, qui se pratiquent sur le corps humain, dernière edition, soigneusement reveüe & enrichie de diverses figures inventées par l'autheur, chez Pierre Ravaud, à Lyon, 1649, 936 pages.

D'ANCENY Poulain (P. D'A.), Auzias-Turenne sa vie son œuvre, in La syphilisation, publication de l'œuvre du docteur Auzias-Turenne faite par les soins de ses amis, Librairie Germer Baillière et Cie, Paris, 1878, pages I-XXIII.

DAREMBERG G. Dr., Le choléra, ses causes, moyens de s'en préserver, Rueff et Cie, Paris, 1892, 189 pages.

DARLUE M., Sur la rage et sur la manière de la guérir, Journal de médecine, chirurgie et pharmacie, 1755, tome III, 2e édition, pages 182-208 et 1756, tome IV, 1re édition, pages 258-280.

DARM ON Pierre, La longue traque de la variole – les pionniers de la médecine préventive, Perrin, Paris, 1986, 503 pages.

DARMON Pierre, Pasteur, Fayard, Paris, 1995, 431 pages.

DARRE H. et MOLLARET P., Etude clinique d'un cas de méningo-encéphalite au cours de la séro-vaccination anti-amarile, Bulletins de la société de pathologie exotique et de ses filiales, 1936, tome XXIX, pages 169-176.

DAVAINE C, Recherches sur les infusoires du sang dans la maladie connue sous le nom de sang de rate, Comptes rendus des séances de l'Académie des sciences, 1863, tome LVII, pages 220-223.

DAVAINE C, Recherches relatives à l'action de la chaleur sur le virus charbonneux, Comptes rendus des séances de l'Académie des sciences, 1873a, tome LXXVII, pages 726-729.

DAVAINE C, Recherches relatives à l'action des substances dites antiseptiques sur le virus charbonneux, Comptes rendus des séances de l'Académie des sciences, 1873b, tome LXXVII, pages 821-825.

de BERG M., Mémoire qui a remporté le prix proposé en 1776 sur les questions suivantes, 1e Déterminer, par une description exacte des symptômes..., Histoires et mémoires de la Société royale de médecine, années 1777 et 1778, chez Didot le jeune, à Paris, 1780, pages 616-648.

DEBRE Patrice, Louis Pasteur, Flammarion, Paris, 1994, 563 pages.

DECAISNE Dr E., Les inoculations anticholériques, L'Univers illustré, numéro 1582 du 18 juillet 1885, pages 455 et 458.

DECAISNE Dr E., Henri Bouley, L'Univers illustré, numéro 1603 du 12 décembre 1885, pages 790-791.

DECAISNE Dr E., Les expériences de M. Pasteur pour la préservation de la rage, L'Univers illustré, 29e année, numéro 1608 du 16 janvier 1886, pages 36 et 38-39.

DE CARRO J., Lettre aux rédacteurs de la... envoyée le 27 juillet 1799, Bibliothèque britannique, tome 11, an VII (1799), Sciences et arts, pages 337-346.

DECHAMBRE A., Dictionnaire encyclopédique des sciences médicales, P. Asselin et Victor Masson et fils puis Asselin & Houzeau et G. Masson, Paris, 1864-1889, 100 volumes.

DECOURT Philippe, Les vérités indésirables volume I première partie Faut-il réhabiliter Galilée – deuxième partie Comment on falsifie l'histoire: le cas Pasteur, Archives internationales Claude Bernard aux éditions La vieille taupe, 1989, Paris, 316 pages.

DEGROISE M.-H., Arrêté municipal du 27 avril 1808, Catalogue de l'exposition "Pauvreté, hygiène et santé à Dijon avant 1914". Archives municipales – Mairie de Dijon, 1990.

de HAEN Antonio, Questiones saepius motae super methodo inoculandi variolas, Typis J.T. Trattner, Vindobone, 1757, pages 235-445.

de KRUIF Paul, Microbe hunters, Harcourt, Brace and Company, New-York, 1926, 363 pages.

de LACERDA J.B. de, De la cause primordiale de la fièvre jaune, Gazette des hôpitaux, 1883, 56e année, pages 821-822.

de LA CONDAMINE, Relation abrégée d'un voyage fait dans l'intérieur de l'Amérique méridionale, depuis la côte de la mer du sud, jusques aux Côtes du Brésil et de la Guiane, en descendant la rivière des Amazones, Histoire de l'Académie royale des sciences, année 1745, pages 391-492.

de LA CONDAMINE, Mémoire sur l'inoculation de la petite vérole, lu à l'assemblée publique de l'Académie royale des Sciences, le mercredi 24 avril 1754, chez F.B. Merande, Avignon, 3e édition, 1755, 74 pages.

de LA CONDAMINE, Réimpression *(name of printer not given)* de la Seconde lettre de M... à M.*** Conseiller a.P.d.D. Pour servir de Réponse à la Seconde Lettre de M. Gaulard & à son défi, publié dans le Mercure d'Août 1759a, 56 pages.

de LA CONDAMINE, Second mémoire sur l'inoculation de la petite vérole contenant son histoire depuis l'année 1754 lu à l'assemblée publique de l'Académie des Sciences du 15 septembre 1758, à Genève, chez Emmanuel du Villard, 1759b, 55 pages.

de LA CONDAMINE, Lettres de M. de La Condamine à M. le Dr Maty sur l'état présent de l'inoculation en France, chez Prault..., Paris, 1764, 207 pages.

de LA COSTE, Docteur en Médecine, Lettre sur l'inoculation de la petite vérole, comme elle se pratique en Turquie & en Angleterre, écrite en 1723 à Monsieur Dodart, Conseiller d'Etat et premier Médecin de S.M.T.C., Recueil de pièces concernant l'inoculation de la petite vérole, et propres à en prouver la sécurité et l'utilité, chez Desaint et Saillant, à Paris, 1756, pages 140-200.

de LA MOTRAYE, Extrait des voyages de la Motraye, sur la manière dont l'inoculation est pratiquée parmi les Circassiens et les Géorgiens, tome II, page 98, in Recueil de pièces concernant l'inoculation de la petite vérole, & propres à en prouver la sécurité et l'utilité, chez Desaint & Saillant, à Paris, 1756, pages 6-41.

de LAROQUE Jacques-Joseph, Préface du traducteur, in Œuvres complètes du docteur Jenner, à Privas, Imprimerie F. Agard, 1805, lvj et 233 pages.

DELAPORTE François, The history of yellow fever An essay on the birth of tropical medicine, The MIT press, Cambridge (USA), 1991, 181 pages.

de L'EPINE G.J., ASTRUC Jean, BOUVARD Mich. Phil., BARON Théodore, VERDELHAN des Moles Jacq., MACQUART Henri Jacq., Rapport sur le fait de l'inoculation de la petite vérole, chez F.A. Quillau, Paris, 1765, 125 pages.

de L'EPINE G.J., BOUVARD, BARON, VERDELHAN, MACQUART, Supplément au rapport fait à la faculté de médecine contre l'inoculation de la petite vérole, chez Quillau, Paris, 1767, 164 pages.

de la VERGNE, Observations sur la rage suivies de réflexions sur cette maladies et sur son traitement, de l'imprimerie de Gabriel Bourel, Saint-Brieuc, 1808, 44 pages.

de LA VIGNE Casimir, Messéniennes et poésies diverses, la découverte de la vaccine, Discours en vers publié en 1815, chez Ladvocat, à Paris, 1826, 13e édition, tome 2, pages 11-27.

DE LOVERDO J., La fièvre aphteuse, une nouvelle application de la sérothérapie, La Nature, numéro 1307 du 18 juin 1898, pages 38-39.

DENIS François, DUBOIS Frédéric, ALAIN Sophie, SIEGRIST Claire-Anne, Immunothérapie passive et vaccination contre l'hépatite B, in Virus des hépatites? et Delta, coordonné par François Denis et Christian Trépo, Elsevier, 2004, pages 155-198.

D'ENTRECOLLES P. Missionnaire de la Compagnie de Jesus, Lettre concernant l'inoculation de la petite Vérole pratiquée à la Chine, Ecrite à Pékin, le 22 Mai 1726, t. XX. Des Lettres édifiantes & curieuses, in Recueil de pièces concernant L'Inoculation de la petite Vérole, & propres à en prouver la sécurité & l'utilité, chez Dessaint & Saillant, à Paris, 1756, pages 288-290.

DENYS J. et LECLEF J., Sur le mécanisme de l'immunité chez le lapin vacciné contre le streptocoque pyogène, La Cellule, 1895, volume XI, pages 177-221.

DEPAUL Docteur, directeur de la vaccine, De la syphilis vaccinale, Projet de rapport à présenter à S. Exe. M. le Ministre de l'agriculture, du commerce et des travaux publics, au nom de la commission de vaccine, Bulletin de l'Académie impériale de médecine. 1864-1865, tome XXX, pages 135-160, 252-271, 276-298, 300-318, 329-365; 1865-1866, tome XXXI, pages 536-553.

DEPAUL M., Communication, Bulletin de l'Académie impériale de médecine, 1866, tome XXXI, pages 590-593.

DEPAUL M., Discussion sur un cas de syphilis vaccinale, Bulletin de l'Académie impériale de médecine. 1866-1867, tome XXXII, pages 486-488 & 1024-1103.

DEPAUL M. Rapporteur, Rapport présenté à son excellence M. le Ministre de l'Agriculture, du commerce et des travaux publiques par l'Académie impériale de médecine sur les vaccinations pratiquées en France pendant l'année 1866, imprimerie impériale, Paris, 1868, 163 pages.

de PONSARD, L'inoculation rectifiée, ouvrage très utile aux pères & mères qui veulent garantir leurs enfants des ravages meurtriers de la petite vérole naturelle, chez G. Bergeret, à Bordeaux, 1776, 102 pages.

de PREVILLE H., Un médecin sans diplôme, Pasteur, Tolra éditeur, Paris, 1897, 216 pages.

DERENNE F., VANDERHEYDEN J.E., BAIN H., JOCQUET Ph., JACQUY J., YANE F., DRUYTS-VOETS E., LAMY M. E., et VANHAEVERBEEK M., Poliomyélite antérieure aiguë maternelle en zone non endémique, Acta neurologica Belgica, 1989, volume 89, pages 358-365.

de ROCHEBRUNE A.-T., Formation de races nouvelles. Recherches d'ostéologie comparée, sur une race de bœufs domestiques observée en Sénégambie, Comptes rendus des séances de l'Académie des Sciences, 1880, tome XCI, pages 304-306.

de ROCHEBRUNE A.-T., Sur le *Bos triceros, Rochbr.*, et l'inoculation préventive de la peripneumonie épizootique, par les maures et les Pouls de la Sénégambie, Comptes rendus des séances de l'Académie des Sciences, 1885, tome C, pages 658-660.

de SAINT-MARTIN A.-F.-C, Monographie sur la rage. Mémoire auquel le cercle médical de Paris décerna la première médaille d'or au concours proposé sur la rage par cette société, depuis 1813 jusqu'à 1817, Chez Mme Huzard et M. Béchet, à Paris, 1823, 394 pages.

DESGUIN M., Un cas de rage après plus de deux ans d'incubation et un traitement à l'Institut Pasteur, Bulletin de l'Académie royale de médecine de Belgique, séance du 25 mai 1889, 1889, 4e série, tome 3, pages 249-251.

DESNOS L., Choléra asiatique, in Nouveau dictionnaire de médecine et de chirurgie pratiques, sous la direction du docteur Jaccoud, Librairie J.-B. Baillière et fils, 1867, tome 7, pages 321-481.

DESPLANTES Fr., Louis Pasteur, le savant et le bienfaiteur de l'humanité, Eugène Ardant, Limoges, vers 1900, 144 pages.

DESPLATS Henri Dr, La Rage, Revue des questions scientifiques, 1886, tome 20, pages 5-29.

de VARIGNY, Les microbes et leur rôle pathogénique d'après des travaux récents, Revue scientifique (revue rose), 1884, tome XXXIV de la collection, 3e série, tome VIII, pages 263-278.

DEVEZE Jean, Mémoire relative à la contagion de la fièvre jaune, Paris, 1820, 513 pages.

DEZOTEUX M., Lettre écrite à M.. .. Médecin à Paris, par M. D..., Médecin & chirurgien Major du Regiment du Roi, Infanterie, Besançon le 14 février 1763; Lettre de M. Middelton de Londres le 12 mars 1763; Lettre de M. Maty de Londres, le 13 mars 1763, in Lettres sur l'inoculation, de l'imprimerie de Jean-Félix Charmet, à Besançon, 1765a, 32 pages.

DEZOTEUX, M. le M. de la P., Mme B., M. ATTHALIN, M. COILLOT, ACTON, Mme BIETRIX, Mlle MARTIN, M. de CHEVIGNEY, M. D., M. le Curé de Pelousey, M. le Curé de Sainte Magdeleine, MM. MOREL & JANNEROT, M. MARET, Pièces justificatives des lettres concernant l'inoculation, Imprimerie Pierre Delhorme, Lons-le -Saunier, 1765b, 51 pages et Réponse à la seconde brochure de M. D*** intitulé Pièces justificatives des lettres concernant l'Inoculation, Imprimerie Cl. Jos. Daclin, Besançon, 1765b, 48 pages.

DEZOTEUX François et VALENTIN Louis, Traité historique et pratique de l'inoculation, chez Agasse, A Paris, l'An 8 de la République (1799), 436 pages.

DICK G.W.A., DANE D.S., FISHER O.D.,CONNOLLY J.H., McKEOWN Florence, BRIGGS Moya, NELSON Robert and WILSON Dermot, Vaccination against poliomyelitis with live virus vaccines 2. A trial of SM type I attenuated virus vaccine, British Medical Journal, 1957, volume 1, pages 65-70.

DICTIONARY OF SCIENTIFIC BIOGRAPHY, Charles Coulston Gillispie editor, Charles Scribner's sons, New York, 1981, 10 volumes.

DIDAY M., Sur un procédé de vaccination préservatrice de la syphilis constitutionnelle, extrait de la Gazette médicale de Paris, 1849, 45 pages.

DIDEROT M. et d'ALEMBERT M., Encyclopédie ou Dictionaire raisonné des sciences, des arts et des métiers, 1751-1772, article contagion, tome IV, chez Briasson &..., Paris, page 110 – article inoculation, tome VIII, à Neuchatel, chez Samuel Faulche et compagnie, libraires et imprimeurs, 1765, pages 755-771.

DIFFLOTH Paul, La lutte contre la tuberculose, L'Illustration européenne, 32e année, numéro 6 du 9 février 1902, page 88.

DIXON C. W., Smallpox, J. & A. Churchill Ldt, London, 1962, 512 pages.

DOLERIS J. Amédée, Rage humaine, in Nouveau dictionnaire de médecine et de chirurgie pratiques, directeur de la rédaction: le docteur Jaccoud, Librairie J.-B. Baillière et fils, Paris 1881, tome 30, pages 421-467.

DOMENJON Augustin, Réflexions historiques sur la petite-vérole et sur son inoculation, Essai présenté et soutenu à l'Ecole de Médecine de Montpellier, le 3 Prairial an IX, à Montpellier, chez Izar et A. Ricard, an IX (1801), 46 pages.

DORLAND's Medical Dictionary, W.B. Saunders Company, Philadelphia, 19th edition, 1942, 1647 pages; 20th edition, 1944, 1668 pages; 28th edition, 1994, 1939 pages; 29th edition, 2000, 2 088 pages.

DOUGLAS R. Gordon Jr and BETTS Robert F., Influenza virus, in Principles and practices of infectious dieases, edited by Gerald L. Mandell, R. Gordon Douglas Jr and John E. Bennette, John Wiley and sons, New-York, 1979, pages 1135-1167.

DUBAIL André, Joseph Meister le premier être humain sauvé de la rage, annuaire 1985 de la société d'Histoire du Val de Ville, pages 93-148.

DUBOIS-HAVENITH Dr, Une page de l'histoire de la syphilis, syphilisation et vaccination syphilitique, Journal de médecine, de chirurgie et de pharmacologie, 1891, 49e année, 92e volume, numéro 19, pages 604-661.

DUBOUE Dr (de Pau), De la physiologie pathologique et du traitement rationnel de la rage, suites d'études de pathogénie, V. Adrien Delahaye et Cie, Paris, 1879, 269 pages.

DUCLAUX E., Ferments et maladies, cours professé à la Sorbonne en 1879-1880, G. Masson éditeur, Paris, 1882, 284 pages.

DUCLAUX Emile, Pasteur, Histoire d'un esprit, Imprimerie Charaire et Cie, Sceaux, 1896, 400 pages – Pasteur, the history of a mind, translated by Erwin F. Smith and Florence Hedges, W.B.Saunders Company, Philadelphia, 1920, 363 pages.

DUCLAUX E., Traité de microbiologie, Masson et Cie, Paris, 1898-1901, 4 tomes.

DUCLAUX Madame Emile, née Mary Robinson, La vie d'Emile Duclaux, L. Barnéoud et Cie, Laval, 1906, 332 pages.

DUCOUT Danielle, Pasteur et Joseph Meister, Autour de Louis Pasteur, Cahiers Dolois, 1995, numéro II, pages 315-338.

DUFFOUR Joseph, Discours préliminaire du traducteur, Preuves de l'efficacité de la vaccine par le docteur John Thornton, Chomel imprimeur libraire, Paris, 1808, xl pages.

DUFRANC, Arrest de la cour de Parlement, sur le fait de l'inoculation, Extrait des registres du Parlement du 8 juin 1763, Chez P.G. Simon, à Paris, 1763, 8 pages.

DUHAUME, Traité de la petite vérole tiré des commentaires de G. van Swieten sur les aphorismes de Boerhaave, chez d'Houry, à Paris, 1776, 330 pages.

DUJARRIC DE LA RIVIERE R., Emile Roux, in Les princes de la médecine, d'Hippocrate à Fleming, Club mondial du livre reproduit avec l'autorisation du Livre contemporain Amiot-Dumont, imprimé à Anvers sur les presses de l'imprimerie Mercurius, *no date given*, pages 329-349.

DUMAY Victor, Notes sur Dijon, imprimé par Frantin, Dijon, 1848, 20 pages.

DUMESNIL René et BONNET-ROY Flavien, sous la direction de... Les médecins célèbres, Editions d'art Lucien Mazenod, Paris, 1999, 628 pages.

DUNGLISON Robley, A dictionary of medical science, Blanchard and Lea, Philadelphia, 1854, 927 pages.

DUNGLISON Robley, A dictionary of medical science, Henri C. Lea, Philadelphia, 1866, 1047 pages.

DUNHAM George C., Military preventive medicine, Military service publishing company, Harrisburg PA., 1940, Third edition, 1198 pages.

DUNLOP Robert H. et WILLIAMS David J., Veterinary medicine, an illustrated history, Mosby-Year Book Inc., St Louis, 1996, 128 pages.

DUPONT Michel, Dictionnaire historique des médecins dans et hors de la médecine, Larousse, Paris, 1999, 628 pages.

DUPUY Edouard, Etude historique, expérimentale et critique sur l'identité de la variole et de la vaccine, G. Steinheil, Paris, 1894, 128 pages.

DUVAL Charles W., Observations upon the nature of the virus of hog cholera, Proceedings of the Society of Biology and Medicine, 1929, volume 27, pages 87-89.

DUVRAC Louis, Question de médecine discutée dans les Ecoles de la Faculté de Médecine de Paris, le 30 décembre 1723, sous la présidence de M. Claude de la VIGNE de FRECHEVILLE: Est-il permis de proposer l'inoculation de la petite vérole? Chez Delaguette, Libraire et Imprimeur, Paris, 1755, 40 pages.

ENCYCLOPAEDIA BRITANNICA, by a Society of Gentlemen in Scoland, printed by A. Bell and C. Macfarquhar, Edinburgh, 1771, in three volumes.

ENCYCLOPAEDIA BRITANNICA new americanized, the Saalfield Publishing Company, Akron, Ohio, U.S., Twentieth Century Edition, 1902, in XII volumes.

EDITEUR, Extrait de trois écrits dont deux sont de M. Jurin & l'autre de M. Scheuzer, de la Société Royale de Londres, contenant la relation du succès de l'inoculation en Angleterre durant les années 1725, 1726, 1727 & 1728, Recueil de pièces concernant l'inoculation de la petite vérole et propres à en prouver la sécurité et l'utilité, chez Desaint et Saillant, à Paris, 1756, pages 126-137.

EDITEUR, Revue-Chronique: La Rage: Rapport de M. Pasteur à l'Académie des sciences, La Science pour tous, numéro 21 du 24 mai 1884, page 161.

EDITORIAL, La Revue scientifique, numéro 34 de la 2e série de la 9e année du 21 février 1880, page 789.

EDITORIAL, Poliomyélite eradication: the endgame, Nature Medicine, 2001, volume 7, page 131.

ELMENDORF John E. Jr and SMITH Hugh H., Multiplication of yellow fever virus in the developing chick embryo, Proceeding Society Experimental Biology and Medicine, 1937, volume 36, pages 171-174.

ELTON Norman W., Public health aspects of the campaign against yellow fever in Central America, American Journal of Public Health, 1952, volume 47, pages 170-174.

EMERY rapporteur, Rapport présenté à M. le ministre du commerce et des travaux publiques par l'Académie royale de médecine sur les vaccinations pratiquées en France pendant l'année 1830, de l'imprimerie royale, Paris, juillet 1832, 59 pages.

EMERY rapporteur, Rapport présenté à M. le ministre des travaux publiques, de l'agriculture et du commerce par l'Académie royale de médecine sur les vaccinations pratiquées en France pendant l'année 1835, de l'imprimerie royale, Paris, septembre 1837, 55 pages.

EMONNOT secrétaire-rapporteur, Premier rapport de la Commission de vaccine, séante au Louvre, à la Société de médecine (extrait du tome XI du Recueil périodique de la Société de médecine, de l'imprimerie de la Société de médecine, à Paris, Prairial an IX, 1801, 40 pages [BANM, n° 33 634 (7)].

ENAUX M. et CHAUSSIER M., Méthode de traiter les morsures des animaux enragés, et de la vipère; suivie d'un précis sur la pustule maligne, chez A. M. Defay, Dijon, 1785, 275 pages.

ENDERS John F., The present status of tissue-culture techniques in the study of the poliomyelitis viruses, in Poliomyelitis, Monograph series, issue 26, World Health Organization, Geneva, 1955, pages 269-294.

ENRIQUEZ Ed. Dr, Traité de médecine de Enriquez, Laffitte, Berge, Lamy, Octave Doin et fils, Paris, 1909, 4 tomes.

ERCOLANI J.-B., Sur l'inoculation des aphthes (sic), traduit et analysé par M. L. Prangé, Recueil de médecine vétérinaire, 1858, volume XXXV ou tome V, 4e série, pages 473-478.

ERNST Harold C., Cholera Asiatique, Reference handbook of the medical sciences, Willial Wood & company, New-York, 1886, volume 2, pages 128-135.

FARRELL L.N., WOOD W., FRANKLIN A.E., SHIMADA F.T., MACMORINE H.G. and RHODES A.J., Cultivation of poliomyelitis virus in tissue culture VI. Methods for quantity production of poliomyelitis viruses in cultures of monkey kidney, Canadian journal of public health, 1953, volume 44, pages 273-280.

FENNER F., HENDERSON D.A., ARITA I., JEZEK Z., LADNYI I.D., Smallpox and its eradication, World Health Organization, Geneva, 1988, 1460 pages.

FELDMAN Burton, The Nobel prizes. A history of genius, controversy and prestige, Arcade Publishing, New-York, 2000, 489 pages.

FERBER Dan, Monkey Virus Link to Cancer Grows Stronger, Science, 2002, volume 296, pages 1012-1015.

FERRAN J., Sur l'action pathogène et prophylactique du bacillus-virgule, lettre de M. J. Ferran, Comptes rendus des séances de l'Académie des sciences, séance du 13 avril 1885a, tome C, pages 959-962.

FERRAN J., Sur la prophylaxie du choléra au moyen d'injections hypodermiques de cultures pures du bacille-virgule, Comptes rendus des séances de l'Académie des sciences, séance du 13 juillet 1885b, tome CI, pages 147-149.

FERRAN J. Dr, Lettre à M. le secrétaire perpétuel, au sujet du procédé de vaccination contre le choléra, Comptes rendus des séances de l'Académie des sciences, séance du 27 juillet 1885c, tome CI, page 367.

FERRAN J. et PAULI L, Le principe actif du Koma-bacille, comme cause de mort et d'immunité, *note presented at the session held Monday 18, 1886*, Comptes rendus des séances de l'Académie des sciences, 1886, tome CII, pages 159-160.

FERRAN, prie l'Académie de tenir compte, dans ses recherches effectuées pour la découverte de la vaccine chimique du choléra asiatique des documents qu'il lui a adressé, Comptes rendus des séances de l'Académie des sciences, 1888, tome CVII, pages 454 & 645.

FERRAN J., A propos de la communication de M. Haffkine, sur le choléra asiatique, [Note de M. J. Ferran (de Barcelone), adressée au Président au début des vacances de la société], Comptes rendus de la Société de biologie, 1892, volume 44, pages 771-773.

FERRAN Jaime, Sur la culture d'un second antigène non acido-résistant et parasite obligé contenu dans le virus tuberculeux naturel, Comptes rendus de la Société de biologie, séance du 13 juillet 1912, tome LXXIII, pages 106-107.

FIGUIER Louis, Le choléra en Europe en 1884, L'année scientifique et industrielle, 28e année (1884), Librairie Hachette, Paris, 1885, pages 378-402.

FIGUIER Louis, Médecine et physiologie. Le choléra en Europe en 1885, L'année scientifique et industrielle, 29e année (1885), Librairie Hachette, Paris, 1886, pages 327-344.

FIGUIER Louis, Médecine et physiologie. Le traitement de la rage par la méthode Pasteur... L'année scientifique et industrielle, 31e année (1887), Librairie Hachette, Paris, 1888a, pages 393-401.

FIGUIER Louis, L'Institut Pasteur, L'année scientifique et industrielle, 31e année (1887), Librairie Hachette, Paris, 1888b, pages 547-548.

FIGUIER Louis, La découverte du vaccin du choléra chez les animaux par un médecin russe, M. Gamaleïa, L'année scientifique et industrielle, 32e année (1888), Librairie Hachette, Paris, 1889, pages 396-400.

FINDLAY G.M. and HINDLE E., Combined use of living virus and immune serum for immunization against virus infections, The British Medical journal, May 2, 1931, pages 740-742.

FINDLAY G.M., Sur l'immunisation contre la fièvre jaune, Bulletin de l'Office international d'hygiène publique, 1933, tome XXV, pages 1009-1014.

FINDLAY G.M. and CLARKE L.P., Reconversion of the neurotropic into the viscerotropic strain of yellow fever virus in Rhesus monkeys, Transactions of the Royal Society of Tropical Medicine and Hygiene, 1935, volume XXVIII, pages 579-600.

FINDLAY G.M., Immunization against yellow fever, Transactions of the Royal Society of Tropical Medicine and Hygiene, 1934a, volume XXVII, pages 437-464.

FINDLAY G.M., Nouvelles expériences concernant l'immunisation contre la fièvre jaune, Bulletin de l'Office international d'hygiène publique, 1934b, tome XXVI, pages 43-51.

FINDLAY G.M., Immunisation against yellow fever with attenuated neurotropic virus, The Lancet, November 3, 1934c, pages 983-985.

FINDLAY G.M., La vaccination contre la fièvre jaune (1932-1936), Bulletin de l'office international d'hygiène publique, 1936a, tome XXVIII, pages 1321-1324.

FINDLAY G.M., Transactions of the society X. Variation in animal viruses. A review, Journal of the Royal Microscopital Society, 1936b, volume 66, pages 213-299.

FINDLAY G.M. and MACKENSIE R.D., Attemps to produce immunity against yellow fever with killed virus, The Journal of Pathology and Bacteriology, 1936c, Volume 43, pages 205-208.

FINDLAY G.M. et MACCALLUM F.O., Note on acute hepatitis and yellow fever immunization, Transactions of the Royal Society of Tropical Medicine and Hygiene, 1937, volume XXXI, pages 297-308.

FINLAY Charles, Yellow fever: its transmission by means of the Culex mosquito, American Journal of medical science, 1886, volume 92, pages 395-409.

FINLAY Charles, Inoculation for Yellow fever by means of contaminated mosquitoes, American Journal of medical science, 1891, volume 92, pages 264-268.

FISHER John D., Description of the distinct, confluent, and inoculated smallpox, varioloid disease, cow pox, and chicken pox, published by Lilly, wait & co, Boston, second edition, 1834, 73 pages.

FISHER Richard B., Joseph Lister, 1827-1912, Macdonald and Jane's, London, 1977, 351 pages.

FISHER Richard B., Edward Jenner, 1749-1823, André Deutsch Limited, London, 1991, 361 pages.

FITZ Reginald H., Zabiel Boylston, inoculator, and the epidemic of smallpox in Boston in 1721, The Johns Hopkins Bulletin, 1911, Volume XXII, issue 247, pages 1-36.

FLECKINGER R., La fièvre aphteuse en France au XXe siècle; Evolution – Moyens de lutte – Résultats – Situation, Edition Bellier, Lyon, 2004, 163 pages.

FLEMING Alexander and PETRIE G.F., Recent advances in vaccine and serum therapy, J. & A. Churchill, London, 1934, 463 pages.

FLÜGGE C. Dr, Les microorganismes étudiés spécialement au point de vue de l'étiologie des maladies infectieuses, traduit de l'allemand d'après la seconde édition par le Dr F. Henrijean, A. Manceaux libraire-éditeur, Bruxelles, 1887, 644 pages.

FLÜGGE C. Dr, Micro-organisms with special reference to the etiology of the infective diseases, translated by W. Watson Cheyne, The new Sydenham society, London, 1890, 826 pages.

FONTAINE Dr et HUGUIER Dr, Nouveau dictionnaire vétérinaire, médecine, chirurgie, thérapeutique, législation sanitaire et sciences qui s'y rapportent, Librairie J.-B. Baillière et fils, Paris, 1921 & 1924, 2 volumes.

FOSTER Eugene, Small-pox in A reference handbook of the medical sciences edited by Albert H. Buck, William Wood & Company, New-York, 1888, volume VI, pages 478-487.

FOUQUET Henri M., Traitement de la petite vérole des enfans, à l'usage des habitans de la campagne, et du peuple dans les provinces Méridionales, à Amsterdam et à Montpellier chez Rigaud et Pons et la veuve Gauthier et Faure, 1772, 276 pages.

FOURNIER Alfred, Inoculation, in Nouveau dictionnaire de médecine et de chirurgie pratique, directeur de la rédaction: le docteur Jaccoud, 1874, tome 19, pages 105-138.

FOURNIER Alfred, Leçons sur la syphilis vaccinale, Lecrosnier et Babé, Paris, 1889, 256 pages.

FOX J.P., LENNETTE E.H., MANSO C. and SOUZA AGUIAS J.B., Encephalitis in man following vaccination against yellow fever. American Journal of Hygiene, 1942, volume 36, pages 117-142.

FRAITOT V., Pasteur (l'œuvre, l'homme, le savant), Librairie Vuibert, 4e édition, Paris, circa 1900, 160 pages.

FRANKLAND Percy and FRANKLAND Mrs Percy, Pasteur, Cassell and Company, London, 1898, 224 pages.

FRANCIS Thomas Jr. and MAGILL T.P., The antibody response of human subjects vaccinated with the virus of human influenza, Journal of experimental medicine, 1937, volume 65, pages 251-259.

FRANCIS Thomas Jr, NAPIER John A., VOIGHT Robert B., HEMPHILL Fay M., WENNER Herbert A., KORNS Robert F., BOISEN Morton, TOLCHINSKY Eva, DIAMOND Earl L, Evaluation of the 1954 field trial of poliomyelitis vaccine, Final report, sponsored by the national foundation for infantile paralysis, University of Michigan, Edwards Brothers, Ann Arbor, 1957, 563 pages.

FRASER Elisabeth T., Manuel d'immunité pour médecins & étudiants, traduit par H. Kufferath, Henri Lamertin libraire éditeur, Bruxelles, 1914, 207 pages.

FREESTONE D.S., Yellow fever vaccine, in Vaccines, Stanley A. Plotkin and Edward A. Mortimer Jr. Editors, 2nd edition, W.B. Saunders company, Philadelphia, 1994, 996 pages.

FREIRE D. et REBOURGEON, Le microbe de la fièvre jaune. Inoculation préventive, Comptes rendus des séances de l'Académie des sciences, 1884, tome XCIX, pages 804-806.

FREIRE Domingos, GIBIER Paul, REBOURGEON C., Du microbe de la fièvre jaune et de son atténuation, Comptes rendus des séances de l'Académie des sciences, 1887a, tome CIV, pages 858-860.

FREIRE Domingos, GIBIER Paul et REBOURGEON C., Résultats obtenus par l'inoculation préventive du virus atténué de la fièvre jaune, à Rio-de-Janeiro, Comptes rendus des séances de l'Académie des sciences, 1887b, tome CIV, pages 1020-1022.

FREIRE Domingos, Sur les inoculations préventives de la fièvre jaune, Comptes rendus hebdomadaires de la Société de biologie, 1891, 9e série, tome III, numéro 26, pages 579-581.

FRENCH George R., PLOTKIN Stanley A., Miscellaneous Limited-use vaccines, in Vaccines edited by Stanley A. Plotkin and Walter A. Orenstein, W.B. Saunders Company, Philadelphia, 1999, 3rd edition, pages 728-733.

FRENKEL H.S., La culture du virus de la fièvre aphteuse sur l'épithélium de la langue des bovidés. Bulletin de l'Office International des Epizootie, 1947, volume 28, pages 155-162.

FRENKEL H. S., Research on Foot-and-Mouth Disease III. The Cultivation of the virus on a practical Scale in Explantations of bovine Tongue Epithelium, American Journal of Veterinary Research, 1951, volume 12, pages 187-190.

FRIERSON J. Gordon, The Yellow fever vaccine: a History, Yale Journal of Biology and Medicine, 2010, volume 83, pages 77-85.

FRIESE F.G., Account of the progress of the Jennerian inoculation upon the continent, The medical and physical journal, 1803, volume IX, pages 128-130.

FROCHOT, Etablissement gratuit pour l'inoculation de la vaccine, Préfecture du département de la Seine, de l'imprimerie de Ballard, Paris, 1801, pages 15-20.

GALISHOFF Stuart, Dictionary of American Medical Biography, editors Martin Kaufman, Stuart Galishoff, Todd L Savitt, Greenwood Press, West port Connecticut, USA, 1984, 2 volumes.

GALTIER V., Traité des maladies contagieuses et de la police sanitaire des animaux domestiques, Imprimerie de Beau jeune & cie, Lyon, 1880, 1re édition, 941 pages – Asselin et Houzeau, Paris, 1891-1892, 2e édition revue corrigée et augmentée, 2 tomes – 1897, 3e édition revue et corrigée, 1283 pages.

GAMALEIA N., Sur la vaccination préventive du choléra asiatique, Comptes rendus des séances de l'Académie des sciences, 1888, tome CVII, pages 432-434.

GANDOGER de FOIGNY M., Traité-Pratique de l'inoculation, dans lequel on expose les règles de conduite relatives au choix de la raison propre de cette opération; de l'âge..., chez J. B. Hyacinthe Leclerc, à Nancy, 1768, 500 pages.

GARDANE J.J., Le secret des Suttons dévoilé ou l'inoculation mise à la portée de tout le monde, A la Haye, chez Ruault à Paris, 1774, 96 pages.

GARNIER M. et DELAMARE V., Dictionnaire des termes techniques de médecine, A. Maloine et fils éditeurs, Paris 1920, 7e édition, 634 pages.

GARRISON Fielding H., An introduction to the history of medicine, W.B. Saunders Company, 4th edition, 1966, 996 pages.

GAUTIER Emile, Les vaccinations anticholériques dans l'Inde, L'année scientifique et industrielle, 39e année (1895), librairie Hachette et Cie, 1896, pages 193-199.

GAUTIER Emile, Nécrologie, Le professeur Grancher, L'année scientifique et industrielle, 51e année (1907), librairie Hachette et Cie, 1908, pages 451-452.

G.C., La grippe en 1959, La Nature, 1960, numéro 3297, page 45 et numéro 3307, page 483.

GEISON Gerald L., The private science of Louis Pasteur, Princeton University Press, Princeton, 1995, 378 pages.

GELL P.G.H. and COOMBS R.R.A., Clinical aspects of immunology, Blackwell Scientific Publications, Oxford, 1962, 883 pages.

GENERAL BOARD OF HEALTH, The history and practice of vaccination, printed by G.E. Eyre and W. Spottiswoode for her majesty stationery office, 1857, 188 + lxxxiii pages.

GEORGEL R. Dr, Vaccination et vaccinothérapie antityphiques par voie gastro-intestinale, Imprimerie Léon Sézanne, Lyon, 1917, 125 pages.

GERSHON Anne A., Varicella Vaccine: Rare Serious Problems but the benefits Still Outweigh the Riks, The journal of Infectious Diseases, 2003, volume 188, pages 945-947.

GERARDIN Auguste secrétaire rapporteur, Rapport présenté à M. le ministre du commerce et des travaux publics par l'Académie royale de médecine sur les vaccinations pratiquées en France pendant l'année 1833, de l'imprimerie royale, Paris, juillet 1835, 79 pages.

GIBIER Paul et VAN ERMENGEN, Recherches expérimentales sur le choléra, Comptes rendus des séances de l'Académie des sciences, séances du 10 août 1885, tome CI, pages 470-472.

GICQUEL Brigitte, Recherche de nouveaux vaccins contre la tuberculose, Bulletin de l'Académie nationale de médecine, 1999, volume 183, pages 53-62.

GILLET Henri Dr, Rage in Traité des maladies de l'enfance, édité par J. Grancher et J. Comby, 2e édition, volume 1, Masson et Cie, éditeurs, Paris, 1904, pages 612-618.

GINTRAC H., Grippe, in Nouveau dictionnaire de médecine et de chirurgie pratiques, directeur de la rédaction: le docteur Jaccoud, 1872, tome 16, pages 728-753.

GIRARD Marc, BANSAL P. Gheetha, PEDROSA-MARTINS Livia, DODET Betty, MEHRA Vijay, SCHITO Marco, MATHIESON Bonnie, DELFRAISSY Jean-François and BRADAC James, Mucosal immunity and HIV-AIDS vaccines. Report of an international workshop, Vaccine, 2008, volume 26, pages 3969-3977.

GIRARD M.P., REED Z.H., FRIEDE M. and KIENY M.P., A review of human vaccine research and development: malaria, Vaccine, 2007, volume 25, pages 1567-1580.

GLENNY A.T., ALLEN K., O'B R.A., The Schich reaction and diphteria prophylactic immunisation with toxin-antitoxin mixture, The Lancet, numéro du 11 juin 1921a, pages 1236-1237.

GLENNY A.T., and SÜDMERSEN H.J., Notes on the production of immunity to diphteria toxin, Journal of hygiene (London), 1921b, volume 20, pages 176-220.

GLENNY A.T., ALLEN K. and HOPKINS Barbara E., Testing the antigenic value of diphtheria toxin-antitoxin mixtures. British Journal of experimental pathology, 1923a, volume 4, pages 19-27.

GLENNY A.T. and HOPKINS Barbara E., Diphtheria toxoid as an immunizing agent, British journal of experimental pathology, 1923b, volume 4, pages 283-288.

GLENNY A.T., POPE C.G., WADDINGTON Hilda and WALLACE U., Immunological notes XVII-XXIV, Journal of pathological Bacteriology, 1926, volume 29, pages 31-40.

GLENNY A.T., Insoluble precipitates in diphtheria and tetanus immunization, The British Medical Journal, August 16, 1930, pages 244-245.

GODINE Jeune, Expériences sur la vaccine dans les bêtes à laine, comme moyen préservatif du claveau, pendant les années X et XI, Journal du galvanisme, de vaccine, etc. an XI (1803a) tome 1, pages 29-48.

GODINE Jeune, Précis d'expériences nouvelles sur la vaccine dans l'espèce humaine et dans les bêtes à laine, Journal du galvanisme, de vaccine, etc., an XII (1803b), pages 226-244.

GOEBEL Walther F. & AVERY Oswald T., Chemo-immunological studies on conjugated carbohydrate-proteins. IV. The synthesis of the p-aminobenzyl ether of the soluble specific substance of type III *Pneumococcus* and its coupling with protein. Journal of experimental medicine, 1931, volume 54, pages 431-436.

GOËTZ, Histoire de l'inoculation pratiquée dans la ville de Strasbourg et la province d'Alsace, Journal de médecine, chirurgie, pharmacie, &c, 1770, volume XXXIII, pages 247-255.

GOODALL E.W. and WASHBOURN J.W., A manual of infectious diseases, H.K. Lewis, London, 1896, 368 pages.

GORDON John E. and HUGUES Thomas P., A study of inactivated yellow fever virus as an immunizing agent, Journal of immunology, 1936, volume 30, pages 221-234.

GORET P., LETARD E. et LE BARS H., L'œuvre scientifique des vétérinaires français, Regards sur la France, Vétérinaires de France, 9e année, octobre 1965, numéro 27, pages 327-366.

GORET Pierre, A propos d'un anniversaire: La vie et l'œuvre de Pierre-Victor Galtier (1846-1908) professeur à l'Ecole vétérinaire de Lyon, Bulletin de l'Académie nationale de médecine, 1969, tome 153, pages 75-77.

GORGAS William C., Sanitation of the tropics with special reference to malaria and yellow fever, The Journal of the American Medical Association, 1909, volume LII, pages 1075-1077.

GOSSELIN rapporteur, commissaires Baron Cloquet, Bouillaud, Sedillot, Vulpian et Marey, Prix Bréant attribué en 1880, Comptes rendus des séances de l'Académie des sciences, tome XCII, 1er semestre, numéro 11, séance du 14 mars 1881a, pages 598-600.

GOSSELIN rapporteur, commissaires Pasteur, Vulpian, Marey et Bouley, Prix Boudet attribué en 1880, Comptes rendus des séances de l'Académie des sciences, tome XCII, 1er semestre, numéro 11, séance du 14 mars 1881b, pages 545-547 et 602-605.

GOSSELIN M., Note, Comptes rendus des séances de l'Académie des sciences, 1885, tome CI, page 227.

GOULD's MEDICAL DICTIONARY, edited by C.V. Brownlow, The Blakiston Company, Philadelphia, 1941, 1528 pages.

GRADLE Dr.H., Bacteria and the germ theory of disease, W.T. Keener, Chicago, 1883, 219 pages.

GRAINGER Thomas H. Jr, A guide to the history of bacteriology, The Ronald Press Company, New York, 1958, 210 pages.

GRANCHER M., La rage et sa prophylaxie, Revue scientifique (revue rose), 1886, tome XXXVIII de la collection, 3e série, tome XII, pages 33-39.

GRANCHER J. et MARTIN H., Tuberculose expérimentale. Sur un mode de traitement et de vaccination, Comptes rendus des séances de l'Académie des sciences, séance du 18 août 1890, tome CXI, pages 333-336.

GRANCHER M., Histoire des sciences, M. Pasteur et la médecine contemporaine, La Revue scientifique (revue rose), tome LII, numéro 22 du 25 novembre 1893, pages 673-685.

GRASSI, GUERIN, ARCHBOLD et CAPELLE, Rapport sur la vaccine, de Pinard, Bordeaux, an X (1801), 42 pages.

GREENSFELDER Liese, Poliomyelitis Outbreak Raises Questions About Vaccine, Science, 2000, volume 290, pages 1867-1869.

GREGORY George, Cursory remarks on smallpox, as it occurs subsequent to vacination, The Medico-Chirurgical Review and Journal of medical science, 1823-4, volume IV, pages 806-811.

GRELLET Isabelle & KRUSE Caroline, Histoires de la tuberculose Les fièvres de l'âme 1800 – 1940, Editions Ramsay, Paris, 1983, 333 pages.

GRODIN M., Historical origins of the Nuremberg Code in "The Nazi doctors and the Nuremberg code. Human Rights in Human Experimentation", edited by Geroge J. Armas and Michael A. Grodin, Oxford University Press, New York, 1992, pages 121-144.

GUERIN M., Suite de la discussion sur la fièvre jaune, Bulletin de L'Académie nationale de médecine, 1862-1863, tome XXVIII, séance du 30 juin 1863, pages 834-864.

GUERSANT et BLACHE, Vaccine in Dictionnaire de médecine ou Répertoire général des sciences médicales, Labé, 1846, 2e édition, tome 30, pages 393-437.

GUILLAUME Pierre, Du désespoir au salut: les tuberculeux aux XIXe et XXe siècles, Aubier, Paris, 1986, 376 pages.

GUIPON J.-J., De la maladie charbonneuse de l'homme, causes, variétés, diagnostic, traitement, ouvrage appuyé sur une enquête médico-administrative concernant la maladie observée chez l'homme et chez les animaux et comprenant huit départements avec cartes et pièces justificatives, J.-B. Baillière et fils, Paris, 1867, 343 pages.

GUIOT M., Mémoire historique sur l'inoculation de la petite vérole, pratiquée à Genève depuis le mois d'octobre 1750, jusqu'au mois de novembre 1752 inclusivement, Mémoires de l'Académie Royale de chirurgie, 1819, tome second, 36e mémoire, pages 387-394.

HAAGEN E. and THEILER M., Studies of yellow fever virus in tissue culture, Proceeding Society Experimental Biology and Medicine, 1932, volume 29, pages 435-436.

HACKS Charles Dr, La guérison de la tuberculose, L'Illustration, numéro 2490 du 15 novembre 1890, pages 415-417. *A summary of this article is reprinted in* : Le docteur Koch et la guérison de la phthisie, La petite revue, 1890, 3e année, 2e semestre, numéro 93, pages 316-318.

HAFFKINE W.-M., Inoculations de vaccins anticholériques à l'homme, Comptes rendus de la Société de biologie, 1892, volume 44, pages 740-741.

HAFFKINE M., Injections against cholera. A lecture, The Lancet, 11 février 1893, pages 316-318.

HAFFKINE W.M., A lecture on inoculation against cholera in India, delivered at the Examination hall, Victoria embankment, on December 18th, 1895, The Lancet, December 21, 1895a, pages 1555-1556.

HAFFKINE W.M., A lecture on vaccination against cholera delivered in the Examination hall of the conjoint board of the Royal College of Physicians of London and Surgeons of England, December, 18th, 1895, The British medical Journal, December 21,1895b, volume II, pages 1541-1544.

HAFFKINE W.M., Remarks on the plague prophylactic fluid, The British Medical Journal, 1897, june 12, pages 1461-1462.

HAIBE A. Dr, La fièvre typhoïde et la vaccination antityphoïdique, Revue des questions scientifiques, 1914, tome LXXVI de la collection, pages 79-95.

HALFORD Henry President, Copy of the Report to the Secretary of State for the Home Department, from the National Vaccine Establishment, dated 12th April 1821, 3 pages.

HALFORD Henry President of the Royal College of Physicians, National Vaccine Establishment, Copies of Reports from the National Vaccine Board to the Right honourable Robert Peel, ordered, by the House of Commons, to be printed, 26 March 1823.

HALFORD Henry President of the Royal College of Physicians, National Vaccine Establishment, A Copy of the last Report of the Vaccine Board to the Secretary of State for the Home Department, dated March 18, 1824, 2 pages.

HALLE rapporteur, BERTHOLLET, PERCY MM., Exposition des faits recueillis jusqu'à présent concernant les effets de la vaccination, et examen des objections qu'on a faites en différens (sic) temps, et que quelques personnes font encore contre cette pratique, Rapport approuvé par la Classe des sciences physiques et mathématiques, le 7 septembre 1812, Institut impérial de France, de l'imprimerie de Firmin Didot, à Paris, 1812, 55 pages.

HALSBAND, New light on Lady Mary Wortley Montagu's contribution to inoculation, Journal of the history of medicine and allied sciences, 1953, volume VIII, pages 390-405.

HAMBURGER Jean, Monsieur Littré, Flammarion, Paris, 1988, 307 pages.

HANNOUN Claude, Les maladies infectieuses in Pasteur, cahiers d'un savant, coordonné par Françoise Balibar et Marie-Laure Prévost, CNRS éditions et Zulma éditions, Paris, 1995, pages 156-180.

HANNOUN Claude, La vaccination, Collection "Que sais-je?", Presses universitaires de France, Paris, 1999, 127 pages.

HANSEN Willy et FRENEY Jean, Des bactéries et des hommes, Editions Privat, 2002, 142 pages.

HARE Ronald, Pomp and Pestilence – Infectious disease, its origins and conquest, Victor Gollancz Ltd, London, 1954, 224 pages.

HAVELBURG Dr. W., The bacteriology of the yellow fever, The British Medical Journal, 1897a, July 31, pages 294-295.

HAVELBURG Dr. W., Recherches expérimentales et anatomiques sur la fièvre jaune, Annales de l'Institut Pasteur, 1897b, tome 11, pages 515-522.

HAWKRIDGE Tony and MAHOMED Hassan, Prospects for a new, safer and more effective TB vaccine, Paediatric Respiratory Reviews, 2011, volume 12, pages 46-51.

HAYDN'S Dictionary of popular medicine and hygiene, edited by Edwin Lankester, E. Moxon, son & co., London, 1874, 646 pages.

HAYGARTH M., Recherches sur les moyens de prévenir la petite-vérole naturelle et Procédés d'une société établie à Chester pour cet objet; & pour rendre l'inoculation générale, traduits de l'Anglois par M. de la Roche, chez Buisson, à Paris, 1786, 216 pages.

HEDIN Fr. Report of the State of Vaccination in Sweden, 10th February 1814, 3 pages.

HENRIJEAN F. Dr, *numerous footnotes signed "?" for "translator"*, in FLÜGGE C. Dr, Les microorganismes étudiés spécialement au point de vue de l'étiologie des maladies infectieuses, traduit de l'allemand d'après la seconde édition par le Dr F. Henrijean, A. Manceaux libraire-éditeur, Bruxelles, 1887, 644 pages.

HERICOURT J. et RICHET Ch., De la transfusion péritonéale, et de l'immunité qu'elle confère, Comptes rendus des séances de 1' Académie des sciences, 1888, tome CVII, pages 748-750.

HERTER Christian Archibald, The influence of Pasteur on medical science, An address delivered before the medical school of Johns Hopkins University, Dodd, Mead & Company, New-York, 1904, 77 pages.

HERVIEUX M., Introduction de la vaccine en France, Bulletin de

l'Académie de médecine, 61e année, 3e série, tome XXX-VII, séance du 16 février 1897, pages 180-187.

HEYMAN Michel, Emile Duclaux et l'affaire Dreyfus, Revue de la Haute-Auvergne, 1992, tome 54, pages 198-210.

HINDLE Edward, A yellow fever vaccine, The British Medical Journal, June 9, 1928, pages 976-977.

HINDLE Edward, An experimental study of yellow fever, Transactions of the Royal Society of Tropical Medicine and Hygiene, 1929, volume XXII, pages 405-484.

HILLEMAN M.R., BUYNAK E.B., WEIBEL R.E., STOKES J., WHITMAN J.E. and LEAGUS M.B., Development and evaluation of the Moraten measles virus vaccine, J.A.M.A., 1968, volume 206, pages 587-590.

HILLEMAN Maurice R., DNA Vectors: Precedents and Safety, in DNA Vaccines A New Era in Vaccinology, Editors Margaret A. Liu, Maurice R. Hilleman, Reinhard Kurt, Annals of the New York Academy of Science, 1995, volume 772, pages 1-14.

HOBLYN Richard D., A dictionary of terms used in medicine, revised by John A. P. Price, thirteenth edition, Whittaker & Co, London, 1899, 838 pages.

HOFT D.F., Tuberculosis vaccine development: goals, immunological design, and evaluation, Lancet, 2008, volume 372, pages 164-175.

HOIN M., De dix-sept personnes mordues par un loup enragé, et Précis des effets du mercure dans la rage, Journal de médecine, chirurgie, pharmacie, &c, 1761, tome XV, pages 99-129.

HOME Francis, Medical facts and experiments, On the measles as they appeared 1758 at Edinburgh, and their inoculation, printed for A. Millar in the Strand and A. Kincaid and J. Bell, at Edinburgh, London, 1759, pages 253-288.

HONORE F., La vaccination contre la tuberculose, L'Illustration, numéro 4244 du 5 juillet 1924, page 16.

HONORE F., La vaccination antituberculeuse, L'Illustration, numéro 4389 du 16 avril 1927, pages 383-384.

HOOPER Robert, A new medical dictionary, E. & R. Parker, M. Carey & son, and Benjamin Warner, Philadelphia, 1817, 870 pages.

HOPKINS Donald R., Princes and pasants. Smallpox in history, The University of Chicago Press, 1983, 380 pages.

HORIOT Louis Joseph, "Louis Pasteur, le berger Jupille", conférence publique faite, à la mairie de Villers-Farlay, le 27 décembre 1922 à 19 heures trente, édité par l'ADAVAL (Association de Développement et d'Aménagement du Val d'Amour), Pouillard Communication, Dole, 1995, 98 pages.

HOSTY ou HOSTI M., Extrait du rapport de M. Hosty, Docteur-Régent de la Faculté de Médecine de Paris, pendant son séjour à Londres, au sujet de l'inoculation, Journal de Médecine, Chirurgie et Pharmacie, tome III, 2e édition, octobre 1755, pages 274-285 et novembre 1755, pages 337-344.

HOWARD Jean, Histoire des principaux lazarets de l'Europe, traduit par Théodore-Pierre Bertin, T.-P. Bertin, Paris, an IX (1801), 181 pages.

HUFELAND Chrétien-Guillaume, Enchiridion medicum ou manuel de médecine pratique fruit d'une expérience de cinquante ans, traduit de l'allemand sur la 4e édition par A.-J.-L. Jourdan, Librairie médicale et scientifique de P. Lucas, Strasbourg, 1841, 813 pages.

HURTREL D'ARBOVAL L.H.J., Dictionnaire de Médecine et de Chirurgie Vétérinaires, chez J-B. Baillière, Paris, 1826-1828, 1re édition, 4 volumes – Dictionnaire de Médecine, de Chirurgie et d'Hygiène Vétérinaires, 1838-1839, 2e édition, chez J-B. Baillière, Paris, 6 volumes.

HURTREL D'ARBOVAL L.H.J. et ZUNDEL A., Clavelisation, in Dictionnaire de Médecine, de Chirurgie et d'Hygiène vétérinaires, J. B. Baillières et fils, 1874-1877, 3 tomes.

HUSSON M., Recherches historiques et médicales sur la vaccine, 1800 (ou 1801), 130 pages.

HUSSON, secrétaire, Note adressée aux médecins, le 4 frimaire de l'an 11 (25 novembre 1802), Comité central de vaccine, 6 pages [BANM, n° 39 612 E(3)].

HUSSON M., Recherches historiques et médicales sur la vaccine ou traité complet sur l'origine, l'histoire, les variétés, les avantages et la pratique de cette nouvelle inoculation, Chez Gabon et Cie, Paris, 3e édition, an XI – 1803a, 396 pages.

HUSSON, secrétaire du Comité central de vaccine, établi à Paris par la Société des souscripteurs pour l'examen de cette découverte, Rapport, Chez Mme Veuve Richard, à Paris, An XI– 1803b, 460 pages.

HUSSON M. secrétaire, Rapport de la séance générale de la société centrale établie pour l'extinction de la petite vérole en France, par la propagation de la vaccine, tenue le 24 frimaire an 13 (15 décembre 1804), de l'imprimerie impériale, à Paris, ventôse an XIII (février-mars 1805), 63 pages.

HUSSON M., Rapport du secrétaire du Comité et de la Société centrale de vaccine de la séance générale de la société centrale, tenue le 12 juin 1806, de l'imprimerie impériale, à Paris, octobre 1806, 130 pages.

HUSSON M. secrétaire, Rapport sur les vaccinations pratiquées en France en 1806 et 1807, de l'imprimerie impériale, à Paris, 1809, 155 pages.

HUSSON M. secrétaire, Rapport du Comité central de vaccine établi à Paris sur les vaccinations pratiquées en France,

... pour les années 1808 & 1809, de l'imprimerie impériale, à Paris, 1811, 143 pages.

... pour l'année 1810, de l'imprimerie royale, à Paris, 1812, 143 pages.

... pour l'année 1812, de l'imprimerie royale, à Paris, 1814, 115 pages.

HUSSON, article Cowpox, in Dictionnaire des sciences médicales, C.L.F. Panckoucke, Paris, 1813, tome 7, pages 239-245.

HUSSON M. secrétaire, Rapport du comité central de vaccine sur les vaccinations pratiquées en France pendant les années 1816, de l'imprimerie royale, à Paris, 1818, 108 pages.

HUSSON M. secrétaire, Rapport du Comité central de vaccine établi à Paris sur les vaccinations pratiquées en France, pour l'année 1817, de l'imprimerie royale, à Paris, 1819, 111 pages.

HUSSON M., article vaccine, in Dictionnaire des sciences médicales, C. L. F. Panckoute, Paris, 1821, tome 56, pages 362-444.

HUSSON J.-B.-E., Rédacteur permanent, De la conviction des vétérinaires belges à propos de l'inoculation de la pleuropneumonie, Annales de médecine vétérinaire, 1857, 6e année, pages 166-167.

HUSSON R.A. et KOERBER R., Le vaccin contre la fièvre jaune préparé par l'Institut Pasteur de Dakar, Annales de l'Institut Pasteur, 1953, tome 95, pages 735-745.

HUTCHEON D., Contagious pleuro-pneumonia in Angora goats, The veterinary journal and Annals of comparative pathology, 1881, volume XIII, pages 171-180.

HUTCHEON D., Contagious pleuro-pneumonia in goats at Cape colony, South Africa, The veterinary journal and Annals of comparative pathology, 1889, volume XXIX, pages 399-404.

HYDE James Nevins, Syphilis in A Reference Handbook of the Medical Sciences, edited by Albert H. Buck, William Wood & Compagny, New-York, 1888, pages 709-736.

IMBS Jean-Louis, DECKER Nicole, WELSCH Marie et le réseau français des centres régionaux de pharmacovigilance, Pharmacovigilance des vaccins contre l'hépatite B, Bulletin de l'Académie nationale de médecine, 2003, volume 187, pages 1489-1500.

ISAAC, Lord Bishop of Worcester, A sermon preached before His Grace Charles Duke of Marlborough, President, the vice-Presidents and Governors of the Hospital for the Small-pox, and for Inoculation, at the St. Andrew Holborn, on Thurday, March 5, 1752, printed by H. Woodfall, London, 1752, 24 pages.

JACCOUD directeur de rédaction, Nouveau dictionnaire de médecine et de chirurgie pratiques, J.-B. Baillières et fils, Paris, 1864-1886, 40 volumes.

JAMES R., A treatise on canine madness, printed for T. Newbury, London, 1760, 254 pages.

JAMES Constantin, La rage, avantages de son traitement par la méthode Pasteur, nécessité de cautérisations préalables, A. Lahure, Paris, 1886, 124 pages.

JAMES S.P. Colonel, Connaissances récemment acquises sur la fièvre jaune, Bulletin de l'Office internationale d'hygiène publique, 1933, tome XXV, pages 46-64.

JAMES S.P., Renseignements sur la fièvre jaune reçus pendant les six mois se terminant au 31 mars 1934, Bulletin de l'Office internationale d'hygiène publique, 1934, tome XXVI, pages 1048-1056.

JARRETT W.F.H., JENNINGS F.W., McINTYRE W.I.M., MULLIGAN W., SHARP N.C.C. and URQUHART G.M., Immunological studies of *Dictyocaulus viviparus* infections in cattle. Double vaccination with irradiated larvae, American Journal of Veterinary Research, 1959, volume 20, pages 522-528.

JEANSELME Ed., Traité de la syphilis, publié sous la direction de..., tome I, Histoire de la syphilis – Etiologie – Expérimentation, G. Doin & Cie, Paris, 1931, 724 pages.

JENNER Edward, Observations on the natural history of the Cuckoo in a letter to J. Hunter, esq., FRS, Philosophical transactions, 1788, volume LXXVII, pages 219-237.

JENNER Edward, An Inquiry into the Causes and Effects of the Variolae Vaccinae, a Disease Discovered in some of the Western Counties of England, particularly Gloucestershire, and know by the Name of the Cow-Pox, printed for the author, London, 1798, 75 pages.

JENNER Edward, Further Observations on the Variolae Vaccinae or Cow-Pox, printed for the author, London, 1799, 64 pages.

JENNER Edward, An Inquiry into the Causes and Effects of the Variolae Vaccinae, a Disease Discovered in some of the Western Counties of England, particularly Gloucestershire, and know by the Name of the Cow-Pox, 1800, 2nd edition, & Further Observations on the Variolae Vaccinae, & A continuation of facts and observations relative to the Variolae vaccinae or cowpox, printed for the author, London, 1800a, 182 pages.

JENNER Edward, Recherches sur les causes et les effets de la variolae vaccinae, maladie découverte dans plusieurs comtés de l'ouest de l'Angleterre, notamment dans le comté de Gloucester, et connue aujourd'hui sous le nom de vérole de vaches, traduit de l'anglais par M. L. C. de L******, Reymann et Ce, Libraires, (1798) 1800b, Lyon, 60 pages.

JENNER Henry, An address to the public on the advantages of vaccine inoculation: with the objections to it refuted, printed and sold by W. Bulgin, London, 1800c, 19 pages, Facsimile edition edited by Akitomo Matsuki and Malcolm F. Beeson and printed by Iwanami Book Service Center, Tokyo, 1998.

JENNER Edward, On the origin of the vaccine inoculation, printed by D.N. Shury, London, 1801, 12 pages. Facsimile edition edited by Akitomo Matsuki and Malcolm F. Beeson and printed by Iwanami Book Service Center, Tokyo, 1998.

JENNER Edward, Œuvres complètes du Docteur Jenner, membre de la Société royale de Londres, &c. sur la découverte de la vaccine, et tout ce qui concerne la pratique de ce nouveau mode d'inoculation, traduit de l'anglais par Jacques-Joseph de Laroque au mois de février 1800, nouvelle édition, revue, corrigée et considérablement augmentée, Imprimerie F. Agard, Privas, 1805 (?), 233 pages.

JENNER Rev. G. C, The evidence at large as laid before the committee of the house of commons respecting Dr. Jenner's discovery of vaccine inoculation; together with the debate which followed; and some observations on the contravening evidence, &c, published by J. Murray, London, 1805, 213 pages, Facsimile edition edited by Akitomo Matsuki and Malcolm F. Beeson and printed by Iwanami Book Service Center, Tokyo, 1998.

JENNEREAN INSTITUTION, The Medical and Physical Journal, 1803, volume IX, pages 192-194.

JESSEN, Inoculation du typhus du bœuf, Annales de médecine vétérinaire, 1859, 8e année, pages 652-653.

JOANNON Pierre, Vaccination antityphoparatyphoidique, L'Année médicale pratique 1941, René Lépine éditeur, Paris, 1941, 20e année, pages 482-485.

JOYEUX Ch. et SICE A., Précis de médecine coloniale, Masson et Cie, Paris, 1937, 2e édition, 1050 pages.

JOYEUX Ch., Précis de médecine coloniale, Masson et Cie, Paris, 3e édition, 1944, 1058 pages.

JOLLIVET Gaston, A M. Pasteur, Le Figaro, numéro 147 du 26 mai 1884, 30e année, 3e série, page de garde.

JONAS Docteur S., 100 portraits de médecins illustres, Masson et Cie, Paris & Academia S.P.R.L., Gand, 1960, 350 pages.

JÖRNVALL Ann-Margreth, The Nobel committee, box 270, SE-171 77 Stockohlm, E-mail du 06 11 2000, *"Dear Prof. Bazin, You sent a question regarding? V Galtier to Dr. Orny which he forwarded to us. The answer is that Pierre Victor Galtier was not nominated for the Nobel Prize in Physiology or Medicine in 1908. Yours sincerely. A. M. J."*

JURIN James, Lettre au D. Caleb Cotesworth, Docteur en Médecine, de la Société Royale de Londres, &c. par M. Jurin, Docteur en Médecine, de la Société Royale de Londres, &c. où l'on fait la comparaison des nombres de ceux qui meurent de la petite Vérole naturelle &c. de l'artificielle ; avec un supplément contenant diverses lettres originales écrites de divers endroits sur l'inoculation (traduite de l'Anglois), Recueil de pièces concernant l'inoculation de la petite vérole et propres à en prouver la sécurité et l'utilité, chez Desaint et Saillant, à Paris, 1722-1723 (1756a), pages 43-79.

JURIN James, Relation du succès de l'Inoculation en Angleterre, avec la comparaison du danger de cette méthode avec celui de la petite Vérole naturelle (traduit de l'Anglois), Recueil de pièces concernant l'inoculation de la petite vérole et propres à en prouver la sécurité et l'utilité, chez Desaint et Saillant, à Paris, 1724 (1756b), pages 80-125.

JURIN James, An account of the success of inoculationg the smallpox for the year 1724 with a comparison between the miscarriages in the practice, and the mortality of the natural small pox, printed for J. Peele, London, 1725, 32 pages.

JURIN Jacques et Scheuzer M., Extrait de trois écrits, dont deux de M. Jurin et l'autre de M. Scheuzer contenant la relation du succès de l'inoculation en Angleterre durant les années 1725, 1726, 1727 & 1728, plus une note de l'éditeur de 1743, Recueil de pièces concernant l'inoculation de la petite vérole et propres à en prouver la sécurité et l'utilité, chez Desaint et Saillant, à Paris, 1732 (1756c), pages126-137.

KAPIKIAN Albert Z., MITCHELdd L., L Reginald H., CHANOCK Robert M., SHVEDOFF Ruth A. and STEWART C. Eleanor, An epidemiologic study of altered clinical reactivity to respiratory syncytial (RS) virus infection in children previously vaccinated with an inactivated RS virus vaccine, American Journal of Epidemiology, 1969, volume 89, pages 405-421.

KATZ S.L., KEMPE C.H., BLACK F.L., LEPOW M.L., KRUGMAN S., HAGGERTY R.J. and ENDERS J.F., Studies on an attenuated measles-virus vaccine, VIII General summary and evaluation of the results of vaccination, The New England Journal of medicine, 1960, volume 263, pages 180-184.

KAUFMAN Martin, GALISHOFF Stuart, SAVITT Todd L. Editors, Dictionary of American biography, Greenwood Press, Westport Connecticut, 1984, 2 volumes.

KAZEEFF W.N., L'immunisation contre la fièvre jaune, L'Illustration, numéro 4769 du 28 juillet 1934, page 421.

KELLY Howard A., Walter Reed and yellow fever, The medical standard book company, Baltimore, 1906, 310 pages.

KENGRAGSAT Sanit, Recherches expérimentales sur les variations de la bactéridie charbonneuse et sur l'immunisation contre le charbon, Thèse pour le doctorat vétérinaire (Diplôme d'Etat) soutenue devant la Faculté de médecine de Paris en 1926, Vigot Frères éditeurs, Paris, 1926, 71 pages.

KENNY J., Procès-verbal de la remise faite par M. le baron Duplantier, Préfet du département du Nord, d'une médaille en or décerné par S. Exe. Le Ministre de l'intérieur, à M. Benjamin Hussey, Quaker du Massachusets, domicilié à Dunkerque, Bulletin sur la vaccine, numéro 17 de mars 1812, pages 14-16.

KERAUDREN, Président, MARC, CHOMEL, DESGENETTES, DUPUYTREN, LOUIS, EMERY, BOISSEAU, DESPORTES, PELLETIER, ITARD, DOUBLE, Rapporteur, Rapport sur le choléra-morbus, lu à l'Académie Royale de médecine, en séance générale, les 26 et 30 juillet 1831, de l'imprimerie royale, Paris, 1831, 199 pages ; translated by John W. Sterling, Report of the Royal Academy of Medicine to the Minister of the interior upon the Cholera-Morbus, Samuel Wood & sons, New-York, 1832, 234 pages.

KESER J., Lettres d'Angleterre, la *Croonian lecture*, La Semaine médicale, 1889, 9e année, pages 182-183.

KEYT Capt. of the 51st regiment, dated Columbo, September 23, 1802, The Medical and Physical Journal, 1803, volume IX, pages 391-392.

KIENY M.-P., LATHE R., DRILLIEN R., SPEHNER S., SKOTY D., SCMITT T., WIKTOR T., KOPROWSKI H., LECOCQ J.-P., Expression of rabies virus glycoprotein from a recombinant vaccinia virus. Nature, 1984, volume 312, pages 163-166.

KILBOURNE Edwin D., A history of Influenza virology, in Microbe Hunters edited by Hilary Koprowsky and Michael B.A. Oldstone, Medi-Ed Press, 1996a, Bloomington, Illinois, pages 187-204.

KILBOURNE Edwin D., A race with evolution – a history of influenza virus, in Vaccinia, vaccination and vaccinology: Jenner, Pasteur and their successors, S. Plotkin, B. Fantini editors, Elsevier, Paris, 1996b, pages 183-188.

KIRKPATRICK D., Extrait du livre: The analysis of inoculation comprizing the history, theory, and practice, of it &c. c'est-à-dire, Analyse de l'Inoculation, contenant son histoire, sa théorie et sa pratique, avec quelques considérations sur les apparences les plus remarquables de la petite vérole, à Londres, 1754, Recueil de pièces concernant l'inoculation de la petite vérole et propres à en prouver la sécurité et l'utilité, chez Dessaint et Saillant, à Paris, 1756, pages 234-270.

KIRKPATRICK Beth D. and ALSTON Kemper W., Current immunizations for travel, Current Opinion on Infectious Diseases, 2003, volume 16, pages 369-374.

KOCH M., La vaccination charbonneuse, La Revue scientifique, 1883a, tome XXXI de la collection, 3e série, tome V, pages 65-74.

KOCH R., L'inoculation préventive du charbon, réplique au discours prononcé à Genève par M. Pasteur, Cassel & Berlin, Chez Théodore Fisher, 1883b, 40 pages.

KOLLE W. et HETSCH H., La bactériologie expérimentale appliquée à l'étude des maladies infectieuses, troisième édition française revue, augmentée et annotée d'après la quatrième édition allemande par H. Carrière, Edition Atar, Genève et Octave Doin et fils, éditeurs, Paris, 1918, 2 tomes.

KOPROWSKI Hilary, JERVIS George A. and NORTON Thomas W., Immune responses in human volunteers upon oral administration of a rodent-adapted strain of poliomyelitis virus, American Journal of Hygiene, 1952, volume 55, pages 108-126.

KOPROWSKI Hilary, Immunization of man against poliomyelitis with attenuated preparations of living virus, in Biology of poliomyelitis, Annals of the New York Academy of sciences, 1955a, volume 61, pages 1039-1049.

KOPROWSKI Hilary, Immunization of man with living poliomyelitis virus, in Poliomyelitis, World Health Organization, Monograph series numéro 26, Geneva, 1955b, pages 335-356.

KOPROWSKI Hilary, Historical aspects of the development of live virus vaccine in poliomyelitis, British medical journal, 1960, volume II, pages 85-91.

KUNTZ P., Les vaccins du charbon, La Nature, 1881, numéro 428 du 13 août 1881, pages 170-171.

LACROIX Frédéric, Le choléra en Sardaigne et en Italie, L'Illustration, numéro 654 du 8 septembre 1855, page 163.

LAGRANGE Emile, Monsieur Roux, AD. Goemaere éditeur, Bruxelles, 1954, 251 pages.

LAIDLAW P.P. and DUNKIN G.W., Studies in dog distemper, V., The immunization of dogs, Journal comparative pathology and therapy, 1928, volume xli, pages 209-227.

LAIGRET J., Recherches expérimentales sur la fièvre jaune (deuxième mémoire), Archives de l'Institut Pasteur de Tunis, 1932, tome XXI, pages 412-430.

LAIGRET J., Recherches expérimentales sur la fièvre jaune (troisième mémoire) ; technique pour la préparation des vaccins amarils, vaccins glycérinés et vaccins secs, Archives de l'Institut Pasteur de Tunis, 1933, tome XXII, pages 198-204.

LAIGRET Jean, Sur la vaccination contre la fièvre jaune par le virus de Max Theiler, 1934a, pages 1593-1594.

LAIGRET Jean, L'organisation de la vaccination contre la fièvre jaune en France, Bulletins de la société de pathologie exotique et de ses filiales, 1934b tome XXVI, pages1078-1082.

LAIGRET J., De l'interprétation des troubles consécutifs aux vaccinations par les virus vivants, en particulier à la vaccination de la fièvre jaune, Bulletins de la société de pathologie exotique et de ses filiales, 1936a, tome XXIX, pages 230-234.

LAIGRET J., Au sujet des réactions nerveuses de la vaccination contre la fièvre jaune, Bulletins de la société de pathologie exotique et de ses filiales, 1936b, tome XXIX, pages 823-828.

LAIGRET J. et BONNEAU E., Longue persistance de l'immunité conférée par la vaccination contre la fièvre jaune, Comptes rendus des séances de l'académie des sciences, 1936c, tome 202, pages 172-175.

LAIGRET Jean, Hommage à Jean Laigret, la petite histoire de la découverte de la vaccination contre la fièvre jaune, conférence donnée à Beyrouth en 1953, La presse médicale, 1966, 5 novembre 1966, pages 2441-2442.

LAIGRET Jean, Résultats de la vaccination contre la fièvre jaune après douze années de pratique, Bulletin de l'Académie de médecine, 1947, tome 131, pages 13-19.

LAMB Captain George and FORSTER Captain W.B.C., On the standardisation of anti-typhoid vaccine, Scientific Memoirs by officers of the medical and sanitary departments of the government of India, Office of the superintendent of government printing, India, Calcutta, 1906, 15 pages.

LANDSTEINER K. & VAN DER SCHEER J. Serological differentiation of steric isomers (antigens containing tartaric acids), Journal of experimental medicine, 1929, volume 50, pages 407-417.

LANE James, On syphilisation (printed from Lancet, January 13, 1866, page 37), the retrospect of pratical medicine and surgery, edited by W. Braithwaite and James Braithwaite, New-York, published by W.A.Townsend, July 1866, volume LIII, pages 171-172.

LAPORTE Dr G., Le vaccin antituberculeux B.C.G., Guérir, numéro 44 du 15 juillet 1934, pages 6 et 12.

LARIVE et FLEURY, Dictionnaire français illustré des mots et des choses ou dictionnaire encyclopédique des écoles, des métiers et de la vie pratique, Georges Chamerot, Imprimeur-Editeur, Paris, 1887-1889, 3 volumes.

LAROUSSE Pierre, Grand dictionnaire universel du XIXe siècle, P. Larousse et Cie, Paris, 1865-1876, 15 volumes plus 2 suppléments 1878 et 1888.

LAROUSSE, Nouveau Larousse illustré, publié sous la direction de Claude Augé, 7 volumes 1897-1904, et 1 supplément 1907.

LAROUSSE, Larousse du XXe siècle, Librairie Larousse, 1928-1930, 6 volumes.

LAROUSSE, Grand dictionnaire encyclopédique, par Auge..., Librairie Larousse, Paris, 1960-1964, 10 volumes, plus 1 supplément, 1969.

LAROUSSE, Grand Larousse en 5 volumes, Librairie Larousse, Paris, 1987-1989.

LARREY Baron, Mémoire sur le Choléra-Morbus, J.-B. Baillière, Paris, 1831, 48 pages.

LARREY M., Discussion du rapport de M. Begin au sujet de la syphilisation, Bulletin de l'Académie nationale de médecine, 16e année, tome XVII, séance du 10 août 1852, pages 967-974.

LATHAM J., Report oft he National Vaccine Establishment for the year 1816, dated 15th May 1817, 6 pages.

LATOUR Dominique, Rapport fait au Citoyen Brun, préfet du département de l'Ariège sur un grand nombre de Vaccinations pratiquées dans l'arrondissement de St Girons, pendant le dernier semestre de l'an onze, chez Guiremand, à Toulouse, an XII (1804), 32 pages [BANM, n° 39 612 E (6)].

LAUMONIER J. Dr, Tuberculine, Larousse mensuel, numéro 170 du mois d'avril 1921, pages 443-444.

LAUMONIER J. Dr, Immunisation contre la tuberculose, Larousse mensuel, numéro 215 du mois de janvier 1925, pages 686-688.

LEAKE J. P., Poliomyelitis following vaccination against this disease, Journal of the American Medical Association, volume 105, december 28, 1935, page 2152.

LECLAINCHE M., Discussion du rapport "Vaccination contre la fièvre aphteuse", séance du 8 septembre (matin), Congrès de Budapest, Compte rendu des travaux du VIIIe Congrès international de médecine vétérinaire, Recueil de médecine vétérinaire publié à l'Ecole d'Alfort, 1905, tome LXXXII, pages 638-640.

LEE Henry, On Syphilis inoculation in 1865 (printed from Lancet, April 14, 1866, page 391), The retrospect of pratical medicine and surgery, edited by W. Braithwaite and James Braithwaite, New-York, published by W.A.Townsend, July 1866a, volume LIII, pages 160-165.

LEE Henry, On the treatment of syphilis (printed from Lancet, April 14, 1866, page 391), The retrospect of pratical medicine and surgery, edited by W. Braithwaite and James Braithwaite, New-York, published by W.A.Townsend, July 1866b, volume LIII, pages 165-171.

LEGER Marcel, Etat actuel de nos connaissances sur l'épidémiologie de la fièvre jaune, Journal de médecine de Bordeaux, 1928, 105e année, pages 970-982.

LEGROUX R., Pasteur et Roux, in Les initiateurs français en pathologie infectieuse, Flammarion, 1942, pages 21-58.

LEMAISTRE Alexis, L'Institut de France et nos grands établissements scientifiques, Collège de France, Muséum, Institut Pasteur, Sorbonne, Observatoire, Librairie Hachette et Cie, Paris, 1896, 336 pages.

LEMERCIER G., GUERIN M. et COLLOMB H., Etude histopathologique de l'encéphalite consécutive à l'inoculation du vaccin antiamaril de l'Institut Pasteur de Dakar, Bulletin de la société médicale d'Afrique noire de langue française, 1966, volume XI, pages 601-609.

L.M. Dr, Le problème de la tuberculose, La vaccination antituberculeuse, Le Cosmos, 1910a, année 59, nouvelle série, tome LXII, 1e semestre, pages 720-721.

L.M. Dr, Les sérums antituberculeux, Le Cosmos, 1910b, année 59, nouvelle série, tome LXII, 2e semestre, pages 12-13.

LE MOIGNIC et PINOY, Les vaccins en émulsion dans les corps gras ou 'lipo-vaccins', Comptes rendus de la Société de biologie, séance du 4 mars 1916, page 201-203.

LEPINE P., Discussion de "Cent cas de vaccination antiamarile (vaccin Laigret) pratiquée à l'Hôpital » Pasteur par R. Martin et AL., Bulletin de la société de pathologie exotique, 1936, tome XXIX, pages 236-238.

LEPINE Pierre, Les vaccinations, Presses universitaires de France, collection "Que sais-je?", Paris, 1975, 128 pages.

LEREBOULLET et JOANNON, Immunisation antidiphtérique de l'enfant par l'anatoxine diphtérique. Allergie et réaction locale, Bulletins et mémoires de la société médicale des hôpitaux de Paris, 1924, 3e série, 40e année, numéro 23, pages 1123-1136.

LESBOUYRIES G., La pathologie des oiseaux, Vigot frères, Paris, 1941, 868 pages.

LETTSOM Docteur, Eloge d'Edouard Jenner, extrait d'un discours prononcé par le docteur Lettsom, en présence de la Société de Médecine de Londres in THORNTON John (docteur), Preuves de l'efficacité de la vaccine, suivies d'une réponse aux objections formées contre la vaccination, contenant l'histoire de cette découverte, etc., traduit par Joseph Duffour, Chomel Imprimeur-Libraire, Paris, 1808, pages 180-214 ou chez Capelle et Renard, à Paris, 1811, 46 pages.

LEUNG Angela Ki-Che, Variolation and vaccination in late Imperial China, ca 1570-1911, in Vaccinia, Vaccination, Vaccinology, Jenner, Pasteur and theirs successors, edited by Stanley A. Plotkin and Bernardino Fantini, Elsevier, Paris, 1996, page 65-71.

LEVADITI C, Virus de la poliomyélite et cultures des cellules *in vitro*, Comptes rendus de la Société de biologie, 1913, volume 75, pages 202-205.

LEVADITI C, KLING C. et HABER P., Est-il possible de vacciner l'homme contre la poliomyélite 1 (séance du 10 mars 1936), Bulletin de l'Académie nationale de médecine, 1936, tome 115, pages 431-440.

LEVADITI C. et LEPINE P., Méthodes de culture, in Les ultravirus des maladies humaines, Librairie Maloine, Paris, 1938, 1182 pages.

LEVADITI C, Précis de virologie médicale, vaccine-variole. Herpès. Encéphalites. Rage..., Masson & Cie, 1945, 250 pages.

LEVIN Myron J., DAHL Karen M., WEINBERG Adriana, GILLER Roger, PATEL Amita and KRAUSE Philip R., Development of Resistance to Acyclovir during Chronic Infection with the Oka Vaccine Strain of Varicella-Zoster Virus, in a immunosuppressed Child, The Journal of infectious diseases, 2003, volume 188, pages 954-959.

LEVY Ofer, ORANGE Jordan S., HIBBERD Patricia, STEINBERG Sharon, LaRUSSA Phillip, WEINBERG Adriana, WILSON S. Brian, SHAULOVAngela, FLEISHER Gary, GEHA Raif S., BONILLA Francisco A. and EXLEY Mark, Disseminated Varicella Infection Due to the Vaccine Strain of Varicella-Zoster Virus, in a Patient with a Novel Deficiency in Natural Killer? Cells, The Journal of infectious diseases, 2003, volume 188, pages 948-953.

L.G., M. Pasteur, L'Illustré pour tous, choix de bonnes lectures, numéro 397 du 20 décembre 1885, page 249.

LISTER Joseph, Remarks on micro-organisms: their relation to disease, Address delivered before the Pathological Section in opening a discussion on the subject at the Annual Meeting of the British Medical Association in Cambridge, August 12th, 1880, The British Medical Journal, september 4, 1880, pages 363-365.

LITTRE E., Œuvres complètes d'Hippocrate, tome 3, Des plaies à la tête, argument, chez J.-B. Baillière, 1841, page 150.

LITTRE E., Dictionnaire de la langue française, Librairie Hachette et Cie, Paris, 1873 & 1879, 4 volumes plus un supplément.

LITTRE Emile et ROBIN Charles, Dictionnaire de médecine, de chirurgie, de pharmacie, des sciences accessoires et de l'art vétérinaire, Librairie J.-B. Baillière et fils, Paris, 1865 (12e édition): 1795 pages, Dictionnaire de médecine, de chirurgie, de pharmacie, de l'art vétérinaire et des sciences qui s'y rapportent, 1873 (13e édition): 1836 pages.

LITTRE Emile, Dictionnaire de médecine, de chirurgie, de pharmacie, de l'art vétérinaire et des sciences qui s'y rapportent, Librairie J.-B. Baillière et fils, Paris, mise à jour reprise par le Dr P. Decaye et des collaborateurs 1884 (15e édition): 1880 pages; 1886 (16e édition): 1876 pages; 1893 (17e édition): 1894 pages; mise à jour reprise par un anonyme et des collaborateurs 1898, (18e édition): 1910 pages; 1902 (19e édition): 1910 pages.

LITTRE E. et GILBERT A., Dictionnaire de médecine, de chirurgie, de pharmacie et des sciences qui s'y rapportent, Librairie J.-B. Baillière et fils, Paris, 1908 (21e édition): 1842 pages.

LLOYD Wray, L'emploi d'un virus cultivé associé à l'antisérum dans la vaccination contre la fièvre jaune, Bulletin de l'office international d'hygiène publique, 1935, tome XXVII, pages 2365-2368.

LLOYD W., THEILER Max and RICCI N.I., Modification of the virulence of yellow fever virus by cultivation in tissues *in vitro*, Transactions of the Royal Society of Tropical Medicine and Hygiene, 1936, volume XXIX, pages 481-502.

LOIR Dr Adrien, L'Institut Pasteur en Australie, La Nature, numéro 997 du 9 juillet 1892, pages 84-87 et numéro 1000 du 30 juillet 1892, pages 134-138.

LOIR A. Dr, Mission au Canada, Compte rendu de la 35e session de l'Association française pour l'avancement des sciences, Lyon, 1906, publié à Paris par le secrétariat de l'association et chez Masson et Cie, 1907, pages 1393-1403.

LOIR Adrien Dr, La question du rat, La Nature, 1930, 1er semestre, pages 551-554.

LOIR Adrien, A l'ombre de Pasteur, le mouvement sanitaire, 1937, 14e année, pages 43-47, 84-93, 135-146, 188-192, 269-282, 328-348, 387-399, 438-445, 487-497, 572-573, 619-621, 659-664, 15e année, pages 179-181, 370-376, 503-508, *these pages are included in a book (with certain minor changes)*: A l'ombre de Pasteur (souvenirs personnels), Le Mouvement sanitaire, Paris, 1938, 171 pages.

LOISEAU G. et LAFFAILLE A., Quelques réflexions sur quinze ans de vaccination antidiphtérique Novembre 1923-Janvier 1939, Le mouvement sanitaire, février 1939, numéro hors série, pages 38-52.

LOPEZ-RIOS Fernando, ILLEI Peter B., RUSCH Valerie and LADANYI Marc, Evidence against a role for SV40 infection in human mesotheliomas and high risk of false-positive PCR results owing to presence of SV40 sequences in common laboratory plasmids, The Lancet, 2004, volume 364, pages 1157-1166.

LÖWY Ilana, Yellow fever in Rio-De-Janeiro and the Pasteur Institute Mission (1901-1905): the transfer of science to the periphery, Medical History, 1990, volume 34, pages 144-163.

LOY John G., An account of some experiments on the origin of the cow-pox, printed by Thomas Webster, Whitby, 1801, reprinted in Crookshank, 1889, tome 2, pages 275-285.

LUCAS-CHAMPIONNIERE Just, Nouvelles recherches de M. Pasteur, Le choléra des poules et sa préservation... Microbes des abcès et de la fièvre puerpérale, choléra des poules et vaccine, Journal de médecine et de chirurgie pratiques, 1880, tome 51, 3e série, art. 11440, pages 243-246.

LUCAS-CHAMPIONNIERE, Vaccination contre la fièvre jaune, Journal de Médecine et de Chirurgie pratiques, 1887, tome 58, 3e série, page 232.

LUCAS-CHAMPIONNIERE, La vie de Pasteur par René Vallery-Radot, Journal de médecine et de chirurgie pratiques, 1901, tome 72, 4e série, pages 401-406.

LUCAS-CHAMPONNIERE, Les méthodes de vaccination anti-typhoïdique. Leur emploi dans l'armée, Journal de médecine et de chirurgie pratiques, 1910, tome 81, 4e série, pages 22-25.

LUCAS-CHAMPIONNIERE, La sérophylaxie diphtérique, Journal de médecine et de chirurgie pratiques, 1914, tome 85, 5e série, pages 215-219.

LUTZKER Edythe and JOCHNOWITZ Carol, Waldemar Haffkine: Pionneer of Cholera Vaccine, American Society for Microbiology News, 1987, volume 53, pages 366-369.

McKIE Robin, Louis Pasteur: Genius, pioneer – and cheat, Historian claims France's greatest scientist was fraud, The Observer magazine, february 14, 1993, page 4.

McLAUGHLIN J.W., Fermentation, Infection and Immunity – a new theory of these processes, Eugene von Boeckmann printer and bookbinder, Austin (Texas), 1892, 240 pages.

MACNAMARA F.N., Reactions following neurotropic yellow fever vaccine given by scarification in Nigeria, Transactions of the Royal Society of Tropical Medicine and Hygiene, 1953, volume 47, pages 199-208.

McSHANE Helen, PATHAN Ansar A., SANDER Clare R., KEATING Sheila M., GILBERT Sarah C, HUYGEN Kris, FLETCHER Helen A. & HILL Adrian V.S., Recombinant modified vaccinia virus Ankara expressing 85A boosts BCG-primed and naturally acquired antimicrobacterial immunity in humans, Nature Medicine, 2004, volume 10, pages 1240-1244.

McVAIL John C, Half a century of small-pox and vaccination being the Milroy lectures delivered before the Royal College of Physicians of London on March 13th, 18th and 20th 1919, E.& S. Livingstone, Edinburgh, 1919, 87 pages.

MADELINE Pierre, La première vaccination antirabique de Pasteur, in L'aventure de la vaccination, sous la direction d'Anne-Marie Moulin, Fayard, 1996, pages 160-167.

MAGNE J.-H. et BAILLET C, Traité d'agriculture pratique et d'hygiène vétérinaire générale, Asselin et Cie et G. Masson, Paris, 1883, 4e édition, tome III, Hygiène vétérinaire générale, 863 pages.

MAILLART Ella, Oasis interdites de Pékin au Cachemire, Editions Bernard Grasset, Paris, 1937, 281 pages.

MAITLAND H.B. and BURBURY Y.M., Further observations on foot and mouth disease section E the part played by serum in immunity to foot and mouth disease, The journal of comparative pathology and therapeutics, 1927, volume xl, pages 93-102.

MAITLAND H.B. and LAING A.W., Experiments on the cultivation of vaccinia virus, British journal of experimental pathology, 1930, volume 11, page 119-126.

MANSON Sir Patrick, Maladies des pays chauds, manuel de pathologie exotique, traduit de l'anglais par Maurice Guibaud, 1re édition, d'après la 2e édition anglaise, 1904, C. Naud, Paris, 776 pages – 2e édition d'après la 4e édition anglaise, Masson et Cie, Paris, 1908, 814 pages.

MANZINI Docteur, Histoire de l'inoculation préventive de la fièvre jaune, analyse du Dr. Onghera, Annales et bulletin de la société de médecine de Gand, 1858, année 24, pages 194-195.

MARCHAL (de Calvi), Vaccine animale, génisses vaccinifères à bord des paquebots de la compagnie transatlantique, Recueil de médecine vétérinaire, 1869, 5e série, tome IV, page 869-871.

MARCHOUX, SALIMBENI et SIMOND, La fièvre jaune Rapport de la mission française, Annales de l'Institut Pasteur, 1903, tome 17, pages 665-731.

MARCHOUX E. et SIMOND P.-L., Etudes sur la fièvre jaune, Deuxième mémoire, Annales de l'Institut Pasteur, 1906, tome 20, pages 16-40.

MARCIGUEY H., Epilepsie et vaccin anti-rabique, Journal des praticiens, 1893, tome VII, page 445.

MARIE Auguste Dr., L'étude expérimentale de la rage, Octave Doin et fils éditeurs, Paris, 1909, 371 pages.

MARRON, Discours prononcé, le 29 septembre 1811, par M. Marron, membre de la Légion d'honneur, et Président du Consistoire de la religion réformée, Comité central de Vaccine, Bulletin sur la vaccine, numéro 12 d'octobre 1811, pages 5-6.

MARTIN Louis, Sur l'immunisation antidipthérique avec l'anatoxine, rapport sur 3 mémoires : 1) De l'immunité antidiphtérique par l'anatoxine diphtérique, recherches cliniques et sérologiques par MM. Darré, G. Loiseau et A. Laffaille ; 2) Résultats obtenus chez l'enfant par MM. Roubenovitch, G. Loiseau et A. Laffaille ; 3) La vaccination antidiphtérique chez l'adulte, par M. Zoeller, Bulletin de l'Académie de médecine, 1924, 88e année, pages 474 and 523-530.

MARTIN René, ROUESSE Gustave et BONNEFOI Antoine, Cent cas de vaccination antiamarile (vaccin Laigret) pratiquée à l'hôpital Pasteur, Bulletins de la société de pathologie exotique et de ses filiales, 1936, tome XXIX, pages 234-238 and 295-313.

MASGANA Michel, de Smyrne, Dissertation sur la rage, présentée et soutenue à la Faculté de médecine de Paris, le 3 avril 1821, pour obtenir le grade de docteur en médecine, Didot le jeune, Paris, 1821, 31 pages.

MASON Patrick, Maladies des pays chauds, traduit de l'anglais par M. Guibaud et J. Brengues, C. Naud, Paris, 1904, pages 170-189.

MASSEY Edmund, A sermon against the dangerous and sinful practice of inoculation, preach'd at St. Andrew's Holborn, on Sunday, July the 8th, 1722, printed for William Meadows, 1722, 30 pages.

MATHIS C., SELLARDS A.W. et LAIGRET J., Sensibilité du *Macacus rhesus* au virus de la fièvre jaune, Comptes rendus des séances de l'académie des sciences, 1928, tome 186, pages 604-606.

MATHIS M., Vaccination antiamarile du singe à l'aide de virus vivant provenant du cobaye mort de la maladie expérimentale, Bulletins de la société de pathologie exotique et de ses filiales, 1934a, tome XXVII, pages 505-510.

MATHIS C., LAIGRET J. et DURIEUX C., Trois mille vaccinations contre la fièvre jaune en Afrique Occidentale Française au moyen du virus vivant de souris, atténué par le vieillissement, Comptes rendus des séances de l'académie des sciences, 1934b, tome 199, pages 742-744.

MATHIS C., DURIEUX C. et MATHIS M., Est-il prudent de se faire vacciner contre la fièvre jaune en Afrique Occidentale Française, Bulletins de la société de pathologie exotique et de ses filiales, 1936, tome XXVII, pages 1042-1046.

MATHIS Constant, Fièvre jaune – virus amaril, in Les ultravirus des maladies humaines, Librairie Maloine, Paris, 1938, pages 747-822.

MATSUKI Akitomo, A brief history of jennerian vaccination in Japan (revised from Medical History 14 :199-201, 1970), Iwanami Book Service Center, 1998, p. 11-20.

MATTHEWS James T., Evolution of the industrial production of inactivated influenza vaccines, in Vaccinia, vaccination and vaccinology: Jenner, Pasteur and their successors, S. Plotkin and B. Fantini editors, Elsevier, Paris, 1996, pages 189-191.

MAUPAS P., COURSAGET P., GOUDEAU A., DRUCKER J., BAGROS P., Immunisation against hepatitis? in man, The Lancet, volume I, june 26, 1976, pages 1367-1370.

MEDECIN, Opinion d'un médecin de la faculté de Paris, sur l'inoculation de la petite vérole, Chez Quillau l'aîné, à Paris, 1768, 24 pages.

MEGLIN docteur, Précis historique de l'établissement de la vaccine dans le département du Haut-Rhin, de l'imprimerie de Decker fils, Colmar, 1811, 144 pages [BANM, n° 39 612 F(2)].

MERIEUX Charles, Le virus de la découverte, avec la collaboration de Louise L. Lambrichs, Editions Robert Laffont, Paris, 1988, 294 pages.

MERIEUX Charles, Avant-propos, in L'aventure de la vaccination, sous la direction d'Anne-Marie Moulin, Fayard, Paris, 1996, pages 7-10.

METCHNIKOFF Elie, L'immunité dans les maladies infectieuses, Masson & Cie, Paris, 1901, 600 pages.

METCHNIKOFF Elie, Trois fondateurs de la médecine moderne, Pasteur-Lister-Koch, Librairie Félix Alcan, 1939, nouvelle édition, Paris, 195 pages ; The Founders of the Modern Medicine – Pasteur, Koch and Lister, translated by D. Berger M.A., Walden publications New-York, 1939, 387 pages.

METSCHNIKOFF (sic) Elie, Sur la lutte des cellules de l'organisme contre l'invasion des microbes, Annales de l'Institut Pasteur, 1887, volume I, pages 321-326.

MEUNIER Stanislas, Comptes-rendus de la séance du 26 octobre 1885 de l'Académie des sciences, La Nature, 1885, 2e semestre, 13e année, pages 351-352.

MEZERETTE Jean, Au Maroc premier barrage à la poliomyélite, Paris Match, numéro 216 du 2 au 9 mai 1953, pages 34-35.

MILBANK Jeremiah, organized by..., Poliomyelitis. A survey made possible by a grant from the International Committee for the study of infantile paralysis, The Williams & Wilkins Company, Baltimore, 1932, 562 pages.

MILLER Geneviève, The adoption of inoculation for small-pox in England and France, University of Pennsylvania Press, Philadelphia, 1957, 355 pages.

MILMAN fr. President, Report of the National Vaccine Establishment, dated 22 April 1813, 13 pages.

MILTON, A collection of papers relative to the transactions of the town of

Milton, in the state of Massachusetts, to promote a general inoculation of the cow pox or kine pox, as a never failing preventive against small pox infection, Boston, 1809, 48 pages.

MOIZARD, Les injections préventives de sérum antidiphtérique, Journal de médecine et de chirurgie, 1901, tome 72, 4e série, pages 568-575.

MOLLARET P. avec la collaboration de G.M. FINDLAY, Etude étiologique et microbiologique d'un cas de méningo-encéphalite au cours de la séro-vaccination anti-amarile, Bulletins de la société de pathologie exotique et de ses filiales, 1936a, tome XXIX, pages 176-185.

MOLLARET P., Discussion of "Cent cas de vaccination antiamarile (vaccin Laigret) pratiquée à l'Hôpital Pasteur » par R. Martin *et al.*, Bulletin de la société de pathologie exotique, 1936b, tome XXIX, pages 234-236.

MOLLARET Henri H. et BROSSOLLET Jacqueline, Alexandre Yersin ou le vainqueur de la peste, Fayard, 1985, 320 pages reédité en Alexandre Yersin 1863-1943, un pastorien en Indochine, Belin, Paris, 1993, 379 pages.

MONATH Thomas P., Yellow fever vaccines: the success of empicism, pitfalls of application, and transition to molecular vaccinology, in Vaccinia, vaccination, vaccinology – Jenner, Pasteur and their successors, edited by A. Plotkin, Bernardino Fantini, Elsevier, Paris, 1996, pages 157-182.

MONATH Thomas P., Milestones in the conquest of yellow fever in Microbe hunters – then and now, edited by Hilary Koprowski and Michael B.A. Oldstone, Medi-ed Press, Blomington ill., 1996, pages 95-111.

MONATH Thomas P., Yellow fever, in Vaccines edited by Stanley A. Plotkin and Walter A. Orenstein, W.B. Saunders Company, 1999, 3rd edition, Philadelphia, pages 815-879.

MONATH Thomas P., CETRON Martin S., TEUWEN Dirk E., Yellow fever vaccine, in Vaccines edited by Stanley Plotkin, Walter Orenstein and Paul Offit, Saunders Elsevier, Fifth edition, 2008, pages 959-1055.

MONATH Thomas P., Yellow Fever in Vaccines, a biography, Andrew W. Artenstein editor, Springer, New York, 2010, pages 159-189.

MONESTIER Emile, Russes de Beloï au laboratoire de M. Pasteur rue d'Ulm, Le Monde illustré, 30e année, numéro 1513 du 27 mars 1886, pages 198-199 et 201.

MONTAGU. Lady M---y W----y M-----e, Letters written during his travels in Europe, Asia and Africa, printed for T. Becket and P.A. De Hondt, London, 1763, 3 volumes and another print: Letters of Lady Mary Wortley Montague, printed by P. Didot the elder, Paris, 1800, 320 pages.

MONTAGU (LADY MARY WORTLEY MONTAGU), L'Islam au péril des femmes, Une Anglaise en Turquie au XVIIIe siècle, Introduction, traduction et notes d'Anne Marie Moulin et Pierre Chuvin, LD/Découverte, Paris, 1991, 254 pages.

MONTEILS E. Dr, Histoire de la vaccination Recherches historiques et critiques sur les divers moyens de prophylaxie thérapeutique employés contre la variole depuis l'origine de celle-ci jusqu'à nos jours, C. Coulet libraire-éditeur à Montpellier et Adrien Delahaye libraire-éditeur à Paris, 1874, 422 pages.

MONTEIRO J. Lemos, Nouvelle technique pour la préparation du vaccin contre la fièvre jaune, Comptes rendus des séances de la société de biologie, 1930, tome 104, pages 695-697.

MOORE James, The history of the small pox, printed for Longman, Hurst, Rees, Orme and Brown, London, 1815, 312 pages.

MOORE James, The history and practice of vaccination, printed for J. Callow, London, 1817, 300 pages.

MOREAU rapporteur, Rapport présenté à son excellence le Ministre de l'intérieur par l'Académie royale de médecine sur les vaccinations pratiquées en France pendant l'année 1823, de l'imprimerie royale, Paris, juillet 1824, 55 pages.

MOREAU Richard, Préhistoire de Pasteur, L'Harmattan, Paris, 2000, 487 pages.

MOREAU Richard, Louis Pasteur: de Besançon à Paris (L'envol), L'Harmattan, Paris, 2003, 283 pages.

MORANGE Michel, sous la direction de..., L'Institut Pasteur – Contributions à son histoire, La Découverte, 1991, 321 pages.

MORREY Charles Bradfield, The fundamentals of bacteriology, Lea and Febiger, Philadelphia & New-York, 1921, 320 pages.

MOUSSU G. Les maladies du mouton, Vigot Frères, Paris, 1923, 332 pages.

MOWAT G.N. and CHAPMAN W.G., Growth of foot-and-mouth disease virus in a fibroblastic cell line derived from hamster kidneys, Nature, 1962, volume 194, pages 253-255.

MOYNAC Léon Dr, Rage chez l'homme in Dictionnaire populaire de médecine usuelle d'hygiène publique et privée par le docteur Paul Labarthe, C. Marpon et E. Flammarion, éditeurs, Paris, 1887-1888, volume 2, pages 849-851.

M.R., Polio: A Lyon, un congrès sur le vaccin vivant laisse prévoir des résultats décisifs, Réalités, numéro 190 de novembre 1961, pages 141-144.

MUNARET Docteur, Iconautographie de Jenner, Germer-Baillière, Paris, 1860, 69 pages.

NATIONAL VACCINE ESTABLISHMENT, Reports from the...1810, 1812, 1816, 1820, 1821, 1822, 1823 et 1824, ordered by the House of Commons to be printed 1st june 1810-17 February 1825.

NETTER, Lutte contre les maladies infectieuses, in Traité de pathologie générale publié par Ch. Bouchard, Masson et Cie, Paris, 1903, tome VI, pages 764-781.

NEUMANN L.-G., Biographies vétérinaires, Asselin et Houzeau, Paris, 1896, 443 pages.

NEWMAN George Sir, The rise of preventive medicine, Oxford University Press, Oxford, 1932, 270 pages.

NEWSHOLME Sir Arthur, Evolution of preventive medicine, The Williams & Wilkins Company, Baltimore, 1927, 226 pages.

NICATI et RIETSCH MM., Atténuation du virus cholérique, Comptes rendus des séances de l'Académie des sciences, 1885, tome CI, pages 186-187.

NICATI W. et RIETSCH M., Recherches sur le choléra, Félix Alcan éditeur, Paris, 1886, 172 pages.

NICHOLAS J.S., Ross Granville Harrison 1870-1959, Biographical memoir, National Academy of sciences, Washington D.C., 1961, pages 130-162.

NICOL Louis, L'épopée pastorienne et la médecine vétérinaire, chez l'auteur, Garches, 1974, 621 pages.

NICOLLE Charles, Biologie de l'invention, Félix Alcan, Paris, 1932, 160 pages.

NICOLLE Charles, Destin des maladies infectieuses, Félix Alcan, Paris, 1933, 301 pages.

NICOLLE Charles et LAIGRET J., La vaccination contre la fièvre jaune par le virus amaril vivant, desséché et enrobé, Comptes rendus des séances de l'Académie des sciences, 1935, tome 201, pages 312-314.

NICOLLE Charles et LAIGRET J., Vaccination contre la fièvre jaune à l'aide d'une seule inoculation d'un virus amaril vivant, desséché et enrobé, Archives de l'Institut Pasteur de Tunis, 1936, tome XXV, pages 28-39.

NOCARD et ROUX, Expériences sur la vaccination des ruminants contre la rage, par injections intra-veineuses de virus rabique, Annales de l'Institut Pasteur, 1888, 2e année, pages 341-353.

NOCARD, Cours de maladies contagieuses, notes prises par les élèves Alglave et Guérin, année 1891-1892, Ecole vétérinaire d'Alfort, Imprimerie Blanc Pascal, Paris, 1892, 517 pages.

NOCARD Ed. et LECLAINCHE E., Les maladies microbiennes des animaux, G. Masson, Paris, 1896, 816 pages.

NOCARD et ROUX avec la collaboration de MM. Borel, Salimbeni et Dujardin-Beaumetz, Le microbe de la péripneumonie, Annales de l'Institut Pasteur, 1898, tome 12, pages 240-262.

NOGUCHI Hideyo, Prophylaxis and serum therapy of yellow fever, Journal American Medical Association, 1921, volume 77, pages 181-185.

NORMAN Jeremy M. edited by... Morton's Medical Bibliography, An Annoted Check-list of Texts Illustrating the History of Medicine (Garisson and Morton), Scolar Press, Aldershot (England), Fifth edition, 1991, 1243 pages.

NORRBY Erling, Yellow fever and Max Theiler: the only Nobel Prize for a virus vaccine, Journal of experimental Medicine, volume 204, pages 2779-2784.

NUTTALL George H.F., On the role of insects, arachnids, and myriapods as carriers in the spread of bacterial and parasitic diseases of man and animals – A critical and historical study, John Hopkins Hospital Reports, 1899, volume VIII, pages 1-154.

NYSTEN P.-H., LITTRE E. et ROBIN Ch., Dictionnaire de médecine, de chirurgie, de pharmacie, des sciences accessoires, et de l'art vétérinaire, chez J.-B. Baillière, Paris, 1855 (10e édition): 1485pages; 1858 (11e édition): 1671 pages.

OAKLEY C.L., A.T. Glenny, Nature, 1966, volume 211, page 1130.

O'BRIEN R.A., EAGLETON A.J., OKELL C.C. and Miss M. BAXTER, The Schick test and active immunisation, British Journal to Experimental Pathology, 1923, volume 4, pages 29-33.

ODIER L., Mémoire sur l'inoculation de la vaccine à Genève, de l'imprimerie de la Bibliothèque britannique, à Genève, an IX (1800), 30 pages [BANM, 33 634 (2)].

OLITSKY Peter K. and COX Herald R., Experiments on active immunization against experimental poliomyelitis, Journal of experimental medicine, 1936, volume 63, pages 109-125.

ONGHENA Dr, Histoire de l'inoculation préservatrice de la fièvre jaune, par le docteur Manzini, Annales et bulletin de la Société de médecine de Gand, juillet et août 1858, 24e année, pages 194-195.

OSLER William, Introduction to The life of Pasteur, written by René Vallery-Radot, translated from the French by Mrs R. L. Devonshire, Garden City Publishing Co., Inc., New-York, undated, 484 pages.

OSLER Sir William, Modern medicine Its theory and practice, edited by William Osler assisted by Thomas McCrae, Lea Brothers & Co., Philadelphia and New-York, 1907-1910, 10 volumes.

OSLER Sir William revised by Christian Henry A. and McCRAE Thomas, The principles and practice of Medicine, D. Appleton-Century Company Inc., New-York & London, 1938, 13e edition, 1424 pages.

OWEN Mr., Yellow fever – A compilation of various publications. Results of the work of Maj. Walter Reed, Medical corps, United States Army, and the yellow fever commission. 61st Congress Document 822, Government printing office, Washington, 1911, 250 pages.

P.A., Comment Pasteur essaya la vaccination contre la rage, Almanach du pèlerin, 1936, page 69.

PAGET James, chairman, M. Pasteur's methods of preventive inoculation (1887), in Œuvres de Pasteur, volume VI, pages 882-883.

PAGET Stephen, Pasteur and after Pasteur, Adam and Charles Black, London, 1914, 152 pages.

PANISSET L., Traité des maladies infectieuses des animaux domestiques, Vigot frères, Paris, 1938, 562 pages.

PANTHIER René, A propos de quelques cas de réactions nerveuses tardives observées chez des nourrissons après vaccinations antiamarile (17D), Bulletin de la société de pathologie exotique, 1956, tome XLIX, pages 477-494.

PANTHIER René, Présentation d'appareils utilisés pour la préparation du vaccin antiamaril (souche 17D de la Fondation Rockefeller), Bulletin de la société de pathologie exotique, 1956, tome XLIX, pages 616-620.

PARFAIT M., Réflexions historiques et critiques sur les dangers de la variole naturelle; sur les différents modes de traitements; sur les avantages de l'inoculation et les succès de la vaccine, pour l'extinction de la variole, chez l'auteur, à Paris, an XIII (1804), 80 pages.

PARISH HJ., Antisera, Toxoids, Vaccines and Tuberculins in Prophylaxis and Treatment, E. & S. Livingstone Ltd, 1954, 3rd edition, 227 pages.

PARISH H. J., A history of immunization, E.&S. Livingstone Ltd, Edinburg and London, 1965, 356 pages.

PARK William H., Toxin-antitoxin immunization against diphteria, Journal of the American Medical Association, 1922, volume 79, pages 1584-1590.

PARK William Hallock, Duration of immunity against diphteria achieved by various methods, Journal of the American Medical Association, 1937, Volume 109, pages 1681-1684.

PARODI Georges, L'œuvre pastorienne et les vétérinaires, thèse de doctorat vétérinaire soutenue devant la Faculté de médecine de Paris, Imprimerie R. Foulon, Paris, 1941, 71 pages.

PARR Bartholomew, London Medical Dictionary, published by Mitchell, Ames and White, Philadelphia, 1819, 2 volumes.

PASTEUR M., Sur les maladies virulentes, et en particulier sur la maladie appelée vulgairement "choléra des poules", Recueil de médecine vétérinaire, 1880, 6e série, tome VI, pages 125-135 et pages 204-206 et Pasteur O.C., tome VI, pages 287-303 (*which, mistakenly, indicates tome VII instead of tome VI for the Recueil de médecine vététérinaire*).

PASTEUR M., Réponse au docteur Koch par M. Pasteur, La Revue scientifique, 1883, tome XXXI de la collection, 3e série, tome V, pages 74-84.

PASTEUR L., Thérapeutique, la rage, La Science illustrée, 1890, tome 6, pages 166-167, 178-179, 195-197 et 211-213.

PASTEUR, Œuvres de... (O.C.) réunies par Pasteur Vallery-Radot, Masson et Cie éditeurs, Paris, 1922-1939, 7 tomes.

PASTEUR, Correspondance, réunie et annotée par Pasteur Vallery-Radot, Flammarion, 1940-1951, 4 tomes.

PASTEUR VALLERY-RADOT, Discours. Jubilé de Jules Bordet, Annales de l'Institut Pasteur, 1950, tome 79, pages 499-506.

PASTEUR VALLERY-RADOT, Préface du catalogue de l'exposition Pasteur, à l'occasion de la donation du professeur Pasteur Vallery-Radot et de madame, à la Bibliothèque nationale, inaugurée le 4 novembre 1964, Paris, 1964.

PASTEUR VALLERY-RADOT, Pages illustres de Pasteur, rassemblées et présentées par... (avec des documents inédits), Hachette, Paris, 1968, 381 pages.

PASTORET P.-P., BLANCOU J., VANNIER P., VERSCHUEREN C, Veterinary Vaccinology, Elsevier, 1997, Amsterdam, 853 pages.

PASTORET P.P., YAMANOUCHI K., MUELLER-DOBLIES U., RWEYEMAMU M.M., HORZINEK M. and BARRETT T., Rinderpest– an old and worldwide story: history to c.1902, in Rinderpest and Peste des petits ruminants Virus plague of large and small ruminants, edited by T. Barrett, P.P. Pastoret & W. Taylor, Elsevier, Amsterdam, 2006, pages 86-104.

PAUL John R., A history of poliomyelitis, Yale University Press, New-Haven and London, 1971, 486 pages.

PAULET J. J., Histoire de la petite vérole avec les moyens d'en préserver les enfans et d'en arrêter la contagion en France, (en 2 tomes) suivie d'une Traduction Française du traité de la petite vérole de Rhasès, sur la dernière Edition de Londres, Arabe et Latine, chez Ganeau, 1768, 2 volumes.

PAYET M., SANKALE M., BOURGEADE A., SOW A.-M. et J.-P. ANCELLE, Les méningo-encéphalites après vaccination antiamarile. Formes observées chez l'adulte (à propos de 7 cas), Bulletin de la société médicale d'Afrique noire de langue française, 1966, volume XI, pages 597-600.

PELLARIN M., Demande d'une instruction sur les précautions à prendre dans la vaccination contre les risques de transmission d'un autre virus, Bulletin de l'Académie impériale de médecine, 1865, tome XXX, pages 505-510.

PELTIER M., DURIEUX C., JONCHERE H. et E. ARQUIE, Pénétration du virus amaril neurotrope par voie cutanée. Vaccination mixte contre la fièvre jaune et la variole, Bulletin de l'académie de médecine, 1939, tome 121, pages 657-660.

PELTIER M., DURIEUX C., JONCHERE H. et E. ARQUIE, Vaccination mixte contre la fièvre jaune et la variole sur des populations indigènes du Sénégal, Bulletin de l'académie de médecine, 1940a, tome 123, pages 137-147.

PELTIER M., DURIEUX C., JONCHERE H. et E. ARQUIE, Vaccination mixte contre la fièvre jaune et la variole sur des populations indigènes du Sénégal, Annales de l'Institut Pasteur, 1940b, tome 65, pages 146-169.

PELTIER Maurice Médecin-Général, Yellow fever vaccination, simple or associated with vaccination against smallpox, of the populations of French West Africa by the method of the Pasteur Institut of Dakar, American Journal of Public Health, 1947, volume 37, pages 1026-1032.

PEPYS Lucas President, Report of the Royal College of Physicians of London on Vaccination, 10th April 1807, 13 pages + attachments.

PEPYS Lucas President, Report from the National Vaccine Establishment, ordered, by the House of Commons, to be printed, 1st June 1810.

PERCHERON Gaston, La rage et les expériences de M. Pasteur, Librairie de Firmin-Didot et Cie, Paris, 1885, 145 pages.

PERDRAU J.R. and TODD C., Canine distemper, the high antigenic value of the virus after photodynamic inactivation by methylene blue, Journal of Comparative Pathology, 1933, volume xlvi, pages 78-89.

PERRY William, The royal standard English dictionary, published by Thomas and Andrews, West and Richardson, and Edward Cotton, Boston, 1777, 491 pages.

PETER M., Réponse de M. Peter à M. Pasteur, Revue scientifique, 1883, tome XXXI de la collection, 3e série, tome V, pages 557-561.

PETIT A., Premier rapport en faveur de l'inoculation, Lu dans l'Assemblée de la Faculté de Médecine de Paris, en l'Année 1764, 1766a, 147 pages.

PETIT A., Second rapport en faveur de l'inoculation, lu dans l'Assemblée de la Faculté de Médecine de Paris, au commencement de l'année 1766, Imprimé par son ordre, chez Dessain Junior, Paris, 1766b, 242 pages. *Excerpts of these reports have been published in the Journal de Médecine, chirurgie, pharmacie, &c*, 1766b, tome XXV, pages 291-310.

PETTIT Auguste et STEFANOPOULO Georges, Le virus de la fièvre jaune, I Discussion sur la nature, Bulletin de l'Académie de Médecine, 1928, 3e série, tome C, pages 921-930.

PETTIT Auguste, STEFANOPOULO Georges et KOLOCHINE Constantin, II Conservation du virus amaril, Bulletin de l'Académie de Médecine, 1929, 3e série, tome CII, pages 98-104.

PETTIT Auguste, Rapport sur la valeur immunisante des vaccins employés contre la fièvre jaune et la valeur thérapeutique du sérum amaril, Bulletin de l'Académie de médecine, 1931, tome CV, pages 522-526.

PETTIT Auguste et STEFAPOULO Georges J., Utilisation du sérum antiamaril d'origine animale pour la vaccination de l'homme, Bulletin de l'Académie de médecine, 1933, tome CX, pages 67-76.

PETTIT Auguste et STEFAPOULO Georges J., La vaccination antiamarile à l'Institut Pasteur, Bulletin de l'office internationale d'hygiène publique, 1934, tome XXVI, pages 1075-1082.

PEUCH M., Quelques mots sur la clavelisation dans le midi de la France; note sur un nouveau procédé de clavelisation, Journal de médecine vétérinaire et de zootechnie, 1882, tome XXXIII de la collection, pages 648-656.

PEUCH F., Rage in Nouveau dictionnaire pratique de médecine, de chirurgie et d'hygiène vétérinaires, commencé par H. Bouley, continué par André Sanson, L. Trasbot et Ed. Nocard, Asselin et Houzeau, Paris, 1890, tome 18, pages 469-545.

PIERRET M., La rage, Les travaux de Pasteur, Discours et conférences faits à l'Université de Lille en 1922-1923 en commémoration du centenaire de Louis Pasteur, premier doyen de la Faculté des sciences, O. Marquant, éditeur, Lille, 1923, pages 181-206.

PIETKIEWICZ M., Circassie in Répertoire des connaissances utiles, Dictionnaire de la conversation et de la lecture, Belin-Mandar, Paris, 1834, tome XIV, pages 355-360.

PILET Charles, Chronique historique Edmond Nocard, un précurseur en microbiologie, en pathologie comparée, en santé publique, Bulletin de l'Académie nationale de médecine, 2003, tome 187, pages 1397-1402.

PIOT M., Inoculation préventive contre le typhus ou peste bovine, repris du Moniteur égyptien, Journal de médecine vétérinaire et de zootechnie, 1883, tome XXXIV, pages 487-488.

PLOTKIN S.A., FARQUHAR J., KATZ M., BUSER F., Attenuation of RA27/3 rubella virus in WI-38 human diploid cells, Am. J. Dis. Child. 1969, volume 118, pages 178-495.

PLOTKIN Stanley A. and MORTIMER Edward A., Vaccines, 2nd edition, W.B. Saunders Company, Philadelphia, 1994, 996 pages.

PLOTKIN Stanley A. & FANTINI Bernardino editors, Vaccinia, vaccination, vaccinology Jenner, Pasteur and their successors, Elsevier, Paris, 1996, 379 pages.

PLOTKIN Stanley A. and ORENSTEIN Walter A., Vaccines, third edition, W.B. Saunders Company, Philadelphia, 1999, 1230 pages and fourth edition, W.B. Saunders Company, Philadelphia, 2004, 1662 pages.

PLOTKIN Stanley, GRENSTEIN Walter and OFFIT Paul, Vaccines, fifth edition, Saunders Elsevier, 2008, 1725 pages.

PORTAL, FOURCROY, HUZARD, HALLE, Rapport fait au nom de la commission nommée par la classe des sciences mathématiques et physiques pour l'examen de la méthode de préserver de la petite vérole par l'inoculation de la vaccine, Journal du galvanisme, de vaccine etc., an XI (1803), tome 1, pages 212-228, 257-277 et 316-328.

POWER M., Précis historique de la nouvelle méthode d'inoculer la petite vérole avec une version abrégée de cette méthode, ouvrage destiné à montrer comment elle s'est établie en Angleterre, les grands succès dont elle a été suivie, & qu'elle est due incontestablement à M. Sutton, à Amsterdam et à Paris, chez Le Breton, 1769, 119 pages.

PRUEN Thomas, Comparative sketch of the effects of variolous and vaccine inoculation, printed for Phillips, Crosby..., Cheltenham, 1807, 102 plus vj pages.

QUID, Tout pour tous par Dominique et Michèle Frémy, Robert Laffont, Paris, 1980, 1589 pages ; 2007, 2190 pages; 2004, 2190 pages.

R. J. (for RAMBOSSON J.?), La syphilisation, La Science pour tous, 2e année, numéro 41 du 17 septembre 1857, page 327.

RAMEAU Alexandre, L'institut Pasteur, La Science illustrée, 1889, tome 3, 1er semestre, numéro 55 (15 décembre 1888), pages 33-35.

RAMON G., Floculation dans un mélange neutre de toxine-antitoxine diphtériques, Comptes rendus de la Société de biologie, 1922, tome LXXXVI, pages 661-663.

RAMON G., Pouvoir floculant et pouvoir toxique de la toxine diphtérique, Comptes rendus de la Société de biologie, 1923a, tome LXXXIX, pages 2-4.

RAMON G., Sur le pouvoir floculant et sur les propriétés immunisantes d'une toxine diphtérique rendue anatoxique (anatoxine), Comptes rendus des séances de l'Académie des sciences, 1923b, tome 178, pages 1338-1340.

RAMON G., Sur la toxine et sur l'anatoxine diphtériques – Pouvoir floculant et propriétés immunisantes, Annales de l'Institut Pasteur, 1924a, 38e année, pages 1-10.

RAMON G., Des anatoxines, Comptes rendus des séances de l'Académie des sciences, 1924b, tome 178, pages 1436-1439.

RAMON G., Sur la production de l'antitoxine diphtérique, Comptes rendus de la Société de biologie, 1925a, tome XCIII, pages 506-507.

RAMON G. et DESCOMBEY P., Sur l'immunisation antitétanique et sur la production de l'antitoxine tétanique, Comptes rendus de la Société de biologie, 1925b, tome XCIII, pages 508-509 et 898-899.

RAMON G. et LAFFAILLE A., Sur l'immunisation antitétanique, Comptes rendus de la Société de biologie, 1925c, tome XCIII, pages 582-584.

RAMON G. & ZOELLER Chr., Les "vaccins associés" par union d'une anatoxine et d'un vaccin microbien (TAB) ou par mélanges d'anatoxines, Comptes rendus de la Société de biologie, 1926a, tome XCIV, pages 106-109.

RAMON G. et ZOELLER Ch., De la valeur antigène de l'anatoxine tétanique chez l'homme, Comptes rendus des séances de l'Académie des sciences, 1926b, tome 182, pages 245-247.

RAMON Gaston, Quarante années de recherches et de travaux, Imprimerie régionale, Toulouse, 1957, 911 pages.

RANBY M., Sur les préparations nécessaires à l'inoculation, & sur la manière de gouverner les inoculés in Recueil de pièces concernant l'inoculation de la petite vérole, & propres à en prouver la sécurité et l'utilité, chez Desaint & Saillant, à Paris, 1756, pages 224-233.

RANQUE H., Théorie et pratique de l'inoculation de la vaccine, précédée d'un tableau comparatif des avantages de l'inoculation ordinaire sur la petite vérole naturelle, et suivie des observations et rapports publiés sur ce sujet, tant en France qu'en Angleterre, chez Mequignon, à Paris, an IX (1801), 139 pages.

RAPPUOLI Rino, Rational design of vaccines; the recombinant pertussis vaccine induces early and long-lasting protection, Nature Medicine, 1997, volume 3, pages 374-376.

RAYNAUD Maurice, Etude expérimentale sur le rôle du sang dans la transmission de l'immunité vaccinale, Comptes rendus des séances de l'Académie des sciences, 1877, tome LXXXIV, pages 453-456.

REDACTION, note de la..., La Presse vétérinaire, avril 1881, 1re année, pages 173-174.

REDI Francesco, Experiments on the generation of insects, translated from the Italian edition of 1688 by Mab Bigelow, The open court publishing company, Chicago, 1909, 160 pages.

REDMAN COXE John, Pratical observations on vaccination : on inoculation for the cow-pox, printed and sold by James Humphreys, Philadelphia, 1802, 152 pages.

REED Walter and CARROLL James, The specific cause of yellow fever. A reply to Dr. G. Sanarelli, The Medical News, 1899a, volume LXXV, pages 321-329.

REED Walter and CARROLL James, Bacillus icteroides and Bacillus cholera suis – A preliminary note, The Medical News, 1899b, volume LXXIV, pages 513-514.

REED Walter and CARROLL James, A comparative study of the biological characters and pathogenesis of bacillus X (Sternberg), bacillus icteroides (Sanarelli), and the hog-cholera bacillus (Salmon and Smith), Journal of experimental medicine, 1900, volume V, pages 215-270.

REGELSPERGER Gustave, Un Français professeur au Canada: Le docteur Loir, Journal des voyages, numéro 601 du 7 juin 1908, page 15.

REICH Warren Thomas, "Encyclopedia of Bioethics", 1978, volume 2, pages 684-690 *(unfortunately, the author (HB) has been unable to find a copy of this encyclopedia and to check the reference)*.

REMLINGER P., Contribution à l'étude du virus rabique fixe. Son innocuité relative pour le chien, Comptes rendus de la Société de biologie, 1904, tome LVII, pages 414-416.

REMLINGER P., Vaccination antirabique, in Bactériothérapie, Vaccination, Sérothérapie par Metchnikoff, Sacquépée, Remlinger, Louis Martin, Vaillard, Dopter, Besredka, Wassermann, Leber, Dujardin-Beaumetz, Salimbeni, Calmette, J.-B. Baillière et fils, Paris, 1909, pages 76-127.

RENAUD-BADET Dr, Les vaccins microbiens, Bibliothèque Larousse, Paris, 1913, 94 pages.

RENAUD François, HANSEN Willy et FRENEY Jean, Dictionnaire des précurseurs en bactériologie, SFM-éditions Eska, 2005, 249 pages.

RENAULT, Extrait des compte-rendu des travaux de l'Ecole d'Alfort pendant l'année scolaire 1851-1852, repris dans les Annales de médecine vétérinaire, 1853, 2e année, pages 383-384.

RENAULT J. Docteur, La vaccination antidiphtérique Historique et Enseignement, Séance du 19 janvier 1939 de la Société de médecine publique, Le Mouvement sanitaire, 16e année, numéro hors série, pages 3-8.

RENGADE Docteur J., Les grands maux et les grands remèdes, traité complet des maladies qui frappent le genre humain, Librairies illustrée et M. Dreyfous, Paris, 1879, 808 pages.

RESPAUT M. le Dr, La vaccination du choléra, L'Illustration, 1885, volume LXXXVI, numéro 2213, pages 49, 52, 62-63.

REY M., SATGE P., COLLOMB H., GUICHENEY A., DIOP MAR I., NIANG I., BERNE C. et NOUHOUAYI A., Aspects épidémiologiques et cliniques des encéphalites consécutives à la vaccination antiamarile (d'après 248 cas observés dans quatre services hospitaliers de Dakar à la suite de la campagne 1965), Bulletin de la société médicale d'Afrique noire de langue française, 1966, volume XI, pages 560-574.

REYNAL J., Traité de police sanitaire des animaux domestiques, P. Asselin, successeur de Béchet Jeune et Labé, Paris, 1873, 1012 pages, pages 31-42.

RHASES, Traduction françoise du traité de Rhasès sur la petite vérole et la rougeole, sur la dernière édition de Londres Arabe & Latine, par M. Paulet, chez Ganeau, à Paris, vers 900 (1778), tome 2, 102 pages.

RICHE M., Le rôle administratif de l'Académie de médecine, Mémoires de l'Académie de médecine, 1906, tome 40, pages 31-42.

RICHELOT G., Syphilisation in Traité des maladies vénériennes par J. Hunter, traduit de l'anglais par le docteur G. Richelot, J.-B. Baillière et fils, Paris, 1859, 3e édition, pages 728-736.

RICHET Charles, L'œuvre de Pasteur, Librairie Félix Alcan, Paris, 1923, 119 pages.

RICORD Ph., Lettres sur la syphilis adressées à M. le rédacteur en chef de l'Union médicale, Aux bureaux de l'union médicale, Paris, 1re édition, 1851, 282 pages et 2e édition, 1856, 472 pages.

RICORD, BEGIN, MALGAIGNE, VELPEAU, DEPAUL, GIBERT, LAGNEAU, LARREY, MICHEL LEVY, GERDY, ROUX, communications à l'Académie nationale de médecine avec les communications de MM. AUZIAS-TURENNE et C. SPERINO à l'Académie des sciences de Paris et à l'Académie de médecine de Turin, De la syphilisation et de la contagion des accidents secondaires de la syphilis, chez J.-B. Baillière, Paris, 1853, 383 pages.

RING John, Mr Ring on vaccine inoculation, The Medical and Physical Journal, 1803, volume IX, pages 296-299.

RIVERS T.M., Cultivation of vaccine virus for Jennerian prophylaxis in man, Journal of Experimental Medicine, 1931, volume 54, pages 453-461.

RIVERS Thomas M. and WARD S.M., Further observations on the cultivation of vaccine virus for Jennerian prophylaxis in man, Journal of Experimental Medicine, 1933, volume 58, pages 635-648.

R. M., Hygiène et santé: L'œuvre de la commission Rockefeller pour la lutte contre la tuberculose en France, La Nature, Supplément au numéro 2519 du 15 juillet 1922, page 17.

RO A, Ferran i Clua Jaume, Gran Enciclopedia Catalana, Edicions 62, Barcelona, (1974?), tome 7, pages 387-388.

ROBERTS Leslie, "Rotavirus vaccines" second chance, Science, 2004, volume 305, pages 890-893.

ROBIN Yves, Lettre à monsieur Pasteur Louis (à l'occasion du centième anniversaire de sa mort), aux France Europe Editions livres, 2002, 249 pages, (www.france-europe-editions.com).

ROCHARD Jules Dr., Traité d'hygiène sociale, Adrien Delahaye et Emile Lecrosnier éditeurs, Paris, 1888, 692 pages.

ROGER H., Les vaccins, La Nature, numéro 2157 du 30 janvier 1915, pages 69-72.

ROGERS L., The treatment of cholera by injections of hypertonic saline solutions with a simple and rapid method of intra-abdominal administration, Philippine J. Sc, 1909, 4, 99, *reprinted in* A bibiography of internal medicine, communicable diseases by Arthur L. Bloomfield, The University of Chicago Press,1958, Chicago, 560 pages.

ROMAN (?), M.L.R., L'inoculation poème en quatre chants, à Amsterdam et à Paris chez Lacombe, 1773, 242 pages.

ROMANES G.-J., La domestication des animaux, Revue scientifique (revue rose), 21e année, 3e série, tome XXXIV, numéro 16 (18 octobre 1884), pages 499-504.

ROMMELAERE M., Discussion d'une présentation de M. V. Desguin, Bulletin de l'Académie royale de médecine de Belgique, séance du 25 mai 1889, 1889, 4e série, tome 3, pages 251-254.

ROSEN de ROSENSTEIN Nils, Traité des maladies des enfans, ouvrage qui est le fruit d'une longue observation, & appuyé sur les faits les plus authentiques, traduit du suédois par M. LeFebvre de Villebrune, chez Pierre-Guillaume Cavelier, Paris, 1778, 582 pages.

ROSSET R., Pasteur et la rage, Informations techniques des services vétérinaires, Revue du syndicat national des vétérinaires inspecteurs du ministère de l'agriculture (SNVIMA), Paris, 1985, 320 pages.

ROSSIGNOL H., Réflexions, La Presse vétérinaire, 1re année, numéro 8 du 31 août 1881a, pages 50-51.

ROSSIGNOL H., Réflexions, La Presse vétérinaire, juin 1881b, 1re année, pages 290-292.

ROSTAND Jean, Charles Richet Prix Nobel de Médecine 1913, in Les Prix Nobel de physiologie et de médecine, Union européenne d'éditions, Monaco, 1962, page 81-87.

ROUX A. M., Mémoire sur l'inoculation de la petite vérole, à Amsterdam et se trouve à Paris chez P. Fr. Didot le jeune, 1765, 26 pages.

ROUX Pierre, Paul, Emile, Des nouvelles acquisitions sur la rage, Thèse de doctorat en médecine de Paris présentée et soutenue le 30 juillet 1883 à 9 heures, A. Parent imprimeur, A. Davy successeur, Paris, 1883, 55 pages.

ROUX et CHAMBERLAND MM., Immunité contre la septicémie conférée par des substances solubles, Annales de l'Institut Pasteur, 1887, tome I, pages 561-572.

ROUX Emile, Louis Pasteur (1822-1895); l'œuvre médicale de Pasteur, L'agenda du chimiste, supplément 1896, librairie Hachette et Cie, Paris, 1896, pages 527-548.

ROUX M.E., II Sur la peste bubonique. Essais de traitement par le sérum antipesteux, à propos d'une note du Dr Yersin, médecin de 2e classe des colonies, directeur de l'Institut Pasteur de Nha-Trang, Bulletin de l'Académie nationale de médecine, 1897, 61e année, 3e série, tome XXXVIII, pages 91-99.

ROUX Emile, Notice sur les travaux scientifiques du Dr Roux. Masson et Cie éditeurs, Paris, 1899, 53 pages.

ROUX M. le Dr, Discours de M. le Dr..., in Inauguration du monument Nocard, Recueil de médecine vétérinaire publié à l'Ecole d'Alfort, tome LXXXIII, numéro 13 du 15 juillet 1906, pages 487-491.

ROUX M., rapport sur les travaux de M. J. Ferran. Prix Bréant, commissaires: MM. Guyon, d'Arsonval, Lannelongue, Laveran, Dastre, Chauveau, Perrier, Giard, Labbé; Bouchard, Roux, rapporteurs, Comptes rendus des séances de l'Académie des sciences, 1907, tome CXLV, pages 1030-1031.

ROUX M., rapporteur de la commission du prix Bréant, composé de MM. Bouchard, Guyon d'Arsonval, Lannelongue, Dastre, Chauveau, Perrier, Labbé, Henneguy; Roux et Laveran rapporteurs, Une partie des arrérages de la fondation est décernée à M. W.-M. Haffkine pour ses travaux sur la vaccination du choléra et de la peste bubonique, Comptes rendus des séances de l'Académie des sciences, séance du 20 décembre 1909, pages 1258-1260.

ROUX Dr, Pasteur et la médecine, Je sais tout, numéro de Noël du 15 décembre 1922, pages 723-729.

ROY C.S., BROWN J.Graham and SHERRINGTON C.S., Preliminary Report on the Pathology of Cholera Asiatica (as observed in Spain, 1885), Proceedings of the Royal Society, 1886, volume 43, pages 173-181.

ROYAL COMMISSION, First and Second report of the Royal Commission appointed to inquire into the subject of vaccination; with minutes of evidence and appendices, 1889-1890, printed for her majesty's stationary office, London, 1889-1890, 132 + 313 pages.

ROYAL COMMISSION, A report on vaccination and its result based on evidence taken by the Royal Commission during the years 1889-1897, volume I, the text of the commission report, 1898, London, The new Sydenham Society, volume 164, 493 pages.

ROYAL JENNERIAN SOCIETY, Address of the Royal Jennerian Society for the extermination of the small-pox with the plan, regulations, and instructions for vaccine inoculations to which is added a list of subscribers, instituted in 1803, printed and sold by W. Phillips, 1803, 70 pages.

SABIN Albert B., Characteristics and genetic potentialities of experimentally produced and naturally occurring variants of poliomyelitis virus, Annals of the New York Academy of Sciences, 1955a, volume 61, pages 924-939.

SABIN Albert B., Immunization of chimpanzees and human beings with avirulent strains of poliomyelitis virus, Annals of the New York Academy of Sciences, 1955b, volume 61, pages 1050-1056.

SABIN Albert B., Immunity in poliomyelitis with special reference to vaccination, in Poliomyelitis, World Health Organization, monograph series numéro 26, Geneva, 1955c, pages 297-334.

SACCO Luigi, Osservazioni pratiche sull'uso del vajuolo vaccine come preservatico del vajuolo umano, Padova, II édizione, 1801, 174 pages.

SACCO Louis, Traité de vaccination avec des observations sur le javart et la variole des bêtes à cornes, traduit de l'italien par Joseph Daquin, chez Michaud frères, Paris 1813, 2e édition, 495 pages.

SALEUN G. et CECCALDI J., Affections ictérigènes suspectes et épreuves de séro-protection de Max-Theiler, Bulletins de la société de pathologie exotique et de ses filiales, 1936, tome XXIX, pages 661-667.

SALMASO Stefania, Pertussis, in The vaccine book, edited by Barry R. Bloom and Paul-Henry Lambert, Academic Press, San Diego, 2003, pages 211-224.

SALMON D.E. and SMITH T., On a new method of producing immunity from contagious diseases, Proceeding of the Biological Society, Washington, 1884-1886, volume 3, pages 29-33.

SALMON D.E. and SMITH Theobald, Infectious diseases of cattle, in Special report on diseases of cattle and on cattle feeding, prepared under the direction of Dr D.E. Salmon, U.S. department of agriculture, reprinted by order of the congress, Government printing office, 1896, pages 371-438. The letter of transmittal is signed from Washington, May 14, 1892.

SAMOÏLOWITZ M. D., Mémoire sur l'inoculation de la peste avec la description de trois poudres fumigatives antipestilentielles, chez les frères Gay, à Strasbourg, 1782, 36 pages.

SAMOÏLOWITZ M. D., Lettre à l'Académie de Dijon avec réponse à ce qui a paru douteux dans le mémoire sur l'inoculation de la peste, chez Le Clerc, à Paris, 1783, 63 pages.

SANARELLI G., A lecture on yellow fever with a description of the bacillus icteroides, The British Medical Journal, July 3, 1897a, pages 7-11.

SANARELLI G., Etiologie et pathogénie de la fièvre jaune, Annales de l'Institut Pasteur, 1897b, 11e année, pages 433-514.

SANARELLI G., Some observations and controversial remarks on the specific cause of yellow fever, The Medical News, 1899, volume LXXV, pages 193-199.

SANKALE M., BOURGEADE A., WADE F. et BEYE B., Contribution à l'étude des réactions vaccinales observées en dehors de Dakar, Bulletin de la société médicale d'Afrique noire de langue française, 1966, volume XI, pages 617-624.

SANSONETTI Philippe J., Un siècle de recherches sur les vaccins contre la fièvre typhoïde, fin du commencement ou commencement de la fin ? In L'aventure de la vaccination, Anne-Marie Moulin éditeur, Fayard, Paris, 1996, pages 210-218.

SASPORTAS M., Circulaire du consistoire central des Israélites, à MM. les membres des divers Consistoires départementaux de l'Empire, les membres du Consistoire central, signé David Sintzheim, président; Abraham Cologna, grand rabbin; B. Cerf-Berr, Ib. Lazard; Bulletin sur la vaccine, numéro 12 d'octobre 1811, pages 6-11.

SATO Y., KIMURAM., FUKUMI H., Development of a pertussis component vaccine in Japan, Lancet, 1984, 1, pages 122-126.

SAUVEUR Docteur D., Compte– rendu des travaux de l'Académie, Mémoires de l'Académie royale de médecine de Belgique, 1857, tome 4, page 79.

SAWYER W.A., KITCHEN S.F. and LLOYD Wray, Vaccination of humans against yellow fever with immune serum and virus fixed for mice, Proceeding of the Society of Experimental Biology and Medicine, 1931a, volume 29, pages 62-64.

SAWYER W.A. and LLOYD Wray, The use of mice in tests of immunity against yellow fever, Journal of Experimental Medicine, 1931b, volume 54, page 533.

SAWYER W.A., The history of yellow fever since the New Orleans epidemic of 1905, Southern Medical Journal, 1932a, volume XXV, pages 291-296.

SAWYER W.A., KITCHEN S.F. and Wray LLOYD, Vaccination against yellow fever with immune serum and virus fixed for mice, Journal of Experimental Medicine, 1932b, volume 54, pages 945-969.

SAWYER W.A., Notre expérience de la vaccination contre la fièvre jaune, Bulletin de l'Office internationale d'hygiène publique, 1934, tome XXVI, page 1072-1074.

SCHAPER A., La fièvre aphteuse, La Nature, numéro 3159 du mois d'août 1948, pages 215-216 et 251-253.

SCHWARZ A.J.F., Premiminary tests of a highly attenuated measles vaccine, American Journal of Diseases of Children, 1962, volume 103, pages 386-389.

SCOFIELD Samuel, A practical treatise on Vaccina or Cowpock, Collins & Perkins, New-York, 1810, 139 pages.

SEATON Edward C, A handbook of Vaccination, J.B. Lippincott & Co., Philadelphia, 1868, 383 pages.

SECRETAIRES PERPETUELS, publiés par... Table générale des comptes rendus des séances de l'Académie des sciences, tomes XCII à CXXI, 5 janvier 1881 à 30 décembre 1895, Gauthier-Villars, Paris, 1900.

SEDILLOT C, De l'influence des découvertes de M. Pasteur sur les progrès de la chirurgie, Comptes rendus des séances de l'Académie des sciences, 1878, volume LXXXVI, 2e semestre, numéro 10, pages 634-640.

SEE M., Histoire et critique. Médecine légale. Propagation de la syphilis par la vaccination, Gazette hebdomadaire, tome II, numéro 10 du 9 mars 1855, pages 176-178.

SELLARDS A.W. and HINDLE Edward, The preservation of yellow fever virus, The British Medical Journal, 1928, April 28, pages 713-714.

SELLARDS A.W. et LAIGRET J., Immunisation de l'homme contre la fièvre jaune par l'inoculation du virus de souris, Archives de l'Institut Pasteur de Tunis, 1932a, tome XXI, pages 229-238.

SELLARS A.W. et LAIGRET J., Vaccination de l'homme contre la fièvre jaune, Comptes rendus des séances de l'Académie des sciences, 1932b, tome 194, pages 1609-1611.

SELLARS A.W. et LAIGRET J., Contrôle, par épreuve sur Macacus rhesus, du pouvoir protecteur du sérum des hommes vaccinés contre la fièvre jaune avec le virus de souris, Comptes rendus des séances de l'Académie des sciences, 1932c, tome 194, pages 2175-2178.

SENET André, La lutte contre la fièvre aphteuse, La Nature, numéro 3211 du mois de novembre 1952, pages 351-352.

SERRES Rapporteur, MAGENDIE, BRESCHET, DUMERIL et ROUX, Rapport sur le prix relatif à la vaccine proposé pour 1842, Comptes rendus des séances de l'Académie des sciences, 1845, tome 20, pages 624-662.

SERRIERES Docteur, Rapport du comité de vaccine du département de la Meurthe au comité central de vaccine, établi près S. Exc. le Ministre de l'intérieur, de l'imprimerie de Delahaye-Haener et Cie, Nancy, 1807, 36 pages [BANM, n° 39 612 E (8)].

SEVESTRE M. et MARTIN Louis M., Diphtérie, in Traité des maladies de l'enfance publié sous la direction de J. Grancher, J. Comby et A.-B. Marfan, Masson et Cie, Paris, 1897, volume 1, pages 516-705.

SHANNON R.C., WHITMAN Loring and FRANCA Mario, Yellow fever virus in jungle mosquitoes, Science, 1938, volume 88, pages 110-111.

SIGERIST Henry E., Letters of Jean de Carro to Alexandre Marcet 1794-1817, The John Hopkins Press, Baltimore, 1950, 78 pages.

SIGNOL M., Présence des bactéries dans le sang, Comptes rendus des séances de l'académie des sciences, tome LVII, 2e semestre, numéro 6, séance du 10 août 1863, pages 348-351.

SILVERSTEIN Arthur M., A history of immunology, Academic Press Inc., San Diego, 1989, 422 pages.

SMITH Theobald and KILBORNE F.L., Investigations into the nature, causation, and prevention of Texas or southern cattle fever, Government printing office, 1893, 301 pages.

SMITH Theobald, Presidential Address to the Society of American Bacteriologists, 1903, reprinted by C.E. Dolman, in Theobald Smith and his presidential address to the society of American Bacteriologists, ASM news, 1981, volume 47, pages 231-235.

SMITH Hugh H. and THEILER Max, The adaptation of unmodified strains of yellow fever virus to cultivation in vitro, Journal of Experimental Medicine, 1937a, 65, pages 801-808.

SMITH Wilson, The influenza problem, St. Mary's Hospital Gazette, 1937b, volume 43, pages 112-120.

SMITH H.H., PENNA H.A. and PAOLIELLO A., Yellow fever vaccination with cultured virus (17D) without immune serum. American Journal Tropical Medicine, 1938, 18, 437-468.

SMORODINTSEV A.A., DROBYSHEVSKAYA A.I., BULYCHEV N.P., VASILIEF K.G., VOTYAKOV V.I., GROISMAN G.M., ZHILOVA G.P., ILYENKO V.I., KANTOROVICH R.A., KURNOSOVA L.M. AND CHALKINA O.M., Immunological and epidemiological effectiveness of live poliomyelitis vaccine, in Poliomyelitis, papers and discussions presented at the Fifth International Poliomyelitis Conference, Copenhagen, Denmark, July 26-28, 1960, compiled and edited for the International Poliomyelitis Congress, J. P. Lippincott company, Philadelphia and Montreal, 1961, pages 240-256.

SNOW John Dr., On the pathology and mode of communication of cholera, Proceeding of Societies, Westminster Medical Society, London Medical Gazette, 1849, volume 44, pages 730-732, 745-752 et 923-929.

SOCIETE DE MEDECINE DE BRUXELLES, Rapport sur la vaccine, par les commissaires de la Société de Médecine de Bruxelles, lu à la séance du 15 thermidor, an 9, de l'imprimerie d'Emmanuel Flon, à Bruxelles, 1800, 15 pages.

SOCIETE DE MEDECINS, Nouveau dictionnaire universel et raisonné de médecine, de chirurgie et de l'art vétérinaire; contenant des connaissances étendues... à Paris, chez la veuve Duchesne libraire, 1772, 6 volumes.

SOCIETE DE MEDECINE PRATIQUE, La vaccination antidiphtérique Est-elle inoffensive ?, Est-elle efficace ? Séance du 19 janvier 1939, Le Mouvement sanitaire, février 1939, numéro hors série, 159 pages.

SOCIETE DE PATHOLOGIE EXOTIQUE, Vœu relatif à la vaccination contre la fièvre jaune, Bulletins de la société de pathologie exotique et de ses filiales, 1936, tome XXIX, page 449-450.

SOPER, Fièvre jaune rurale et sylvatique. Un nouveau problème d'hygiène publique en Colombie, Editorial Minerva S.A., Bogota, 1935 in Office internationale d'hygiène publique, 1935, tome XXVII, page 2404.

SOREL Médecin Général Inspecteur, La vaccination anti-amarile en Afrique occidentale française. Mise en application du procédé de vaccination Sellards-Laigret, Office internationale d'hygiène publique, 1936, tome XXVIII, pages 1325-1356.

SPENCER Steven M., Where are we now on polio? The Post'science editor reports on the Salk vaccine, its triumphs and troubles, in the light of what we have learned since last spring's historic rhubarb. The Saturday September 10, 1955, pages 19-21, 152-153, 156-157.

SPERINO Casimiro, Sifilizzazione nell'uomo, Giornale delle Scienze Mediche della Reale Academia Medico-Chirurgica di Torino, 23 maggio 1851, pages 1-9. *This text is reproduced in French*: Mémoire sur la syphilisation de l'homme, lu à l'Académie royale de médecine et de chirurgie de Turin, le 23 mai 1851 dans RICORD, 1853a, page 205.

SPERINO C, La syphilisation étudiée comme une méthode curative et comme moyen prophylactique des maladies vénériennes, Librairie J. Bocca, Turin et Chamerot, Paris, traduit de l'italien par A. Tresal, 1853b, 821 pages.

STANWELL-SMITH Rosalind, Immunization : celebrating the past and injecting the future, Journal of the Royal Society of Medicine, 1996, volume 89, pages 509-513.

STEFANOPOULO G.-J., Sur la vaccination contre la fièvre jaune, Bulletins de la société de pathologie exotique, 1936, tome XXIX, pages 359-360.

STEINHARDT Edna, ISRAELI C. and LAMBERT R.A., Studies on the cultivation of the virus of vaccinia, Journal of Infectious Diseases, 1913, volume 13, pages 294-300.

STEINHARDT Edna and LAMBERT Robert A., Studies on the cultivation of the virus of vaccinia II, Journal of Infectious Diseases, 1914, volume 14, pages 87-92.

STEINBRENNER Ch.-Ch., Traité sur la vaccine ou recherches historiques et critiques sur les résultats obtenus par les vaccinations et revaccinations, Labé libraire, Paris, 1846, 844 pages.

STERNBERG George M., A manual of bacteriology, William Wood & company, New-York, 1892, 886 pages.

STERNBERG George M., Immunity – Protective inoculations in infectious diseases and serum-therapy, William Wood and Company, New-York, 1895, 325 pages.

STIENON L., Une épidémie d'ictère par Lurman (Berliner Klinische Wochenschrift, 1885, p. 20), in Journal de Médecine, de Chirurgie et de Pharmacologie, Bruxelles, 43e année, 80e volume, mars 1885, pages 123-124.

STOKES Adrian, BAUER Johannes H. and HUDSON N.Paul, Experimental transmission of yellow fever to laboratory animals, The American Journal of Tropical Medicine, 1928a, volume VIII, pages 103-164.

STOKES Adrian, BAUER J.H. and HUDSON N. Paul, The transmission of yellow fever to Macacus rhesus – Preliminary notes, Journal of the American Medical Association, 1928b, volume 90, pages 253-254.

STOLL Maximilien, Aphorismes sur la connoissance et la curation des fièvres, traduits en français par J.N.Corvisart, avec le texte latin, chez Régent et Bernard, à Paris, l'an V de la république française (1797), 581 pages; *the same text has been translated by P.-A.-O. Mahon, new edition*, Gabon libraire, Paris, 1809, 240 pages.

STRAUSS Paul, Paris ignoré, librairies-imprimeries réunies, ancienne maison Quantin, Paris, *undated (refers to an event that occured in April 1892)*, 484 pages.

SURGEON-GENERAL'S OFFICE, Cholera epidemic of 1873 in the United States, Government Printing Office, Washington, 1875, 1025 pages.

SUZOR Renaud, Hydrophobia, an account of the Pasteur's system containing a translation of all his communications on the subject, the technique of his method, and the latest statistical results, Chatto & Windus, London, 1887, 231 pages.

SVEDIAUR M., Observations pratiques sur les maladies vénériennes, les plus opiniâtres & les plus invétérées, traduit de l'anglais de monsieur Svédiaur, docteur en médecine, chez Cuchet Librairie, Paris, 1790, 328 pages.

TAKAHASHI M., OTSUKA T., OKUNO Y., ASANO Y., YAZAKI T., ISOMURA S., Live vaccine used to prevent the spread of varicella in children in hospital, The Lancet, 1974, volume 2, pages 1288-1290.

TARDIEU Ambroise Dr, Etude medico-légale sur les maladies accidentellement et involontairement produites par imprudence, négligence ou transmission contagieuse comprenant l'histoire médico-légale de la syphilis et de ses divers modes de transmission, Annales d'hygiène publique et de médecine légale, 1864, 2e série, tome XXI, pages 340-379.

TAYLOR R.M., Studies on survival of influenza virus between epidemics and antigenic variants of the virus, American Journal of public health, 1949, volume 39, pages 171-178.

TESSIER Abbé, Mémoire sur l'inoculation de la clavelée, Histoire de la Société royale de médecine, année 1786, publié en 1790, pages 379-386.

TETRY Andrée, L'atténuation de la virulence du virus rabique dans l'expérience de Pasteur, et son interprétation moderne, Revue scientifique (revue rose illustrée), 1941, 79e année, page 386.

THACHER James, Observations on hydrophobia produced by the bite of a mad dog, or other rabid animal..., published by Joseph Avery, Plymouth (Mass.), 1812, 302 pages.

THACHER James, Dr Dalhonde deposition, in American Medical Biography, an unabridged republication of the first edition published in Boston, 1828, Volume 1, Da Capo Press reprint edition, New-York, 1967, pages 42-43.

THACHER James, Zabdiel Boyston, in American Medical Biography, an unabridged republication of the first edition published in Boston, 1828, Volume 1, Da Capo Press reprint edition, New-York, 1967, pages 185-192.

THAISS Christoph A. and KAUFMANN Stefan H.E., Toward Novel Vaccines Against Tuberculosis: Current Hopes and Obstacles. Yale Journal of Biology and Medicine, 2010, volume 83, pages 209-215.

THE COLONIAL SOCIETY OF MASSACHUSETTS, Medicine in Colonial Massachusetts, 1620-1820, distributed by The University Press of Virginia, The Stinehour Press, Boston, 1980, 425 pages.

THE MERK VETERINARY MANUAL, Anthrax, Merk and Co. Inc., Rahway (USA), 6th edition, 1986, pages 359-362.

THEILER Max, Susceptibility of the white mice to the virus of yellow fever, Science, April 4, 1930a, volume 71, page 367.

THEILER Max, Studies on the action of yellow fever virus in mice, Annals of Tropical Medicine and Parasitology, 1930b, volume 24, pages 249-272.

THEILER Max, A yellow fever protection test in mice by intracerebral injection, Annals of Tropical Medicine and Hygiene, 1933, volume 27, pages 57-77.

THEILER Max, Spontaneous encephalomyelite of mice – a new virus disease, Science, 1934a, volume 80, page 122.

THEILER Max and WHITMAN Loring, Quantitative studies of the virus and immune serum used in vaccination against fever, The American Journal of Tropical Medicine, 1934b, volume 15, pages 347-356.

THEILER Max and WHITMAN Loring, Le danger de la vaccination par le virus amaril neurotrope seul, Office international d'hygiène publique, 1935, tome XXVII, pages 1342-1347.

THEILER Max et SMITH H.H., L'emploi du sérum hyperimmun de singe dans la vaccination humaine contre la fièvre jaune, Bulletin de l'office international d'hygiène publique, 1936, tome XXVIII, pages 2354-2357.

THEILER Max and SMITH Hugh H., The effects of prolonged cultivation in vitro upon the pathogenicity of yellow fever virus, Journal of Experimental Medicine, 1937a, volume 65, pages 767-786.

THEILER MAX and SMITH Hugh H., The use of yellow fever virus modified by in vitro cultivation for human immunization, Journal of Experimental Medicine, 1937b, volume 65, pages 787-800.

THEODORIDES Jean, Un précurseur de Pasteur: Pierre-Victor Galtier (1846-1908), Archives internationales Claude Bernard, numéro 2 du 1er trimestre 1972, pages 167-171.

THEODORIDES Jean, Histoire de la rage *Cave* Canem, Masson, Paris, 1986, 289 pages.

THIAUCOURT, 2000, Personal communication.

THIERRY E., Prophylaxie de la rage chez l'homme. Diagnostic de la rage chez le chien et le chat. Conseils pratiques, Journal des praticiens, 1897, 11e année, numéro 44, pages 692-696 et 710-712.

THOMAS Joseph, Universal pronouncing dictionary of biography and mythology, J.P. Lippincott company, Philadelphia, 1893, 2549 pages.

THOMSEN Oluf og JENSEN VILH., Louis Pasteur Minderskrift, Levin & Munkgaards Forlag, Kobenhavn, 1922, 297 pages.

THOMSON John, An account of the varioloid epidemic, which was lately prevaled in Edinburgh and others parts of Scotland..., printed for Longman, Hurst, Rees, Orme, and Brown, Edinburgh, 1820, 322 plus 78 pages.

THOMSON W.O., Encephalitis in infants following vaccination with 17 D yellow fever virus: report of a further case, British Medical Journal, July 16, 1955, volume 2, pages 182-183.

THORNTON John (docteur), Preuves de l'efficacité de la vaccine, suivies d'une réponse aux objections formées contre la vaccination, contenant l'histoire de cette découverte, etc., traduit par Joseph Duffour, Chomel Imprimeur-Libraire, Paris, 1808, 214 pages.

THUILLIER, Correspondence of... Pasteur & Thuillier concerning Anthrax and swine Fever Vaccinations, translated and edited by Robert M. Frank et Denise Wrotnowska, University of Alabama Press, 1968, 240 pages.

TIBURCE, Causeries de la semaine:. ..La préparation des sérums à l'Institut de Garches, le cheval de bataille du général Canrobert, Les Veillées des chaumières, 20e année, numéro 1162 du 19 juin 1897, pages 524-526.

TIGERTT W.D., Anthrax William Smith Greenfield, M.D., F.R.C.P., Professor Superintendent, The Brown Animal Sanatory Institution (1878-1881) concerning the priority due to him for the production of the first vaccine against anthrax, Journal of Hygiene (Cambridge), 1980, volume 85, pages 415-420.

TIMONE Emmanuel Dr, Dissertation historique sur l'inoculation de la petite vérole suivie de Sur l'inoculation de la petite vérole, concernant l'histoire de cette méthode et adressée à la Société Royale de Londres & à M. Skragenstierna, premier médecin de S.M. le Roi de Suède, écrites vers 1714, Recueil de pièces concernant l'inoculation de la petite vérole et propres à en prouver la sécurité et l'utilité, chez Desaint et Saillant, à Paris, 1756, pages 11-20 & 20-29.

TIOLLAIS Pierre et DEJEAN Anne, Le virus de l'hépatite B, La recherche, 1985, volume 16, pages 1324-1333.

TISSANDIER Gaston, L'Institut Pasteur, La Nature, numéro 807 du 17 novembre 1888, pages 402-406.

TISSOT Mr., L'inoculation justifiée ou dissertion pratique et apologétique sur cette méthode, chez Marc-Michel Bousquet et compagnie, à Lausane, 1754, 179 pages.

TISSOT M., Avis au peuple sur sa santé, chez Benoit Duplain libraire, Lyon, 1768, 3e édition, 2 tomes, 464 pages.

TODD Charles, Experiments on the virus of fowl plague, Journal of Experimental Pathology, 1928, volume IX, pages 101-106.

TOPLEY W.W.C. and WILSON G.S., The principles of bacteriology and immunity, Edward Arnold & Co., London, 1931, 1300 + XX pages in 2 volumes.

TOUSSAINT M., Recherches expérimentales sur la contagion du charbon, La Revue scientifique de la France et de l'étranger, 1879, tome XXIII de la collection, pages 1143-1144.

TOUSSAINT H., De l'immunité pour le charbon, acquise à la suite d'inoculations préventives, Comptes rendus des séances de l'Académie des sciences, 1880a, tome XCI, pages 135-137.

TOUSSAINT M., in BOULEY M., Observations à l'occasion du procès verbal, Bulletin de l'Académie nationale de médecine, 44e année, 2e série, tome IX, séance du 27 juillet 1880b, pages 753-756.

TOUSSAINT H., Académie de médecine: De l'immunité pour le charbon acquise à la suite d'inoculations préventives, Journal de médecine vétérinaire et de zootechnie, 1880c, tome XXXI, pages 574-584.

TOUSSAINT H., Identité de la septicémie aiguë et du choléra des poules, Comptes rendus des séances de l'Académie des sciences, 1880d, tome XCI, pages 301-303.

TOUSSAINT Dr., Anthrax vaccinations Thurday, August 12th, in 48e annual meeting of the British Medical Association held in Cambridge, Aug. 10th, 11th, 12th, and 13th, 1880, The British Medical Journal, september 4, 1880e, page 385.

TOUSSAINT H. Dr, Vaccinations charbonneuses, Association française pour l'avancement des sciences, 9e session, Reims, séance du 19 août 1880, au secrétariat de l'association, Paris, 1881a, pages 1021-1025.

TOUSSAINT H., Sur la culture du microbe de la clavelée, Comptes rendus des séances de l'Académie des sciences, 1881b, tome XCII, pages 362-364.

TOUSSAINT H., Sur quelques points relatifs à l'immunité charbonneuse, Comptes rendus des séances de l'Académie des sciences, 1881c, tome XCIII, pages 163-164.

TOUSSAINT H., Sur un procédé nouveau de vaccination du choléra des poules, Comptes rendus des séances de l'Académie des sciences, 1881d, tome XCIII, pages 219-221.

TOUSSAINT H., Contribution à l'étude de la transmission de la tuberculose. Infection par les jus de viandes chauffés, Comptes rendus des séances de l'Académie des sciences, 1881e, tome XCIII, pages 281-284.

TOUSSAINT H., Infection tuberculeuse, par les liquides de sécrétion et la sérosité des pustules de vaccin, avec une remarque de M. Vulpian Sur la contagion de la tuberculose, Comptes rendus des séances de l'Académie des sciences, 1881f, tome XCIII, pages 322-324.

TOUSSAINT H., Sur le parasitisme de la tuberculose, Comptes rendus des séances de l'Académie des sciences, 1881g, tome XCIII, pages 350-353.

TOUSSAINT H., Sur la contagion de la tuberculose, Comptes rendus des séances de l'Académie des sciences, 1881h, tome XCIII, pages 741-743.

TOUSSAINT M., Mémoire sur l'immunité pour le charbon, acquise à la suite d'inoculations préventives (récompensé par l'Académie des sciences, mention honorable, prix Montyon (Médecine et chirurgie 1881), et l'Académie de Médecine (prix Barbier, 1881), Revue vétérinaire, Journal mensuel publié à l'Ecole vétérinaire de Toulouse, 1883, 2e série, tome III, pages 207-216, 256-265 et 297-310.

TRONCHIN M., article inoculation, Encyclopédie ou dictionnaire raisonné des sciences, des arts et des métiers, tome VIII, chez Samuel Faulche & Cie à Neufchatel, 1765, pages 755-771.

TRONCHIN Henry, Un médecin du XVIIIe siècle, Théodore Tronchin (1709-1781) d'après des documents inédits, Librairie Pion, Paris, 1906, 417 pages.

TROUESSART Dr E.-L., Les microbes, les ferments et les moisissures, Félix Alcan, éditeur, Paris, 1886, 1re édition, 304 pages et 1891, 2e édition, 282 pages.

TROUESSART E.-L., La fièvre jaune et ses inoculations préventives, Revue scientifique (revue rose), 1887, 3e série, tome XIII, tome XXXIX de la collection, pages 49-52.

TROUSSET Jules, Nouveau dictionnaire encyclopédique universel illustré, répertoire des connaissances humaines, à la librairie illustrée, Paris, 1886-1891, 5 volumes plus 1 supplément.

TURNBULL Peter C.B., Anthrax in Vaccines a Biography, edited by Andrew W. Artenstein, Springer, New-York, 2010, pages 57-71.

VAISSAIRE J., MOCK M., LE DOUJET C, LEVY M., Le charbon bactéridien. Epidemiologie de la maladie en France, Médecine Maladies infectieuses, 2001, tome 31 supplément 2, pages 257-271 et Vaissaire, communication personnelle.

VALENTIN Louis, Résultats de l'inoculation de la vaccine dans les départements de la Meurthe, de la Meuse, des Vosges et du Haut-Rhin précédés d'un discours préliminaire, et suivis de ceux de la vaccination sur divers animaux, se trouve à Nancy chez Haener et Delahaye, Messidor an X (Juillet 1802), 85 plus 15 pages.

VALLAT François, Le chirurgien Thomas Bates et les vaches malades: une heureuse gestion anglaise de l'épizootie de peste bovine en 1714 Bulletin de la société française d'histoire de la médecine et des sciences vétérinaires, 2006, numéro 6, pages 40-51.

VALLAT François, Les bœufs malades de la peste, Presses universitaires de Rennes, Rennes, 2009, 360 pages.

VALLEE H. et PANISSET J., Les tuberculoses animales, Librairie Octave Doin-Gaston Doin éditeur, Paris, 1920, 528 pages.

VALLEE H., CARRE H., and RINJARD P. Vaccination against Foot-and-mouth by means of formalinised virus. Journal of Comparative Pathology and Therapy, 1926, volume 39, pages 326-329.

VALLEIX F. L. L, Guide du médecin praticien ou résumé général de pathologie interne et de thérapeutique appliquées, J.-B. Baillière et fils, 4e édition revue par V.-A. Racle et P. Lorain, Paris, 1860-1861, 5 tomes.

VALLERY-RADOT René, Journal d'un volontaire d'un an, J. Hetzel et Cie, 1874, 226 pages.

VALLERY-RADOT René, M. Pasteur, histoire d'un savant par un ignorant, J. Hetzel et Cie, Paris, 1884, 389 pages, translated in English by Lady Claude Hamilton, Louis Pasteur his life and labours by his son-in-law, D. Appleton and Company, New-York, 1885, 374 pages.

VALLERY-RADOT René, La vie de Pasteur, Flammarion, Paris, 1re édition, 1900, 692 pages.

VAN ERMENGEM E., Recherches sur le microbe du choléra asiatique, Georges Carré à Paris et A. Manceaux à Bruxelles, 1885, 374 pages.

VAN ERMENGEN E., Les sciences bactériologiques et parasitologiques, in Le mouvement scientifique en Belgique, 1830-1905 sous la direction de van Overbergh, Oscar Schepens et Cie éditeurs, Bruxelles, 1907-1908, 2 tomes.

VAPEREAU G., Dictionnaire universel des contemporains, Hachette, 6e édition, 1893, 1620 + 103 pages.

VERDUNOY chanoine, Pasteur 1822-1895, Publications "Lumen", Collection "Les grands catholiques des XIXe et XXe siècles", Dijon, 1922, 156 pages.

VERGE J., Fièvre aphteuse, in Levaditi C, Lépine P. et Verge J., Les ultravirus des maladies animales, Librairie Maloine, Paris-Montpellier, 1943, pages 265-353.

VERMEERSCH Etienne, Ethical-philosophical aspects of human and animal experimentation in "The ethics of animal and human experimentation", edited by P.P. De Deyn, John Libbey and Company Ldt, London, 1994, pages 3-12.

VERMEY Dr A., Sciences médicales, le dernier congrès contre la tuberculose, La Science illustrée, 1902, tome XXIX, pages 182-183 et 198-199.

VERMENOUZE Pierre, Emile Duclaux (1840-1904), Revue de la Haute-Auvergne, 1992, tome 54, pages 111-136.

VEZARD Y., MOYEN E.-N. et BOIRON, Recherches sur l'immunité antiamarile de quelques habitants d'un quartier de Dakar, Bulletin de la société médicale d'Afrique noire de langue française, 1966, volume XI, pages 557-559.

VIAUD Louis Dr., La défense contre la variole, La médecine internationale illustrée, numéro 10 du mois d'octobre 1907, page 681.

VICQ-D'AZYR M., Exposé des moyens curatifs & préservatifs qui peuvent être employés contre les maladies pestilentielles des bêtes à cornes, chez Mérigot l'aîné, à Paris, 1776, 728 pages.

VICQ-D'AZYR M., Examen impartial des avantages de l'inoculation de la maladie épizootique a produits en Hollande & en Allemagne, & de ceux que l'on peut en attendre en France, Histoire de la société royale de médecine, 1780, pages 163-184.

VICQ-D'AZYR, Instructions et observations sur les maladies des animaux domestiques... par CC. Chabert, Flandrin et Huzard, an 3e de la République Françoise (1795, vieux style), pages 233-268.

VIETTE M., Vallée A. et Chabert Y., Vaccins et sérums, l'Encyclopédie par l'image, Hachette, Paris, 1963, 63 pages.

VIETS Henry R., A brief History of Medicine in Massachussetts, Houghton Mifflin Co., Boston and New-York, 1930, 194 pages.

VIGAROUS J.M.J., Rapport sur l'inoculation de la vaccine, fait à l'Ecole de Médecine de Montpellier, à Montpellier, chez G. Izar et A. Ricard, an IX (1801), 56 pages.

VILLEMIN J.-A., Etudes sur la tuberculose. Preuves rationnelles et expérimentales de sa spécificité et de son inoculabilité, J.-B. Baillière et fils, Paris, 1868, 640 pages.

VIOLLE H., Le choléra, in Infections à germe connu, tome XV, par Pr Hutinel, Darré, Lenglet, Ayrignac... Traité de pathologie médicale et de thérapeutique appliquée, Editions médicales Norbert Maloine, Paris, 1928, 2e édition, pages 388-429.

VISEUR J., La clavelée ou petite vérole des moutons dans le département du Pas-de-Calais, Recueil de médecine vétérinaire, 5e série, tome X, numéro 9 du mois de septembre 1873, pages 662-687.

VOISIN F., Mémoire sur la vaccination des bêtes à laines, lu à la Société libre d'Agriculture de Seine et Oise, séance de la Société du 25 messidor an 12 (14 juillet 1804) et de sa mission intermédiaire du 4 thermidor suivant (23 juillet 1804), de l'imprimerie de la Société d'Agriculture de Seine et Oise, à Versailles, 19 pages [BANM, no 39 612 D (1)].

VOISIN F., Rapport fait à la commission de vaccine sur le plan d'expériences qui doit être exécuté incessamment à Versailles, sous les auspices..., Société d'Agriculture du département de Seine et Oise, de l'imprimerie de la Société d'Agriculture, à Versailles, 1805a, 14 pages [BANM, n° 39 612 D (3)].

VOISIN F., Rapports d'expériences sur la vaccination des bêtes à laine et sur le claveau fait à la Société d'Agriculture du Département de Seine et Oise, dans sa séance du 25 fructidor an 13 (12 septembre 1805) chez Jacob, à Versailles, an 13 (1805b), 100 pages [BANM, n° 39 612 D (3)].

VOLNEY C.-F., Voyage en Syrie et en Egypte pendant les années 1783, 1784, & 1785 avec deux cartes géographiques... chez Volland libraire et Desenne libraire à Paris, 1787, pages 222-229.

VOLTAIRE, Douzième lettre (écrite en 1727), Sur l'insertion de la petite vérole, in Lettres philosophiques, in Œuvres complètes, chez Th. Desoer, Paris, 1817, pages 18-20. Translation from: Letters concerning the English Nation, ed. Nicholas Cronk, Oxford University Press, 1994, page 44.

VRANCKEN L.H.J., Notice historique et statistique sur la vaccine depuis son introduction à Anvers en 1801 jusqu'à nos jours, Imprimerie de la veuve J.S. Schoesetters, Anvers, 1851, 150 pages.

VULPIAN, rapporteur, Rapport sur des communications récentes relatives à l'épidémie actuelle de choléra, Comptes rendus des séances de l'Académie des sciences, 1884, tome IC, pages 175-176.

VULPIAN, Observation au sujet de la lettre à M. le secrétaire perpépuel, au sujet du procédé de vaccination contre le choléra par le Dr J. Ferran, Comptes rendus des séances de l'Académie des sciences, séance du 13 juillet 1885, tome CI, page 367.

VULPIAN Professeur, Pasteur et la rage, La Chronique médicale, 27e année, numéro 20 du 15 octobre 1895, pages 621-624.

WALKER's critical pronouncing dictionary, The English language, Cooperstown, USA, 1828, 400 pages.

WALLACE E. Marjorie, The first vaccinator, Benjamin Jesty of Yetminister and Worth Matravers and his family, 1981, Anglebury-Bartlett Ldt, Wareham, 20 pages.

WATERHOUSE Benjamin, Certificate number 6, to the Committee of the town of Milton, appointed to consider the subject of vaccination, in A collection of papers relative of Milton in the state of Massachussetts to promote A General Inoculation of the cow pox or kine pock, printed by J. Belcher, Boston, 1809, pages 18-19.

WARLOMONT E., Traité de la vaccine et de la vaccination humaine et animale, J.-B. Baillière et fils, Paris, 1883, 384 pages.

WEBBY Richard J. and WEBSTER Robert G., Are We Ready for Pandemic Influenza? Science, 2003, volume 302, pages 1519-1522.

WEBSTER Noah, A brief history of epidemic and pestilential diseases with... printed by Hudson & Goodwin, Hartford, 1799, 2 volumes.

WEBSTER Noah, An American dictionary of the English language, revised by Chauncey A. Goodrich, Harper & Brothers Publishers, New-York, 1849, 1152 + 113 pages.

WEBSTER Noah, An American dictionary of the English language, revised by Chauncey A. Goodrich, George and Charles Merriam, Springfield, 1854, 1367 pages.

WEBSTER Noah, A dictionary of the English language, George and Charles Merriam, Springfield, Mass., 1883, 1928 pages.

WEIGL Rudolf, Faits d'observation et d'expériences démontrant l'efficacité du vaccine à Rickettsia pour la prévention du typhus, Archives de l'Institut Pasteur de Tunis, 1933, tome XXII, page 315-320.

WEIJER Charles, The future of research into rotavirus vaccine – Benefits of vaccine may outweigh risks for children in developing countries, British Medical Journal, 2000, volume 321, pages 525-526.

WEYLAND Dr, article Rage, in Nouveau dictionnaire de la conversation ou répertoire universel, publié par Auguste Walhen, à la librairie historique-artistique, Bruxelles, 1844, tome 23, pages 86-87.

WIKTOR T.-J., MacFARLAN K.J., REAGAN K.J., DIETZSCHOLD B., CURTIS P.J., WUNNER W.H., KIENY M.P., LATHE R., LECOCQ J.P., MACKETT M., MOSS B., KOPROWSKI H, Protection from rabies by a vaccinia virus recombinant containing rabies virus glycoprotein gene, Proceeding of the National Academy of Sciences (Wash.), 1984, volume 81, pages 7194-7198.

WILKINSON Lise, Animals & Disease An introduction to the history of comparative Medicine, Cambridge University Press, 1992, 272 pages.

WILLEMS Louis, Mémoire sur la pleuropneumonie épizootique du bétail, adressé à M. le Ministre de l'intérieur, Imprimerie de Th. Lesigne, Bruxelles, 1852, 33 pages.

WILLEMS M. le docteur, Rapports et documents officiels relatifs à l'inoculation de la pleuropneumonie exsudative d'après le procédé de. .., Ministère de l'Intérieur, imprimerie de A. Labroue et compagnie, Bruxelles, 1853, 176 pages.

WILLEMS Louis, Correspondance, Inoculation de la pleuropneumonie, réclamation de M. le docteur Willems, relative à un article de notre numéro de décembre 1856 (page 669), Annales de médecine vétérinaire, 1857, 6e année, pages 107-110.

WILLIAMS Dawson, Recent researches on attenuation of virus and protective vaccination, in Recent essays by various authors on bacteria in relation to disease, selected and edited by W. Watson Cheyne, New Sydenham Society, London, 1886, pages 549-647.

WILLIAMS Trevor, Biographical dictionary scientists – Collins, Harper-Collins Publishers, Glasgow, 1994, 602 pages.

WILSON John Rowan, Margin for safety, a doctor tells the controversial story of the development of poliomyélite vaccines, Doubleday & Company Inc., New-York, 1963, 258 pages.

WINSLOW C.-E. A., The life of Hermann M. Biggs, M.D., D.Sc, LL.D., physician and statesman of the public health, Lea & Febiger, Philadelphia, 1929, 432 pages.

WINSLOW Charles-Edward Amory, The conquest of epidemic disease, a chapter in the history of ideas, Princeton University Press, Princeton, new Jersey, 1943, 411 pages.

WONE I., CORNET M., CIRE LY., LARIVIERE M., MICHEL R., GUISSE Sidi, BRES P., Fièvre jaune : étude d'ensemble de l'épidémie du Sénégal de 1965, Bulletin de la société médicale d'Afrique noire de langue française, 1966, volume XI, pages 500-511.

WOODRUFF Alice Miles and GOODPASTURE Ernest W., The susceptibility of the chorio-allantoic membrane of chick embryos to infection with the fowl-pox virus, American Journal of pathology, 1931, volume 7, pages 209-222.

WOODVILLE W., Reports of a series of inoculations for the variolae vaccinae, or cow-pox with remarks and observations on this disease, considerate as a substitute for the small-pox. Printed and sold by James Philipps and son, London, 1799, 43 pages, reprinted in Crooshrank (1889), pages 93-154.

WOODVILLE W., Observations on the cow-pox, printed and sold by William Phillipps, London, 1800, 43 pages.

WOODWARD Samuel Bayard, The story of smallpox in Massachusetts, The annual discourse delivered before the Massachusetts Medical Society at the hundred and fifty-first reunion, held in Boston June 8 to 10, 1932, The New England Journal of Medicine, volume 206, issue 23 (June 9, 1932), 32 pages.

WORLOCK M., Lettre écrite au sujet de la méthode suttonienne d'inoculation, pratiquée depuis peu à Paris par M. Worlock, Médecin anglois, & beau-père du célèbre M. Daniel Sutton, tirée du Journal Encyclopédique du mois d'Août 1770, 4 pages plus 14 pages de témoignages.

WORTLEY, *see* MONTAGU.

WRIGHT A.E. and BRUCE D., On Haffkine's method of vaccination against choléra, The British Medical Journal, February 4, 1893, pages 227-231.

WRIGHT A.E., On the association of serous haemorrhages with conditions of defective blood-coagulability, The Lancet, September 19, 1896, pages 807-809.

WRIGHT A.E. and SEMPLE Surg.-Maj. D., Remarks on vaccination against typhoid fever, The British Medical Journal, January 30, 1897, pages 256-259.

WRIGHT A.E.and LEISHMAN W.B., Remarks on the results which have been obtained by the antityphoid inoculations and on the methods which have been employed in the preparation of the vaccine, The British Medical Journal, January 20, 1900, pages 122-129.

WRIGHT A.E. and DOUGLAS Stewart R., An Experimental Investigation of the Rôle of Blood Fluids in connexion to Phagocytosis, Proceedings of the Royal Society (London), 1903-1904, volume 72, pages 357-370.

WRIGHT A.E. and DOUGLAS Stewart R., Further Observations on the Rôle of the Blood Fluids in connexion to Phagocytosis, Proceedings of the Royal Society (London), 1904, volume 73, pages 128-142.

WROTNOWSKA Denise, Le vaccin anti-charbonneux, Pasteur et Toussaint d'après des documents inédits, Histoire des Sciences médicales, 1975, volume 12, pages 261-290.

XXX, Plus de rage! Le Figaro, numéro 140 du lundi 19 mai 1884, page 1 dite de garde.

XXX, La peste et le remède, L'Illustration européenne, 26e année, numéro 41 du 8 octobre 1899, page 654.

ZINSSER Hans, Infection and resistance, an exposition of the biological phenomena underlying the occurrence of infection and the recovery of the animal body from infectious disease, The Macmillan Company, 1918, second edition revised, New York, 585 pages.

Index

* Pasteur always referred to his laboratory as: "*laboratoire de l'Ecole Normale*". His nephew Adrien Loir, in his Memoires, uses the expression : "*le laboratoire de la rue d'Ulm™ mon arrivée rue d'Ulm…*".

V

Achevé d'imprimer par Corlet, Imprimeur, S.A.
14110 Condé-sur-Noireau
N° d'Imprimeur : 130930 - Dépôt légal : mars 2011
Imprimé en France